VITAMIN D
The Calcium Homeostatic Steroid Hormone

NUTRITION: BASIC AND APPLIED SCIENCE

A SERIES OF MONOGRAPHS

WILLIAM J. DARBY, Editor
Professor of Biochemistry (Nutrition)
Vanderbilt University School of Medicine
Nashville, Tennessee
and
President, The Nutrition Foundation
New York, New York

Anthony W. Norman. *Vitamin D: The Calcium Homeostatic Steroid Hormone*, 1979.

VITAMIN D

The Calcium Homeostatic Steroid Hormone

ANTHONY W. NORMAN

Department of Biochemistry
University of California
Riverside, California

ACADEMIC PRESS New York San Francisco London 1979
A Subsidiary of Harcourt Brace Jovanovich, Publishers

ACADEMIC PRESS, INC.
111 Fifth Avenue, New York, New York 10003

United Kingdom Edition published by
ACADEMIC PRESS, INC. (LONDON) LTD.
24/28 Oval Road, London NW1 7DX

Library of Congress Cataloging in Publication Data

Norman, Anthony W Date
Vitamin D : the calcium homeostatic steroid hormone.

Bibliography: p.
Includes index.
1. Vitamin D. 2. Vitamin D metabolism.
3. Calcium metabolism. 4. Homeostasis. I. Title.
[DNLM: 1. Vitamin D. QU173 N842v]
QP772.V53N67 612'.399 79-6941
ISBN 0-12-521050-7

PRINTED IN THE UNITED STATES OF AMERICA

79 80 81 82 9 8 7 6 5 4 3 2 1

Contents

CHAPTER 3
The Vitamins D

CHAPTER 4
Biological and Chemical Assay of Vitamin D, Its Metabolites, and Analogs

CHAPTER 5
Vitamin D Metabolites and Analogs

CHAPTER 6
Metabolism of Vitamin D

CHAPTER 7

The Tissue and Subcellular Localization of Vitamin D and Its Metabolites: A Basis for Their Hormonal Mode of Action

CHAPTER 8

Binding Proteins and Receptors for Vitamin D and Its Metabolites

CHAPTER 9
Interrelationships between Vitamin D and Other Hormones

CHAPTER 10
Intestinal Effects of Vitamin D

CHAPTER 11
Vitamin D Actions in the Kidney (Excluding Vitamin D Metabolism)

CHAPTER 12
Vitamin D Actions on Bone

CHAPTER 13
Vitamin D and Its Clinical Relationships

Appendix

Foreword

There are no more exciting basic scientific developments with immediate applications in preventive medicine and therapy than the fascinating unfolding of the story of provitamin—vitamins D—hormone interconversions. Elucidation of the chemical and metabolic phenomena has been especially rapid during the past decade. The current developments are based on the brilliant earlier investigations of rickets, its distinction from scurvy, the structural identification of the steroids, and the vitamin–precursor activation by ultraviolet irradiation. Our scientific knowledge of this important area of nutrition is authoritatively summarized in this monograph.

This book, therefore, fittingly introduces a new technical series of publications in the field of nutrition entitled "Nutrition: Basic and Applied Science." It will provide a continuing coordinated group of edited critiques of the dynamic state of the science and art of nutrition. The most recent basic advances will be reviewed within the broad framework of the scientific knowledge of food and nutrition, including its application to man, individually and societally.

Each volume will be a self-contained treatise of appropriate breadth, depth, and length to warrant a permanent place in the library of the individual scholar or institution. The subjects in a volume will range from consideration of a single nutrient or process to wider concepts such as clinical nutrition, nutrition requirements and standards, nutritional toxicology, or history of the science.

The volumes, authored singly or by invited contributors, will appeal to serious scholars concerned with pure or applied nutrition. For the advanced scholar and investigator they will serve as authoritative, correlative reviews of current advances. For the younger scholar, they will provide background necessary to develop a perspective to discriminate between new discovery and rediscovery, between conceptionally important and feasibly "researchable" inquiry and less creative investigations that often are described as "further refinement of knowledge" or "collecting more data." They will facilitate recognition and correlation of related developments and applications in different disciplines, thereby promoting interdisciplinary understanding. Selected editorial committees will advise on content and authors assuring, thereby, the quality of the individual treatises.

Another volume projected for the immediate future is on nutritional toxicology. A definitive multivolume history of nutrition science is in preparation.

It is a privileged responsibility to serve as editor of this series and to introduce it with this monograph by Anthony W. Norman.

William J. Darby

Preface

The need for a book which comprehensively reviews all aspects of vitamin D has been apparent for many years. The last such comprehensive treatise to appear on this subject was Reed, Struck, and Steck's monograph in 1939.* Indeed, the author of the Preface of that book, D. J. Davis, concluded his remarks with the comment "... one feels additional exciting discoveries in this field may be made at any moment...." In retrospect, now some four decades later, this was an understatement.

An explosion of new information, concepts, hypotheses and vitamin D metabolites has occurred. The "vitamin D problem" has challenged many: clinicians, biochemists, physiologists, chemists, and anthropologists all have made important contributions. A conservative estimate is that, in the past fifteen years, 1800 papers have been published, all bearing some relationship to the resolution of the vitamin D problem. Out of these endeavors has emerged a major new concept: not only is vitamin D chemically a steroid, but its mode of action is akin to that of classic steroid hormones. We now visualize the existence of an endocrine system for vitamin D in which the kidney serves as the endocrine gland producing the metabolites 1,25-dihydroxyvitamin D and 24,25-dihydroxyvitamin D.

Thus, in preparing this book, it has been my objective to provide a comprehensive but discriminating review of the stream of developments related to vitamin D that have occurred in the past two decades, including chemical, nutritional, and clinical topics, and to place them in the context of the earlier literature. This book will be of value to clinicians—both research and practice oriented—endocrinologists, physiologists, nutritionists, biochemists, analytical chemists, organic chemists, and researchers concerned with dental problems.

The major thesis of this book is that vitamin D and its metabolites should be

*Reed, C. I., Struck, H. C., and Steck (1939). "Vitamin D: Physiology, Pharmacology, Pathology, Experimental Clinical Investigations." University of Chicago Press, Chicago, Illinois.

considered collectively as steroid hormones. Certainly in terms of its chemical structure the parent vitamin D is a seco steroid, albeit a molecule in which one of the four cyclopentanoperhydrophenanthrene rings has been broken. Hence, the terminology "seco." The physical and chemical properties of vitamin D and its metabolites are certainly similar to those of steroids. Functionally, much evidence has been accumulated to support the view that 1,25-dihydroxyvitamin D_3 induces many of its biological responses through genome activation in selected target tissues; similar models have been supported for classic steroid hormones, e.g., aldosterone, estradiol, glucocorticoids, progesterone, and testosterone. As with the classic hormones, it is still unclear whether or not the complete spectrum of biological responses of vitamin D and its metabolites is produced via steroid–receptor complex formation followed by genome activation. Certainly the intricate metabolic pathway for vitamin D, coupled with the unique properties of the conformationally mobile A-ring of these seco steroids, may confer upon this clan of molecules the capability of inducing biological responses by a variety of mechanisms.

The organizational scheme of this book is first to set the stage with a historical review of the nutritional/clinical and chemical background. Then the chemistry of vitamin D and its metabolites and analogs is discussed, including current chemical, bioassay, and steroid competition analytical methodology. This is then followed by a systematic analysis of vitamin D metabolism, and the physiological and biochemical actions of these steroids in intestine, kidney, and bone. The book concludes with an assessment of the relationship of these developments to the maintenance of good health.

This project has been a labor of love. Virtually all my scientific career has been devoted to vitamin D. It has been a delight to observe and participate in the unraveling of these problems. In addition, the creation of this book has been, in its own way, one of my most interesting educational experiences. There are few subjects which touch upon so many other disciplines and techniques. I have made a sincere effort to be comprehensive without being voluminous, to cite all viewpoints while indicating my preference, and to cite as many relevant papers as possible.

This book would not have been possible without the intellectual stimulation of many, including Drs. J. W. Coburn, W. H. Okamura, A. S. Brickman, A. N. Taylor, D. J. Hartenbower, H. C. Tsai, D. A. Procsal, S. Christakos, R. M. Wing, W. Hunziker, J. Merke, N. Ohnuma, and particularly H. L. Henry as well as my students, Drs. A. Foung, M. R. Haussler, T. H. Adams, J. F. Myrtle, R. G. Wong, A. M. Spielvogel, R. J. Midgett, R. L. Johnson, T. Osborn, W. Wecksler, E. J. Friedlander, J. O. Putkey, B. Miller, L. Wen, and P. Siebert. Also without the tireless efforts of P. A. Roberts and J. Bishop, who coped with proofreading literature citations and sorting and filing reprints, this project could not have been brought to fruition. Mrs. Wendy Reid is responsible for many of the scientific illustrations and help with the jacket design. Mrs. J. Fast, S. Staton, and N. Nobles performed the herculean task of generating both the rough drafts and final copy of the manuscript. Ms. M. Johnson and Ms. R. Lanier played indispensable roles in proofreading and in generating the index. Also, I wish to acknowledge the continuing support of the National Institutes of Arthritis, Metabolism, and Digestive Diseases for the research endeavors in my laboratory.

Finally, without the support, patience, and love of my wife Helen and interludes with Thea, Jacqueline, and Derek, this book would not have been possible.

Anthony W. Norman

CHAPTER

1

Vitamin D—Cholecalciferol: From Vitamin to Steroid Hormone

I. HISTORICAL REVIEW

A. Opening Comments

Vitamin D is essential for life in higher animals. It is one of the most important biological regulators of calcium metabolism. Along with the two peptide hormones calcitonin and parathyroid hormone, vitamin D is responsible for the minute-to-minute as well as the day-to-day maintenance of calcium homeostasis. These three substances also play an important role in phosphorus homeostasis.

In the absence of vitamin D a host of problems arise, ranging from those that affect the whole organism (e.g., inhibition of growth), to those that affect particular organs (e.g., development of rickets or osteomalacia by the skeletal system), to those that affect particular cell types (e.g., the columnar epithelial and/or goblet cells of the intestinal mucosa), and ultimately to those that are manifest at the subcellular level (e.g., alteration of the morphology of kidney mitochondria). In view of the obvious dependence of normal life in higher animals on the continued presence of vitamin D, it is not surprising that scientists have exerted a major effort to understand the physiological, cellular, subcellular, and molecular mode of action of this vital substance.

Man is reported to have been aware in a general sense of vitamin D since early antiquity (Solecki, 1971a,b). The first scientific description of rickets was provided by both Dr. Daniel Whistler (1645) and Professor Francis Glisson (1650a,b) in the seventeenth century. These developments set the stage for the brilliant formulation of the vitamin concept by Sir Gowland Hopkins and the era of experimental nutrition fostered in the vitamin D field by Sir Edward Mellanby.

It is apparent that today vitamin D plays an important multidisciplinary role. This ranges from its indispensable role in general nutrition (both human and agricultural) and in human disease states to its important economic position in the pharmaceutical industry and to the implications of its involvement at the anthropological–sociological level.[1] What is surprising, then, in view of the amazing accomplishments of modern biological science, is that a half a century passed between the specific recognition of the existence of vitamin D (Mellanby, 1921) and the formulation of a theory of the "mode of action" of vitamin D consistent with many if not all of the known facts. This hypothesis states that vitamin D is in reality a steroid and that its mode of action is akin to that of steroid hormones. The purpose of this book is to review comprehensively the vitamin D-related literature, both old and new, and to include clinical, biological, and chemical topics.

B. History

1. Prior to 1700

There is no unanimity of agreement as to when the first effects of a vitamin D deficiency were manifest in man. Solecki (1971a,b) and Loomis (1967) report and postulate, respectively, on the basis of paleontological evidence, that Neanderthal man's (circa 50,000 B.C.) stooped appearance may have been the result of disease rather than low evolutionary status. Kjerrulf (1922) claims that human skeletons from the Neolithic age (circa 8000 B.C.) were deformed by rickets. Similarly, Hansen (1924) purported to show rickets in bones originating from the first settlers in Greenland.

[1]Loomis (1967) proposed a theory that the known differences in the skin pigmentation of man result from adaptive evolutionary efforts on his part to avoid the dangers of toxic doses of vitamin D, on the one hand, and the deformities of rickets, on the other. In this theory the evolutionary pressure is presumed to be the increasing intensity of solar ultraviolet light as one approaches the latitude of the equator. This results in an adaptation of the epidermal stratum corneum to regulate the transmission of solar uv to the photochemical site of production of vitamin D_3 from 7-dehydrocholesterol in the underlying stratum granulosum.

A detailed discussion of the problem of definitely ascertaining the scientific priority of the first description of rickets is given in Chapter 1 of the scholarly treatise by Hess (1929). Although the archaelogical records of the early Egyptians (circa 1500 B.C.) contain hints of and allusions to afflictions reminiscent of some of the clinical symptoms of rickets, the writings of Soranus of Epheus, a physician in the Greco-Roman era (circa 100–200 A.D.), are, in the opinion of Hess (1929), the first to give a clearly recognizable description of rickets. Soranus was claimed by Hess to be "the most eminent obstetrician in antiquity."

The first precise written descriptions of rickets can be attributed to Dr. Daniel Whistler of Leiden, the Netherlands, in 1645 and to Professor Francis Glisson of London in 1650. Both were written in the scholarly language characteristic of that period—Latin (Whistler, 1645; Glisson, 1650a,b). In view of the communication problems of that time and the lack of more modern scientific communication aids such as *Current Contents* and *Medlars,* it is only fair and reasonable to give both authors credit for first priority. The publication by Whistler was a concise monograph of only 14 pages and was written when the author was 20 years old. It represented the thesis required for his degree of doctor of medicine. Glisson (1597–1677) was one of the original fellows of the Royal College of Physicians and a noted orthopedic surgeon. He was quite thorough in his written description of rickets (some 200 pages) and covered all aspects of the disease. The frontispiece from his book is reproduced as Fig. 1-1. A detailed evaluation of Glisson's treatise was provided by Moore in 1884.

2. *From 1700 to 1920*

The eighteenth century provided little in the way of specific advances. It can be most properly characterized as a period of recognition and acceptance of the views of Glisson, i.e., that there was a distinct disease state termed rickets. However, major strides were made in the nineteenth century which set the stage for the magnificent work of Sir Edward Mellanby.

The 1800's included the first formal description of bone by Marchand (1842), Bibra (1844), and Friedleben (1860). The most thorough histological and pathological description of the rachitic skeleton was that provided by Pommer (1885). Trousseau and Laseque (1849) appreciated that osteomalacia and rickets were different expressions of the same malady.

Also of importance was the recognition that rickets was not confined to England or even the European continent. Hirsch (1886) and particularly Palm (1890) pioneered a quantitative geographic study of the worldwide distribution of rickets, especially in all European countries, China, Japan, India, West Indies, and the United States. Hess eventually commented (1929, p. 29) that "in general a map of the incidence of rickets is . . . the practical equivalent of a map . . . of deficiency of sunlight."

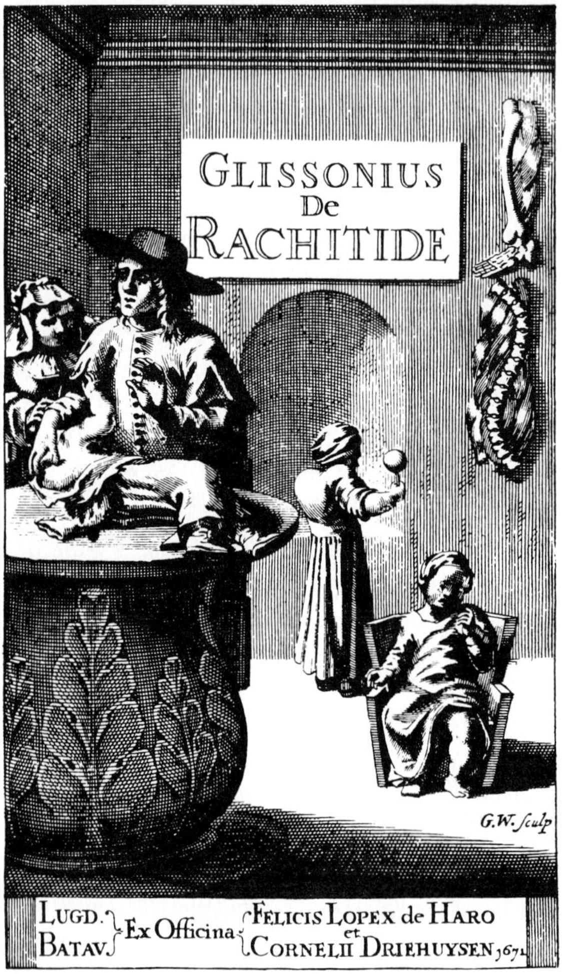

Figure 1-1. Frontispiece of F. Glisson's book entitled "De Rachitide," published first in London in 1650.

In view of these developments it was only natural that various theories would be put forth to explain the etiology of rickets. A chronological summary of many of these suggestions is given in Table 1-1.

Clearly the two most important proposals concerned the relationship between lack of sunlight and incidence of rickets and the possibility that rickets was induced by a lack or deficiency of a nutritional factor. However, at this time, the close interdependency of these two relationships was not at all appreciated or even intimated.

TABLE 1-1
Proposed Causative Factors of Rickets

Factor	Comment	Reference
Lack of fresh air	Some held that rickets came about from infants breathing the "noxious gasses" of badly ventilated rooms	Kassowitz (1881)
Congenital factor	Nutritional errors of the mother during pregnancy could produce congenital defects in the offspring; not to be confused with a primary genetic aberration	Kassowitz (1881), Korenchevsky (1922)
Malfunction of endocrine glands	Osteomalacia was proposed to be due to an overactivity of the ovaries; also, it was appreciated that osteomalacia could occur during lactation; some workers implicated the thymus (Basch) and adrenals (Biedl)	Fehling (1894), Basch (1906), Biedl (1910), Stoeltzner (1900)
Heredity	A study of two generations of families with a high incidence of rickets suggested that "heredity was the most important etiological factor in this disorder" and presupposed a specific alteration in the germ plasm	Siegert (1903)
Age	Congenital rickets was noted to never occur before the ninth month or scarcely after the second year	Boerhaave (cited in Hess, 1929, p. 90)
Syphilis	For years congenital syphilis and rickets were considered the same disease	Parrot (1897)
General infection	Rickets were claimed to be induced in rats by injecting them with cultures of *Diplococcus* (Morpurgo) or *Streptococcus longus* (Koch)	Morpurgo (1902), Koch (1911)
Lack of exercise or domestication	In the absence of regular exercise there is a predisposition for rickets to develop; this view has been put forth at various times since 1700, but most prominently supported by Findlay; an interesting variation of this causative factor is the "domestication concept" put forth by von Hansemann; he noted that wild animals when confined in a zoo often develop rickets	Findlay (1922), von Hansemann (1906)
Ultraviolet rays	A correlation between lack of sunlight and the incidence of rickets (Palm) was followed by a demonstration of the calcifying effect of ultraviolet rays (Huldschinsky) and the curative effect of sunshine on rickets (Hess and Ungar)	Palm (1890), Huldschinsky (1919), Hess and Ungar (1921)
A vitamin factor	The concept of a nutritional factor or vitamin being associated with rickets was first suggested by Funk and then experimentally verified by Mellanby	Funk (1914), Mellanby (1919, 1921)

The major breakthrough in understanding the causative factors of rickets was the development of nutrition as an experimental science and the appreciation of the existence of vitamins. In this respect the leadership roles of Sir F. Gowland Hopkins and Professor C. Funk should be acknowledged. In 1914 Funk wrote in his classic "Die Vitamine": "It is very probable that rickets occurs only when certain substances in the diet essential for normal metabolism are lacking or are supplied in insufficient amounts. The substances occur in good breast milk, also in cod-liver oil, but are lacking in sterilized milk and in cereals" (translated by Hess, 1929, p. 66).

These views were not overlooked by Sir Edward Mellanby. In a landmark series of studies (Mellanby, 1919, 1921) involving the feeding of a plethora of scientifically devised diets to more than 400 dogs over a period of 5 years, Mellanby unequivocably established that rickets was caused by a deficiency of a trace component present in the diet. In 1921 he wrote, "The action of fats in rickets is due to a vitamin or accessory food factor which they contain, probably identical with the fat-soluble vitamin" (Mellanby, 1921, p. 68).[2] Furthermore, he established that cod-liver oil was an excellent antirachitic agent.

In the discussion section of his definitive monograph, Mellanby (1921) stated that the following conditions "inhibit calcification or increase growth relative to calcification so that defectively calcified bone results: (1) a deficiency of calcium and phosphorus in the diet; (2) a deficiency of fat containing the *anti-rachitic vitamine* in the diet; (3) excess of bread, other cereals, and carbohydrates; (4) absence of meat; (5) excess of the protein moiety of casein-enogen free from calcium; (6) confinement." He also noted that the following conditions "tend to prevent rickets in puppies: (1) plenty of calcium and phosphorus in the diet; (2) something associated with certain fats probably identical with the *fat-soluble vitamine;* (3) meat; (4) the possibility of exercise" (Mellanby, 1921, p. 75; italics added).

Mellanby was acutely aware of the complicated nature of rickets and understood how the existence of a specific antirachitic substance could have been previously overlooked. He stated, "It has been shown that many of the food elements exert a potent influence on the operation of bone calcification or growth, and moreover, that there is great interplay among the dietetic elements that a condition which appears of prime importance at any one time may sink into relative insignificance at another time" (Mellanby, 1921, p. 74). In retrospect it is easy to appreciate and respect the prescience and wisdom of Mellanby's comment. Some 40–50 years have elapsed between his brilliant work and the development of a true understanding of the mode of action of vitamin D.

[2]Actually, Mellanby felt that the antirachitic substance was fat-soluble A. However, it should be appreciated that it was not until 1922 that a clear distinction was made between vitamins A and D.

3. From 1920 to 1960

Although many would argue that the prime accomplishment of Mellanby was the unequivocal demonstration that a true dietary component was the causative agent of rickets, in retrospect his accomplishments were much more far-reaching. Of far greater value was his application of the scientific technique to the infant field of nutrition so that it was possible to routinely raise a vitamin D-deficient animal. This great stride forward made it possible for scientists the world over to use the scientific technique to unravel the mode of action of the elusive "antirachitic factor." On the biological front, work from the laboratories of Goldblatt and Soames (1923), Hess and co-workers (Hess and Unger 1920, 1921; Hess *et al.* 1921a,b,c; Hess and Gutman, 1922), Hopkins (1920), Huldschinsky (1919), Korenchevsky (1922), McCollum and co-workers (1921, 1922a,b), and Steenbock and Black (1924) should not be overlooked. On the chemical fronts, the laboratories of Windaus, Askew, and Crowfoot-Hodgkin all made solid contributions to the elucidation of the chemical structure of the fat-soluble vitamin D.

As with all phases of rapid development, it is difficult in retrospect to unravel the precise order of discovery of the many facets of the total problem. There were three areas in which progress had to be made: (a) separation of vitamin A and D activities; (b) appreciation that uv light and cod-liver oil could both effect the same cure of rickets; and (c) demonstration that irradiation of food (in the absence of the animal) produces the same effect as irradiation of the animal.

However, the most significant advance undoubtedly was an appreciation of the importance of ultraviolet light or radiant energy to the cure and etiology of rickets. Huldschinsky (1919, 1919–1920) first showed that the uv rays from a mercury-vapor lamp were quite effective in increasing the degree of calcification of the epiphysis of rachitic infants. Even today the illustrations included in his paper are remarkably convincing. These results were quickly reproduced in experimental animals. Accounts of these experiments can be found in the work of Hess (1922) and Hess and Gutman (1922).

In 1920 Hopkins reported that vitamin A activity could be destroyed by both heat and oxygen. This observation was the basis for the breakthrough made in McCollum's laboratory which ultimately led to a resolution of the "fat-soluble vitamin problem." Next, Hess *et al.* (1921a) stated, "We are of the opinion that this vitamin [vitamin A] cannot be regarded as the anti-rachitic vitamin and that if the diet is otherwise adequate, this deficiency does not bring about rickets." At approximately the same time (July 1921) McCollum and co-workers (Shipley *et al.*, 1921) pointed out: "We have not found it possible to demonstrate experimentally a difference between the effects of cod-liver oil and butterfat when the content of the diet in calcium and phosphorus is near the optimum. . . . These results suggest the possibility that a dietary essential [i.e., vitamin D] distinct from the anti-xerophthalmic substance (fat-soluble A) may exist.'' Thus, the stage was set for the definitive proof that vitamins D and A were separate entities.

In their historic paper, McCollum *et al.* (1922a) demonstrated that the antirachitic activity of cod-liver oil could survive both aeration and heating to 100°C for 14 hr, whereas the antixerophthalmic factor, or vitamin A, was inactivated by this process. They stated: ''*The evidence set forth in this paper demonstrates that the power of certain fats to initiate the healing of rickets depends on the presence of a substance which is distinct from fat-soluble A. These experiments clearly demonstrate the existence of a fourth vitamin whose specific property, as far as we can tell at present, is to regulate the metabolism of the bones*'' (italics added). McCollum named the new substance vitamin D.

It is interesting to note in retrospect that Mellanby (1921, p. 36) had carried out virtually the identical experiment.[3] He concluded that the antirachitic component of the fat-soluble vitamin was not destroyed. Unfortunately, he did not assay the xerophthalmic component of the fat-soluble vitamin or he undoubtedly would have reached the same conclusion as McCollum.

Although the correlation between ultraviolet light and cod-liver oil in terms of their equivalent efficacy in preventing rickets was appreciated by most of the workers of that period, there was no simple explanation put forth for the observation. Both ultraviolet light and cod-liver oil were found to be equivalently effective in reversing the roentgenographic evidence of the ravages of rickets upon the skeleton. However, until the work of Goldblatt and Soames (1923) and Steenbock and Black (1924), no connection was made between the mysterious curative powers of ultraviolet light on rickets and the presence of an equally effective molecular species in cod-liver oil.

In 1923 Goldblatt and Goldblatt and Soames (1923) irradiated with uv light livers that had been excised from rachitic rats and found that when the irradiated tissue was ground and fed to other rachitic rats there was a remission of the D deficiency. In parallel studies carried out at the same time, Steenbock and Black (1924) found that food which was irradiated and subsequently fed to rachitic rats had acquired the property of being ''antirachitic.''[4] In short, both groups had for the first time produced *in vitro* the elusive vitamin D component of the fat-soluble vitamin. Without a doubt the specific effect of light was no longer mysterious; it simply had produced a permanent chemical change in a component in the rat diet.

[3]Mellanby heated cod-liver oil to 120°C for 4 hr while oxygen was passed through it.

[4]This observation ultimately led to several patents by which the antirachitic properties of foods such as grains, oils, butter, yeast, cereals, and particularly milk could be dramatically increased. The Wisconsin Alumni Research Foundation (WARF), was created to administer this patent. According to Fieser and Fieser (1959, p. 90), this patent generated, up to 1945, some $14 million.

Hess and Weinstock (1925a,b,c) in an elegant experiment confirmed the dictum that "light equals vitamin D." They excised a small portion of skin, irradiated it with uv light, and then fed it to groups of rachitic rats. The skin that had been irradiated provided an absolute protection against rickets, whereas the unirradiated skin provided no protection whatsoever.

Hess and Weinstock (1925a,b,c) as well as Steenbock and Black (1925) quickly followed up on their observations that ultraviolet light could generate antirachitic activity in various foods, including rat diet. Both groups showed conclusively that the antirachitic factor was confined to the nonsaponifiable fraction of these substances and that it resided exclusively in the phytosterol or cholesterol fractions that they contain. Thus, another major stride forward was made. It was apparent that the antirachitic factor was associated with nonsaponifiable lipids, particularly sterols. The stage was now set for the next era of unraveling the vitamin D web. However, there was still a dilemma. Nelson and Steenbock (1925) observed that the antirachitic activity of cod-liver oil or "activatable" cholesterol isolated from the cod-liver oil could not be precipitated by digitonin.[5]

From this point a description of the evolution of our understanding of vitamin D becomes largely chemical in nature. What was unappreciated initially was that Steenbock and Black (1924) had produced vitamin D_2 from irradiation of the ergosterol in a yeast component of their rat diet, whereas Hess and Weinstock (1925a,b,c) had generated vitamin D_3 via irradiation of the skin. Also, the relation of both of these substances to the antirachitic component of cod-liver oil remained to be established. A further complication was that for a period of time many workers felt that it was cholesterol, rather than a trace component in it, that was rendered antirachitic by uv irradiation.[6]

In 1926 Professor A. F. Hess, a clinical professor of pediatrics at the Medical College of New York City, went to Göttingen, Germany, to study in the laboratory of Professor A. Windaus. Hess felt intuitively that the provitamin of D was a sterol. The highlights of the herculean efforts to chemically characterize the key provitamin, ergosterol, are described in Chapter 2, and those of the efforts required to elucidate the structure of vitamins D_2 and D_3 are described in Chapter 3. Suffice it to say that Professor Windaus had some 55 doctoral and postdoctoral associates who worked on the "vitamin D project" at one time or another.[7]

These studies culminated in 1932 when Windaus *et al.* and Askew *et al.* simultaneously identified the structure of vitamin D_2. The puzzling inability of

[5]By 1928 the use of digitonin to selectively precipitate sterols was widespread. The use of digitonin to precipitate cholesterol and other sterols was introduced by Windaus in 1909. The question was, How could the antirachitic substance both be a sterol and yet not be precipitable by digitonin?

[6]Hess and Rosenbaum and Webster reportedly crystallized cholesterol 15–20 times without eliminating the provitamin of the antirachitic substance (taken from Fieser and Fieser, 1959, p. 91).

[7]A listing of the co-workers of Professor Windaus is given in Fieser and Fieser (1959, p. 96).

digitonin to precipitate the "antirachitic sterol" was now solved; the antirachitic sterol, vitamin D, was actually a secosterol.[8]

Vitamin D_3 was not chemically characterized until 1936, when Windaus *et al.* determined the structure of the antirachitic factor that resulted after uv irradiation of 7-dehydrocholesterol. Virtually simultaneously, the elusive antirachitic component of cod-liver oil was shown to be identical to the newly characterized vitamin D_3 (Brockmann, 1936, 1937). Brockmann isolated 2 g of crystalline vitamin D_3 from 150 kg of tuna-liver oil. At last all was clear: Natural vitamin D from cod-liver oil is identical to vitamin D_3, and 7-dehydrocholesterol, not ergosterol, is the true provitamin of the "natural" vitamin.

Of equal importance, it was unmistakably clear that the antirachitic substance, vitamin D, was a steroid, more specifically a secosteroid. The implications of this fact were largely unappreciated for another 25–30 years.

Thus, the close of the "modern history era" of vitamin D was virtually at hand. All that remained was for Dr. Dorothy Crowfoot-Hodgkin to carry out her elegant X-ray crystallographic analysis of the vitamin D molecule (Crowfoot and Dunitz, 1948; Crowfoot-Hodgkin *et al.,* 1963). Her results also emphasize the seco nature of vitamin D. Because the 9–10 carbon bond of ring B of the provitamin is broken upon irradiation, ring A is free to assume a more extended configuration (see Fig. 3-7). However, in all other respects, the X-ray picture of vitamin D is like that of other steroids. The studies of Wing *et al.* (1974), which determined the shape of vitamin D secosteroids in solution, further emphasized that the A ring is conformationally mobile (see Chapter 4).

II. THE PRESENT (1960 TO 1979)

A. Biological Facts Related to Vitamin D

The focus of many workers from 1930 to 1960 was the role of vitamin D in mineral metabolism, i.e., calcium and phosphate absorption and excretion and bone formation and mobilization. In addition, many studies dealt with the role of the vitamin in organic acid metabolism, i.e., citric acid, and also in membrane permeability and animal growth. It was quite difficult to integrate all these diverse studies into an organized scheme that would adequately explain the biochemical mechanism of action of vitamin D. The overriding influence on the conduct of many of these studies was the concept that vitamin D was acting as a cofactor in some particular reaction. However, in each of the instances cited, the

[8]Secosteroids are those in which one of the rings has undergone fission; in vitamin D, this is ring B, and it is indicated by the inclusion of "9,10-seco" in the nomenclature. Thus, the official name of vitamin D_3 is 9,10-secocholesta-5,7,10(19)-trien-3β-ol.

observation being investigated was apparently several steps removed from the first fundamental action of vitamin D.

One of the hallmarks of vitamin D action, largely unrecognized until the work of Irving (1944), is the apparent time lag between the time of administration of the vitamin and the initiation of every one of its physiological responses. It is likely that the latency in action of vitamin D was not universally recognized because of the necessity for biological assays to determine the effects of the vitamin. The end points usually employed to indicate the presence of the vitamin were gross morphological, histological, or roentgenographic observations, which of necessity required a significant period of time to develop.

It was not until the advent of radioisotopes that the investigator was potentially capable of measuring instantaneous metabolic changes or fluxes. Lindquist (1952), who studied the effect of vitamin D on radioactive calcium metabolism, claimed that a maximal effect of 15 IU[9] (325 ng; 0.97 nmole) of vitamin D_2 on rat intestinal calcium absorption could be observed in 4 hr and on serum calcium levels in 6 hr and upon deposition of $^{45}Ca^{2+}$ in the skeleton in 36–48 hr. Since this report, a lag in the action of dietary vitamin D has been found for the following responses to the vitamin: (a) skeletal deposition of calcium after an oral dose of $^{45}Ca^{2+}$ to chicks (Patrick and Schweitzer, 1955; Migicovsky, 1957); (b) intestinal absorption of calcium as measured by the appearance of $^{45}Ca^{2+}$ in the serum of chicks and rats (Migicovsky and Nielson, 1951; Coates and Holdsworth, 1961; Sallis and Holdsworth, 1962; Norman, 1966); (c) increased level of serum calcium as measured by total serum calcium (Carlsson and Lindquist, 1955; Zull *et al.*, 1966); (d) apparent energy-dependent accumulation of $^{45}Ca^{2+}$ into rat intestinal slices (Schachter *et al.*, 1961) or across everted intestinal sacs (Dowdle *et al.*, 1960); (e) apparent increased permeability of intestinal mucosa as determined by $^{45}Ca^{2+}$ transfer with everted rat intestinal sacs (Harrison and Harrison, 1965); (f) bone resorption or solubilization (Carlsson, 1952); (g) increased levels of citric acid in serum, bones, and incisors (Carlsson and Hollunger, 1954); and (h) increased incorporation of $^{32}P_i$ into rat intestinal mucosal phospholipids (Thompson and DeLuca, 1964).

A direct comparison of the length of the lag in each observation is severely complicated by widely varying dosage levels of the vitamin and the assay techniques utilized. It is very important though, to note that there is a lag in the action of vitamin D for every known physiological response to the vitamin. As a consequence, *in vitro* effects of vitamin D must be carefully assessed with regard to their relationship to the normal physiological effects of the vitamin.

Figure 1-2 shows an example of the lag in action for mediation of one of the prime responses of vitamin D: stimulation of intestinal calcium absorption. It is

[9]One international unit (IU) of vitamin D_3 is 0.025 μg, or 65.0 pmoles. See Chapter 4 for a detailed discussion.

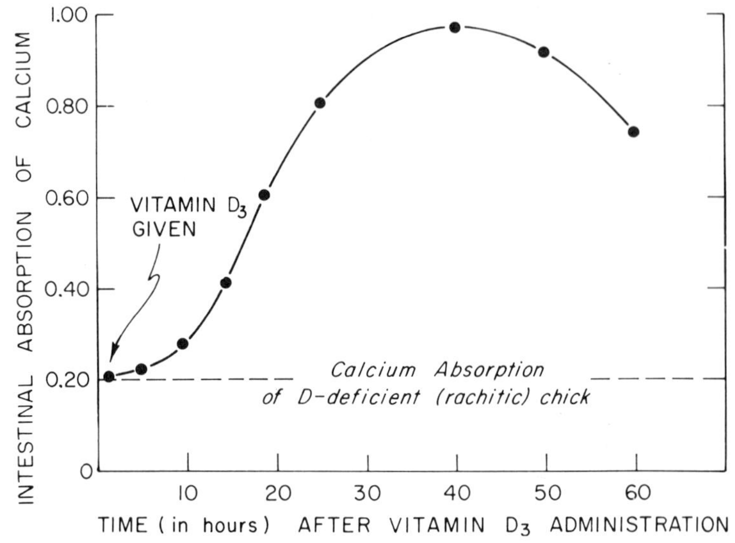

Figure 1-2. Slow onset of biological response (intestinal calcium absorption) after administration of vitamin D_3 to rachitic chicks. A dose of 100 IU (6.5 nmoles) was administered intracardially to groups of rachitic chicks at the indicated time points prior to assay of the biological response of intestinal calcium absorption. From Norman (1965).

quite apparent that 36–48 hr are required for generation of the maximal response in the rachitic chick.

It was found (Norman, 1966) that the duration of the lag and the magnitude of response are proportional to the size of the dose of vitamin D. With oral, intraperitoneal, or intracardial doses of 20,000,100, or 10 IU of vitamin D_3, the lag in response of chick intestinal calcium absorption was 5–8, 10–15, or 15–25 hr, respectively. This suggested that there was possibly a competition among specific and nonspecific receptor sites in the intestinal mucosa, bone, kidney, and perhaps other tissues. Only at higher dosage levels could all the receptor sites in all target organs become rapidly saturated.

There are several possible explanations for the lag in action of vitamin D. (a) Metabolic conversion to an "active" form may be necessary before the vitamin can perform its biochemical role, as was originally suggested by Raoul and Gounelle (1958) and Sallis and Holdsworth (1962). (b) The lag may be due to a slow absorption and transportation of the vitamin to the target organ and subsequent association with its receptor site(s). (c) The lag may reflect some as yet undefined induction process involving expression of genetic information that is ultimately utilized to elicit the expected effect(s).

As a consequence of intensive efforts in many laboratories, a new model emerged for the mechanism of action of the fat-soluble vitamin D. The development of this model was based on the concept that, in terms of its structure and mode of action, vitamin D (calciferol) is similar to the classic steroid hormones, e.g., aldosterone, testosterone, estrogen, hydrocortisone, and ecdysterone. This model was also based on the results obtained from experiments in which actinomycin D [an inhibitor of DNA-directed RNA synthesis (Reich *et al.*, 1961)] was shown to block the intestinal and skeletal responses of the rachitic rat or chick to vitamin D (Eisenstein and Passavoy, 1964; Zull *et al.*, 1965, 1966; Norman, 1965, 1966). It was further observed (Norman, 1965) that actinomycin D was capable of inhibiting the response to a dose of vitamin D_3 that was 4000 times that of a physiological dose. If vitamin D were functioning as an enzyme cofactor, this amount of the vitamin would be more than that necessary to saturate any receptor sites on an enzyme. Apparently, any manifestation of the vitamin's activity is strictly dependent on the actinomycin D-sensitive events involving the conversion from the deficient to a normal state.

The concept that an understanding of the mechanism of action of steroid hormones (estradiol, testosterone, aldosterone, hydrocortisone, ecdysterone, progesterone) must be sought in terms of hormonal interactions with genetic information is now firmly established (O'Malley and Schrader, 1976). The concept that the biological actions of vitamin D could be explained by a hormone-like action of calciferol was first reviewed in depth by Norman (1968).

The most notable advance in our current understanding of the mechanisms of action of vitamin D has been the elucidation of the complex metabolic pathway for the production of the biologically active form (Fig. 1-3). It is now agreed that the biologically active form of vitamin D is the steroid 1α,25-dihydroxycholecalciferol [$1,25(OH)_2D_3$]. Vitamin D_3, which may be ingested dietarily or produced in the skin via a photochemical reaction, is first transported to the liver, where it is hydroxylated on C-25. 25-Hydroxycholecalciferol [$25(OH)D_3$] is next transported to the kidney, where it undergoes further metabolism to $1,25(OH)_2D_3$. In this respect it should be appreciated that $1,25(OH)_2D_3$ is a steroid hormone produced by an endocrine gland, the kidney, and acts distally in a variety of target organs, particularly the intestine and bone, to elicit the characteristic responses formerly attributed to the molecular species, vitamin D.

B. The Steroid Hormone Mode of Action of Vitamin D

What evidence is there to support the thesis that 1α,25-dihydroxycholecalciferol is a hormone? It is not sufficient to simply have a mode of action similar to that of other steroid hormones. A hormone is classically defined as a systemic-acting substance produced by a specialized cell in response to a specific set of physiological stimuli or signals. Very small amounts of the substance are then released into the circulation and transported to distal target organs, where the

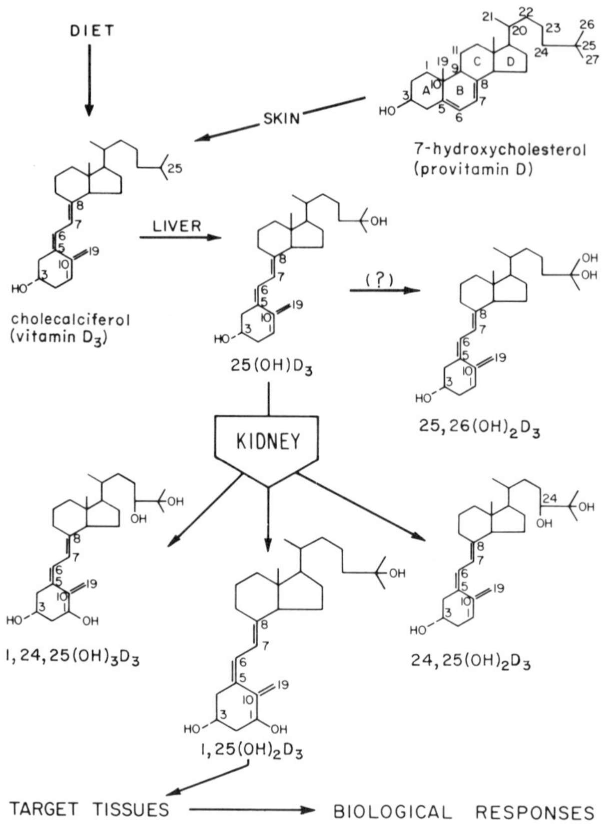

Figure 1-3. Metabolic pathway for the production of the hormonally active form of vitamin D_3, 1α,25-dihydroxycholecalciferol. The vitamin (calciferol) may be acquired either by the photochemical reaction occurring in the skin that converts 7-dehydrocholesterol to cholecalciferol or from nutritional sources in the diet.

substance interacts to elicit a set of specific physiological responses. It is the lack of these responses which usually generates indirectly the signal that results in the secretion of the hormone. Normally, an endocrine system has a method of self-regulation; i.e., once the physiological response that is produced by the presence of the hormone is manifested, there is an autoregulation or homeostasis such that the secretion or production of the hormone is "feedback" regulated.

The classic method of demonstrating that an organ has an endocrine role in the economy of the organism is to create a deficit of the hormone by surgical removal or chemical inactivation of the organ in question. With reference to calciferol, there were suggestions in the literature as early as 1943 that the kidney was related in some crucial way to the biological actions of the vitamin. Specifically, Liu and Chu (1943) and more recently Avioli *et al.* (1970) and Lumb *et al.* (1971) suggested there was a relationship between chronic renal failure or renal osteodystrophy and vitamin D. Patients who suffer from chronic renal failure often exhibit many symptoms of a classic vitamin D deficiency, e.g., reduced intestinal absorption of calcium, lowered bone ash, and chronic hypocalcemia. In retrospect, it can be appreciated that in chronic renal disease there is an impairment of the production of the biologically active form of vitamin D: $1,25(OH)_2D_3$.

A direct demonstration of the renal production of $1,25(OH)_2D_3$ was first provided by Fraser and Kodicek (1970), who found that a nephrectomized rat could not produce a polar metabolite (subsequently identified as $1,25(OH)_2D_3$) of vitamin D. This observation was quickly confirmed by Norman *et al.* (1971a) and Gray *et al.* (1971). Furthermore, Wong *et al.* (1972) clearly demonstrated that a nephrectomized, vitamin D-deficient rat was unable to respond to moderate doses of either vitamin D_3 or $25(OH)D_3$. In marked contrast, these same vitamin D-deficient, nephrectomized rats gave a completely normal response to $1,25(OH)_2D_3$. These observations unequivocally demonstrated that a deficit of the biologically active (hormonally active) form of vitamin D could be created by surgical removal of the kidney and that this deficit could be overcome by administration of the hormone $1,25(OH)_2D_3$. Thus, these results collectively support the concept that the kidney is an endocrine organ for the production of the biologically/hormonally active form of vitamin D.

Another critical step which contributed to the realization that $1,25(OH)_2D_3$ was the biologically active form of calciferol was a thorough evaluation of its biological activity. It was reported that a single dose of $1,25(OH)_2D_3$ was 13–15 times as effective as cholecalciferol in stimulating the intestinal absorption of calcium and 5–6 times as effective as cholecalciferol in stimulating serum calcium elevation (Myrtle and Norman, 1971; Haussler *et al.*, 1971; Norman and Wong, 1973). In experiments in which $1,25(OH)_2D_3$ was administered daily, the results indicated that it was at least as active, if not more active, than the parent vitamin D in terms of every parameter tested (bone ash, serum calcium, and rate of growth) (Norman and Wong, 1973; Tanaka *et al.*, 1973).

These results support the contention that 1α,25-dihydroxycholecalciferol is the most biologically active form of vitamin D presently known. There is a possibility that this steroid is capable of meeting all the nutritional and physiological requirements that are known to be met by calciferol. It is already apparent that $1,25(OH)_2D_3$ may have application in certain clinical disorders that arise from the alterations in the metabolism of vitamin D or in the production of $1,25(OH)_2D_3$ (see Chapter 11).

Figure 1-4 is a flow chart analysis of the multiple steps involved in the postulated hormonal mechanism of action of the steroid $1,25(OH)_2D_3$. The sum

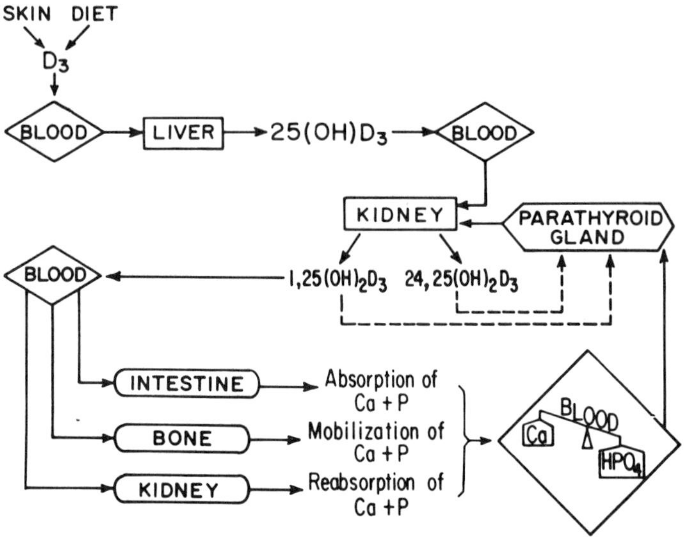

Figure 1-4. Proposed endocrine system related to vitamin D action.

of these steps constitutes the integrated endocrine system for the action of vitamin D, which is discussed in detail in this book. There are a variety of potential target tissues to which the hormone 1,25$(OH)_2D_3$ may be transported. The two most obvious are the intestinal mucosa and the skeletal system.

In the intestine there are two major problems facing the biochemist who wishes to clarify the detailed mechanism of action of this steroid: (a) elucidation of the steps of interaction of the hormone with its target tissue and understanding of how the presence of the steroid hormone initiates the classic physiological response of increased calcium transport and (b) understanding of the molecular basis of calcium translocation across the intestinal mucosal cell, i.e., study of the uptake of calcium into the cell across the intestinal brush border membranes, and elucidation of its translocation across the interior of the intestinal mucosal cell or its possible movement out of the cell into intercellular spaces, and exit of calcium through the basal membrane of the cell and movement through the capillary membranes into the plasma.

The approach pioneered in the laboratories of DeLuca, Kodicek, and Norman, which permitted for the first time the possibility of developing a biochemical description of the action of cholecalciferol, was to administer *small physiological doses* of radioactive vitamin D and to trace the appearance of the radioactive label in the target tissue. In the course of these studies (Haussler *et al.*, 1968; Lawson *et al.*, 1969), it became apparent not only that there was a specific localization of radioactivity within the target intestinal nuclear and chromatin fraction, but also that this radioactivity was not chemically identical to that of the parent vitamin D. Further extensive studies eventually resulted in the unequivocal demonstration that this substance which selectively localized in the target intestine and its nuclear fraction was chemically distinct from both cholecalciferol and the intermediate 25-hydroxycholecalciferol (Myrtle *et al.*, 1970; Kodicek *et al.*, 1970). With the concomitant demonstration that this polar metabolite had a highly significant amount of biological activity in terms of stimulating the intestinal transport of calcium (Haussler *et al.*, 1968, 1971; Myrtle *et al.*, 1970; Norman *et al.*, 1971b), the extensive effort necessary to chemically characterize the substance was undertaken. This resulted in simultaneous, yet independent, reports from three laboratories that the chemical structure of this calciferol metabolite was 1,25-dihydroxycholecalciferol (Lawson *et al.*, 1971; Norman *et al.*, 1971b; Holick *et al.*, 1971).

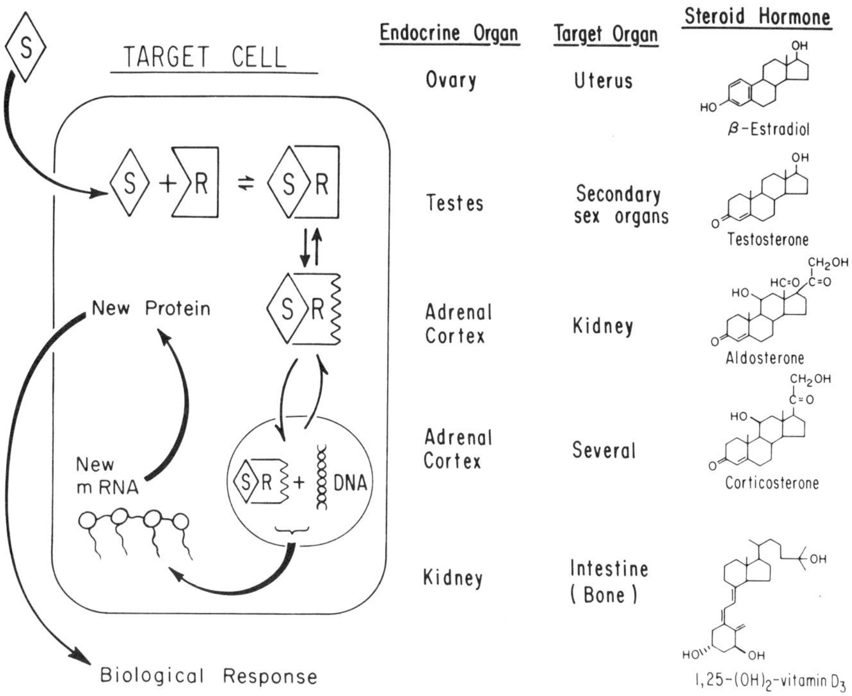

Figure 1-5. Generalized two-step model of the action of steroid hormones in their target tissues. The left panel indicates how steroid hormones [including $1,25(OH)_2D_3$] are believed to interact in the target tissue [for $1,25(OH)_2D_3$, the intestinal mucosa]. Abbreviations: R, a protein receptor localized in the cytoplasmic portion of the cell; SR, the steroid–receptor complex, which undergoes a temperature-dependent activation step prior to its entry into the nucleus of the cell. The right panel illustrates the structural similarities of many steroid hormones, including $1,25(OH)_2D_3$.

TABLE 1-2

Hormone-like Action of 1α,25-Dihydroxycholecalciferol—Evolution of Nutritional Component (Vitamin D) to Steroid (Calciferol) to Hormone (1,25-Dihydroxyvitamin D)

Date	Observation	Laboratory[a]	Reference
I. *Evidence for an antirachitic nutritional component (vitamin D)*			
50,000 B.C.	Occurrence of rickets in Neanderthal man	—	Solecki (1971a,b) *Time* magazine (1971)
1645	First formal description of rickets as a disease	Leiden	Whistler (1645)
1650	First authoritative description of rickets and recognition that it was a distinct disease	London	Glisson (1650a,b)
1820	Correlation between incidence of rickets and lack of sunshine	—	Sniadecki (cited by Mozolowski, 1939)
1885	A thorough and precise morphological description of the effects of rickets on the skeleton	—	Pommer (1885)
1919	First experimental dietary production of rickets	London	Mellanby (1919)
1919	Demonstration of the calcifying and hence curative effect of uv light on rickets	—	Huldschinsky (1919)
1922	Identification of "vitamin D" as the antirachitic factor	New York, Baltimore	Hess and Gutman (1922), McCollum *et al*. (1922a,b; 1925)
1923	Prevention of rickets via uv irradiation of food	London	Goldblatt and Soames (1923)
1923	Production of vitamin D by uv irradiation	Madison	Steenbock (1924); Steenbock and Black (1924)
II. *Chemical determination that vitamin D is a steroid (cholecalciferol)*			
1932	Chemical characterization of synthetic vitamin D_2 as a secosteroid	Göttingen London	Windaus *et al*. (1932) Askew *et al*. (1932)
1934	Chemical characterization of synthetic vitamin D (D_4) as a secosteroid	Göttingen	Windaus and Langer (1934)
1936	Chemical characterization of natural vitamin D_3 as a secosteroid	Göttingen	Brockmann (1936), Brockmann and Busse (1938)
1948	X-ray crystallographic analysis of vitamin D_3 (evidence for open-ring structure)	Oxford	Crowfoot and Dunitz (1948), Crowfoot-Hodgkin *et al*. (1963)

III. *Evidence that vitamin D functions as a steroid hormone*			
1964	Detection of a polar metabolite fraction with some biological activity	Madison	Norman *et al.* (1964)
1966	Time lag for the biological action of administered vitamin D emphasized	Riverside, Madison	Norman (1966), Zull *et al.* (1966)
1966	Chemical characterization of $25(OH)D_3$; claimed to be biologically active form	Madison	Blunt *et al.* (1968)
1967	Discovery of biologically active metabolite in intestine (chromatin fraction)—more polar than $25(OH)D_3$	Riverside	Haussler *et al.* (1968)
1969	Metabolite more polar than $25(OH)D_3$ undergoing tritium loss at the carbon 1 position	Cambridge	Lawson *et al.* (1969)
1970	Demonstration of rapid biological effect of $1,25(OH)_2D_3$	Cambridge	Kodicek *et al.* (1970)
		Riverside	Myrtle and Norman (1971)
		Philadelphia	Haussler *et al.* (1971)
1971	Identification and confirmation of the kidney as site of production of $1,25(OH)_2D_3$-like compound	Cambridge	Fraser and Kodicek (1970)
		Riverside	Norman *et al.* (1971a)
		Madison	Gray *et al.* (1971)
1971	Demonstration that metabolite produced by kidney is identical to that found in intestinal mucosa	Riverside	Norman *et al.* (1971), Midgett *et al.* (1973)
1971	Chemical identification of $1,25(OH)_2D_3$	Cambridge	Lawson *et al.* (1971)
		Riverside	Norman *et al.* (1971b)
		Madison	Holick *et al.* (1971)
1972	Biological activity of $1,25(OH)_2D_3$ in uremic and normal human beings	Los Angeles–Riverside	Brickman *et al.* (1972)
1973	Demonstration that $1,25(OH)_2D_3$ stimulates intestinal RNA synthesis	Riverside	Tsai and Norman (1973b)
		Cambridge	Emtage *et al.* (1973)
1974	Conformation of calciferol in solution	Riverside	Wing *et al.* (1974)
1974	Radiocompetition assay for $1,25(OH)_2D_3$	Tucson	Brumbaugh *et al.* (1974)

[a] In some cases laboratories whose major focus was vitamin D have been specified. These include Leiden, the Netherlands; Göttingen, Germany; London; Oxford; Cambridge, England; New York; Baltimore; Madison, Wisconsin; Los Angeles; Riverside, California; Philadelphia; Tucson, Arizona.

It could be shown that irrespective of whether radioactive vitamin D_3, 25(OH)D_3 or 1,25$(OH)_2D_3$ was given to a rachitic chick, 20, 8, or 4 hr later there was a maximal localization of radioactivity in the intestinal nuclear fraction. In each instance, the nuclear fraction had associated with it approximately 70–80% of the total radioactivity present within the target tissue. Extraction and chromatographic evaluation of the radioactivity resulting from the separate administration of the three steroids indicated that it was exclusively in the chemical form 1,25$(OH)_2D_3$. Further evaluation of the localization of the radioactivity in the crude nuclear fraction of the intestine revealed that it was also present when purified nuclei were prepared (Haussler *et al.*, 1968) or when the subnuclear chromatin fraction was prepared (Haussler and Norman, 1969). It was then possible to correlate the dose of calciferol steroid necessary to saturate intestinal chromatin receptors with the dose of calciferol steroid required to give a maximal stimulation of intestinal calcium transport.

The nuclear and chromatin localization of 1,25$(OH)_2D_3$ in intestinal tissue that resulted under *in vivo* conditions was duplicated under *in vitro* conditions (Tsai and Norman, 1973a; Chen and DeLuca, 1973; Brumbaugh and Haussler, 1974). This was followed shortly by reports from Emtage *et al.* (1973) that they had isolated a messenger RNA in the intestinal mucosal polysomes that was capable of synthesizing a specific calcium-binding protein (see Chapter 7). Also, it was reported that the administration of 1,25$(OH)_2D_3$ to rachitic chicks stimulated the incorporation of [^{3}H]uridine into intestinal mucosal RNA (Tsai and Norman, 1973b) and that actinomycin D was capable of blocking the biological responses in the intestine to 1,25$(OH)_2D_3$ (Tsai *et al.*, 1973).

Thus, it appears that there is almost complete confirmation of the genome-activation theory for the mechanism of action of vitamin D, at least with regard to the synthesis of calcium-binding protein. A general mechanism of the steroid hormone-like action of 1,25$(OH)_2D_3$ is presented in Fig. 1-5. It is quite apparent that the analogy of the hormone action of 1,25$(OH)_2D_3$ with that of other classic steroid hormones is now on a firm footing. What is not resolved, however, is whether the complete action of vitamin D (calciferol) in the intestinal mucosa is dependent on gene activation or whether the exclusive route of action of the biologically active hormone, 1,25-dihydroxycholecalciferol, is through its association with nuclear binding proteins. Extensive efforts are now being directed in a number of laboratories toward providing definitive answers to these questions.

It can now be appreciated that the prohormone, cholecalciferol, became a trace dietary constituent, i.e., a vitamin, only because of man's predilection for clothing, industrial air pollution, and indoor activities away from a source of ultraviolet irradiation. Table 1-2 is a listing of the significant events that have occurred in the evolution of man's understanding of the transformation of the fat-soluble vitamin D to the steroid hormone cholecalciferol. It is now apparent that, when adequate amounts of ultraviolet irradiation are present, ample quantities of the prohormone, cholecalciferol, are produced via normal endogenous endocrine mechanisms, thereby obviating the necessity for a dietary source of vitamin D and permitting its normal steroid hormone mode of action.

REFERENCES*

Askew, F., Bourdillon, R. B., Bruce, H. M., Callow, R. K., Philpot, J., and Webster, T. A. (1932). *Proc. R. Soc., London, Sec. B.* **109,** 448.

Avioli, L. V., Birge, S. J., and Slatopolsky, E. (1970). *Proc. Int. Congr. Nephrol., 4th, 1969* Vol. 2, p. 175.

Basch, K. (1906). Beitraege Physiologie und Pathologie des Thymus. *Jahrb. Kinderheilkd Phys. Erzieh.* [n.s.] **64,** 285.

Bibra, E. (1844). "Chemische Untersuchungen über Knochen und Zähne." Schwenfurt (cited by A. Hess, 1929).

Biedl, A. (1910). "Innere Sekretion," Urban & Schwarzenberg, Berlin.

Blunt, J. W., DeLuca, H. F., and Schnoes, H. K. (1968). *Chem. Commun.* p. 801.

Brickman, A. S., Coburn, J. W., and Norman, A. W. (1972). *N. Engl. J. Med.* **287,** 891.

Brockmann, H. (1936). *Hoppe-Seyler's Z. Physiol. Chem.* **241,** 104.

Brockmann, H. (1937). *Hoppe-Seyler's Z. Physiol. Chem.* **245,** 96.

Brockmann, H., and Busse, A. (1938). *Naturwissenschaften* **26,** 122.

Brumbaugh, P. F., and Haussler, M. R. (1974). *J. Biol. Chem.* **249,** 1251.

Carlsson, A. (1952). Tracer experiments of the effect of vitamin D on the skeletal metabolism of calcium and phosphorus. *Acta Physiol. Scand.* **26,** 212–220.

Carlsson, A., and Hollunger, G. (1954). The effect of vitamin D in the citric acid metabolism. *Acta Physiol. Scand.* **31,** 317–333.

Carlsson, A., and Lindquist, B. (1955). Comparison of intestinal and skeletal effects of vitamin D in relation to dosage. *Acta Physiol. Scand.* **35,** 53–55.

Chen, T. C., and DeLuca, H. F. (1973). *J. Biol. Chem.* **248,** 4890.

Coates, M. E., and Holdsworth, E. S. (1961). Vitamin D_3 and the absorption of calcium in the chick. *Br. J. Nutr.* **15,** 131–147.

Crowfoot, D., and Dunitz, J. (1948). *Nature (London)* **162,** 608.

Crowfoot-Hodgkin, D., Rummer, B. M., Dunitz, J. D., and Trueblood, K. (1963). *J. Chem. Soc.* p. 4945.

Dowdle, E. B., Schachter, D., and Schenker, H. (1960). Requirement for vitamin D for the active transport of calcium by the intestine. *Am. J. Physiol.* **198,** 269–274.

Eisenstein, R., and Passavoy, M. (1964). Actinomycin D inhibits parathyroid hormone and vitamin D activity. *Proc. Soc. Exp. Biol. Med.* **117,** 77–79.

Emtage, G. S., Lawson, D. E. M., and Kodicek, E. (1973). *Nature (London)* **246,** 100.

Fehling, H. (1894). Ueber Osteomalacia. *Z. Geburtschilfe Gynaekol.* **30,** 471.

Fieser, L. F., and Fieser, M. (1959). "The Steroids." Van Nostrand-Reinhold, Princeton, New Jersey.

Findlay, L. (1922). Etiology of rickets. *Lancet* **1,** 825.

Fraser, D. R., and Kodicek, E. (1970). *Nature (London)* **228,** 764.

Freudenthal, P. (1917). "Experimental Rickets." Munksgaard, Copenhagen.

*For key historical citations in the first chapter only, the title of the paper or book is provided.

Friedleben, A. (1860). "Physikalische und chemische Konstitution wachsender und rachitischer Knochen." Wien (cited by A. Hess, 1929).

Funk, C. (1914). "Die Vitamine." Bergmann, Wiesbaden.

Glisson, F. (1650a). "De Rachitide sive Morbo Puerili, qui Vulgo 'The Rickets' Diciteur," London.

Glisson, F. (1650b). "De Rachitide." London (editions II and III of this same treatise were published in 1660 and 1670). This source has been cited by both Freudenthal (1917), Korenchevsky (1922), and A. Hess (1929). A photocopy is available in the Library of the Surgeon General of the United States.

Goldblatt, H. (1923). Studies on the fat-soluble growth promoting factor. *Biochem. J.* **17**, 446.

Goldblatt, H., and Soames, K. N. (1923). A study of rats on a normal diet irradiated daily by the mercury vapor quartz lamp or kept in darkness. *Biochem. J.* **17**, 294.

Gray, R., Boyle, I., and DeLuca, H. F. (1971). *Science* **172**, 1232.

Hansen, F. C. C. (1924). *Medd. Groenl.* **67**, 36.

Harrison, H. E., and Harrison, H. C. (1965). Vitamin D and permeability of intestinal mucosa to calcium. *Am. J. Physiol.* **208**, 370–374.

Haussler, M. R., and Norman, A. W. (1969). *Proc. Natl. Acad. Sci. U.S.A.* **62**, 155.

Haussler, M. R., Myrtle, J., and Norman, A. W. (1968). *J. Biol. Chem.* **243**, 4055.

Haussler, M. R., Boyle, D. W., Littledike, E. T., and Rasmussen, H. (1971). *Proc. Natl. Acad. Sci. U.S.A.* **68**, 177.

Hess, A. F. (1922). Influence of light in the prevention and cure of rickets. *Lancet* **2**, 1222.

Hess, A. F. (1929). "Rickets, Osteomalacia and Tetany." Lea & Febiger, Philadelphia, Pennsylvania.

Hess, A. F., and Gutman, M. G. (1922). *J. Am. Med. Assoc.* **78**, 29.

Hess, A. F., and Unger, L. J. (1920). The clinical role of the fat soluble vitamine. Its relation to rickets. *J. Am. Med. Assoc.* **74**, 217.

Hess, A. F., and Unger, L. J. (1921). The cure of infantile rickets by sunlight. *J. Am. Med. Assoc.* **77**, 39.

Hess, A. F., and Weinstock, M. (1925a). The antirachitic activity of irradiated cholesterol and phytosterol. *J. Biol. Chem.* **64**, 181.

Hess, A. F., and Weinstock, M. (1925b). Evidence of chemical change as shown by absorption spectra. *J. Biol. Chem.* **64**, 193.

Hess, A. F., and Weinstock, M (1925c). The antirachitic value of irradiated cholesterol and phytosterol. II. Further evidence of a change in biological activity. *J. Biol. Chem.* **64**, 1181.

Hess, A. F., McCann, G. F., and Pappenheimer, A. M. (1921a). The failure of rats to develop rickets on a diet deficient in vitamin A. *J. Biol. Chem.* **47**, 395.

Hess, A. F., Unger, L. J., and Pappenheimer, A. M. (1921b). The prevention of rickets in rats by exposure to sunlight. *Proc. Soc. Exp. Biol. Med.* **19**, 8.

Hirsch, A. (1886). "Handbook of Geographical and Historical Pathology." New Sydenham Soc., London.

Holick, M. F., Schnoes, H. K., DeLuca, H. F., Suda, T., and Cousins, R. J. (1971). *Biochemistry* **10**, 2799.

Hopkins, F. G. (1920). Effects of heat and aeration upon the fat soluble vitamin. *Biochem. J.* **14**, 725.

Huldschinsky, K. (1919). Heilung von Rachitis durch kuenstliche Hohensonne. *Dtsch. Med. Wochenschr.* **45**, 712.

Huldschinsky, K. (1919–1920). Die Behandlung der Rachitis durch ultraviolett Bestrahlung. *Z. Orthop. Chir.* **39**, 426.

Irving, J. T. (1944). The action of vitamin D upon the incisor teeth of rats consuming diets with a high or low Ca:P ratio. *J. Physiol. (London)* **103**, 9–26.

Kassowitz, M. (1881). "Die normale Ossifikation und die Erkrankungen des Knochensystems bei Rachitis und hereditaerer Syphylis." Braumueller, Wien.

Kjerrulf, H. (1922). *Hygeia* **84,** 530.

Koch, J. (1911). Untersuchungen über die Lokalisation der Bakterien, etc. *Z. Hyg. Infektionskr.* **69,** 486.

Kodicek, E., Lawson, D. E. M., and Wilson, P. W. (1970). *Nature (London)* **228,** 763.

Korenchevsky, V. (1922). The aetiology and pathology of rickets from an experimental point of view. *Med. Res. Counc. (G.B.), Spec. Rep. Ser.* **SRS-71.**

Lawson, D. E. M., Wilson, P. W., and Kodicek, E. (1969). *Biochem. J.* **115,** 269.

Lawson, D. E. M., Fraser, D. M., Kodicek, E., Morris, H. R., and Williams, D. H. (1971). *Nature (London)* **230,** 228.

Lindquist, B (1952). The effect of Vitamin D on the metabolism of radiocalcium in rachitic rats. *Acta Paediat. (Stockholm)* **41,** Suppl. 86, 1-80.

Liu, S. H., and Chu, H. I. (1943). *Medicine (Baltimore)* **22,** 103.

Loomis, W. F. (1967). *Science* **157,** 501.

Lumb, G. A., Mawer, E. G., and Stanbury, S. W. (1971). *Am. J. Med.* **50,** 421.

McCollum, E. V., Simmonds, N., Parsons, T. H., Shipley, P. G., and Park, E. A. (1921). The production of rachitis and similar diseases in the rat by deficient diets. *J. Biol. Chem.* **45,** 332.

McCollum, E. V., Simmonds, N., Becker, J. E., and Shipley, P. G. (1922a). Studies on experimental rickets. XXI. An experimental demonstration of the existence of the vitamin which promotes calcium deposition. *J. Biol. Chem.* **53,** 293.

McCollum, E. V., Simmonds, N., Becker, J. E., and Shipley, P. G. (1922b). *Bull. Johns Hopkins Hosp.* **33,** 229.

McCollum, E. V., Simmonds, N., Becker, J. E., and Shipley, P. G. (1925). *J. Biol. Chem.* **65,** 97.

Marchand, R. F. (1842). *J. Prakt. Chem.* **27,** 83-97 (cited by Korenchevsky, 1922).

Mellanby, E. (1919). The present state of knowledge concerning accessory food factors. *Med. Res. (G.B.), Spec. Rep. Ser.* **SRS-38.**

Mellanby, E. (1921). Experimental rickets. *Med. Res. Counc. (G.B.), Spec. Rep. Ser.* **SRS-61.**

Midgett, R. J., Spielvogel, A. M., Coburn, J. W., and Norman, A. W. (1973). *J. Clin. Endocrinol. Metab.* **36,** 1153.

Migicovsky, B. B. (1957). Influence of vitamin D on Ca^{++} resorption and accretion. *Can. J. Biochem. Physiol.* **35,** 1267-1275.

Migicovsky, B.B., and Nielson, A. M. (1951). *Arch. Biochem. Biophys.* **34,** 104.

Moore, N. (1884) "The History of the First Treatise on Rickets." St. Bartholomew Hospital Reports, London.

Morpurgo, B. (1902). Durch Infection hervorgerufene malacische und rachitische Skelettveraenderungen an jungen Ratten. *Zentralbl. Allg. Pathol. Pathol. Anat.* **13,** 113.

Mozolowski, W. (1939). *Nature (London)* **143,** 121.

Myrtle, J. F., and Norman, A. W. (1971). *Science* **171,** 78-82.

Myrtle, J. F., Haussler, M. R., and Norman, A. W. (1970). *J. Biol. Chem.* **245,** 1190.

Nelson, E. M., and Steenbock, H. (1925). The non-precipitability of the antiopthalmic and antirachitic properties from cod liver oil by digitonin. *J. Biol. Chem.* **64,** 299.

Norman, A. W. (1965). Actinomycin D and the response to vitamin D. *Science* **149,** 184-185.

Norman, A. W. (1966). Actinomycin D effect on lag in vitamin D-mediated calcium absorption in the chick. *Am. J. Physiol.* **211,** 829-834.

Norman, A. W. (1968). The mode of action of vitamin D. *Biol. Rev. Cambridge Philos. Soc.* **43,** 97-137.

Norman, A. W., and Wong, R. G. (1973). *J. Nutr.* **102,** 1709.

Norman, A. W., Midgett, R. J., Myrtle, J. F., and Nowicki, H. G. (1971a). *Biochem. Biophys. Res. Commun.* **42,** 1082.

Norman, A. W., Myrtle, J. F., Midgett, R. J., Nowicki, H. G., Williams, V., and Popjak, G. (1971b). *Science* **173,** 51.

O'Malley, B. W., and Schrader, W. T. (1976). *Sci. Am.* **234,** 32.

Palm, T. A. (1890). The geographical distribution and etiology of rickets. *Practitioner* **45,** 270.

Parrot, J. (1897). The osseous lesions of hereditary syphilis. *Lancet* **1,** 696.

Patrick, H., and Schweitzer, G. K. (1955). Usage of Ca^{45} in determination of vitamin D depletion and response time in chicks. *Poult. Sci.* **34,** 832–833.

Pommer, G. (1885). "Untersuchungen über Osteomalacia und Rachitis." Vogel, Leipzig.

Raoul, Y., and Gounelle, J. C. (1958). Localization surrenalienne initiale de la vitamine D_3 après injection intravéinuse chez le Rat. *C.R. Heled. Seances Acad. Sci.* **247,** 161–163.

Reich, E., Franklin, R. M., Shatkin, A. J., and Tatum, E. L. (1961). Effect of actinomycin D on cellular nucleic acid synthesis and virus production. *Science* **134,** 556–557.

Sallis, J. D., and Holdsworth, E. S. (1962). Influence of vitamin D on calcium absorption in the chick. *Am. J. Physiol.* **203,** 497–505.

Schachter, D., Kimberg, D. V., and Schenker, H. (1961). Active transport of calcium by intestine: action and bioassay of vitamin D. *Am. J. Physiol.* **200,** 1263–1271.

Shipley, P. G., Park, E. A., McCollum, E. V., and Simmonds, N. (1921). The relative effectiveness of cod liver oil as contrasted with butter fat for protecting the body against insufficient calcium in the presence of a normal phosphorus supply. *Am. J. Hyg.* **1,** 512.

Siegert, F. (1903). Beitraege zen Lehre von der Rachitis. *Jahrb. Kinderheilkd. Phys. Erzieh.* [n.s.] **58,** 929.

Solecki, R. S. (1971a). *Smithson.* May 17.

Solecki, R. S. (1971b). "Shanidar: The Humanity of Neanderthal Man." Knopf, New York.

Steenbock, H. (1924). The induction of growth promoting and calcifying properties in a ration by exposure to light. *Science* **60,** 224.

Steenbock, H., and Black, A. (1924). Fat soluble vitamins. XXIII. The induction of growth-promoting and calcifying properties of a ration by exposure to ultraviolet light. *J. Biol. Chem.* **61,** 405.

Steenbock, H., and Black, A. (1925). The induction of growth promoting and calcifying properties in fats and their unsaponifiable constituents by exposure to light. *J. Biol. Chem.* **64,** 263.

Steenbock, H., and Nelsen, M. T. (1924). The induction of calcifying properties in a rickets-producing ration by radiant energy. *J. Biol. Chem.* **62,** 209.

Stoeltzner, W. (1900). Ueber Behandlung der Rachitis mit Nebennierensubstanz. *Jahb. Kinderheilkd. Phys. Erzieh.* [n.s.] **51,** 73 and 199.

Tanaka, Y., Frank, H., and DeLuca, H. F. (1973). *Endocrinology* **92,** 417.

Thompson, V. W., and DeLuca, H. F. (1964). Vitamin D and phospholipid metabolism. *J. Biol. Chem.* **239,** 984.

Time magazine (1971). Author unknown, May 17 issue, p. 75.

Trousseau, A., and Laseque, C. (1849). *Arch. Gen. Med.* **19,** 257.

Tsai, H. C., and Norman, A. W. (1973a). *J. Biol. Chem.* **248,** 5967.

Tsai, H. C., and Norman, A. W. (1973b). *Biochem. Biophys. Res. Commun.* **54,** 622.

Tsai, H. C., Midgett, R. J., and Norman, A. W. (1973). *Arch. Biochem. Biophys.* **157,** 339.

von Hansemann, (1906). *Berl. Klin. Wochenschr.* **43,** 1201.

Whistler, D. (1645). "Morbo puerli Anglorum, quem patrio idiomate indigenae vocant *the rickets.*" Lugduni Batavorum.

Windaus, A. (1909). *Ber. Dtsch. Chem. Ges.* **42,** 238.

Windaus, A., and Langer, R. (1934). *Justus Liebigs Ann. Chem.* **508,** 105.

Windaus, A., Linsert, O., Luttringhaus, A., and Weidlich, A. (1932). *Justus Liebigs Ann. Chem.* **492,** 276.

Windaus, A., Schenck, F., and von Werder, F. (1936). *Hoppe-Seyler's Z. Physiol. Chem.* **241,** 100.

Wing, R. M., Okamura, W. H., Pirio, M. R., Sine, S. M., and Norman, A. W. (1974). *Science* **186,** 939.

Wong, R. G., Norman, A. W., Reddy, C. R., and Coburn, J. W. (1972). *J. Clin. Invest.* **51,** 1287–1291.

Zull, J. E., Czarnowska-Misztal, E., and DeLuca, H. F. (1965). Actinomycin D inhibition of vitamin D action. *Science* **149,** 182–183.

Zull, J. E., Czarnowska-Misztal, E., and DeLuca, H. F. (1966). On the relationship between vitamin D action and actinomycin sensitive processes. *Proc. Natl. Acad. Sci. U.S.A.* **55,** 177–184.

CHAPTER 2

The Provitamins D

I. BACKGROUND CONSIDERATIONS

A. Definition of a Provitamin

As discussed in Chapter 1 concerning the historical events pertaining to the discovery of vitamin D, a major breakthrough occurred with the identification of the effect of ultraviolet irradiation in curing rickets. The simultaneous demonstration by Hess and Weinstock (1924, 1925) and Steenbock and Black (1924) that antirachitic activity could be imparted to foods by ultraviolet irradiation provided the key to the ultimate isolation and chemical characterization and then chemical synthesis of vitamin D. It was quickly appreciated that a precursor of vitamin D existed in these foods that could be converted after ultraviolet irradiation to the substance termed vitamin D. Thus, the definition of provitamin D simply implies a substance that can be converted to a compound with vitamin D-like activity during the process of ultraviolet irradiation.

The chief structural prerequisite of a provitamin D is that it be a sterol with a $\Delta_{5\text{-}7}$-diene double-bond system in ring B (see Fig. 2-1). The conjugated double-bond system in this specific location of the molecule allows the absorption of light quanta at certain specific wavelengths in the ultraviolet range. This initiates a complex series of transformations (see Fig. 3-9), which ultimately produces the secosteroid known as precalciferol.[1]

Thus, it is apparent that a host of steroid compounds may satisfy the prerequisite of being a provitamin D; it is essential only that they have a $\Delta_{5\text{-}7}$-diene system in ring B (see Table 2-3). The two most prevalent provitamins D are ergosterol (provitamin D_2) and 7-dehydrocholesterol (provitamin D_3).

B. Identification of the Concept of a Provitamin

The concept of "provitamin D" originated as a result of studies done by Goldblatt and Soames (1923), who irradiated rat liver extracts, Steenbock and Black (1924, 1925; Steenbock, 1924), who irradiated rat food, and Hess and Weinstock (1924, 1925), who irradiated both vegetable oils and human skin. These workers observed that, although the unirradiated control sample had no antirachitic activity, the irradiated samples were capable of ameliorating the deficiency syndrome of rickets in experimental rats. Shortly thereafter, Hess and Weinstock (1924, 1925) and Hess *et al.* (1925) determined that the activatable substance present in vegetable oils that was capable of producing an antirachitic substance was a constituent of the nonsaponifiable fraction, which was known to consist mainly of phytosterol.[2] In control experiments employing cholesterol as a comparison steroid, it was found, surprisingly, that ultraviolet irradiation of cholesterol, as well as phytosterol, generated antirachitic activity. Parallel studies by Steenbock and Black (1925), as well as by Rosenheim and Webster (1925) at the National Institute for Medical Research in England, indicated that cholesterol could be converted to an antirachitic substance after ultraviolet irradiation.

The fact that cholesterol (a chemically defined substance at this time, (1920–1925) could be converted to an antirachitic substance was a puzzling observation which took some six to eight years to resolve. It took much hard work and laborious experimentation to definitively establish that the antirachitic activity generated upon ultraviolet irradiation was not produced from cholesterol but

[1]Provitamin D compounds are derivatives of such sterol-like structures as cholesterol or cholestanol. These compounds are comprised of a hydrogenated 1,2-cyclopentanoperhydrophenanthrene system with angular methyl groups at C-10 and C-13 and a side chain of varying length at C-17 (see Table 2-3). The term "calciferol" or "vitamin D" is reserved for the class of compounds produced by the ultraviolet irradiation of provitamins (sterols containing a $\Delta_{5\text{-}7}$ double-bond system in ring B). This process ruptures the carbon bond between C-9 and C-10 to produce a sterol containing an intact A, C, and D ring but a broken B ring. According to the official IUPAC nomenclature system, this steroid is referred to as a "secosteroid," where the prefix "seco" indicates that one of the rings has been opened or broken. In particular, calciferol is a seco-B-steroid.

[2]"Phytosterol" is the name given to a mixture of plant sterols.

from a contaminating substance present in the "pure" cholesterol preparations available at the time. For example, both Windaus and Hess (1926) and Rosenheim and Webster (1925, 1927) recrystallized cholesterol some 15–20 times without eliminating the provitamin that could be rendered antirachitic via uv irradiation. Progress was hampered by the laborious, time-consuming bioassays involving the rat line test (see Chapter 4), which were employed to follow the presence of the antirachitic substance. Another important discovery was the observation that, although the provitamin compound could be precipitated by digitonin, the active material produced via uv irradiation could not be precipitated by digitonin. Eventually, Windaus, Hess, and their co-workers (Windaus *et al.*, 1927; Rosenheim and Webster, 1927) reached the following conclusion: "From our studies it follows with certainty that ergosterol, or a sterol which corresponds completely with ergosterol in u.v. absorption spectrum and in physiological properties, is the antirachitic provitamin."

Thus, chemists of this period were frustrated in their attempts to determine the chemical structure of the provitamins D and to appreciate the subtle difference in structure between that of 7-dehydrocholesterol and ergosterol. The problem was ultimately resolved only after the isolation and chemical characterization of vitamin D_2 and vitamin D_3 (ergocalciferol and cholecalciferol, respectively) in the early 1930's.

C. Chemical Characterization of Provitamins

Developments pertaining to the identification of the provitamins D date back to 1889, when the Parisian apothecary Charles Tanret isolated from the ergot of rye a sterol bearing a close resemblance to cholesterol, which he named ergosterol.[3] It is interesting that the physical constants (melting point, optical rotation, and elemental composition analysis of C, 84.75, H, 11.75) for ergosterol that Tanret reported (1889) were verified in the laboratory of Windaus (Windaus and Grosskopf, 1923; Windaus and Luttringhaus, 1932) over 30 years later.

Many students and postdoctoral fellows in Professor Windaus' laboratory in the decade from 1922 to 1933 were involved with the structural determination of ergosterol. However, it was only at the end of this interval that the relationship of ergosterol to vitamin D was established. As was determined in Windaus' laboratory in 1932 (Windaus and Luttringhaus, 1932), the correct elementary formula for ergosterol was $C_{28}H_{44}O$. An important point to emphasize in retrospect, however, is that the compound ergosterol was recognized by chemists of the era

[3]Ergot is a disease of rye and other cereal grasses caused by a fungus of the genus *Claviceps purpurea* which replaces the affected grain with a long, hard, hornlike, dark-colored sclerotial body. Thus, ergosterol is not produced principally by the plant itself but by a fungus living on it (see Table 2-1).

1905–1935 as a substance of definite chemical composition different from that of cholesterol. As pointed out in Chapter 3, this fact caused some confusion as the tangled web of developments leading to the determination of the chemical structure of vitamin D was unraveled.

The fact that esters of the provitamin (Windaus and Luttringhaus, 1932) in a molar ratio of 1 : 1 could be prepared with acetic acid and benzoic acid suggested that the oxygen present in the steroid was in the form of an alcohol hydroxyl group. When ergosterol was subjected to catalytic hydrogenation, it was found to absorb precisely 3 moles of gas to produce the saturated compound ergostanol; this indicated the presence of three double bonds in the original molecule (Windaus and Luttringhaus, 1930). Since the product was a saturated alcohol, it also was inferred that four rings were present. When the fully saturated compound ergostanol was reduced further with sodium in amyl alcohol, the parent hydrocarbon ergostane was obtained (Chuang, 1933). It was known at this time (1930–1933) that the ring system of ergostane was identical in structure and configuration to that of cholestane. Thus, this established the identity of the structure of the steroid ring nucleus of ergosterol with that of cholesterol (Windaus *et al.*, 1934).

The positioning of the hydroxyl group in ergosterol on C-3 was determined by oxidation of ergostanol acetate with chromic acid to yield a product that was identical in structure to that obtained from the chromic acid oxidation of dihydrocholesteryl acetate; therefore, the alcoholic hydroxyl group of ergostanol had to be on C-3 and in the β configuration (Fernholz and Chakravorty, 1934). A further bit of supporting information pertaining to the orientation of the hydroxyl group was derived from the knowledge that ergosterol could be precipitated with digitonin, which is specific for three β-hydroxyl-containing steroids. The elucidation of the complete skeletal structure of ergosterol should be attributed to Chuang (1933), who was a colleague of Windaus in the Göttingen laboratory.

The structure of the side chain of ergosterol was not established unequivocally until 1948, when X-ray analysis and infrared spectroscopy indicated that the configuration of the double bond in the side chain was in the *trans* orientation (Crowfoot and Dunitz, 1948). These studies were preceded by the work of Reindel and Kipphan (1932), who carried out ozonolysis of the side chain. This helped to identify the presence of the 22–23 double bond.

The precise location of the double bonds in the B ring also posed a particular challenge. The ultraviolet spectrum of ergosterol (see Fig. 2-2) is characteristic of a diene. Furthermore, it was known that ergosterol readily formed a Diels–Alder adduct with maleic anhydride (Windaus and Luttringhaus, 1931). The position of the double bonds in the B ring was established via treatment of ergosterol with perbenzoic acid, which yielded a doubly unsaturated triol monobenzoate. Since only two of the hydroxyl groups of the triol could be acetylated, it was apparent that one of the hydroxyls had to be tertiary. Furthermore, the fully saturated triol reacted with 1 mole of lead tetraacetate, indicating that there was an α-glycol system present in the molecule. The subsequent oxidation of the saturated triol with chromic acid produced a hydroxy diketone, which readily lost water; through a series of complicated deductive reasoning steps it was ultimately possible to conclude that one of the double bonds of ergosterol was 4-5, that the second was 22-23, and that the third double bond must be conjugated with the first and therefore must be 7-8 (Windaus *et al.*, 1934).

The provitamin 7-dehydrocholesterol was isolated and chemically characterized by Windaus and Bock (1937); some 100 kg of pig skins were utilized to supply 30 g of crude sterol containing 4% of the provitamin.

II. OCCURRENCE

In contrast to the rather limited biological occurrence of vitamin D, the provitamins D are widely distributed in nature, in both the plant and animal kingdoms. Bills and co-workers (Bills, 1935, 1954; Bills *et al.*, 1939) carried out extensive evaluations of the precise levels of provitamin D in the sterol fractions of various plant and animal species. A representative cross section of their extensive determinations in nonvertebrates is given in Table 2-1. It is apparent that provitamins of vitamin D are present in the plant world. The phanerogams and the cryptogams, particularly the mold *Aspergillus niger* and brewer's yeast, *Saccharomyces cerevisiae*, have essentially their complete sterol component present as ergosterol. This has proved to be of major economic importance in obtaining sufficient quantities of the provitamin D_2 necessary for the industrial production of vitamin D_2 (ergocalciferol). According to Bills (1954) the ergosterol content of *Saccharomyces cerevisiae* or *Aspergillus niger* can be as high as 10% of the dry weight of the sample.

The exact significance of the distribution of provitamins D in the Porifera, Coelenterata, Annelida and Arthropoda, Mollusca, and Echinodermata is not known. It is not apparent whether the substance that is capable of functioning as a provitamin upon irradiation plays a unique structural rọle in the biological events or calcium-related processes of these organisms. However, an understanding of the widespread biological occurrence of the provitamins in nonvertebrates may be of some value in explaining the biological distribution of vitamin D.

7-Dehydrocholesterol is the most common provitamin D occurring in higher animals, including man. Thorough studies by Bills (1935, 1954; Bills *et al.*, 1939) demonstrated that provitamin D, principally 7-dehydrocholesterol, is present in the skin of many species of vertebrates and to a minor extent in the liver, brain, and other tissues. Pigskin has been a commercial source for obtaining provitamin D_3 for industrial preparations. However, it is clear that the concentra-

TABLE 2-1
Representative Distribution of Provitamins D in Nonvertebrates[a]

Systematic name (common name)	Provitamins D (parts per 1000 total steroid)
Phanerogams	
Cottonseed oil	28
Ryegrass	15
Carrot	2
Cryptogams	
Aspergillus niger	1000
Saccharomyces cerevisiae	800
Fucus vesiculosces (alga)	<1
Porifera	
Cliona celata (boring sponge)	<10
Coelenterata	
Metridium dianthus (snowy or red sea anemone)	86
Madreporaria (commercial corals)	10
Annelida	
Tubifex (waterworm)	210
Lumbricus terrestris (earthworm)	170
Arthropoda	
Tenebrio molitor (mealworm)	120
Musea domestica (housefly)	7
Homaris vulgaris (European spring lobster)	2
Mollusca	
Arcuatula demissa (ribbed mussel)	370
Ostrea virginica (American oyster)	80
Echinodermata	
Asterias rubens (''five-finger'' red starfish)	4

[a]These values were abstracted from more extensive tables given by Sebrell and Harris (1954).

tion of provitamin D in the sterol fraction of vertebrates (Table 2-2) is a much lower proportion of the total steroid present than is the case in nonvertebrates and plants (Table 2-1).

It is not apparent even today how the high concentrations of vitamin D in cod-liver oil are produced. This is particularly puzzling since the cod is a deep-water fish, and the most effective wavelength of light for conversion of provitamin D to vitamin D (280 nm) would be transmitted through only approximately 1 meter of water. Thus, it is not tenable to hypothesize that the cod or other ocean-dwelling fish with high liver levels of vitamin D produce the vitamin via ultraviolet irradiation processes. One possible alternative explanation relates to the unusually high content of provitamins D in a variety of the algae or mollusks that normally dwell in the ocean (see Table 2-1). A particularly likely source of provitamin D, as advanced by Darby and Clarke (1937), is the floating

TABLE 2-2
Representative Distributions of Provitamins D in Various Tissues of Vertebrates[a]

Tissue	Animal	Provitamins D (parts per 1000 total sterol)
Skin	Pig	46
	Chicken (feet)	25
	Rat	19
	Human being (adult)	4
	Human being (infant)	1
	Cow	2
	Chicken (trunk)	<0.1
Liver	Tuna (Japanese)	17
	Cod (Atlantic)	4
	Pig	1
Brain	Human being (fetus)	0.5
	Sheep	0.4
	Human being (adult)	<0.1
Eggs	Duck (Chinese)	60
	Chicken	2
Milk	Cow	2
Blood serum	Cow	2
Heart	Calf	0.3
Gallstones	Human being	0.25

[a]These values were abstracted from a more extensive table given by Bills (1954).

brown alga *Sargassum,* which accumulates in enormous quantities in the clear waters of the West Indies. Quantities of this material are known to break off and be transferred as far north as Iceland via the Gulf Stream. If, in the process, the drifting weed were to become irradiated and at the same time cohabited with other invertebrates also containing significant levels of provitamin D, it is possible to envision a photochemical irradiation process occurring in these biological substances that might produce prodigious quantities of vitamin D and that might be consumed as a source of food by the appropriate species of ocean-dwelling fish. However, at present there is no substantiation of this hypothesis.

III. CHEMISTRY

A. Structural Requirement for Activity

The chief structural prerequisite of a sterol to be classed as a provitamin D is its ability to be converted upon ultraviolet irradiation to a vitamin D, i.e., a substance with antirachitic activity. Thus, a consideration of the allowable structures for provitamins D can be deferred until the next chapter, where the chemistry of vitamin D as well as the reactions involved in the ultraviolet irradiation process are considered in detail.

For a substance to be classified as a provitamin D, it is sufficient, first, that it be some kind of sterol and, second, that it have in its B ring a $\Delta_{5\text{-}7}$ unconjugated double-bond system. These relationships are emphasized in Fig. 2-1A, which shows the planar two-dimensional representation of the generic class of provitamins D. It is apparent that the structures and configurations of provitamins D are related to the ring structures of the parent compounds, cholesterol and cholestanol. Rings A, B, C, and D comprise a hydrogenated 1,2-cyclopentanoperhydrophenanthrene system. Joined to this nucleus are angular methyl groups at C-10 and C-13 and an eight-carbon side chain at C-17. In cholesterol, the secondary

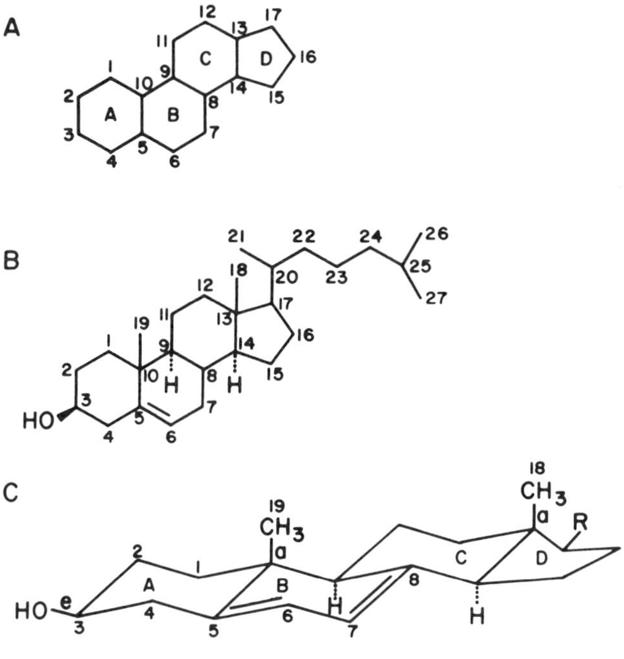

Figure 2-1. Representation of the ring structures of provitamins D. (A) The ring structure is derived, as with all steroids, from the saturated hydrocarbon cyclopentanoperhydrophenanthrene. The lettering of the four rings and the numbering of the carbon positions are in accordance with the standard IUPAC system for steroids. The side chain R of various provitamins is given in Table 2-3. (B) Structure of the parent cholesterol in planar view. (C) Conformational view of a provitamin. Rings B and C are rigidly fused to the A and D rings, respectively. Ring A preferentially assumes a chair conformation. The lowercase letters a and e refer to the axial and equatorial orientation, respectively. Ring C is fused to ring D in the *trans* configuration. The $\Delta_{5\text{-}7}$-double bonds of ring B tend to make that ring quite planar.

hydroxyl group is at C-3, and the double bond is between C-5 and C-6. The two angular methyl groups in the side chain are known to project toward the front of the molecule and thus they are described as β oriented and are drawn as solid-line bonds. The C-3 hydroxyl group and C-8 hydrogen atom are also β oriented, but the hydrogens of C-9 and C-14 are α oriented and project to the underside and their carbon bonds are indicated by dotted lines. The ring junctions B—C and C—D are *trans* fused. The numbering system of the carbons is indicated in Fig. 2-1.

Quite a wide variety of steroids have been found to have vitamin D or antirachitic activity. Accordingly, it must be inferred that there are an equal number of different steroids that are capable of serving as provitamins D. In particular, at least seven different specific provitamins D are known to exist (see Table 2-3). All of the provitamins D have the same structure for rings A, B, C, and D and differ only in the length and stereochemistry of their side chain. One provitamin whose structure has never been chemically characterized is the provitamin D_M reported by Petering and Waddell (1951). The "M" refers to *Modiolus,* a form of ribbed mussel. The steroid is believed to have 29 carbons.

As discussed in Chapter 1, one of the key aspects in elucidating the structure of vitamin D and determining the existence of a steroid with "provitamin D status" was the complete dependence of the interconversion of the two species on the presence of ultraviolet light. In retrospect, it is easy to understand the requirement for ultraviolet light to mediate the transition of provitamin D to vitamin D. Figure 2-2 shows the ultraviolet spectrum of any provitamin D. Provitamins D have a characteristic ultraviolet absorption spectrum with four maxima at 293,

TABLE 2-3
Side Chains of Provitamins D[a]

Provitamin trivial name	Vitamin D produced upon irradiation	Empirical formula (complete steroid)	Side-chain structure
Ergosterol	D_2	$C_{28}H_{44}O$	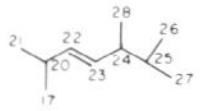
7-Dehydrocholesterol	D_3	$C_{27}H_{44}O$	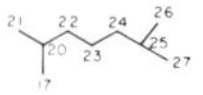
22,23-Dihydroergosterol	D_4	$C_{28}H_{46}O$	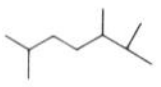
7-Dehydrositosterol	D_5	$C_{29}H_{48}O$	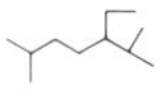
7-Dehydrostigmasterol	D_6	$C_{29}H_{46}O$	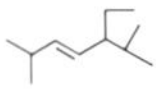
7-Dehydrocampesterol	D_7	$C_{28}H_{46}O$	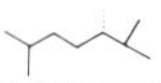

[a]Note that 22,23-dihydroergosterol and 7-dehydrocampesterol are epimers at C-24.

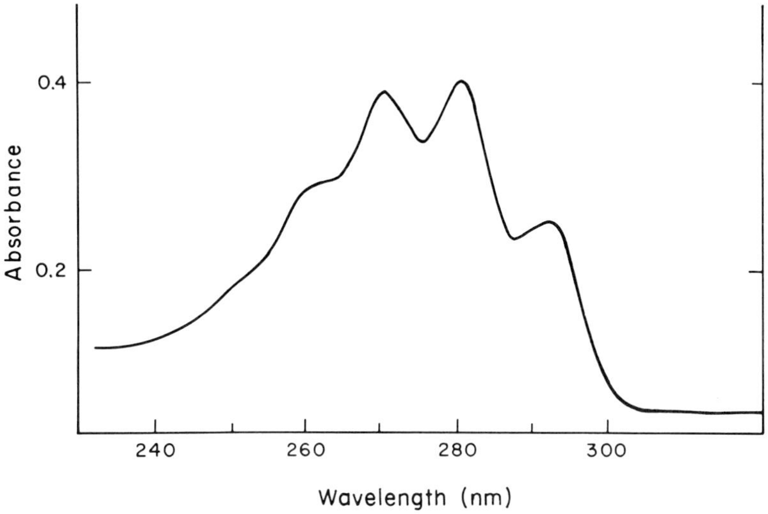

Figure 2-2. Characteristic ultraviolet absorption spectrum of provitamins. The wavelengths of the several absorption maxima (for 7-dehydrocholesterol) are (in nanometers) 262, 271, 282, and 293. The molar extinction coefficient at 282 nm is 11,500.

282, 271, and 262 nm. The molar extinction coefficient at 282 nm is 11,300. The two double bonds of the B ring form a homoannular diene unit, which explains the ability of provitamins D to form Diels–Alder adducts with such compounds as maleic or citraconic anhydride.

B. Chemical Synthesis

A challenging and significant problem for the organic chemist has been to chemically synthesize the provitamins appropriate for the particular vitamin D under investigation. However, as a rule the objective of the synthesis has been to produce a vitamin rather than the provitamin and, accordingly, the discussion of the chemical synthesis of the provitamins D and vitamin D itself is deferred until Chapter 3. However, these reactions are also of economic interest in that the industrial production of the prodigious quantities of vitamin D_2 or D_3 required worldwide requires a ready source of the appropriate provitamin. Although a significant fraction of this provitamin may be isolated from natural sources, i.e., either pigskin (7-dehydrocholesterol) or yeast or mold (ergosterol), it is still attractive industrially to envision a chemical synthesis of the required provitamins. Also, with the appreciation of the clinical efficacy of $1,25(OH)_2D_3$ in certain disease states, there have been renewed efforts by synthetic chemists to devise new methods of producing the provitamin of this D metabolite.

REFERENCES

Bills, C. E. (1935). *Physiol. Rev.* **15,** 1.

Bills, C. E. (1954). *In* "The Vitamins" (W. H. Sebrell, Jr. and R. S. Harris, eds.), 1st ed., Vol. 2, 149. Academic Press, New York.

Bills, C. E., Nassengale, O. N., and Prickett, P. S. (1939). *J. Biol. Chem.* **87,** 259.

Chuang, C. K. (1933). *Justus Liebigs Ann. Chem.* **500,** 270.

Crowfoot, D., and Dunitz, J. (1948). *Nature (London)* **162,** 608.

Darby, H. H., and Clarke, H. T. (1937). *Science* **85,** 318.

Fernholz, E., and Chakravorty, P. N. (1934). *Ber. Dtsch. Chem. Ges. A.* **67,** 2021.

Goldblatt, H., and Soames, K. N. (1923). *Biochem. J.* **17,** 294.

Hess, A. F., and Weinstock, M. (1924). *J. Biol. Chem.* **62,** 301.

Hess, A. F., and Weinstock, M. (1925) *J. Biol. Chem.* **63,** 297.

Hess, A. F., Weinstock, M., and Helman, F. D. (1925) *J. Biol. Chem.* **63,** 305.

Petering, H. G., and Waddell, W. (1951) *J. Biol. Chem.* **191,** 765.

Reindel, F., and Kipphan, A. (1932). *Justus Liebigs Ann. Chem.* **493,** 181.

Rosenheim, O., and Webster, T.A. (1925). *Lancet* **1,** 1025.

Rosenheim, O., and Webster, T. A. (1927). *Biochem. J.* **21,** 389.

Sebrell, W. H., Jr., and Harris, R. S., eds. (1954). "The Vitamins," 1st ed., Vol. 2, p. 149. Academic Press, New York.

Steenbock, H. (1924). *Science* **60,** 224.

Steenbock, H., and Black, A. (1924). *J. Biol. Chem.* **61,** 405.

Steenbock, H., and Black, A. (1925). *J. Biol. Chem.* **64,** 263.

Tanret, C. (1889). *C. R. Hebd. Seances Acad. Sci.* **108,** 98.

Windaus, A., and Bock, F. (1937). *Hoppe-Seyler's Z. Physiol. Chem.* **245,** 168.

Windaus, A., and Grosskopf, W. (1923). *Hoppe-Seyler's Z. Physiol. Chem.* **124,** 8.

Windaus, A., and Hess, A. F. (1926). *Nachr. Ges. Wiss. Goettingen, Math.-Phys. Kl.* p. 175.

Windaus, A., and Luttringhaus, A. (1930). *Justus Liebigs Ann. Chem.* **481,** 119.

Windaus, A., and Luttringhaus, A. (1931). *Ber. Dtsch. Chem. Ges. A.* **64,** 850.

Windaus, A., and Luttringhaus, A. (1932). *Nachr. Ges. Wiss. Goettingen, Math-Phys. K1.* p. 4.

Windaus, A., Hess, A. F., Rosenheim, O., Pohl, R., and Webster, T. (1927). *Chem.-Ztg.* **51,** 113.

Windaus, A., Inhoffen, H. H., and von Reichel, S. (1934). *Justus Liebigs Ann. Chem.* **510,** 248.

CHAPTER

3

The Vitamins D

I. BACKGROUND CONSIDERATIONS

A. Minimal Structural Requirements for Activity

The chemical structure of vitamin D_3, or cholecalciferol, is closely related to that of its provitamin, 7-dehydrocholesterol, from which it is produced by a photochemical reaction (Fig. 3-1). An important point is that the chemical compound vitamin D is therefore closely related structurally to the four-ring nucleus

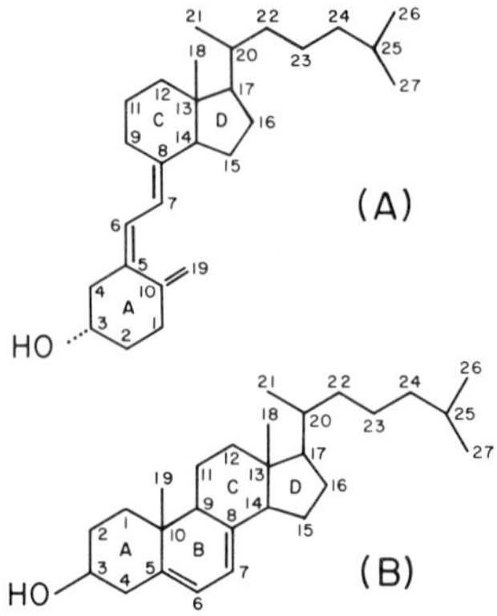

Figure 3-1. Structural relation of vitamin D_3 (A) to its provitamin, 7-dehydrocholesterol (B). The hydroxyl at C-3 is in the β (or "up") configuration. In the provitamin this is designated conventionally by a solid line; the α (or "down") orientation would be indicated by a dotted line. In the vitamin structure (A) the orientation of the hydroxyl is still β; however, due to the rotation around the bond between C-7 and C-8 that occurs upon irradiation, the configuration of the 3β-hydroxyl in the A ring is now indicated by a dotted line. In the provitamin, rings A and B are *cis*-fused, and rings B and C *trans*-fused. Rings C and D in both the provitamin and vitamin are *trans*-fused.

of other steroids that are derived from the cyclopentanoperhydrophenanthrene ring system (see Fig. 2-1). The official nomenclature proposed for vitamin D by the International Union of Pure and Applied Chemistry (IUPAC) relates it to the steroid nucleus, which is numbered as shown in Fig. 3-1B for the provitamin. The same carbons in vitamin D retain the same number (Fig. 3-1A).

No vitamin D activity in a biological sense becomes apparent until ring B of the provitamin is opened (usually by a photochemical reaction) to form the structure given for cholecalciferol. Thus, vitamin D is simply a steroid with a broken B ring; in particular the bond between C-9 and C-10 is broken. The fact that the B ring is broken in the steroid nucleus is officially designated by the term "seco." The formal chemical name for vitamin D_3 is 9,10-secocholesta-5,7,10(19)-trien-3β-ol, and the formal chemical name for vitamin D_2 is 9,10-secoergosta-5,7,10(19),22,23-tetraen-3β-ol (see Appendix C). Detailed discussions of the structural features required in the biologically active form of vitamin D_3, 1,25$(OH)_2D_3$, for optimal interaction with its intestinal receptor to generate biological responses are given in Chapters 5 and 7. It has been found that vitamin D cannot be altered by replacement of the hydroxyl at position 3 with a sulfhydryl (Bernstein and Sax, 1951), keto (Windaus and Buckholz, 1938), or halogen group (Bernstein *et al.*, 1949) and still retain biological activity. Thus, the presence of a 3β-hydroxyl group is highly desirable.

The location of the conjugated double bonds also markedly affects the biological activity of vitamin D. The preferred location is at the 10–19,5–6,7–8 positions. As will be discussed in Section III, C, there is a family of secosteroids produced that differ in the position of these double bonds. It is quite clear that maximal biological activity is attained only when the location of the double bonds is the same as in vitamin D_3. For example, Meunier and Thibaudet (1946) noted that tachysterol, which has its double bonds all shifted one position to yield a 5–10,6–7,8–9 triene system, has little if any biological activity.

A side chain of a length at least equivalent to that of cholesterol or ergosterol is necessary for vitamin D activity. When the side chain is replaced by a hydroxyl group (Dimroth and Paland, 1939) or by a bile acid side chain (Haslewood, 1939), the compounds are devoid of vitamin D activity. Furthermore, it has been well known for a number of years that, whereas in rats vitamin D_2 and vitamin D_3 have equivalent biological activities, in the chick vitamin D_2 has only one-tenth the activity of vitamin D_3 (Massengale and Nussmeier, 1930; Chen and Bosmann, 1964; Hibberd and Norman, 1969).

B. Chemical Characterization

1. *Vitamin D_2*

A detailed summary of the series of events that led to the discovery of the "antirachitic" factor has been presented in Chapter 1 (see also Hess, 1929). A further description of this complicated story from the standpoint of the chemical characterization of the provitamin has been given in a Section I,C of Chapter 2. The present section is concerned solely with the structural determination of vitamin D itself.

The two most important factors that provided key insights into the structure of vitamin D (both D_2 and D_3) were the realizations (a) that there were two distinct provitamins, i.e., ergosterol and 7-dehydrocholesterol, and (b) that vitamin D activity was generated from these provitamins only by ultraviolet light in a process that resulted in some chemical transformation of the steroid nucleus. The only difference in chemical structure between the provitamins 7-dehydrocholesterol and ergosterol (or the vitamins D_3 and D_2) is the presence in ergosterol of a double bond between C-22 and C-23 and an additional methyl group at C-24 (see Table 2-3). Considering the state of the art of analytical organic chemistry in the 1930's, it is easy to understand how these differences posed such severe problems to the natural products chemist of that day.

A key contribution to the elucidation of this problem was the realization by Pohl (1926), Heilbron *et al.* (1926, 1928), and Bills *et al.* (1928) that the provitamin D absorbed light in the ultraviolet region; this led to the development of techniques to both detect and quantitate the provitamin. Prior to this discovery, it had been necessary to use Lieberman–Burchard type of color tests to follow the sterol with antirachitic activity. It became apparent, however, that this color assay was not unique for sterols with antirachitic activity and thus was not of particular utility as a tool in the purification of "the antirachitic substance." The new ultraviolet absorption assay provided scientists with the ability to follow the purification of both provitamins. Ultimately, it also became apparent that the ultraviolet spectrum of the provitamin was strikingly altered upon exposure to ultraviolet light, a process that also produced antirachitic activity. Thus, in time it was possible to identify the ultraviolet absorption spectrum of vitamin D itself and use it as an assay for both purification and quantitation. The ultraviolet spectrum of a provitamin is given in Fig. 2-2, and that of vitamin D is given in Fig. 3-2.

By 1928–1929 it was apparent that antirachitic factors could be produced by the irradiation of partially purified cholesterol or ergosterol; it was also known that antirachitic activity was present—without irradiation—in cod-liver oil. Furthermore, the antirachitic substance was known to be a sterol that was not precipitated by digitonin. The final determination of the chemical structure of vitamin D, however, was dependent on the elucidation of the structure of ergosterol (see Chapter 2).

The focus of many investigations in the Göttingen laboratory of Professor Windaus in 1928–1931 was the search for some method other than that of ultraviolet irradiation that could convert the provitamin to an antirachitic substance. In this regard Windaus' group subjected ergosterol to photosensitive oxidation, hydrogenation, dehydrogenation, dehydration, and acid isomerization—all to no avail. By 1930 it was concluded that ultraviolet irradiation was

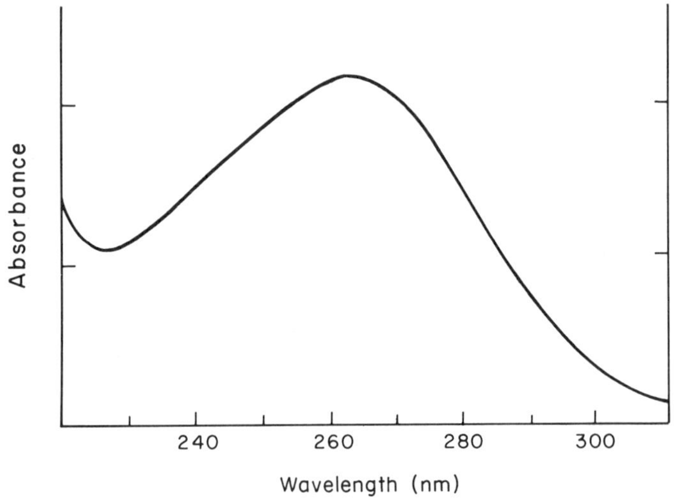

Figure 3-2. Ultraviolet spectrum of vitamin D. The molar extinction coefficient at the 264–265 nm absorption maximum is 18,300.

the primary means of converting the provitamin to an antirachitic substance. Also, the product was annoyingly resistant to efforts to effect its crystallization, and it was, as well, extremely sensitive to air oxidation.

By this time the biological importance of the antirachitic substance had attracted enough workers so that major efforts were carried out simultaneously in the Göttingen laboratory under the direction of Windaus and at the National Institute for Medical Research in London under the direction of F. A. Askew, T. A. Webster, and R. K. Callow. The efforts of these laboratories were surprisingly similar in their approach. Both groups focused first on the chemical characterization of vitamin D_2. The molecular formula of the antirachitic substance was determined to be $C_{28}H_{44}O$ (Windaus *et al.*, 1932b), and hence the vitamin was isomeric with ergosterol. Windaus *et al.* (1931) carried out irradiation of ethereal solutions of ergosterol under nitrogen for 1–9 hr. The unirradiated provitamin was then removed by precipitation with digitonin, which resulted in a supernatant solution enriched in the antirachitic substance. A time-consuming difficulty was the necessity of carrying out biological assays to learn in which fraction the antirachitic substance was located. It should be recalled that at this time the art of bioassay in the rat was not developed or refined to any great extent; thus, the results from such an assay were qualitative rather than quantitative. A further complication was that some fractions, instead of being antirachitic in activity, were "toxic" in their effect; accordingly, Windaus, for a period of time, entertained the possibility that the vitamin D activity was related to one steroid component of the irradiation mixture and the toxicity to another steroid component.

In the course of these studies in Windaus' laboratory a comparison was made of the differential rate at which steroids with a conjugated diene system present in the irradiation mixture might enter into a Diels–Alder reaction with either maleic or citraconic anhydride. An ethereal solution of the ergosterol-free irradiation product was reacted with citraconic anhydride at room temperature for 10 days. The Diels–Alder adduct with interfering non-antirachitic sterols could then be saponified with alcoholic KOH and extracted. As a result, an unreacted steroid remained in the neutral fraction. After standing, this steroid crystallized completely (m.p. 125°C; $\alpha_D + 140°$). The final purified substance was found to be isomeric with ergosterol and to possess high antirachitic potency; it was appropriately designated vitamin D_1 by Windaus and collaborators (1931).

At exactly the same time a similar crystalline substance was isolated by the workers at the National Institute for Medical Research (Angus *et al.*, 1931). Their crystalline steroid was produced via irradiation of an ethereal solution of ergosterol with a mercury-vapor lamp in an atmosphere of nitrogen. The unchanged ergosterol was also removed by digitonin precipitation, and the resulting oily solution was distilled under high vacuum in a very elaborate 1.5-meter still. The fraction condensing over the temperature range 100°–125°C was crystallized from a solution of methanol and water and had a final melting point of 125°C and an α rotation of α_{5461} +260°. Angus *et al.* named their steroid calciferol. It was apparent that it corresponded closely in terms of melting point and biological potency to the vitamin D_1 of Windaus' laboratory.

As a result of a comparison of the published physical properties of the crystalline steroids of Windaus *et al.* (1931) and of Angus *et al.* (1931), it was deduced that the two preparations were not identical. Ultimately, it was established that each was a molecular complex of the antirachitic vitamin with a number of other inactive steroids.[1] Further work resulted in two additional, virtually simultaneous publications, one from the group in Germany (Windaus *et al.*, 1932a) and one from England (Askew *et al.*, 1932). Both groups now reported identical physical properties for their steroid: m.p. 115°–116°C; α_D +102°, ethanol; uv absorption maximum at 264 nm; and a protective dose for rats against rickets of as little as 25 ng/day. Windaus and co-workers named their second crystalline antivitamin substance vitamin D_2, whereas the British workers retained the name calciferol for their new preparation.

The isolation and crystallization of the "antirachitic substance" in reasonable quantities afforded the opportunity of determining its complete chemical structure. This challenging project was carried out principally under the direction of Professor Windaus with important contributions from Heilbron's group in England.

It was the fact that the first preparations containing an antirachitic steroid were mixed crystals of the vitamin and inactive steroids that led in 1932 to Professor J. D. Bernal's first crystallographic studies of the sterols as a group of compounds. He was asked by Rosenheim and King[2] if he could establish that the new crystalline vitamin D preparations contained a single chemical species. The X-ray photographs he took showed that the actual crystal structure of calciferol was complicated; there were four molecules in the crystallographic asymmetric unit. It was only by comparison with other sterol-containing crystals and particularly with that of the original pyrocalciferol–calciferol that Bernal (1932) was able to conclude that calciferol itself was almost certainly a single chemical entity.[3]

Figure 3-3 is a reproduction of the diffraction pattern from the first crystals of calciferol obtained by Bernal's student, Dr. Dorothy Crowfoot-Hodgkin. Her

[1]The Windaus preparation was found to be mainly lumisterol and vitamin D, whereas the Askew preparation was determined to be pyrocalciferol and vitamin D.

[2]As described by Hodgkin (1976) in a symposium held at Dubrovnik, Yugoslavia, on May 31, 1976.

[3]An interesting sidelight to these studies is that, as a consequence of Bernal's X-ray analysis of these calciferol crystals, he was unable to support the then currently accepted structure of cholesterol (Hodgkin, 1976). The molecular dimensions of the 1928 Wieland–Windaus cholesterol structure were inconsistent with Bernal's measurements. Accordingly there ensued a rapid rethinking of the sterol chemistry, which led to the adoption of the structure we know today (see Fig. 2-1B).

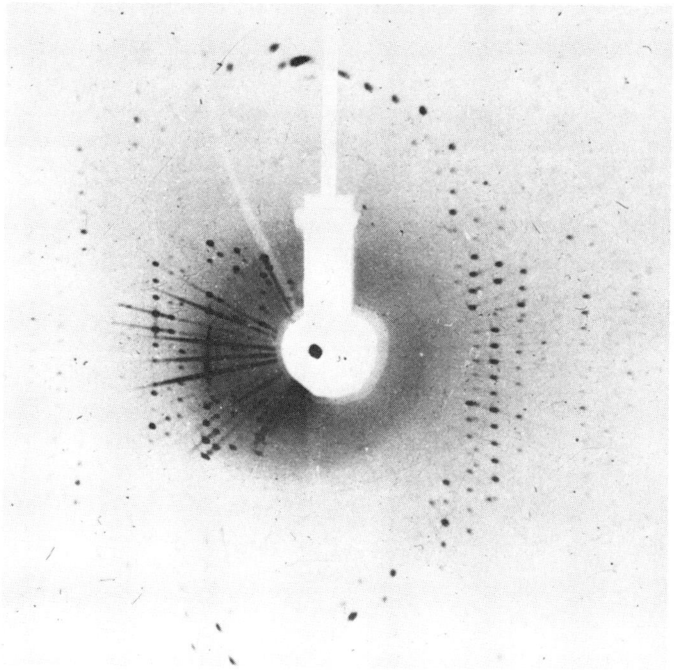

Figure 3-3. Reproduction of a typical diffraction pattern obtained from early crystals of calciferol. (Kindly provided by Dr. Dorothy Crowfoot-Hodgkin from work she carried out in the 1930's.)

Ph.D. dissertation was concerned with the X-ray crystallographic determination of the structure of calciferol. Thus, the structure determination of vitamin D was vigorously pursued both by natural products chemists and by X-ray crystallographers. Professors Bernal and Windaus, while in competition with one another, were clearly on good terms. Figure 3-4 is a copy of a letter written in 1935 by Windaus to Bernal in which he proposes a structure for the derivative dihydrocalciferol and encourages Bernal to learn as much as possible from the crystal structures.

Windaus' approach to the structure determination of vitamin D was based on the usual complex series of wet chemistry manipulations that were available to the organic chemists of that era. The starting point involved the catalytic hydrogenation of calciferol. Windaus' group found that the steroid absorbed precisely 4 moles of hydrogen to give the fully saturated steroid $C_{28}H_{52}O$. Further reduction of ergocalciferol with alcohol and sodium produced a dihydro compound, which reacted with 3 moles of perbenzoic acid. Collectively, these results showed that the vitamin contained only four double bonds, indicating that the molecule was tricyclic. In agreement with this hypothesis it was noted that

DER DIREKTOR
DES ALLGEMEINEN CHEMISCHEN
UNIVERSITÄTS-LABORATORIUMS

GÖTTINGEN, DEN 12. XI. 1935
HOSPITALSTRASSE 8/9

Sehr geehrter Herr Dr Bernal,

ich danke Ihnen verbindlich für Ihre Mitteilungen, die mich sehr interessiert haben. Ich habe nun unsere Arbeit über Vitamin D_2 (Calciferol) zur Publikation gegeben.

Ergosterylacetat krystallisiert sehr schön und ist sehr leicht zu machen, ebenso die Dihydro-, Tetrahydro- und Hexahydro-acetate. Calciferol-acetat habe ich nicht zur Krystallisation gebracht, ebensowenig Pyro-calciferol-acetat.

Dihydro-calciferol wird aus „Calciferol" bereitet durch Hydrierung mit Natrium und Alkohol. Als wahrscheinlichste Formel sehe ich die folgende an

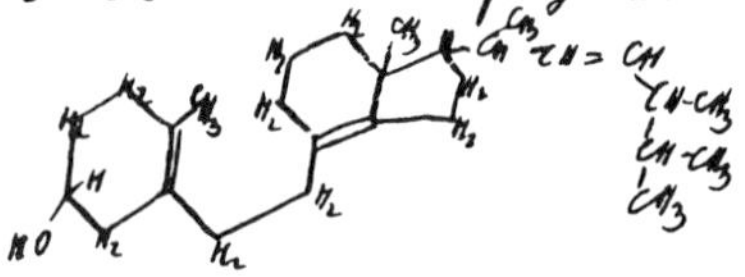

Es gibt 2 verschiedene Dichlorcholestane in der Literatur: eines durch Anlagerung von HCl an Cholesterylchlorid,

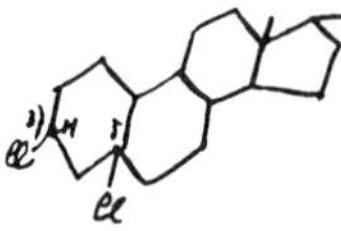

es hat die Chloratome wohl an C_3 und C_5,

ein anderes aus dem Cholestan-3,6 diol mit PCl_5, es hat die Chloratome in 3 und 6.

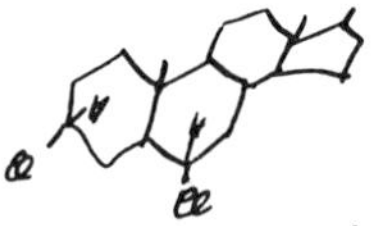

Wenn diese Stoffe Sie interessieren, lasse ich Proben darstellen.

Mit den besten Grüßen
Ihr sehr ergebener A. Windaus

Figure 3-4. Reproduction of a letter from Professor Windaus to Professor Bernal in 1935. In this letter Professor Windaus proposes a structure for dihydrocalciferol. (Kindly provided by Dr. Dorothy Crowfoot-Hodgkin.)

selenium dehydrogenation of ergocalciferol did not yield a Diels hydrocarbon.[4] Thus, it was apparent that the irradiation of ergosterol resulted in the cleavage of one of the steroid rings with the concomitant introduction of a double bond. It was not, however, immediately apparent which ring was broken to generate the secosteroid.

It was known that the side chain of ergosterol survived the irradiation reaction, since ozonolysis of calciferol gave the product 2,3-dimethylbutanol (Fig. 3-5). From this it was concluded that no modification of the side chain had occurred under irradiation.

It was also known that vitamin D_2 formed a mono adduct with maleic anhydride and that this could be hydrolyzed to a dicarboxylic derivative. After this compound was further processed by acetylation of hydroxyls and esterification of the carboxyls, a derivative was obtained which upon hydrogenation and further ozonolysis gave a saturated ketone, $C_{19}H_{34}O$ (Fig. 3-5). Since no aldehyde fragment was apparent, the hydrogenation must have saturated the side-chain double bond. From the molecular formula it was known that the saturated ketone must be bicyclic and contain the intact side chain of the original vitamin. Accordingly, it was felt that this derivative must represent the C and D rings of the original steroid nucleus and that its structure must be that shown in Fig. 3-5. It was deduced that there must be a $\Delta^{7,8}$ unsaturation in vitamin D_2 and that this was the only linkage between rings C and D and the remainder of the molecule present in the A ring. Accordingly, ring B of ergosterol must have been opened by the photolytic cleavage of the bond between C-9 and C-10.

Further information on the precise location of the double bonds in vitamin D_2 was obtained by treating the maleic anhydride adduct in a dehydrogenation process with platinum or palladium. It was possible to detect the presence of naphthalene and β-naphthoic acid, but when dehydrogenation with selenium was carried out only 2,3-dimethylnaphthalene was detected. The formation of β-naphthoic acid implied that the original adduct possessed a hydronaphthalene structure with a β-carboxyl substituent. This could occur only by addition of the maleic anhydride molecule to a diene system that extended from C-19 to C-6. Thus, the structure of vitamin D_2 shown in Fig. 3-5 was supported by the work of both the British and German laboratories (Windaus and Grundmann, 1936; Heilbron *et al.*, 1936).

The evidence accumulated by Windaus and others about the structure of vitamin D_2 was surprising to Bernal. The crystal form of calciferol was so closely similar to that of pyrocalciferol–calciferol he felt sure that vitamin D should be based on the same steroid nucleus as cholesterol, which was shown to be present in pyrocalciferol. The formula with ring B broken seemed to require an extended diene system and very different stereochemistry from that of cholesterol or

[4]When ergosterol is dehydrogenated with selenium a principal product is 3′-methyl-1,2-cyclopentanophenanthrene. This contains the four-ring structure characteristic of steroids.

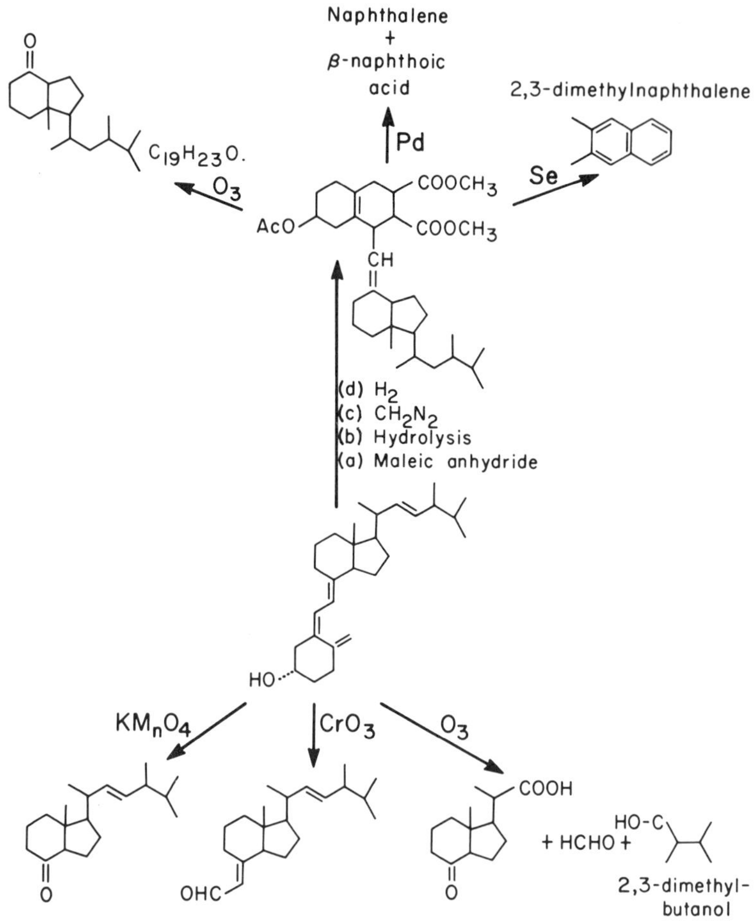

Figure 3-5. Key steps in the structural identification of the "antirachitic substance," vitamin D_2, as carried out by Windaus and co-workers in the 1930's. Vitamin D_2 was subjected to a series of degradation steps, which resulted in the generation of known compounds.

pyrocalciferol. Bernal, however, in correspondence with Windaus agreed that he could not rule out the proposed structure for calciferol. A detailed X-ray analysis of the calciferol structure was not taken up until after the war by Dorothy Crowfoot-Hodgkin and Jack Dunitz. Their analysis of a calciferol derivative, the nitroiodobenzoate, showed that in this crystal the diene system in calciferol from C-5 to C-8 was transoid and coplanar, whereas the diene system from C-6 to C-19 was cisoid and the side chain existed in an extended conformation (Crowfoot and Dunitz, 1948; Hodgkin *et al.*, 1963).

2. *Vitamin* D_3

The actual isolation and chemical characterization of vitamin D_3 was an entirely separate chapter in the history of vitamin D, and was not accomplished until 5 years after the characterization of vitamin D_2. In this intervening period, it was possible to determine the relationship between the antirachitic activities of irradiated cholesterol, irradiated ergosterol, and cod-liver oil. From these studies (Hess and Supplee, 1929–1930; Massengale and Nussmeier, 1930; Steenbock *et al.*, 1932) it was found that ergosterol was not as "antirachitic in the chick" as it was in the rat. However, an intriguing complication was that one could most effectively protect chicks against the ravages of rickets by simple irradiation of the total animal.

At this time (1932–1935) it was generally agreed that the provitamin present in trace quantities in cholesterol was not ergosterol. Also during this time the Norwegian investigators Ender (1933, 1934) and Rygh (1935) concentrated some 20,000-fold the antirachitic activity present in tuna-liver oil and cod-liver oil, respectively. Rygh (1935) found that one rat unit of his cod-liver oil preparation was at least 100 times more potent in chicks than was one rat unit of the chemically characterized vitamin D_2. This permitted him to conclude that the two factors were not identical. It could be calculated, however, on the basis of the biological assay data that 1 ton of cod-liver oil would contain only 2–3 g of the vitamin.

Ultimately, Brockmann (1936) achieved the isolation of a pure crystalline derivative of vitamin D_3 that was present in tuna-liver oil. The procedure consisted of the following steps: (a) saponification and separation of the unsaponifiable fraction of the oil; (b) partial separation of the vitamin D from the vitamin A present by partitioning between alcohols and hydrocarbons; (c) purification via chromatography on columns of alumina gel; (d) removal of other sterols by crystallization from methanol and precipitation with digitonin; (e) preparation of the 3,5-dinitrobenzoate ester; (f) chromatographic purification of the esters on alumina columns; (g) recrystallization of the esters; (h) saponification of the highly purified crystalline ester to the free vitamin; and (i) final crystallization of the free vitamin. The properties of the crystalline 3,5-dinitrobenzoate esters as well as those of the free vitamin differed from those of the previously chemically characterized vitamin D_2 but proved to be identical to the physical properties of the dinitrobenzoate esters of vitamin D_3, which had been produced by uv irradiation of 7-dehydrocholesterol and then chemically characterized by Windaus *et al.* (1936). Thus, the natural vitamin D present in tuna-liver oil was identical to vitamin D_3. Two years later Brockmann and Busse (1938) were able to isolate vitamin D_3 itself in the crystalline state from tuna-liver oil. Subsequently, vitamin D_3 was also isolated as the dinitrobenzoate ester from halibut oil (Brockmann, 1937) and from blue fin tuna oil (Brockmann and Busse, 1937).

Thus ended the era of vitamin D natural products chemistry which was concerned with the determination of the structure of the provitamins and the vitamins D.

II. NATURAL OCCURRENCE OF VITAMINS D

As noted in Chapter 2 there is a universal occurrence of the provitamins D in all phyla, extending from the phanerogams to the invertebrates and vertebrates. In contrast, the distribution of vitamin D is very limited in the biosphere (Table 3-1). Especially notable is the absence of free vitamin D in the plant kingdom.[5] Clover hay, when cured in the dark, contains no endogenous vitamin D activity but when dried in the sun acquires some antirachitic activity (Steenbock *et al.*, 1925). There is no evidence supporting the role of seasonal participation of vitamin D in any aspect of plant physiology or growth; thus, it is not surprising that there are few if any reports of the presence of antirachitic activity in live plant tissue.

The highest concentrations of vitamin D found in nature are those present in fish oils, particularly fish-liver oils. This was first noted in a Ph.D. dissertation by Bills (1924) and subsequently studied by him in much greater detail (Bills 1929, 1930, 1954; Bills *et al.*, 1928). The function of vitamin D in various fish species is unknown but presumably is related to their calcium and phosphorus homeostatic mechanisms. However, an intriguing aspect is that not only do osseous fish or animals with a calcified skeleton have prodigious quantities of vitamin D, but, as also reported in the studies of Bills, cartilaginous fish in some instances store even higher quantities of vitamin D.

In view of the high concentrations of vitamin D in certain fish tissues, particularly liver oil extracts, much attention has been focused on the possible biogenesis of this vitamin. It has been suggested that these high levels of vitamin D may not be produced metabolically by the fish in question, but rather represents a substance that they have acquired nutritionally. Steenbock and Black (1925) and Drummond and Gunther (1930, 1934) found little or no vitamin D activity associated with phytoplankton harvested from the ocean. Similarly, Johnson and Levring (1947) reported that there was no vitamin D present in two species of higher algae. A different view was expressed by Darby and Clarke (1937), who evaluated the possible vitamin D activity of the floating ground algae *Sargassum*. This alga grows prodigiously in the tropical regions near the Tortugas Islands, and it was suggested by these workers that this alga might supply a

[5] A possible exception to this generalization is the presence of vitamin D-like biological activity in various species of Solanaceae, particularly *Solanum glaucophyllum, Cestrum diurnum,* and *Tricetum flavescens*. See Chapter 10 for a discussion of recent developments. It has been determined in one instance that in leaves of *Solanum glaucophyllum* a steroid sugar glycoside of $1,25(OH)_2D_3$ (Haussler *et al.*, 1976; Peterlik *et al.*, 1976) is present that has antirachitic activity.

TABLE 3-1
Distribution of Vitamin D Activity[a]

Sample	Amount[b]	Reference
Phytoplankton	0	Drummond and Gunther (1930, 1934)
Sargassum (a gulfweed)	Some activity	Darby and Clarke (1937)
Clover hay		
Sun-cured	"Slight"	Steenbock *et al.* (1925)
Dark-cured	0	Steenbock *et al.* (1925)
Mushrooms, *Agaricus campestris*	0.21 IU/g	Scheunert *et al.* (1935)
Milk		
Winter (bovine)	5 IU/quart	Campion *et al.* (1937)
Summer (bovine)	50 IU/quart	Campion *et al.* (1937)
Milk (human)	60 IU/quart	Drummond *et al.* (1939)
Milk colostrum (human)	300–600 IU/quart	Drummond *et al.* (1939)
Egg yolk	150–400 IU/g	Heinz (1950)
Butter	4–8 IU/g	Coward and Morgan (1935)
Fish-liver oils[c]	50–45,000 IU/g	Bills *et al.* (1934), Bills (1954)

[a]See Table 13-2 for a tabulation of the important sources of vitamin D in human nutrition, as well as Booher *et al.* (1942).

[b]One international unit (IU) of vitamin D is 25 ng. (See Chapter 4 for a detailed discussion.)

[c]Bills (1954) and Bills *et al.* (1934) studied and tabulated the vitamin D activity in liver extracts of over 100 species of fish.

portion of the vitamin D activity to various forms of marine life. It has been documented that large portions of the *Sargassum* are able to break away from their habitat and migrate via the Gulf Stream as far north as Iceland. The antirachitic activity of *Sargassum* was claimed to be of the same magnitude as that found in some fish-liver oils (Darby and Clarke, 1937). In the animal kingdom, vitamin D is much more prevalent, with significant levels in the liver and milk of mammals and in egg yolks of birds (Daniel and Munsell, 1937).

It is known that although vertebrate tissues contain vitamin D activity this cannot be a consequence of enzymatic or metabolic production of the secosteroid. The vitamin was originally discovered because of its absence and the resulting deficiency syndromes. Under appropriate (or, more correctly, inappropriate) circumstances, cholecalciferol is truly a vitamin; that is, mammals, birds, and probably reptiles are unable to biosynthesize any quantities of this important substance to meet their calcium and phosphorus metabolic needs. The fact that significant quantities of vitamin D are noted in various vertebrate tissues is a reflection of "storage" of the vitamin when it has been available in excess amounts. In fact this storage phenomenon was the basis of the "stosstherapie," which was a clinically accepted technique of preventing rickets in children in the 1930's and 1940's. It involved the administration of massive doses of vitamin D at intervals of several months prior to the onset of the cold, long winter (Harnapp, 1940; Uflacker, 1949). It should be noted that the successful application of "stosstherapie" meant that massive doses of vitamin D activity were accumulated by the body tissues without such deleterious effects as hypercalcemia or formation of kidney stones. In retrospect, with an understanding of the endocrine system concerned with the metabolism of vitamin D (see Chapter 6), it can be appreciated that in reality one was storing a precursor form of the active molecule, $1,25(OH)_2D_3$.

Certainly one obvious mechanism for production of vitamin D in vertebrates is via the photochemical conversion of the precursor, 7-dehydrocholesterol, present in the epidermis. Huldschinsky (1919, 1920) was the first to note the therapeutic properties of sunlight and the light of the quartz mercury arc. This observation was substantiated by Goldblatt and Soames (1923), who discovered that the livers of irradiated rats when fed to nonirradiated rats produced a biological response typical of the fat-soluble vitamin D.

It should be recalled that Windaus and Bock (1936) isolated and chemically characterized 7-dehydrocholesterol from organic solvent extracts of pigskin. Ponsold and Pfennigsdorf (1954) demonstrated in very thorough studies that the antirachitic sterol is produced directly in the skin itself and is not utilized by licking and ingestion; apparently it is absorbed through the basal epidermis and is in that manner made available to the physiological system.

III. CHEMISTRY OF VITAMINS D

A. Structure and Physical Properties of Vitamin D and Related Steroids

1. Vitamin D_3 or Cholecalciferol ($C_{27}H_{44}O$)

Three double bonds; m.p. 84°–85°C; uv absorption maximum at 264–265 nm with a molar extinction coefficient of 18,300 in alcohol or hexane; α_D^{20} +84.8° in acetone (Huber and Barlow, 1943).

2. Vitamin D_2 or Ergocalciferol ($C_{28}H_{44}O$)

Four double bonds; m.p. 121°C; uv absorption maximum at 265 nm; molar extinction coefficient of 19,400; α_D^{20} +106° (Penau and Hagemann, 1946).

Under normal circumstances crystalline vitamin D_3 is somewhat more stable than crystalline vitamin D_2; both compounds undergo oxidation when exposed to air for periods of 24 to 72 hr. Both compounds may be stored adequately in evacuated amber ampules at refrigerated temperatures (Huber and Barlow, 1943). For both vitamin D preparations, the 3,5-dinitrobenzoate esters are unusually stable and have been reported not to lose biological activity or to undergo

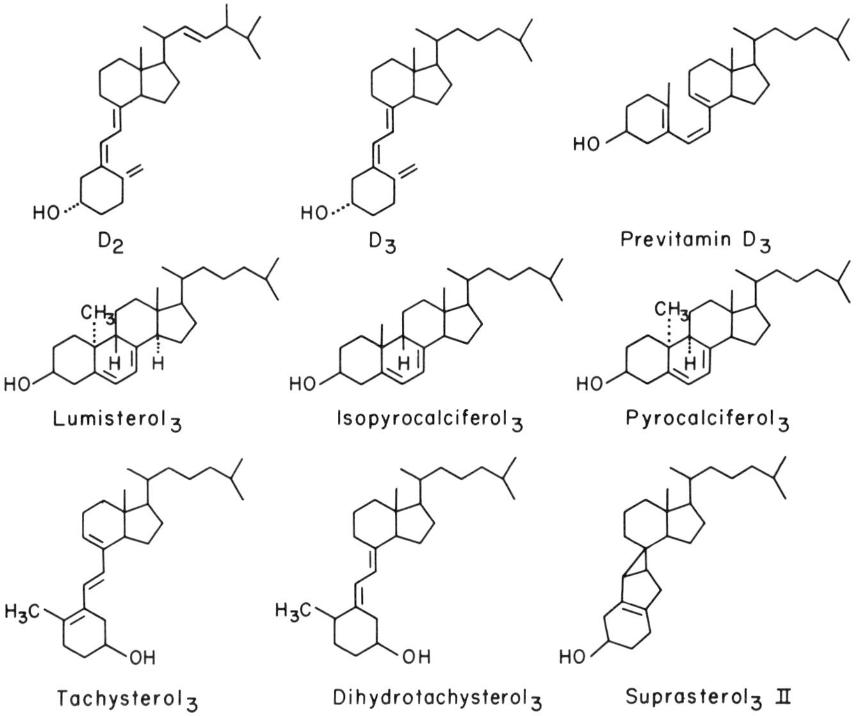

Figure 3-6. Structures of vitamin D and related compounds.

alteration of chemical properties when stored in the dark and cold for periods of up to 5 years.

3. Lumisterol$_2$ *(Derived from Ergosterol)*[6] *(*$C_{28}H_{44}O$*)*

Three double bonds; m.p. 118°C; uv absorption maxima at 265 and 279 nm; molar extinction coefficient at 279 nm is 8500; α_D^{19} +192°. Lumisterol is one of the phototransformation products of either ergosterol or 7-dehydrocholesterol and was first isolated by Windaus *et al.* (1932a) and Askew *et al.* (1932). Lumisterol is epimeric with the provitamin at C-10, where the methyl group is α rather than β.

4. Pyrocalciferol and Isopyrocalciferol

The four compounds ergosterol, lumisterol, isopyrocalciferol, and pyrocalciferol are all epimers of one another at C-9 and C-10 (Fig. 3-6). Isopyrocal-

[6]The subscript 2 indicates that this sterol has a side chain identical to that of ergosterol (the precursor of vitamin D_2), whereas a subscript 3 indicates that the sterol has a side chain identical to that of 7-dehydrocholesterol (the precursor of vitamin D_3).

ciferol is the 9β,10β isomer; ergosterol is the 9α,10β isomer; lumisterol is the 9β,10α isomer; and pyrocalciferol is the 9α,10α isomer. Isopyrocalciferol and pyrocalciferol are products of overirradiation of the provitamin. These steroids do not have biological activity since they are not secosteroids.

5. *Tachysterol$_2$ (Derived from Ergosterol) ($C_{28}H_{44}O$)*

Four double bonds; m.p. of 3,5-dinitro-4-methylbenzoate 154°C; uv absorption maximum at 280 nm; molar extinction coefficient is 24,000; α_D^{18} −70°. Tachysterol was first isolated from irradiation products of ergosterol by Windaus *et al.* (1932a), and its physical properties were described in detail by Windaus *et al.* (1932c). The name tachysterol is derived from the Greek *tachys,* which signifies the rapidity of its reaction with maleic anhydride to form a Diels–Alder adduct. Lugtenburg and Havinga (1969) carried out a 220-MH_z NMR study of tachysterol. Their results support the structure given in Fig. 3-9 (see later).

6. *Previtamin D$_2$ ($C_{28}H_{44}O$)*

Three double bonds; m.p. of 3,5-dinitrobenzoate 103°–104°C; molar uv absorption maximum at 265 nm; molar extinction coefficient at 265 nm is 9600. Precalciferol is one of the principal products of the irradiation of the provitamin; it is in thermoequilibrium with vitamin D.

The thermodynamics and kinetics of the thermal interconversion of previtamin D and vitamin D have been studied by Legrand and Mathieu (1957), Hanewald *et al.* (1961), as well as by Velluz and Amiard (1961). The isomerization of previtamin D to vitamin D is an exothermic reaction; the reaction follows first-order kinetics in a straightforward fashion. Thus, the vitamin D/previtamin D equilibrium ratio depends on the temperature and can be calculated from the appropriate equilibrium constants and kinetic constants as published by Hanewald *et al.* (1961). Table 3-2 shows the equilibrium ratio of these two

TABLE 3-2
Equilibrium Ratio of Vitamin D to Previtamin D at Various Temperatures[a]

Temperature (°C)	Percentage at Equilibrium: Vitamin D_3	Percentage at Equilibrium: Previtamin D_3	Equilibrium constant vit. D_3/previt. D_3
100	71.5	28.5	2.5
80	78	22	3.5
40	89	11	8.1
20	93	7	13.2
0	96	4	24.0
−20	98	2	49.0

[a]Abstracted from Hanewald *et al.* (1961).

steroids at different temperatures. It is apparent that when vitamin D is stored in the cold the equilibrium constant hinders the conversion to previtamin D.

The precise determination of the biological activity of pure previtamin D is complicated in that at 37°–40°C there is a reasonably rapid interconversion of the previtamin to vitamin D. Thus, when previtamin D is administered to deficient animals, in view of the time lag necessary to produce a biological response to vitamin D, there is an inherent problem in determining whether the biological activity that one observes is due to vitamin D or previtamin D. Hanewald *et al.* (1961) approached this problem in a quantitative fashion by carrying out biological assays in the chick and determining antirachitic activity via the prophylactic test (discussed in Chapter 4). They reported that the apparent antirachitic activity of previtamin D was 35% of that of pure vitamin D_3.

Holick *et al.* (1977) clearly demonstrated that previtamin D is formed *in vivo* as an obligatory intermediate between 7-dehydrocholesterol and vitamin D_3 after ultraviolet irradiation of rat epidermis.

7. *Suprasterol I and Suprasterol II*

Both suprasterol I and suprasterol II are known to be products of extreme overirradiation of the provitamin. They were first identified by Windaus *et al.* (1930). The structure of suprasterol II was established by Dauben *et al.* (1958); it is interesting that this steroid has a cyclopropane ring (see Fig. 3-6).

8. *Toxisterol*

Prolonged uv irradiation of previtamin D or any of its photoisomers (tachysterol, lumisterol, 7-dehydrocholesterol) eventually leads to the disappearance of the dienes and trienes in favor of a number of overirradiation products. These are referred to as toxisterols. The structures of the toxisterols have only recently been determined (Jacobs *et al.*, 1977).

Toxisterol was referred to in some older papers as "substance 248"; this reflected its maximal ultraviolet absorption at 248 nm. It was known to be a product of overirradiation of ergosterol and was claimed to have toxic properties while having no antirachitic activity (Laquer and Linsert, 1933). Some attention was focused on this steroid for a period of time. Indeed, according to Harris (1954) toxisterol was very likely the "chief vitamin D component" of the I. G. Farbenindustrie patent of 1928, which was sold under the brand name of Vigantol (Farbenindustrie Aktiengesellschaft, 1928). This was also patented in the United States by Zimmermann and Frankenburger (1933). Both patents claimed that the substance had "blood calcium raising activity."

9. *Dihydrotachysterol (Antitetany Compound 10, AT-10)*

The steroid is obtained by the reduction of the 10,19 double bond of vitamin D, followed by inversion of the A ring. Dihydrotachysterol$_2$(DHT_2), $C_{28}H_{46}O$;

m.p. 125°–127°C; α_D^{22} +97.5°; uv absorption maxima at 242, 251, and 261 nm. Von Werder (1939, 1941) first described the physical and biological properties of this DHT_2. It has been used clinically since approximately 1940 because of its highly useful biological property of elevating blood calcium in parathyroid tetany. It is now appreciated that the biological effectiveness of dihydrotachysterol is due to its ability to mimic certain structural features of the biologically active form of vitamin D, $1,25(OH)_2D_3$. (See Chapters 5 and 13 for a detailed discussion of this point.) Dihydrotachysterol$_3$ can readily be obtained by a lithium metal reduction of tachysterol$_3$ or vitamin D_3 in liquid ammonia (Westerhof and Keverling-Buisman, 1956).

B. Conformation

The structure of vitamin D was determined largely by the classic organic techniques available to the natural products chemists in the period from 1930 to 1940. The traditional means of designating the structure of vitamin D by chemists and biologists of that period is shown in Fig. 3-7A. In this representation the seco nature of the steroid was certainly apparent; however, the remainder of the ring structure and the relative orientation of ring A to rings C and D was implied to be identical to that present in the provitamin or in cholesterol. Dr. D. Crowfoot-Hodgkin (Crowfoot and Dunitz, 1948; Hodgkin *et al.*, 1963) felt that a more accurate depiction of the vitamin D molecule as deduced from their

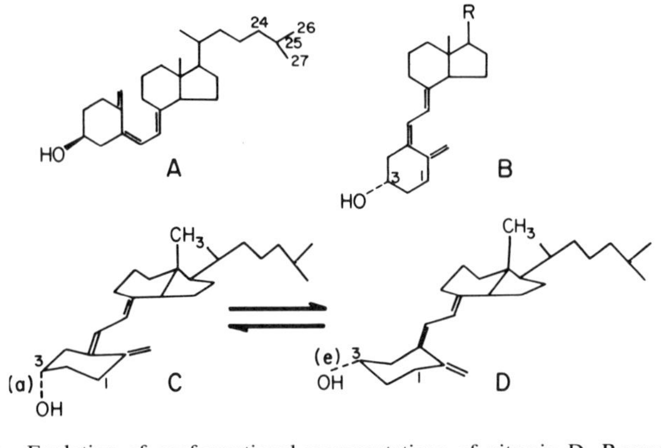

Figure 3-7. Evolution of conformational representations of vitamin D. Representation A resulted from the original chemical structure determination. The first X-ray crystallographic analysis indicated the presence of a single A-ring chair conformation as shown in C, but this was normally simplified to that shown in B. More recent studies emphasize that in solution there is a rapid equilibration between the two A-ring chair conformations, as shown in C and D. In structures C and D, the (e) and (a) refer, respectively, to the equatorial and axial orientations of the 3-hydroxyl, which in both instances is geometrically β.

thorough X-ray crystallographic studies was that shown in Fig. 3-7B. The stereochemistry of vitamin D_2 was determined by the X-ray analysis of Crowfoot and Dunitz (1948) of a heavy-atom derivative, the 4-iodo-5-nitrobenzoate of vitamin D_2. They determined that the diene system extending from C-5 to C-8 was transoid and coplanar, whereas that extending from C-6 to C-19 was cisoid. However, the X-ray data also indicated that the C-7–C-19 cisoid system was not coplanar but that the 5,10 bond was twisted with a corresponding reduction of steric strain. Their X-ray crystallographic analysis indicated the presence of a single A-ring chair conformation, as shown in Fig. 3-7C, but this was normally simplified to the representation shown in Fig. 3-7B. This structure more clearly emphasizes the seco aspects of calciferol molecules. In particular, the A ring is inverted out, down, and away from rings C and D, with rotation occurring around the bond between C-7 and C-8. As a result the α and β designations for substituent groups on the A ring must be drawn with reverse notation due to the inversion of the A ring.

Okamura, Wing, and colleagues evaluated the topology of vitamin D_3, its metabolites, and its analogues in solution by high-resolution proton magnetic resonance spectroscopy in conjunction with lanthinide-induced shift studies (Okamura *et al.*, 1974; Wing *et al.*, 1974, 1975). Figure 3-8 shows the high-resolution proton NMR spectra obtained for vitamin D_3 and dihydrotachysterol$_3$. A similar study was also independently reported by LaMar and Budd (1974).

The studies of Wing, Okamura, and colleagues emphasize that in solution the secosteroid vitamin D undergoes a dynamic equilibration between the two chair conformers (see Fig. 3-7C and D). It is their view that this is the most accurate molecular representation of vitamin D secosteroids; it is currently the most preferred means of illustrating the structure of vitamin D. As discussed in the paper by Okamura *et al.* (1974), any detailed understanding of the structure–function relationship of vitamin D demands consideration of the consequences of this dynamic interchange between the two "chairlike" conformers of the A ring. One interesting feature of this study is that it is apparent that the conformational equilibrium of the two chair conformers depends substantially on the nature of substituent functional groups on the A ring. Thus, for vitamin D the equilibrium ratio is 55 : 45 where the 3β-hydroxyl is oriented equatorial versus axial. In contrast, the A ring of dihydrotachysterol exists in solution preferentially, if not completely (within the limits of detectability), with its 3β-hydroxyl as well as the C-19 methyl in the equatorial orientation. This result would be clearly predictable since the other conformers require that both the 3β-hydroxyl and the methyl group be in the energetically less favorable diaxial orientation. As a consequence of these studies Okamura and Norman proposed (Okamura *et al.*, 1974) that vitamin D-like molecules, particularly "active metabolites" that have their 1α-OH relatively more equatorial than axial, should be relatively more biologically active. As yet this theory has not been confirmed. (A further discussion

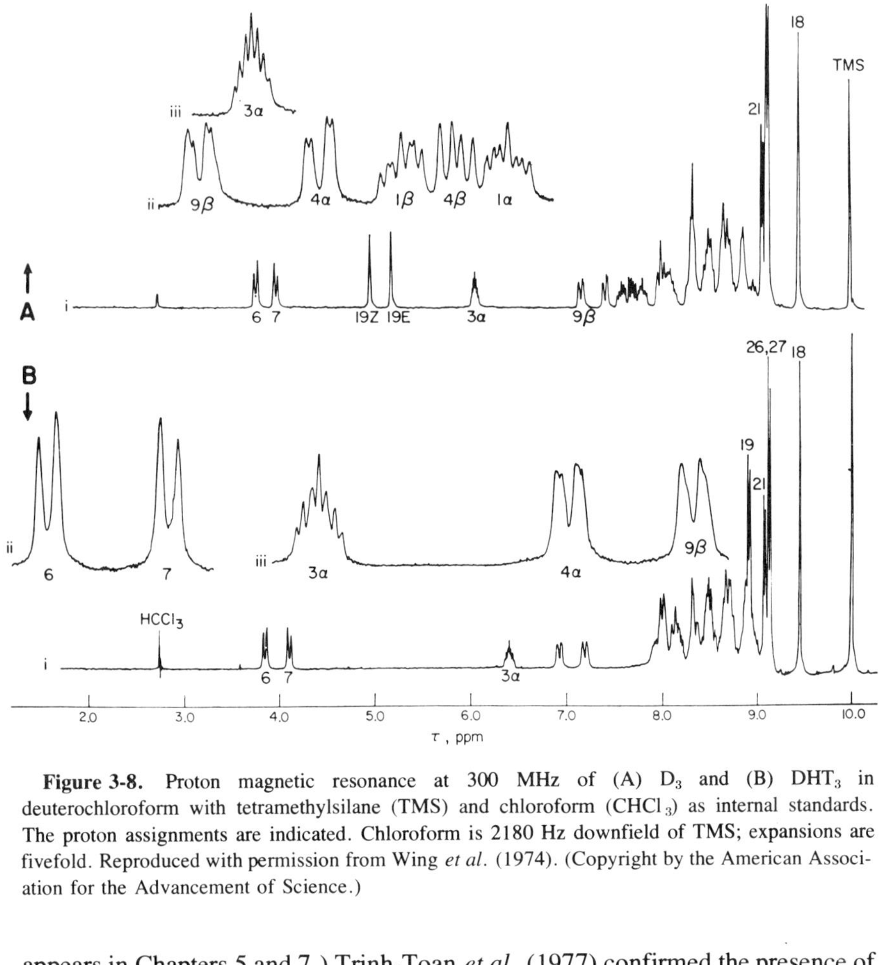

Figure 3-8. Proton magnetic resonance at 300 MHz of (A) D_3 and (B) DHT_3 in deuterochloroform with tetramethylsilane (TMS) and chloroform ($CHCl_3$) as internal standards. The proton assignments are indicated. Chloroform is 2180 Hz downfield of TMS; expansions are fivefold. Reproduced with permission from Wing *et al.* (1974). (Copyright by the American Association for the Advancement of Science.)

appears in Chapters 5 and 7.) Trinh-Toan *et al.* (1977) confirmed the presence of both the equatorial and axial chair species of vitamin D via X-ray crystallographic evaluation of vitamin D crystals that had both chair conformers cocrystallized.

C. Photochemical Production

The important role of ultraviolet irradiation in the production of vitamin D was recognized as early as 1924 by Steenbock and Black (1925), Hess and Weinstock (1924, 1925), and Hess *et al.* (1925). As indicated previously this was the key insight that ultimately permitted Windaus and his collaborators as well as Callow and collaborators to carry out the chemical characterization of vitamin D. In the course of these studies several substances were discovered, isolated, and chemically characterized; they include lumisterol, tachysterol, precalciferol, as well as the suprasterols I and II. (The structures of many of these are given in Fig. 3-6.) An intriguing chemical problem both theoretically and structurally was to deduce the sequence of events that intervened between the interaction of quanta of light with the provitamin and the appearance of vitamin D and other related compounds.

Windaus originally suggested (Windaus *et al.*, 1932c) that the sequence of events was ergosterol→lumisterol→tachysterol→calciferol→suprasterol. In this scheme they assumed that the production of calciferol was a stepwise process involving sequential conversion through the series of compounds previously indicated; furthermore, each step was thought to be irreversible.

Subsequently, this irradiation process was studied in great detail by Velluz and associates (Velluz and Amiard, 1949a,b,c; Velluz *et al.*, 1955) as well as Havinga and co-workers (1955, 1960; Havinga and Schlactman, 1961; Sanders and Havinga, 1964). Both groups employed radioisotope and heavy isotope (deuterium) labels and carried out quantitative measurements of quantum yields in the individual photochemical steps. It soon became apparent that the pathway was a direct photochemical reaction from the provitamin to the previtamin and that tachysterol and lumisterol were products of subsequent side reactions.

The original Velluz scheme supporting this view is given in Fig. 3-9. The principal contribution of Velluz and Amiard (1949a,b,c; 1961; Velluz *et al.*, 1949) was in establishing that the reactions in the irradiation process were reversible and that the conversion of previtamin D to vitamin D was a thermal process that could occur in the dark, completely in the absence of light quanta. Furthermore, through the use of the radiotracer technique they established that neither tachysterol nor lumisterol was an obligatory intermediate in the conversion of ergosterol to vitamin D. This conclusion was also supported by the work of Koevoet *et al.* (1955), who were able to convert previtamin D to tachysterol in the dark simply by the addition of iodine; this method is known to effect the conversion of a *cis*-diene system to a *trans*-diene system.

The molecular events associated with a photochemical reaction include the molecule in its ground state (which possesses a minimum of electronic energy) absorbing a discrete quantum of light, which perturbs the molecule so that it is no longer in thermodynamic equilibrium with its surroundings. The resulting excited, unstable molecule has a higher electronic energy; ultimately this molecule must lose energy to its environment in the form of either (a) fluorescence or phosphorescence, (b) chemical energy, or (c) thermal energy so that the molecule is again in the ground state. If in the ground state the molecule has undergone a change in its chemical energy, it will now be a new compound with a different structure. The ability of a molecule to absorb quanta of light is determined by chromophoric groups present in the molecule; in the case of the provitamins D

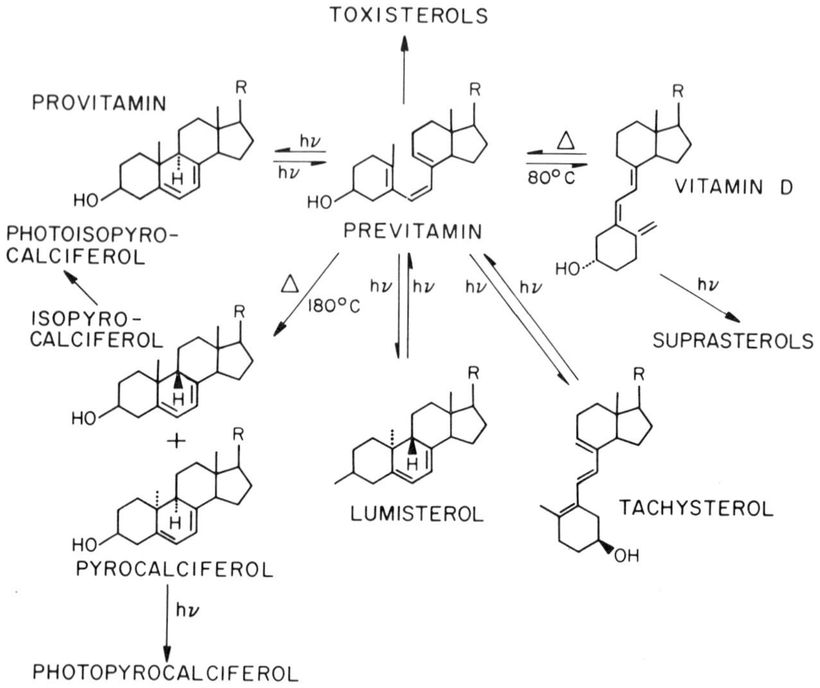

Figure 3-9. Photochemical pathway of production of calciferol.

these are the 5,7-diene double-bond system. Only the light absorbed by the provitamin is effective in producing a photochemical change in that molecule. Furthermore, there is a one-to-one relationship between the absorbed photon or quantum of energy and any given molecule; the energy-rich, excited species may then undergo secondary reactions that either lead back to the ground state of the original molecule or to molecules with new chemical structures.

Thus, it should be noted (see Fig. 3-9) that the intermediate precalciferol can, upon irradiation, be converted to three products: tachysterol, lumisterol, and provitamin. Similarly, these three products can, upon irradiation, be converted to precalciferol and generate any of the other steroids in the pathway. However, the only molecule in thermal equilibrium with precalciferol that does not require incident radiant energy is calciferol or vitamin D. Thus, if conditions can be found that optimize the production of previtamin D from the provitamin, then this steroid in a second, separate manipulation may be thermally converted to vitamin D in a very efficient way without the concomitant production of other contaminating steroids.

The conversion of previtamin D to vitamin D involves an intermolecular hydrogen transfer from C-19 to C-9. This transfer was postulated by Verloop *et al.* (1957) and Legrand and Mathieu (1959) and was confirmed by Autrey *et al.* (1961) and Akhtar and Gibbons (1965), who irradiated 7-dehydrocholesterol that was labeled in the C-19 position with tritium and obtained tritium-labeled vitamin D_3. From their analysis of the distribution of radioactivity between C-19 and C-9, Akhtar and Gibbons (1965) determined that the intermolecular hydrogen transfer was not stereospecific in the course of the conversion of previtamin D to vitamin D.

D. Chemical Synthesis

There have been two basic methods of approach to the total synthesis of vitamin D. One involves total synthesis of a compound that can be chemically converted to a provitamin and then irradiated to generate vitamin D. The second approach is independent of any photochemical transformation.

The first total synthesis of vitamin D was in reality accomplished with the first total synthesis of cholesterol; cholesterol is readily converted to 7-dehydrocholesterol, the provitamin D_3. The first total synthesis of cholesterol was reported virtually simultaneously by Woodward and collaborators (Woodward *et al.*, 1952) and Robinson and colleagues (Cardwell *et al.*, 1953). The Woodward synthesis involved the 20-step conversion of the starting material 4-methoxy-2,5-toluquinone to a progesterone derivative, specifically ($\pm$)-$\Delta^{9(11)16}$-bisdehydro-20-norprogesterone. This progesterone derivative was subsequently converted in several steps to progesterone, testosterone, cortisone, and cholesterol.

Robinson's synthesis (Cardwell *et al.*, 1953) used the starting material 1,6-dihydroxynaphthalene, which was ultimately converted to the B and C rings of the steroid. This was followed by attachment of ring A and then ring D in a further series of laborious chemical transformations. The final product in the Robinson synthesis was epiandrosterone and, since epiandrosterone had been previously converted to cholesterol, Robinson's synthesis constituted a formal total synthesis of cholesterol and, in turn, vitamin D_3.

A variation of the Robinson synthesis was carried out by Johnson and colleagues, who used the same starting material, 1,6-dihydroxynaphthalene. However, in this synthesis the starting material became rings C and D, and this was followed by the attachment of ring B and finally ring A (Johnson, 1956).

The first total synthesis specifically of vitamin D_2 was accomplished by Inhoffen (1958; Inhoffen *et al.*, 1957). Inhoffen used as the starting material vitamin D_2 itself. This was subjected to a series of oxidative degradations to yield the starting material which was a C-$_{19}$ ketone of rings C and D plus the intact side chain. This molecule was then built back up to a 5,6-*trans*-ergocalciferol. Independently, this C_{19} ketone was itself totally synthesized in a 15- to 18-step series of transformations. Thus, *in toto* Inhoffen had effected a total synthesis of vitamin D_2.

Lythgoe has pioneered a synthesis of the vitamin D molecule directly, without the use of any photochemical irradiation steps (Bruck *et al.*, 1967; Davidson *et al.*, 1967). Thus, this is the first truly pure chemical synthesis in the vitamin D field and represents a major accomplishment. This is a continuing area of investigation for Lythgoe and co-workers and potentially represents attractive ways to produce metabolites and analogues of vitamin D without the necessity of going through the photochemical irradiation process. Inasmuch as the yield of vitamin D from the irradiation process is usually 10% or less, the results of Lythgoe and co-workers provide encouraging alternatives for the future.

E. Synthesis of Radioactive Vitamin D and Metabolites

In recent years it has become increasingly important for the study of the metabolism of vitamin D to have available specific techniques for the preparation of highly radioactive cholecalciferol or ergocalciferol. Several papers have appeared describing techniques for preparing these steroids. In general, the procedures rely on the preparation of either tritium- or ^{14}C-labeled cholesterol followed by the conversion of cholesterol to the provitamin 7-dehydrocholesterol. These techniques have been pioneered largely by the laboratory of DeLuca and co-workers. Table 3-3 summarizes the preparations of radioactive vitamin D and its metabolites that are currently available and indicates the specific activities that have been obtained.

F. Industrial Production of Vitamin D

It is pertinent to consider the economic aspects of vitamin D manufacture. The largest commercial production of vitamin D has been for the supplementation of animal feeds: poultry feeds with vitamin D_3 and cattle and swine feeds with vitamin D_2. Usually the supplement is in the form of a "resin" rather than a pure crystalline calciferol. As discussed earlier in this chapter, irradiation of the provitamin produces a family of closely related compounds that are particularly difficult on an industrial scale to cleanly separate from one another. Therefore, economic considerations have mandated the use of resins rather than pure steroids. There is at present a trend away from the incorporation of vitamin D_2 in the animal field industry.

Vitamin D is also used commercially in the supplementation of foods for human consumption (milk, both homogenized and evaporated; margarine; and breads) and in the pharmaceutical area (mixed vitamin preparations and as pure vitamin D_2 or D_3). In this regard it is a curious anomaly that at the present time there are no preparations of crystalline vitamin D_3 approved by the U.S. Food and Drug Administration (FDA) for human use. As a result a physician in the

TABLE 3-3
Methods for Preparation of Radioactive Vitamin D: Metabolites and Analogs

Steroid	Specific activity	Reference
Vitamin D (tritum-labeled)		
[3-^{3}H]D_2	1.2 Ci/mmole	Jones *et al.* (1975)
	0.15 Ci/mmole	Callow *et al.* (1966)
[*G*-^{3}H]D_2	3.2 mCi/mmole	Norman and DeLuca (1963b)
[1-^{3}H]D_2	1.3 Ci/mmole	Pelc and Kodicek (1971)
[*G*-^{3}H]D_3	7.2 mCi/mmole	Norman and DeLuca (1963b)
[1,2-^{3}H]D_3	180 mCi/mmole	Neville and DeLuca (1966)
[1,2-^{3}H]D_3	1–10 Ci/mmole	See footnote *a*
[1-^{3}H]D_3	21.1 mCi/mmole	Callow *et al.* (1966)
[6-^{3}H]D_3	0.21 mCi/mmole	Callow *et al.* (1966)
[7-^{3}H]D_3	0.35 mCi/mmole	Callow *et al.* (1966)
[24,25,26,27-^{3}H]D_3	0.15 mCi/mmole	Callow *et al.* (1966)
[22,23-^{3}H]D_4	0.7 Ci/mmole	DeLuca *et al.* (1968)
Vitamin D (^{14}C-labeled)		
[*G*-^{14}C]D_3	Very low	Kodicek (1955)
[*G*-^{14}C]D_3	4 mCi/mmole	Blumberg *et al.* (1960)
[4-^{14}C]D_3	25 mCi/mmole	See footnote *a*
Vitamin D metabolites		
25(OH)[23,24-^{3}H]D_3	70 Ci/mmole	Yamada *et al.* (1978)
25(OH)[26,27,-*methyl*-^{3}H]D_3	1–10 Ci/mmole	See footnote *a*
25(OH)[26,27-^{14}C]D_3	50 mCi/mmole	See footnote *b*
1,25$(OH)_2$[1-^{3}H]D_3[c]	1–10 Ci/mmole	Wong and Norman (1972)
1,25$(OH)_2$[23,24-^{3}H]D_3	100 Ci/mmole	See footnote *a*
Vitamin D analogs		
1(OH)[6-^{3}H]D_3	Not reported	Holick *et al.* (1975)

[a] This steroid is available from New England Nuclear Corporation or the Amersham Searle Corporation.

[b] This steroid is available from New England Nuclear Corporation.

[c] This preparation of tritium labeled 1,25$(OH)_2D_3$ is made biosynthetically using chick kidney homogenates.

United States may prescribe only vitamin D_2. Most of the vitamin D content of the ubiquitous vitamin pill also is in the form of ergocalciferol.

It is difficult to precisely state what is the current worldwide production of vitamin D. Due to the competitive nature of the market, individual manufacturers are reluctant to disclose exact figures on the amount they have produced. However, the U.S. Trade Commission has an annual publication entitled *Synthetic Organic Chemicals,* which reports on a per annum basis the number of billion units of vitamin D manufactured, the number of billion units sold, and their sales value. These figures are tabulated in Table 3-4. It should be noted that the

TABLE 3-4
Production and Market Value of Vitamin D in the United States

Year	Production (10^{12} IU)	Sales (10^{12} IU)	Sales value (million dollars)
1956[a]	46.8	—	1.3
1970[b]	243.9	137.6	1.129
1971[b]	250.7	136.3	1.089
1973[b]	288.8	195.7	2.318
1975[b]	225.5	140.5	2.782

[a]Taken from statements made by Fieser and Fieser (1959).
[b]Taken from U.S. International Trade Commission (USITC) (1975).

amount of vitamin D manufactured is reported as international units (IU) rather than as kilograms or pounds. This reflects the impure nature of the resin. Both chemical measurements and biological assay determinations are usually made on the resin preparations to determine in international units the actual vitamin D content.

The principal American producers of vitamin D_3 include Dawes Laboratories, Diamond Shamrock, and Vitamins Incorporated. Prior to 1971, the Peter Hand Foundation also produced a small share of the U.S. vitamin D_3 market; they have recently been acquired by Thompson Hayward. Vitamin D_2 is produced largely by the R. P. Sherer Corporation.

As indicated in Table 3-4, in 1973, in the United States, some 289,000 billion IU of vitamin D were manufactured. If this were chemically pure, it would be equivalent to 8.22×10^6 g, i.e., 7220 kg, or 7.94 tons.[7]

In Canada, vitamin D is manufactured by Canada Packers Limited, and, in England, Peboc is the principal source of the vitamin D steroids. The world's largest producer of vitamins is Philips-Duphar of the Netherlands; unfortunately, their production figures are not available. However, if one estimated the combined production and sales outside the United States (principally Philips-Duphar) to be 1.25–1.5 times that produced in the United States, then the total world production of vitamin D in 1973 might have approached 7.22×10^{14} IU, or, if pure, 198 tons with an approximate market value of $5.8 million.

The current prices in 1976 for crystalline vitamin D_3 were $1.38 per gram and for vitamin D_2 $1.13 per gram. This contrasts most favorably with 1958 costs of $8.00 per gram ($D_3$) and $1.40 per gram ($D_2$). Clearly, the technical advances within the industry have more than offset the ravages of inflation.

[7]One gram of pure crystalline D_3 supplies 40 million IU, and 1 lb supplies 18.2 billion IU.

The cost of vitamin D reflects, on the one hand, the effort required to irradiate the provitamin and the subsequent laborious work-up necessary to obtain the crystalline calciferol secosteroid. On the other hand, an important cost consideration relates to the market price of the provitamin D_2.

Ergosterol is obtained largely from the growing of suitable yeasts (see Table 2-1); some 300–400 lb of compressed yeast are required to obtain 1 lb of ergosterol. The current market price of ergosterol is \$95–\$130/lb, or 20–30 cents/g. In the past decade the availability of ergosterol has been curtailed, which of necessity limits the amount of vitamin D_2 that can be produced.

The commercial production of vitamin D_3 is dependent on the supply of 7-dehydrocholesterol. This can be obtained via organic solvent extraction and purification of animal skins or via laborious (on an industrial scale) chemical synthesis from cholesterol. However, the chemical production of the provitamin is becoming increasingly a dominant fact. The current market price of cholesterol is \$20/lb, or 4.7 cents/g, whereas an estimate of the cost of 7-dehydrocholesterol is \$400/lb, or \$1/g. The exact details of the chemical conversion of cholesterol to 7-dehydrocholesterol and the method of large-scale photolysis of the provitamin and subsequent work-up are closely held topics for which there have been many patents.

IV. METHODS OF CHROMATOGRAPHIC SEPARATION OF VITAMIN D COMPOUNDS

Over the years a wide variety of chromatographic techniques have been used to separate vitamin D from its structurally related family of compounds, particularly irradiation products and, more recently, metabolites. These include column, paper, thin-layer, and gas chromatographic methods. These techniques and their applications are summarized in Table 3-5.

As indicated in Table 3-5 a number of paper chromatographic techniques have been devised for the separation of vitamin D employing either quinoline-impregnated paper or reversed-phase paper. These methods are characterized by unsatisfactory resolutions, long development times, and, more importantly, a limited capacity.

Accordingly, column chromatographic techniques have been developed. The supports employed have included alumina, Floridin, celite, Sephadex LH-20, and silicic acid. Often, these methods were devised for the separation of classes of compounds rather than individual components (Hirsch, 1963). This has been of particular importance in the industrial fields related to vitamin D or in the analysis of vitamin D in that it has often been important to separate vitamin D compounds from vitamin A compounds. Studies on the metabolism of vitamin D (see Chapter 6) could not have been carried out without the routine availability of

TABLE 3-5
Methods for Chromatographic Separation of Vitamin D and Related Steroids

Method	Comment	Reference
Paper chromatography		
Quinoline-impregnated paper		Davis *et al.* (1952), Kritchevsky and Kirk (1952)
Reversed-phase paper		Kodicek and Ashby (1954), Terepka *et al.* (1961), Michalec and Strasek (1960), Chen *et al.* (1963)
Column chromatography		
Alumina		Festenstein and Morton (1955)
Floridin		Green (1951)
Celite		DeWitt and Sullivan (1946), Ewing *et al.* (1954), Fujita and Numata (1958), Jones *et al.* (1959)
	Useful for multivitamin tablets	Theiragt and Campbell (1959)
Silicic acid	Useful for metabolites	Norman and DeLuca (1963a), Fischer and Kabara (1964), Mawer and Backhouse (1969)
Factice	Can resolve D_2 and D_3	Dollwet and Norman (1968)
Sephadex LH-20	Highly useful for metabolites	Holick and DeLuca (1971)
High-pressure liquid chromatography		
Zorbax-Sil support	Useful for D_2 in capsules	Tomkins and Tscherne (1974)
	Separates $24(R),25(OH)_2D_3$ from $24(S),25(OH)_2D_3$	Ikekawa and Koizumi (1976)
	Assay of 25(OH)D	Koshy and Vanderslik (1976), Bjorkhem and Holmberg (1976)
ODS-Permaphase	Useful for vitamin D metabolites	Matthews *et al.* (1974)
	Useful for metabolites	Jones and DeLuca (1975)
Silica gel		Hofsass *et al.* (1976)
Thin-layer chromatography		
Silicic acid	Effective for irradiation mixtures	Norman and DeLuca (1963a)
Silica gel G	Two-dimensional	Fraser and Kodicek (1971)
Silicic acid		Fisher *et al.* (1972a,b), Parekh and Wasserman (1965)
Gas chromatography		Ziffer *et al.* (1960)
	Separates trimethylsilyl ethers of D_3	Evans (1972)
	Cyclizes D_3	Murray *et al.* (1966), Avoili and Lee (1966)
	Useful for $25(OH)D_3$	Sklan *et al.* (1973)
	Useful for multivitamin tablets	Edlund and Filippini (1973)
	Useful for D_2 in milk	Bell and Christie (1974)

silicic acid column chromatography (Norman and DeLuca, 1963a) and particularly Sephadex LH-20 column chromatography (Holick and DeLuca, 1971). The latter technique provided the necessary resolution to separate many closely related metabolites in rapid fashion.

Until the advent of gas chromatography the major criticism of all the methods of separation was their inability to resolve and distinguish vitamin D_2 from vitamin D_3. Thus, a primary attribute of gas chromatography is the ability to carry out this separation. However, it should be noted that most gas chromatography techniques do not chromatograph the vitamin D molecule per se. Instead, a thermal conversion occurs at the time of introduction of the sample into the column such that vitamin D as the secosteroid is cyclized to give an equilibrium mixture of pyrocalciferol and isopyrocalciferol. Accordingly, the one compound, vitamin D, generates two peaks in the chromatogram profile.

One noteworthy technological advance is the application of high-pressure liquid chromatography (HPLC) to the separation of vitamin D from other steroids or from its metabolites. This is an exceedingly powerful separation technique that is only beginning to come into general application. Figure 3-10 is a chromatogram showing the HPLC resolution of vitamin D and its metabolites. It is obvious

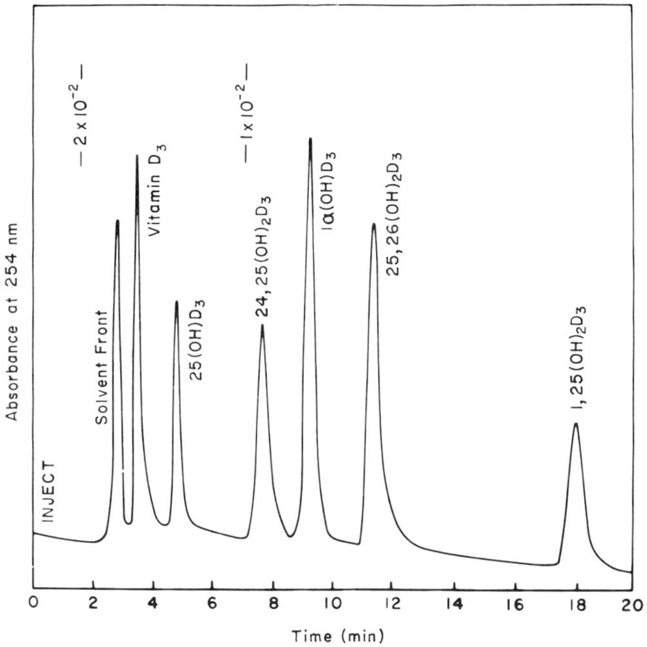

Figure 3-10. High-pressure liquid chromatography separation of vitamin D_3 and its metabolites. Taken from Jones and DeLuca (1975); reproduced by permission of the authors and publisher.

that this technique has the capacity for fine resolution not readily obtained by other chromatographic techniques.

REFERENCES

Akhtar, M., and Gibbons, C. J. (1965). *Tetrahedron Lett.* p. 509.

Angus, T. C., Askew, F. A., Bourdillon, R. B., Bruce, H. M., Callow, R. K., Fischmann, C., Philpot, J. St. L., and Webster, T. A. (1931). *Proc. R. Soc. London, Ser. B* **108,** 340.

Askew, F. A., Bourdillon, R. B., Bruce, H. M., Callow, R. K., Philpot, J. St. L., and Webster, T. A. (1932). *Proc. R. Soc. London, Ser. B* **109,** 488.

Autrey, R. L., Barton, D. H. R., Ganguly, A. K., and Reusch, W. H. (1961). *J. Chem. Soc., London* p. 3313.

Avioli, L. V., and Lee, S. W. (1966). *Anal. Biochem.* **16,** 193.

Bell, J. G., and Christie, A. A. (1974). *Analyst* **99,** 385.

Bernal, J. D. (1932). *Nature (London)* **129,** 277.

Bernstein, S., and Sax, K. J. (1951). *J. Org. Chem.* **16,** 685.

Bernstein, S., Oleson, J. J., Ritter, H. B., and Sax, K. J. (1949). *J. Am. Chem. Soc.* **71,** 2576.

Bills, C. E. (1924). "Studies on the Antiricketic Vitamin: Dissertation." Johns Hopkins Press, Baltimore, Maryland.

Bills, C. E. (1929). *J. Biol. Chem.* **72,** 751.

Bills, C. E. (1930). U. S. Patent 1,775,548.

Bills, C. E. (1954). *In* "The Vitamins" (W. H. Sebrell, Jr. and R. S. Harris, eds.), 1st ed., Vol. 2, p. 132. Academic Press, New York.

Bills, C. E., Honeywell, E. M., and MacNair, W. A. (1928). *J. Biol. Chem.* **76,** 251.

Bills, C. E., McDonald, F. G., Massengale, O. N., Imboden, M., Hall, H., Hergert, W. O., and Wallenmeyer, J. C. (1934). *J. Biol. Chem.* **109,** proc. vii.

Bjorkhem, I., and Holmberg, I. (1976). *Clin. Chim. Acta* **68,** 215.

Blumberg, A., Aebi, H., Hurni, H., and Schonholzer, G. (1960). *Helv. Physiol. Pharmacol. Acta* **18,** 56.

Booher, L. R., Hortzler, E. R., and Hewston, E. M. (1942). "Vitamin Values of Foods." Chem. Publ. Co., New York.

Brockmann, H. (1936). *Hoppe-Seyler's Z. Physiol. Chem.* **241,** 104.

Brockmann, H. (1937). *Hoppe-Seyler's Z. Physiol. Chem.* **245,** 96.

Brockmann, H., and Busse, A. (1937). *Hoppe-Seyler's Z. Physiol. Chem.* **249,** 176.

Brockmann, H., and Busse, A. (1938). *Naturwissenschaften* **26,** 122.

Bruck, P., Clark, R. D., Davidson, R. S., Gunther, W. H. H., Littlewood, P. S., and Lythgoe, B. (1967). *J. Chem. Soc. C,* p. 2529.

Callow, R. K., Kodicek, E., and Thompson, G. A. (1966). *Proc. R. Soc. London, Ser B* **164,** 207.

Campion, J. E., Henry, K. M., Skon, S. K., and Mackintosh, J. (1937). *Biochem. J.* **31,** 81.

Cardwell, H. M. E., Cornforth, J. W., Duff, S. R., Holterman, H., and Robinson, R. (1953), *J. Chem. Soc.* p. 361.

Chen, P. S., and Bosmann, H. (1964). *J. Nutr.* **83,** 133.

Chen, P. S., Terepka, A. R., and Remsen, N. (1963). *Anal. Chem.* **35,** 2030.

Coward, K. H., and Morgan, B. G. E. (1935). *Br. Med. J.* **2,** 1041.

Crowfoot, D., and Dunitz, J. D. (1948). *Nature (London)* **162,** 608.

Daniel, E. P., and Munsell, H. E. (1937). *U.S., Dep. Agric., Misc. Publ.* **275; also see Booher** *et al.* (1942), p. 109.

Darby, H. H., and Clarke, H. T. (1937). *Science* **85,** 318.

Dauben, W. G., Bell, I., Hutton, T. W., Laws, G. F., Rheiner, A., and Urscheler, A. (1958). *J. Am. Chem. Soc.* **80,** 4117.
Davidson, R. S., Waddington-Feather, S. M., Williams, D. H., and Lythgoe, B. (1967). *J. Chem. Soc. C,* p. 2534.
Davis, R. B., McMahon, J. M., and Kalnitsky, G. (1952). *J. Am. Chem. Soc.* **74,** 4483.
DeLuca, H. F., Weller, M., Blunt, J. W., and Neville, P. E. (1968). *Arch. Biochem. Biophys.* **124,** 122.
DeWitt, J. B., and Sullivan, M. X. (1946). *Anal. Chem.* **18,** 117.
Dimroth, K., and Paland, J. (1939). *Ber. Dtsch. Ver. Volkshyg.* **72,** 187.
Dollwet, H. H. A., and Norman, A. W. (1968). *Anal. Biochem.* **25,** 297.
Drummond, J. C., and Gunther, E. R. (1930). *Nature (London)* **126,** 398.
Drummond, J. C., and Gunther, E. R. (1934). *J. Exp. Biol.* **11,** 203.
Drummond, J. C., May, C. H., and Richardson, N. E. G. (1939). *Br. Med. J.* **2,** 757.
Edlund, D. O., and Filippini, F. A. (1973). *J. Assoc. Agric. Chem.* **56,** 1374.
Ender, F. (1933). *Z. Vitaminforsch.* **2,** 241.
Ender, F. (1934). *Z. Vitaminforsch.* **3,** 161.
Evans, J. R. (1972). *Clin. Chim. Acta* **42,** 167.
Ewing, D. T., Schlabach, T. D., Powell, M. J., Vaitkus, J. W., and Bird, O. D. (1954). *Anal. Chem.* **26,** 1406.
Farbenindustrie Aktiengesellschaft, I. G. (1928). British Patent 296,093.
Festenstein, G. N., and Morton, R. A. (1955). *Biochem. J.* **60,** 22.
Fieser, L. F., and Fieser, M. (1959). "Steroids," p. 103. Van Nostrand-Reinhold, Princeton, New Jersey.
Fischer, G. A., and Kabara, J. J. (1964). *Anal. Biochem.* **9,** 303-309.
Fisher, A. L., Parfitt, A. M., and Lloyd, H. M. (1972a). *J. Chromatogr.* **65,** 493.
Fisher, A. L., Parfitt, A. M., and Lloyd, H. M. (1972b). *J. Chromatogr.* **65,** 571.
Fraser, D. R., and Kodicek, E. (1971). *Biochem. J.* 59P.
Fujita, A., and Numata, K. (1958). *J. Vitaminol.* **4,** 299.
Goldblatt, H., and Soames, K. M. (1923). *Biochem. J.* **17,** 446.
Green, J. (1951). *Biochem. J.* **49,** 45.
Hanewald, K. H., Rappoldt, M. P., and Roborgh, J. R. (1961). *Recl. Trav. Chim. Pays-Bas* **80,** 1003.
Harnapp, G. O. (1940). *Wien. Klin. Wochenschr.* **53,** 698.
Harris, R. S. (1954). *In* "The Vitamins" (W. H. Sebrell, Jr. and R. S. Harris, eds.), 1st ed., Vol. 2, p. 199. Academic Press, New York.
Haslewood, G. A. D. (1939). *Biochem. J.* **33,** 454.
Haussler, M. R., Wasserman, R. H., McCain, T. A., Peterlik, M., Bursac, K., and Hughes, M. R. (1976). *Life Sci.* **18,** 1049.
Havinga, E., and Schlatmann, J. L. M. A. (1961). *Tetrahedron* **16,** 146.
Havinga, E., Koevoet, A. L., and Verloop, A. (1955). *Recl. Trav. Chim. Pays-Bas* **74,** 1230.
Havinga, E., DeKock, R. J., and Rappoldt, M. P. (1960). *Tetrahedron* **11,** 276.
Heilbron, I. M., Kamm, E. D., and Morton, R. A. (1926). *Chem. Ind. (Berlin)* **45,** 932.
Heilbron, I. M., Morton, R. A., and Sexton, W. A. (1928). *J. Chem. Soc.* p. 47.
Heilbron, I. M., Jones, R. N., Samant, K. N., and Spring, F. S. (1936). *J. Chem. Soc.* p. 905.
Heinz, H. J. (1950). "Nutritional Data." H. J. Heinz Co., Pittsburgh, Pennsylvania.
Hess, A. F. (1929). "Rickets, Osteomalacia and Tetany," p. 92. Lea & Febiger, Philadelphia, Pennsylvania.
Hess, A. F., and Supplee, G. C. (1929-1930). *Proc. Soc. Exp. Biol. Med.* **27,** 609.
Hess, A. F., and Weinstock, M. (1924). *J. Biol. Chem.* **62,** 301.
Hess, A. F., and Weinstock, M. (1925). *J. Biol. Chem.* **63,** 297.

Hess, A. F., Weinstock, M., and Helman, F. O. (1925). *J. Biol. Chem.* **63,** 305.
Hibberd, K. A., and Norman, A. W. (1969). *Biochem. Pharmacol.* **18,** 2347.
Hirsch, J. (1963). *J. Lipid Res.* **4,** 1.
Hodgkin, D. C. (1976). *Izvj. Jugoslav. Centr. Krist. (Zagreb)* **11,** 5.
Hodgkin, D. C., Rimmer, B. M., Dunitz, J. D., and Trueblood, K. N. (1963). *J. Chem. Soc.* p. 4945.
Hofsass, H., Grant, A., Alicino, N. J., and Greenbaum, S. B. (1976). *J. Assoc. Agric. Chem.* **59,** 251.
Holick, M. F., and DeLuca, H. F. (1971). *J. Lipid Res.* **12,** 460–465.
Holick, M. F., Holick, S. A., Tavela, T., Gallager, B., Schnoes, H., and DeLuca, H. F. (1975). *Science* **190,** 576.
Holick, M. F., Frommer, J. E., McNeill, C. S., Richtand, N. M., Henley, J. W., and Potts, J. T., Jr. (1977). *Biochem. Biophys. Res. Commun.* **76,** 107.
Huber, W., and Barlow, O. W. (1943). *J. Biol. Chem.* **149,** 125.
Huldschinsky, K. (1919). *Dtsch. Med. Wochenschr.* **45,** 712.
Huldschinsky, K. (1920). *Z. Orthop. Chir.* **39,** 426.
Ikekawa, N., and Koizumi, N. (1976). *J. Chromatogr.* **119,** 227.
Inhoffen, H. H. (1958). *Angew. Chem.* **70,** 576.
Inhoffen, H. H., Kath, J., Sticherling, W., and Bruckner, K. (1957). *Justus Liebigs Ann.* **603,** 25.
Jacobs, H. J. C., Boomsma, F., Havinga, E., and VanderGen, A. (1977). *In* "Vitamin D: Biochemical, Chemical and Clinical Aspects Related to Calcium Metabolism" (A. W. Norman *et al.*, eds.), p. 15. de Gruyter, Berlin.
Johnson, N. G., and Levring, T. (1947). *Sven. Hydrogr.-Biol. Komm. Skr., Ser. 3* **1,** No. 3, 7.
Johnson, W. S. (1956). *J. Am. Chem. Soc.* **78,** 6278.
Jones, G., and DeLuca, H. F. (1975). *J. Lipid Res.* **16,** 448.
Jones, G., Schnoes, H. K., and DeLuca, H. F. (1975). *Biochemistry* **14,** 1250.
Jones, S. W., Morris, W. W., and Wilkie, J. B. (1959). *J. Assoc. Agric. Chem.* **42,** 180.
Kodicek, E. (1955). *Biochem. J.* **60,** 25.
Kodicek, E., and Ashby, D. R. (1954). *Biochem. J.* **57,** XII.
Koevoet, A. L., Verloop, A., and Havinga, E. (1955). *Recl. Trav. Chim. Pays-Bas* **74,** 788.
Koshy, K. T., and Vanderslik, A. L. (1976). *Anal. Biochem.* **74,** 282.
Kritchevsky, D., and Kirk, M. R. (1952). *J. Am. Chem. Soc.* **74,** 4484.
LaMar, G. N., and Budd, D. L. (1974). *J. Am. Chem. Soc.* **96,** 7318–7324.
Laquer, F., and Linsert, O. (1933). *Klin. Wochenschr.* **12,** 753.
Legrand, M., and Mathieu, J. (1957). *C. R. Hebd. Seances Acad. Sci.* **245,** 2502.
Lugtenburg, J., and Havinga, E. (1969). *Tetrahedron Lett.* **28,** 2391.
Massengale, O. N., and Nussmeier, M. (1930). *J. Biol. Chem.* **87,** 415 and 423.
Matthews, E. W., Byfield, P. G. H., Colston, K. W., Evans, K. M. A., Galante, L. S., and MacIntyre, I. (1974). *FEBS Lett.* **48,** 122.
Mawer, E. B., and Backhouse, J. (1969). *Biochem. J.* **112,** 255.
Meunier, P., and Thibaudet, G. (1946). *C. R. Hebd. Seances Acad. Sci.* **223,** 172.
Michalec, C., and Strasek, J. (1960). *J. Chromatogr.* **4,** 254.
Murray, T. K., Day, K. C., and Kodicek, E. (1966). *Biochem. J.* **98,** 29P.
Neville, P. F., and DeLuca, H. F. (1966). *Biochemistry* **5,** 2201.
Norman, A. W., and DeLuca, H. F. (1963a). *Anal. Chem.* **35,** 1247.
Norman, A. W., and DeLuca, H. F. (1963b). *Biochemistry* **2,** 1160.
Okamura, W. H., Norman, A. W., and Wing, R. M. (1974). *Proc. Natl. Acad. Sci. U.S.A.* **71,** 4194–4997.
Parekh, C. K., and Wasserman, R. H. (1965). *J. Chromatogr.* **17,** 261.
Pelc, E., and Kodicek, E. (1971). *J. Chem. Soc.* p. 3415.
Penau, H., and Hagemann, G. (1946). *Helv. Chim. Acta* **29,** 1366.

Peterlik, M., Bursak, K., Haussler, M. R., Hughes, M. R., and Wasserman, R. H. (1976). *Biochem. Biophys. Res. Commun.* **70,** 797.
Pohl, R. (1926). *Nachr. Ges. Wiss. Goettingen, Math.-Phys. Kl.* pp. 142 and 185.
Pohl, R. (1927). *Naturwissenschaften* **15,** 433.
Ponsold, W., and Pfennigsdorf, G. (1954). *Strahlentherapie* **95,** 468.
Reindel, F., and Kipphan, H. (1932). *Justus Liebigs Ann. Chem.* **493,** 181.
Rygh, O. (1935). *Nature (London)* **136,** 396.
Sanders, G. M., and Havinga, E. (1964). *Recl. Trav. Chim. Pays-Bas* **83,** 665.
Scheunert, A., Schieblich, M., and Reschke, J. (1935). *Hoppe-Seyler's Z. Physiol. Chem.* **235,** 91.
Sklan, D., Budowski, P., and Katz, M. (1973). *Anal. Biochem.* **56,** 606–609.
Steenbock, H., and Black, A. (1925). *J. Biol. Chem.* **64,** 263.
Steenbock, H., Hart, E. B., Elvehjem, C. A., and Kletzien, S. W. F. (1925). *J. Biol. Chem.* **66,** 425.
Steenbock, H., Kletzien, S. W. F., and Halpin, J. G. (1932). *J. Biol. Chem.* **97,** 249.
Terepka, A. R., Chen, P. S., and Jorgensen, B. (1961). *Endocrinology* **68,** 996.
Theiragt, J. G., and Campbell, D. J. (1959). *Anal. Chem.* **31,** 1375–1377.
Tomkins, D. F., and Tscherne, R. J. (1974). *Anal. Chem.* **46,** 1602–1604.
Trinh-Toan, DeLuca, H. F., and Dahl, L. F. (1977). *J. Org. Chem.* **41,** 3476.
Uflacker, H. (1949). *Z. Kinderheilkd.* **67,** 350.
U.S. International Trade Commission (1975). *Synth. Org. Chem., Publ.* **804.**
Velluz, L., and Amiard, G. (1949a). *C. R. Hebd. Seances Acad. Sci.* **228,** 692.
Velluz, L., and Amiard, G. (1949b). *C. R. Hebd. Seances Acad. Sci.* **228,** 853.
Velluz, L., and Amiard, G. (1949c). *C. R. Hebd. Seances Acad. Sci.* **228,** 1037.
Velluz, L., and Amiard, G. (1961). *C. R. Hebd. Seances Acad. Sci.* **253,** 603.
Velluz, L., Amiard, G., and Petit, A. (1949). *Bull. Soc. Chim. Fr.* **16,** 501.
Velluz, L., Amiard, G., and Goffinet, B. (1955). *Bull. Soc. Chim. Fr.* **22,** 1341.
Verloop, A., Koevoet, A. L., and Havinga, E. (1957). *Recl. Trav. Chim. Pays-Bas* **76,** 689.
von Werder, F. (1939). *Hoppe-Seyler's Z. Physiol. Chem.* **260,** 119.
von Werder, F. (1941). U. S. Patent 2,228,491.
Westerhof, P. J., and Keverling-Buisman, J. A. (1956). *Recl. Trav. Chem. Pays-Bas* **75,** 453.
Windaus, A., and Bock, F. (1936). *Hoppe-Seyler's Z. Physiol. Chem.* **245,** 168.
Windaus, A., and Buckholz, K. (1938). *Hoppe-Seyler's Z. Physiol. Chem.* **256,** 273.
Windaus, A., and Grundmann, H. (1936). *Justus Liebigs Ann. Chem.* **524,** 295.
Windaus, A., Gaede, J., Koser, J., and Stein, G. (1930). *Justus Liebigs Ann. Chem.* **483,** 17.
Windaus, A., Luttringhaus, A., and Deppe, M. (1931). *Justus Liebigs Ann. Chem.* **489,** 252.
Windaus, A., Linsert, O., Luttringhaus, A., and Weidlick, G. (1932a). *Justus Liebigs Ann. Chem.* **492,** 226.
Windaus, A., Dithmar, K., and Fernholz, E. (1932b). *Justus Liebigs Ann. Chem.* **493,** 259.
Windaus, A., von Werder, F., and Luttringhaus, A. (1932c). *Justus Liebigs Ann. Chem.* **499,** 188.
Windaus, A., Schenck, F., and von Werder, F. (1936). *Hoppe-Seyler's Z. Physiol. Chem.* **241,** 100.
Wing, R. M., Okamura, W. H., Pirio, M. R., Sine, S. M., and Norman, A. W. (1974). *Science* **186,** 939.
Wing, R. M., Okamura, W. H., Rego, A., Pirio, M. R., and Norman, A. W. (1975). *J. Am. Chem. Soc.* **97,** 4980.
Wong, R. G., and Norman, A. W. (1972). *J. Nutr.* **102,** 1709.
Woodward, T. B., Sondheimer, F., Taub, D., Heusler, K., and McLamore, W. M. (1952). *J. Am. Chem. Soc.* **74,** 4223.
Yamada, S., Schnoes, H. K., and DeLuca, H. F. (1978). *Anal. Biochem.* **85,** 34.
Ziffer, H., VandenHeuvel, W. J., Haahti, E. O., and Horning, E. C. (1960). *J. Am. Chem. Soc.* **82,** 6411.
Zimmermann, W., and Frankenburger, W. (1933). U. S. Patent 1,896,191.

CHAPTER

4

Biological and Chemical Assay of Vitamin D, Its Metabolites, and Analogs

I. INTRODUCTION

A. Types of Methods and Their Sensitivity

This chapter is concerned with older methods for the determination of vitamin D activity as well as newer physical techniques for analysis of both the parent vitamin and its metabolites and analogs. Until recent years, when the metabolic pathways associated with the biological action of vitamin D were uncovered, most analytical efforts were directed toward devising reliable and sensitive means for the estimation of concentrations of the parent steroid. Chapter 8 presents information pertaining to the quantitative evaluation of some of the biologically active forms of vitamin D, e.g., $25(OH)D_3$, $24,25(OH)_2D_3$, and $1,25(OH)_2D_3$, by steroid competition assay.

A wide variety of biological assays and chemical determinations are capable of quantitating with some precision the amount of vitamin D present in a test sample. Tables 4-1 and 4-2 show that the biological assays are, as a rule, capable of detecting smaller quantities of vitamin D than are the direct chemical or physicochemical methods. The mean amount of vitamin D detectable by all the biological methods is 120 ng, or 0.3 nmole, whereas by chemical methods the mean detectable level is approximately 1000 ng, or 2.6 nmoles. Two notable exceptions are the ultraviolet absorption analysis after separation by high-pressure liquid chromatography, which can detect 5 ng, and the electron capture detector associated with a gas chromatography apparatus, which can detect as little as 50 pg of calciferol. However, these methods are not as yet routinely available or accepted by individuals concerned with the measurement of biologically relevant levels of vitamin D.

With the exception of vitamin B_{12}, vitamin D is the most potent of the vitamins. Accordingly, biological samples and animal tissues usually contain exceedingly low concentrations of vitamin D, which are virtually undetectable by physical or chemical methods. For example, the circulating plasma level of vitamin D_3 in man is only 10–20 ng/ml, i.e., $2\text{–}5 \times 10^{-8} M$ (Belsey *et al.*, 1971). Thus, it was only through the development of laborious biological assays that information was gained on the tissue levels of vitamin D or the vitamin D content of foodstuffs.

B. Definition and Standardization of Activity

The Health Organization of the League of Nations in 1931 adopted an international standard of reference for vitamin D: "the vitamin D activity of 1 mg of international standard solution of irradiated ergosterol" (League of Nations, 1931). Since at that time the precise chemical properties of ergocalciferol (i.e., irradiated ergosterol) had not yet been elucidated, this definition was dependent on certain specified conditions of irradiation. In 1935 the definition of one international unit (IU) was modified to be "the activity of 1 mg of the international standard solution of irradiated ergosterol, which has been found equivalent to 0.025 μg of crystalline vitamin D" (League of Nations, 1935). Note that, although the definition makes reference to irradiated ergosterol, it was not identified as vitamin D_2. Furthermore, the Health Organization stated that "if the present standard solution were to be exhausted or if it becomes unsatisfactory for any reason, it should be replaced by a solution of pure crystalline vitamin D

TABLE 4-1
Comparison of Sensitivity and Working Range of Biological Assays for Vitamin D

Assay	Time required for assay	Minimal level detectable in assay: ng	Minimal level detectable in assay: nmoles	Usual working range	Reference
Rat line test	7 days	12	0.03	25–25 ng	Association of Official Agricultural Chemists (1960, 1975)
AOAC chick test	21 days	50	0.13	50–1250 ng	Association of Official Agricultural Chemists (1960, 1975)
Intestinal Ca^{2+} absorption,					
In vivo					
$^{45}Ca^{2+}$	1 day	125	0.33	0.125–25 μg	Hibberd and Norman (1969)
$^{47}Ca^{2+}$	1 day	125	0.33	0.125–25 μg	Wasserman and Taylor (1962)
In vitro					
Everted sacs	1 day	250	0.65	250–1000 ng	Schachter and Rosen (1959) Martin and DeLuca (1969b)
Duodenal uptake of $^{45}Ca^{2+}$	1 day	250	0.65	250–1000 ng	Martin and DeLuca (1969a)
Bone Ca^{2+} mobilization					
In vivo	24 hr	125	0.32	0.125–25 μg	Hibberd and Norman (1969)
In vitro[a]	None available				
Body growth	21–28 days	50	0.06	50–1250 ng	Hibberd and Norman (1969)
Immunoassay for calcium-binding protein	1 day	12	0.03	125–3125 ng	Wasserman *et al.* (1974)

[a]There are no methods for measuring bone calcium mobilization *in vitro* that are responsive to the parent vitamin D; however, the method of Reynolds (1974) is applicable to vitamin D metabolites.

(calciferol) in olive oil, of such strength that 1 mg (of the oil) contains 0.025 gamma of crystalline vitamin D."

This definition of the League of Nations was widely accepted and is usually given as the official statement of vitamin D activity. According to the U.S. Pharmacopoeia (USP) (1955), "one United States Pharmacopoeia Unit of vitamin D is equal in antirachitic potency for the rat, to one International Unit of vitamin D as defined and adopted by the Conference of Vitamin Standards of the Permanent Commission on Biological Standardization of the League of Nations in June 1934."[1] However, the USP also maintained a reference cod-liver oil solution that was used by the Association of Official Agricultural Chemists (AOAC) as their standard (1940). One AOAC chick unit of vitamin D was stated by them to be equal in biological activity for the chick to one unit of vitamin D in the USP reference cod-liver oil (World Health Organization, 1950).

Thus, there is the paradoxical situation that, although the original definition of one international unit made reference to irradiated ergosterol, i.e., vitamin D_2, the reference standard maintained by the USP in cod-liver oil is vitamin D_3. As a result of these conflicting statements it was not clear whether 1.0 IU should be considered to be 0.025 μg of ergocalciferol or of cholecalciferol or the biological activity of a specified amount of "standard" cod-liver oil solution. Also, it was not obvious which "reference solution" of vitamin D was considered to be the ultimate standard.

Then, in 1949, the World Health Organization stated that "the International Unit of vitamin D recommended for adoption is the vitamin D activity of 0.025 μg of the international standard preparation of crystalline vitamin D_3" (World Health Organization, 1950). At that time only 14 g of crystalline vitamin D_3 was available for storage at the National Institute for Medical Research in London, and procedures for its replacement were indicated. However, today crystalline vitamin D_3 of high purity is readily available from several commercial organizations.

The first official standard of vitamin D activity in the United States was described by the U.S. Pharmacopoeia (1934). This was a reference solution of cod-liver oil whose vitamin D content was stated in USP units; one USP unit was defined "as being equal in antirachitic potency for the rat to one IU as defined and adopted by The League of Nations Conference on Vitamin Standards in June 1931."

The current USP standard for vitamin D was defined by Nelson (1949) to be vitamin D_3 rather than the previously employed irradiated solutions of ergosterol. Standardized quantities of vitamin D_3 for biological assays are available as a solution of cottonseed oil, where 1.0 g of oil contains 10.0 μg, or 400 USP units,

[1]This statement made in 1934 was published in 1935 (League of Nations, 1935).

TABLE 4-2
Comparison of Sensitivity and Working Range for Chemical Determinations of Vitamin D

Method	Minimal level detectable in assay		Usual working range (nmoles)	Reference
	ng	nmoles		
Ultraviolet absorption[a]	1000	2.6	2.6–52	Fieser and Fieser (1959)
Colorimetric methods				Haftman and Mosettig (1960)
Aniline–HCl reagent				Shear (1925)
Phosphorus pentachloride				Stoeltzner (1928)
Alcoholic solution of vitamin D + HCl				Cruze-Coke (1930)
Alcoholic solution of vitamin D + anhydrous $AlCl_3$ + pyrogallol				Halden and Tzoni (1936)
Alcoholic solution of vitamin D + $NaNO_2$ and acetic acid				Robinson (1937)
Antimony trichloride[b,c]	1250	3.2	3.2–6.5	Brockmann and Chen (1936), Nield *et al.* (1940), Association of Official Agricultural Chemists (1940), DeWitt and Sullivan (1946), Wilkie *et al.* (1958)[c], Mulder *et al.* (1965), Panalaks (1971), Wardynska *et al.* (1973), U.S. Pharmacoeoeia (1975)[c]

Boron trifluoride[b]		No values provided		Kobayashi and Adachi (1973)[b]
Trifluoroacetic acid[b]	1000	2.6	1–80	Clements *et al.* (1967), Gharbo and Gosser (1974)[b]
Acetyl chloride[b]	1000	2.6	1–80	Sheppard *et al.* (1965)
Ultraviolet, fluorescence	1000[d]	2.6	2.6–26	Chen *et al.* (1964)[d], Passannante and Avioli (1966)[d]
Gas chromatography (GC)	0.05[e]	0.1 pmole	0.01–10	Sklan *et al.* (1973)[e]
	500[f]	1.30	2–10	Evans (1972)[f]
High-pressure liquid chromatography (HPLC)	5	0.01	0.05–100	Tompkins and Tscherne (1974), Jones and DeLuca (1975), Hofsass *et al.* (1976), Koshy and Vanderslik (1976)
Mass spectrometry (MS)	500			Eismann *et al.* (1977)
Mass fragmentography	5	12 pmoles	0–10	Bjorkhem and Holmberg (1976)
GC—MS[g]	<1			Tsukida and Saiki (1972)[h], Cruye and de Leenheer (1974)

[a] A solution with 2.1 μg/ml (84 IU/ml; 5.47 nmoles/ml) of vitamin D will have an absorbance at 264 nm of 0.10. See Fig. 3-2 for the uv spectrum of vitamin D.

[b] The procedure is based on the isomerization of vitamin D to isotachysterol. Method employs a uv detector with 0.01 OD sensitivity.

[c] This procedure is now used primarily to determine the vitamin D content of pharmaceutical preparations.

[d] The procedure is based on the property of (acetic anhydride–sulfuric acid)-induced fluorescence of vitamin D or dihydrotachysterol.

[e] Method employs an electron capture detector. The steroids were derivatized with DF_3COOH prior to analysis (Sklan *et al.*, 1973).

[f] Method employs a flame ionization detector. The steroids were derivatized as trimethylsilyl ethers prior to analysis after extensive preliminary purification by column chromatography.

[g] Authors state that if derivatization as a heptafluorobutyl ester were carried out, assay at the subnanogram level should be possible.

[h] This method is capable of detecting vitamin D_2 in the presence of D_3.

of vitamin D_3. Also, capsules containing 2.5 μg, or 100 USP units, are available. Both are distributed by the Board of Trustees of the U.S. Pharmacopoeia Convention, Inc., principally for use in the rat line test or other bioassays. For chemical assays of vitamin D the USP also has available ampules containing 30 mg of vitamin D_3.

II. BIOLOGICAL DETERMINATION

A. Official Assays

1. Rat Line Test

The only official method for the determination of the vitamin D content of pharmaceutical products or foodstuffs from 1922 to 1958 was the "rat line test" (U.S. Pharmacopoeia, 1934, 1950, 1955). This assay is still widely employed to determine and document the vitamin D content of many foods, particularly milk. In 1958, an alternative chemical method was adopted which is appropriate for samples that contain 10,000 IU (250 μg, or 651 nmoles) or levels that are often present in pharmaceutical preparations (U.S. Pharmacopoeia, 1960, 1975).

The "line test" was first described by McCollum *et al.* (1922) and has since been referred to in some circles as the Johns Hopkins line test. The term "official" in reference to the assay indicates that the reproducibility and accuracy of the assay when conducted according to the procedures described by the U.S. Pharmacopoeia (1934, 1950, 1955) or the Association of Official Agricultural Chemists (1960, 1975) are such that the results can be accepted legally.

The "line test" for vitamin D is conducted in recently weaned, rachitic rats. Weanling rats are fed the classic rachitogenic Steenbock ration 2965 (see Appendix A) for 19 to 25 days. After the development of florid rickets, a 7-day assay period ensues. During this time 9 groups of 7 to 10 animals receive in their diet either a graded series of known amounts of cholecalciferol or the unknown test sample. One week is adequate to demonstrate the "curative effect" of dietary vitamin D. At this time the animals are killed; the radii and ulnae are dissected, cleaned of adhering muscle and fat tissue, sliced longitudinally, and placed in a solution of silver nitrate. The basis of the assay is the deposition of silver in areas of bone where new calcium has recently been deposited. These regions turn black upon exposure to light. (See Fig. 4-1 for typical results.) The black line across the cartilage plate of unknown samples is visually "scored" in relation to the intensity and width of lines generated by the vitamin D_3 standards.

The "line test" assay is capable of detecting 1–12 IU (25–300 ng; 65–780 pmoles) of vitamin D. Since the assay is conducted in the rat, there is no

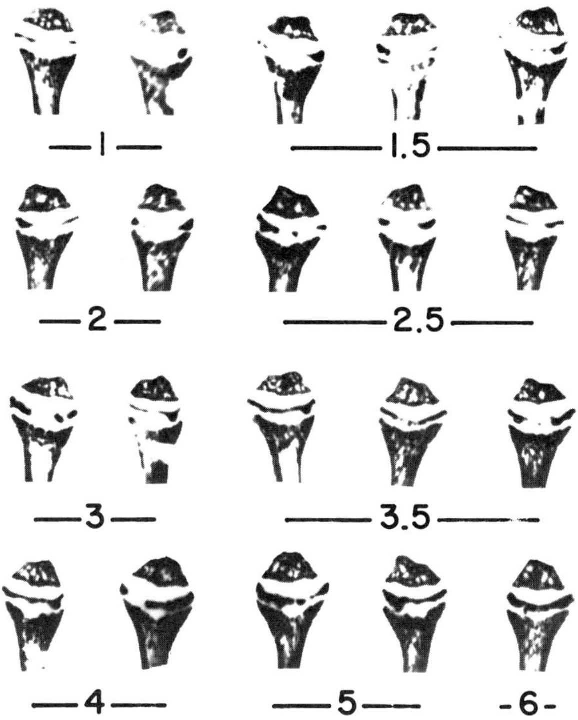

Figure 4-1. Typical results from the rat line test assay for vitamin D activity. Reproduced by permission of the Association of Official Analytical Chemists and taken from the 12th edition of "Official Methods of Analysis" (1975).

discrimination between vitamin D_2 and vitamin D_3; both give identical results. When only one level of test sample is bioassayed, the results are commonly reported on a "pass-or-fail" basis; however, if two or more levels of test samples are evaluated, the results can be expressed quantitatively.

Some sample preparation is normally required before assay. Whereas vitamin D oils can be assayed directly, milk, vitamin tablets, and vitamin D-fortified foods must be saponified and the residue taken up into a suitable oil vehicle prior to assay.

Although considerable progress has been made in the development of chemical or physical means for the determination of vitamin D, these lack both the specificity and sensitivity achieved by the biological assays, particularly the rat line test, for the routine determination of steroid levels. It is anticipated that the development of the steroid competition assays described in Chapter 8 will offer some attractive alternatives in the future.

2. *AOAC Chick Test*

An official description of the AOAC chick assay is given by the Association of Official Agricultural Chemists (1960, 1975). The principal use of the AOAC chick test is to assess quantities of vitamin D_3 as distinct from vitamin D_2. Whereas in the rat vitamins D_2 and D_3 are equivalently active, in the chick vitamin D_3 is some 10 times more potent than D_2 (Waddell, 1934; Rygh, 1935; Hibberd and Norman, 1969). Thus, the availability of the AOAC chick test is vital for the accurate determination of the cholecalciferol levels of poultry feeds.

The assay is conducted by placing groups of 20 newly hatched chicks on the specified vitamin D-deficient diet (see Appendix A) containing added levels of D_3 (1–10 IU; 25–250 ng; 65–650 pmoles) or test substance. After 3 weeks of feeding, the percent bone ash of dried lipid-free tibias is determined. A rachitic bird typically has 25–27% bone ash, whereas a vitamin D-supplemented bird has 40–45% bone ash. Typical results from the assay are shown in Fig. 4-2. Due to the 3-week duration of the assay and the time-consuming processing of the bones, the assay is expensive and not frequently employed.

B. Other Assays

1. *Stimulation of Intestinal Calcium Absorption*

Certainly the most extensively studied action of vitamin D is its potent ability to effect the stimulation of calcium absorption across the small intestine. It is therefore not surprising that this characteristic aspect of vitamin D action has been utilized to develop biological assays that are capable of detecting physiological quantities of this steroid. There are two basic types of assays available: those employing techniques *in vivo* and others employing manipulations of the intestine *in vitro*. Each is capable of detecting approximately equivalent amounts, i.e., 2–50 IU (50–1250 ng; 0.13–3.2 nmoles), of vitamin D. As discussed in Chapter 1 there is a time lag of approximately 36 to 48 hr prior to the development of maximal response to vitamin D. Thus, both assays have the same general design. The test dose or standard dose of vitamin D is administered to the animal 24–48 hr prior to assessment of the calcium-transporting ability of the small intestine.

The technique *in vivo* for quantitating calcium absorption in the chick was originally described in detail by Coates and Holdsworth (1961). A somewhat modified version of the assay was given by Hibberd and Norman (1969). The method involves utilization of rachitic chicks that have been raised on a test diet containing low levels of available calcium, e.g., 0.6% (see Appendix A). In the event that a simultaneous assay *in vivo* of "mobilization of bone calcium" is to be carried out, the birds must be switched to a rachitogenic diet containing zero

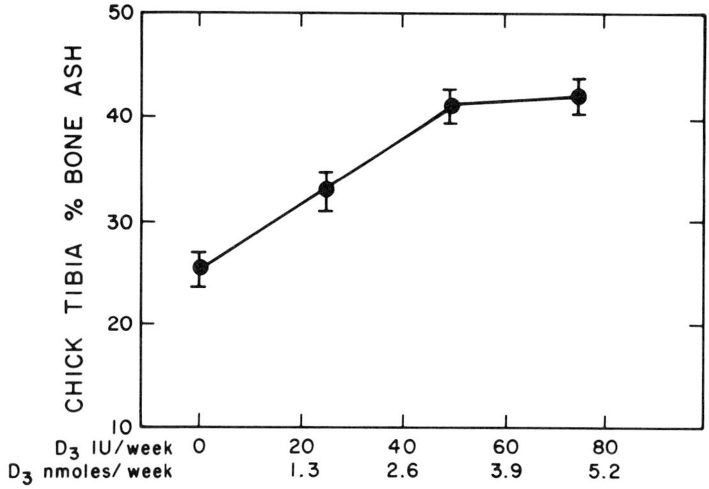

Figure 4-2. Typical results from AOAC 21-day prophylactic chick assay for vitamin D_3. White Leghorn cockerels were fed a rachitogenic diet for 21 days and supplemented three times weekly with oral doses of vitamin D_3. Replotted from Hibberd and Norman (1969).

added calcium 3 days before assay. The chicks then receive one dose (oral, intraperitoneal, or intracardial) of the test compound in a vehicle, usually 0.2 ml of 1,2-propanediol. Twenty-four or, more appropriately for vitamin D_3, 48 hr later, the chicks are anesthetized and a small incision is made on the abdomen of each bird. The duodenal loop is lifted out, injected with 0.2 ml of a solution containing 4.0 mg $^{40}Ca^{2+}$ as the chloride and approximately 6×10^6 dpm $^{45}Ca^{2+}$. The loop is then returned to the peritoneal cavity and the opening closed with a wound clip. Thirty minutes after receiving the $^{45}Ca^{2+}$, the chicks are killed by decapitation, and blood is collected. Serum is prepared from the whole blood, and small aliquots are taken for $^{45}Ca^{2+}$ determination in either a thin window gas flow Geiger–Muller counter or a liquid scintillation counter. Total serum calcium concentration (for bone calcium mobilization evaluation) can be determined by atomic absorption spectrometry.

Results from a typical bioassay are shown in Fig. 4-3. The assay is linear over the dose range of approximately 2 to 50 IU (50–1250 ng; 0.13–3.2 nmoles). It is apparent that a vitamin D-deficient, rachitic chick has a significant baseline absorption of calcium. However, it is possible to stimulate this basal level approximately three- to fivefold by the administration of vitamin D. As such, this constitutes the most meaningful way of assessing the activity of vitamin D or an analogue present in a sample. This technique has been widely employed for such determinations (Hibberd and Norman, 1969; Myrtle and Norman, 1971; Sallis and Holdsworth, 1962; Haussler *et al.*, 1973; Norman *et al.*, 1975).

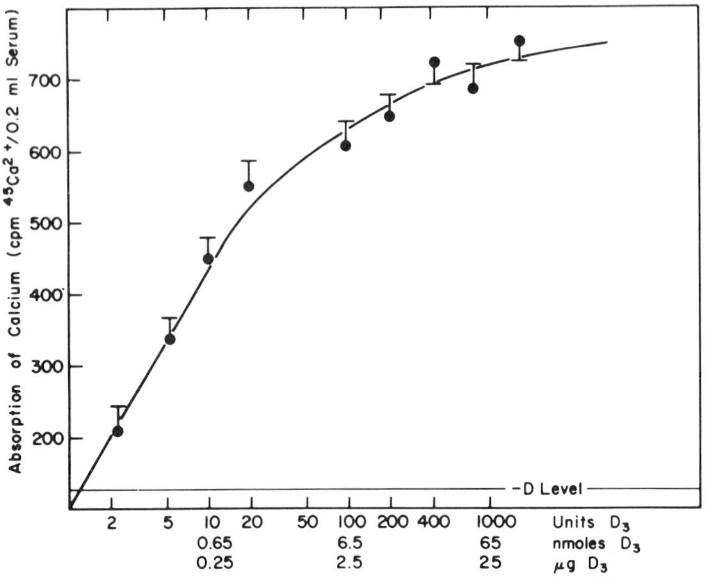

Figure 4-3. Dose-response study of the stimulation of intestinal calcium absorption in the rachitic chick by vitamin D_3. Replotted from Hibberd and Norman (1969).

It is also possible to carry out the same assessment of vitamin D activity in terms of stimulation of intestinal calcium transport by using preparations of intestinal loops that have been everted and incubated under *in vitro* conditions with solutions of radioactive calcium. This technique was pioneered by Schacter and Rosen (1959). Their method of preparing everted intestinal sacs was a modification of the earlier procedure of Wilson and Wiseman (1954).

The prime reason for employing the *in vitro* technique has been that it facilitates inquiry into the biochemical mechanisms concerned with calcium absorption. However, it has also been possible to develop the technique precisely enough so that a quantitative determination of vitamin D can be carried out. Under the conditions of the assay, the everted intestinal loop or sac has a fluid medium of identical calcium concentration on both the mucosal and serosal sides of the tissue. The principle of the assay is dependent on the fact that the mucosal surface of the tissue will actively transport the calcium through the tissue to the serosal side; thus, a determination of the ratio of calcium concentration in the mucosal and serosal fluid compartments will provide a measure of the "active" transport of calcium. In a vitamin D-deficient animal the serosal/mucosal fluid flux ratio is approximately 1–2.5, whereas in an animal that has received vitamin D the ratio can be as high as 6–7 (Martin and DeLuca, 1969b).

This technique has been employed largely in studies in mammals rather than birds (Martin and DeLuca, 1969b). A vitamin D standard or test compound is given either orally or intraperitoneally 24–48 hr in advance of the assay. At the time of assay the animals are killed, the upper small intestine is dissected free, and a 10-cm length of duodenum is removed from the animal and turned inside out. The everted intestine is then washed in ice-cold Krebs Ringer solution, and a gut sac with the mucosal surface on the outside and the serosal surface on the inside is prepared from each segment by tying off with suture each end of the intestinal segment. The inside of the sac is filled with 0.4–0.6 ml of the standard medium of Krebs Ringer–bicarbonate containing radioactive $^{45}Ca^{2+}$. These sacs are then placed in an incubation flask containing 2–5 ml of the standard incubation medium, which contains the radioactive calcium. The gas phase is normally replaced with 95% O_2, 5% CO_2, and the flask is incubated for a standard period of time, usually 2–3 hr. At the end of the incubation, equal aliquots are taken from the inside (serosal) and outside (mucosal) media and are transferred to planchets or liquid scintillation vials for determination of radioactivity content. The data are expressed as a ratio of concentration of $^{45}Ca^{2+}$ in counts per minute/milliliter medium, i.e., inside/outside.

The ratio of radioactivity in the serosal/mucosal fluid varies with the segment of the small intestine examined; in rabbits and rats the highest ratios have been consistently observed with the duodenum. The assay is capable of detecting 10–100 IU (25–250 ng) of vitamin D_3. In comparison to the chick *in vivo* assay, this technique suffers from the fact that it is considerably more time-consuming due to the tedious nature of preparing the everted intestinal sacs and the duration of the incubation period. This technique has been employed by a number of laboratories (Schachter and Rosen, 1959; Harrison and Harrison, 1960; Martin and DeLuca, 1969a,b).

2. *Mobilization of Bone Calcium*

As indicated above in the discussion of the technique for measurement *in vivo* of the intestinal absorption of calcium in chicks, it is possible to simultaneously determine the vitamin D-mediated elevation of serum calcium. If the chicks employed in the assay have been raised on a diet devoid of calcium for a period of at least 3 days prior to the time of assay, when a compound with vitamin D activity is administered there is a highly characteristic elevation of serum calcium, which is proportionate to the dose of steroid administered. Since there is no dietary calcium available under the conditions of the assay, the only source of calcium for elevation of serum calcium during the 24- to 48-hr test period is bone. The serum calcium level of a rachitic 21-day-old chick is usually 4.5–5.0 mg per 100 ml of serum. Within 24–48 hr after administration of 5–500 IU (125–12,500 ng) of vitamin D_3, the serum calcium levels can rise by 4–5 mg of

Ca per 100 ml of serum to a value of 9.5–10.0 mg Ca per 100 ml. The interesting advantage of the determination of bone calcium mobilization simultaneously with that of intestinal calcium absorption is that the assays measure different aspects of the animals' response to vitamin D. If the intestinal absorption of $^{45}Ca^{2+}$ has been conducted simultaneously, only a negligible portion of the 4.0 mg of $^{40}Ca^{2+}$ placed in the duodenum is transferred to the blood in the 30-min test period (Coates and Holdsworth, 1961). It cannot be presumed that these responsive systems—the intestinal absorption system and the bone calcium mobilization system—have an identical set of response patterns to various structural modifications of vitamin D. In fact, Hibberd and Norman (1969) and Johnson (1975) noted that the intestinal calcium absorption system was less tolerant of modification of the side chain than was the bone calcium mobilizing system. We have suggested that these results might be an indication of differences in the properties of the receptors for vitamin D and/or its metabolites in these two systems.

3. *Stimulation of Growth*

It has long been known that administration of vitamin D to animals results in an enhanced rate of growth. The exact relationship between this effect of vitamin D and growth per se and dietary calcium, phosphorus, and other nutritional factors was extensively studied by Steenbock and Herting (1955) and more recently by Adams *et al.* (1975). In a series of experiments with young rats, Steenbock and co-workers found that a low-calcium diet adequately supplied with phosphorus and other essentials provided optimal conditions for eliciting a maximal growth differential between vitamin D-deficient and treated animals. Vitamin D always tended to normalize the serum phosphorus from either high or low levels; on the other hand, the only action of vitamin D on serum calcium was to mediate an elevation. It was impossible to duplicate the marked growth-promoting effects of vitamin D by varying either the amount or the proportion of calcium and phosphorus in the diet. It was concluded that the weanling rat and, by inference, other species require adequate levels of vitamin D for optimal growth and performance.

As shown in Fig. 4-4, it is possible to develop an assay for vitamin D activity in the chick utilizing the growth-promoting properties of the steroid. The results shown were obtained using the procedures of Hibberd and Norman (1969). One-day-old hatchling chicks were placed on a rachitogenic diet and given standard amounts of vitamin D_3 or the test compound three times weekly. Groups of birds were weighed periodically, and their weight was plotted versus age. Figure 4-4 shows the growth response data for chicks receiving various levels of vitamin D for a period of 4 weeks. In the absence of vitamin D the rate of growth essentially plateaus by the fourth week, but it can be seen that 5–10 IU (125–250 ng; 0.32–0.65 nmoles) per day or 50 IU (1250 ng) of vitamin D_3 per week is

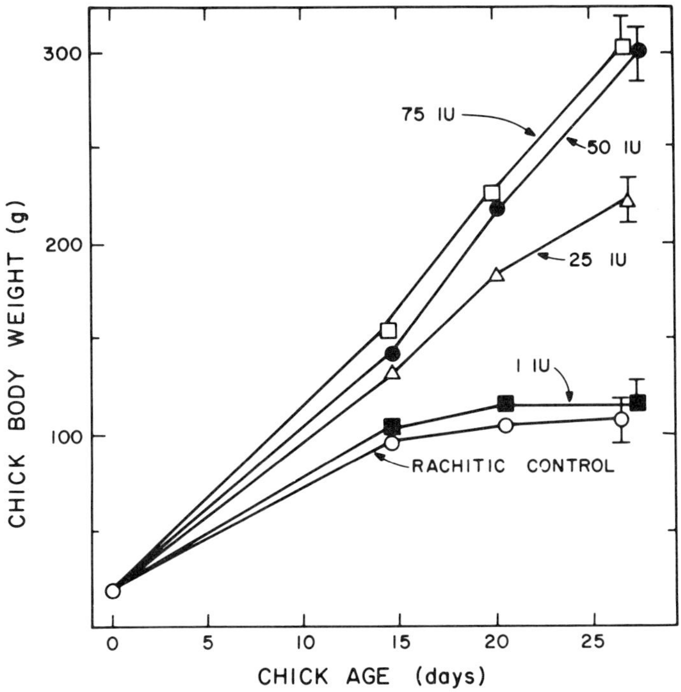

Figure 4-4. Growth response curves of chicks fed various amounts of vitamin D_3. The level of steroid indicated is the total amount in international units that was administered orally (in equivalent doses) per week. Values reported are the mean ± S.D. (n = 10). Replotted from Hibberd and Norman (1969).

sufficient to maintain a maximal growth rate of the chick. These data are consistent with the earlier results of Chen and Bosmann (1964). The disadvantage of this assay is the rather lengthy 21-day period required for precise determination of the rate of growth. However, this assay has a sensitivity comparable to that of the rat line test or the 21-day prophylactic assay of vitamin D activity in the chick.

4. Immunoassay for Calcium-Binding Protein

One additional biological assay that has some potential in terms of its sensitivity and specificity concerns the utilization of an immunoassay that is specific for the vitamin D-dependent calcium-binding protein. A brief discussion has appeared in a review article by Wasserman *et al.* (1974). The vitamin D-dependent calcium-binding protein (CaBP) is not present in the intestinal mucosa of vitamin D-deficient chicks and is synthesized only in response to the administration of a compound containing vitamin D activity (see Chapter 10). Thus, it is possible to use the presence of CaBP as an end point in a vitamin D bioassay. Figure 4-5 shows typical standard curves of linear increases in intestinal CaBP which result from the chronic administration of D_3, 25(OH)D_3, or 1,25$(OH)_2D_3$. The assay is highly sensitive (as little as 0.5–1.0 μg of CaBP per gram mucosa can be detected) while having a linear range of 1–50 μg of CaBP which results from the administration of 1–200 IU of vitamin D_3.

A principal advantage of the immunoassay for calcium-binding protein is that in the absence of vitamin D there is a zero baseline; i.e., no calcium-binding protein is present. All the other bioassays capable of detecting vitamin D have significant nonzero baselines, which often fluctuate over rather wide limits.

Murray *et al.* (1974) and Christakos and Norman (1979) developed a radioimmunoassay for porcine and chick intestinal CaBP, respectively. The unusual sensitivity of this procedure (it can detect nanogram quantities) has made possible, for the first time, the determination of the presence of trace quantities of CaBP in the blood. This technique undoubtedly will provide new opportunities for investigating the roles of vitamin D-dependent CaBP in calcium metabolism.

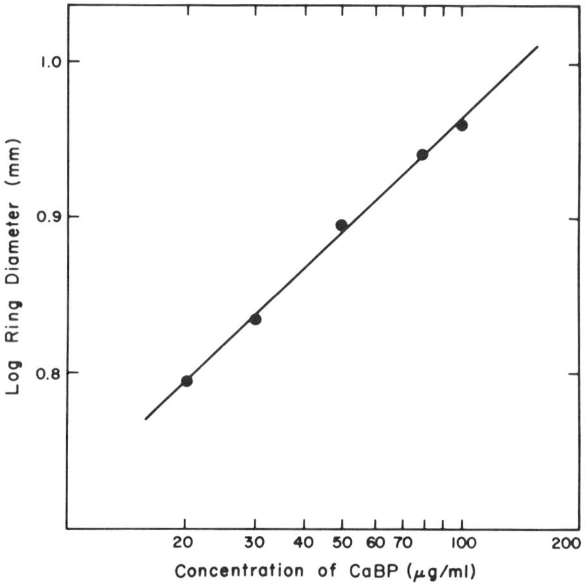

Figure 4-5. Radial immunoassay for vitamin D-dependent chick intestinal calcium-binding protein (CaBP). Fourteen-day-old vitamin D-deficient chicks raised on a diet containing 0.6% Ca, 0.4% P were fed on a daily basis oral doses of the indicated steroid for a period of 7–10 days. Homogenates of the intestinal mucosa were then prepared and the radial immunodiffusion assay conducted with antiserum specific to chick intestinal CaBP (as described by Wasserman *et al.*, 1974). Data presented are the unpublished observations of E. J. Friedlander and A. W. Norman (1975).

III. CHEMICAL DETERMINATION

A. Ultraviolet Absorption

One of the most characteristic features of the vitamin D secosteroids is the conjugated triene system of double bonds. Accordingly, these molecules have highly characteristic ultraviolet absorption spectra. The first techniques available for quantitating vitamin D were based on the measurement of the ultraviolet absorption at 264 nm. At this wavelength the molar extinction coefficient of vitamins D_2 and D_3 is 18,300 (see Fig. 3-2). Thus, a solution with 2.1 μg/ml of vitamin D will have an absorbance at 264 nm of 0.10 in a cuvette with a 1.0-cm light path. Several published analytical procedures are based on this technique (Fuchs and Beck, 1933; Topelmann and Schuhknecht, 1935; Marcussen, 1939). However, the chief disadvantage of these procedures is that the sample must be scrupulously purified prior to assay to remove potential uv absorbing contaminants.

B. Colorimetric Methods

Over the years a variety of colorimetric methods have been proposed which have some applicability to the quantitative estimation of vitamin D. Many of these are listed in Table 4-2. However, until the method of Brockmann and Chen (1936) appeared there was no satisfactory method of detecting the presence of vitamin D, even in relatively high concentrations, in biological samples.

The method of Brockmann and Chen (1936) is based on the principle that a chloroform solution of antimony trichloride will form a fleeting pink color in the presence of vitamin D which absorbs at 400 nm. This analytical procedure was employed by Brockmann in his pioneering effort to isolate in crystalline form vitamin D_3 from several tons of tuna-liver oil (Brockmann, 1936). In spite of the importance of this first applicable chemical assay for vitamin D_3, it was still subject to much further improvement. Wolf (1938) claimed that the error of the procedure in its original form was $\pm 19\%$. Nield *et al.* (1940) subsequently modified the original Brockmann–Chen procedure by adding acetyl chloride as a color stabilizer.

The first practical spectrophotometric procedure for determining the concentration of vitamin D in pharmaceutical preparations was that of DeWitt and Sullivan (1946). They replaced the chloroform solvent of the $SbCl_3$–acetyl chloride reagent with ethylene chloride. This reagent yields readily reproducible results and is stable for several weeks; it reacts with vitamin D to give a salmon pink solution with an absorption maximum at 500 nm, which is stable for 5 to 10 min (Fig. 4-6). The molar extinction coefficient is 2200, and the assay follows Beer's law over a concentration range of 500 to 4000 ng/ml (1.3–10.4 nmoles/ml).

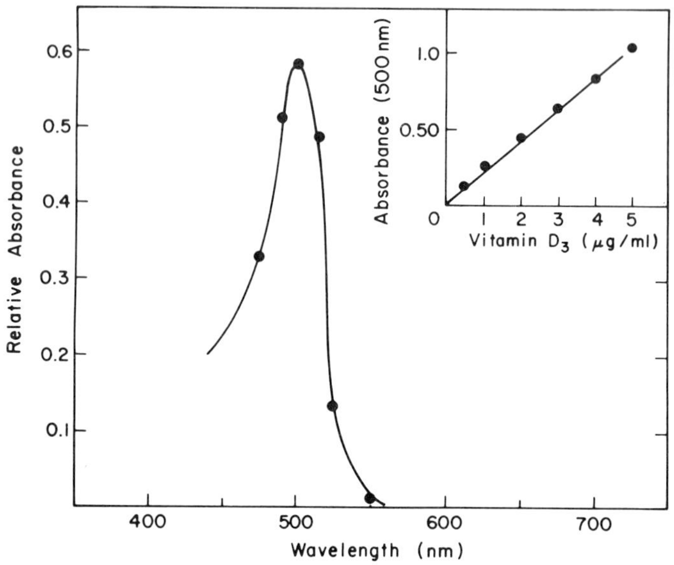

Figure 4-6. Antimony trichloride colorimetric procedure for the determination of vitamin D. The absorption curve of the salmon pink color was replotted from the data of Nield *et al.* (1940), and the standard curve was plotted from the data of DeWitt and Sullivan (1946).

The antimony trichloride colorimetric assay for vitamin D_3 has been of value principally in determining the amount of this steroid in pharmaceutical preparations, i.e., samples that contain quite high levels of vitamin D (1–1000 μg). In these pharmaceutical samples, the vitamin D is usually admixed with other vitamins, particularly vitamin A, a fact that often poses complications to the analyst. This technique was officially adopted by the U.S. Pharmacopoeia in 1960 and has been described in the AOAC ''Official Methods of Analysis'' (1960, 1975).

The official USP method consists of four consecutive steps: (a) isolation of the unsaponifiable lipids, i.e., the elimination of all water-soluble vitamins and oils; (b) partition chromatography on siliceous earth, which is designed to separate vitamin A compounds from vitamin D compounds; (c) adsorption chromatography employing celite or Fuller's earth, which is designed to eliminate decomposition products of vitamin A from vitamin D; (d) the colorimetric determination of the putative vitamin D using antimony trichloride carried out in a solvent of ethylene dichloride.

For the colorimetric step three assay tubes are normally prepared, one containing the standard calciferol or unknown sample plus color reagent, one tube containing only the solvent, ethylene chloride, plus the color reagent, and a third tube containing ethylene chloride plus acetic anhydride plus the color reagent.

Forty-five seconds after the addition of the color reagent, the absorbance at 500 nm is measured. The concentration of vitamin D in the sample is proportionate to the absorbance of the first tube corrected for the blank absorbance and the absorbance of the tube containing the acetic anhydride. Beer's law has been found to apply for solutions containing 50–1000 IU (1.2–25 μg; 3.1–65.0 nmoles), of vitamin D per milliliter of assay solution (Wilke *et al.*, 1958). The smallest deviations were observed in solutions that were of a concentration of 100–400 IU/ml.

The principal disadvantage of the official USP procedure is obviously the laborious multistep nature of the assay. However, it is the only direct chemical method currently available and as such has widespread industrial application. Another obvious disadvantage is the necessity for careful timing of the reaction because the time required for the appearance of the maximal intensity of color is very short. Mulder *et al.* (1971) have reviewed the problems associated with the chemical determination of vitamin D in multivitamin preparations.

The antimony trichloride component of the Wilkie *et al.* (1958) assay procedure has been replaced by boron trifluoride (Kobayashi and Adachi, 1973) or trifluoroacetic acid or acetyl chloride (see Table 4-2 for reference citations). Of these procedures the method of Gharbo and Gosser (1974) employing trifluoroacetic acid is perhaps the most valuable. Their assay is based on mixing a chloroform solution containing vitamin D with appropriate amounts of trifluoroacetic acid and measuring the subsequent yellow color produced within a time interval of 1 to 3 min at 490 nm. Appropriate corrections for interference by contaminating substances can be carried out by addition of hydrogen peroxide to the cuvette, which will specifically quench the color produced by the vitamin D and will leave absorbance due to interfering contaminants. The principal advantages of the trifluoroacetic acid method are as follows: (a) the color produced is more intense and more stable than that of the simple antimony trichloride procedure; (b) the utilization of hydrogen peroxide to correct for interfering contaminants can be carried out directly in every sample tube; (c) the color produced by the addition of trifluoroacetic acid is stable for a longer period of time, i.e., 1–10 min.

The other methods listed in Table 4-2 employ acetyl chloride and boron trifluoride and have not yet been widely adopted; accordingly, they are not described in detail here.

There is one attractive alternative to the utilization of antimony trichloride or related solutions to develop a colorimetric assay for vitamin D. This is the technique of fluorescence spectroscopy, wherein vitamin D is reacted with a substance that is capable of fluorescing. There have been two reports in the literature describing possible assays dependent on this principle (Chen *et al.*, 1964; Passannante and Avioli, 1960). Both of these procedures are based on the fact that an acetic anhydride-sulfuric acid solution containing vitamin D is capable of fluorescence if the solution is activated by light of the appropriate wavelength. However, the limits of detectability of the fluorescent vitamin D solutions are not markedly lower than those for the traditional antimony trichloride-induced color reaction, i.e., approximately 1000 ng. Also many of the same compounds that interfere with the antimony trichloride assay, such as vitamin A and carotene, also interfere with the fluorescence assay. Thus, although the technique is theoretically interesting, it has yet to be adopted for the analytical determination of vitamin D concentration.

C. Gas Chromatography

In principle, gas chromatography should have strong potential for the development of assays capable of detecting physiological quantities of vitamin D. However, due to some of the problems discussed in Chapter 3 concerning the isomerization of vitamin D compounds, which occurs when the sample is vaporized for introduction into the gas chromatography column, these procedures have as yet to be widely adopted for the analytical determination of vitamin D. Gas chromatography separation processes inherently have an exceedingly high resolving capability due to the high number of theoretical plates present in a typical column. However, the value of gas chromatography to an analytical determination of vitamin D cannot be assessed simply on the basis of resolving power. Of much more interest and concern is the sensitivity of the assay. That is, what is the sensitivity of the detector used in the gas chromatographic procedure? In this respect, the procedure of Sklan *et al.* (1973) is potentially very attractive in that the electron capture detector employed in their method is capable of responding to as little as 50 pg of vitamin D. In their procedure it was necessary to derivatize vitamin D or its metabolites as esters of trifluoroacetic acid, which resulted in only one elution peak. One awaits with interest the application of this potentially useful technique to the analytical determination of vitamin D.

D. Gas Chromatography–Mass Spectrometry

One of the most powerful modern techniques available to steroid chemists for the analytical determination of samples containing mixtures of steroids is mass spectrometry or mass spectrometry coupled with prior separation via gas chromatography. The mass spectrometer with its multiple ion detector can be used as a very sensitive detector for the gas chromatographic separation of steroids. The intermittent focusing in the instrument on selected ions can give a very high specificity to the assay. When the gas chromatography–mass spectrometry technique is coupled with the use of an on-line computer to collect information on the fragmentation patterns of steroids in the mass spectrometer, one is capable of developing an incredibly sophisticated and sensitive quantitative assay for the simultaneous evaluation of a wide range of steroid structures. These assays often approach the sensitivity and selectivity of radioimmunoassay techniques. The ideal internal standards for this type of assay are the relevant steroids labeled with stable isotopes. These allow corrections to be made for any losses in the initial procedures preceding gas chromatographic separation.

To date, only two published procedures have appeared describing either the mass spectrometric analysis of vitamin D (Tsukida and Saiki, 1972) or gas chromatography coupled with mass spectrometry (Cruye and de Leenheer, 1974). Both of these techniques are presently in developmental stages, and it is not possible to state what their possible sensitivity and reproducibility may ultimately be.

E. High-Pressure Liquid Chromatography

Several papers have appeared describing the separation of vitamin D and related metabolites by the procedure of high-pressure liquid chromatography (see Table 4-2). In principle the same considerations apply to this technique as to gas chromatography. What is not of critical importance is the inherent high resolving power of the separation technique; what is important is the sensitivity of the detector used for observing the presence of the separated compounds. Thus, the published procedures (see Table 4-2) use a uv detector, and their sensitivity is accordingly limited to approximately 5 ng. The chief advantage of these techniques, however, is the major saving in labor normally required to carry out the separation procedures. For example, the present official USP procedure for the determination of vitamin D involves two laborious prepurifications of the sample prior to the colorimetric determination. These purification procedures require up to 8 hr and thus preclude the assay of large numbers of samples. In contrast, high-pressure liquid chromatography can, within 1 hr, result in a highly reproducible and amazingly sensitive separation of closely related compounds (see Fig. 3-10). The method of Eisman *et al.* (1977) employs high-pressure liquid chromatography to carry out the simultaneous determination in plasma samples of D_2, D_3, 25(OH)D_2, and 25(OH)D_3. Clearly, these procedures have much potential, and one must await further developments to see how they are specifically applied to individual problems.

IV. SUMMARY

It is apparent that there are a wide variety of techniques that depend on either biological evaluation or chemical analysis for determination of the amount of vitamin D in a sample. Although considerable progress has been made in the development of chemical or physical means for determination of vitamin D, these lack both the specificity and sensitivity of the biological assays—particularly the rat line test—for routine determination of steroid levels. As a rule, for samples that contain low concentrations of vitamin D, it is necessary to rely on rather time-consuming biological assays for accurate estimation of the concentration, whereas for determination of the rather high amounts of vitamin D normally present in pharmaceutical samples, it is adequate and appropriately accurate to rely on the rather more insensitive chemical determination of vitamin D. However, it is apparent that a new era is dawning with regard to techniques and procedures for determination of vitamin D. The techniques of high-pressure liquid chromatography and gas liquid–mass spectrometry have great potential, at least from a theoretical viewpoint, for the development of specific assays that can satisfy the need for both a rapid separation of contaminating substances and a highly sensitive detection of low concentrations of vitamin D. Also, the development of the steroid competition assays (see Chapter 8) for vitamin D and its metabolites may be of value in some circumstances.

REFERENCES

Adams, P. H., Fyans, P., Hill, L. F., Lumb, G. A., Mawer, E. B., and Taylor, C. M. (1975). *In* "Calcium Regulatory Hormones" (R. V. Talmage, M. Owens, and J. Parsons, eds.), Int. Congr. Ser. No. 346, p. 391. Found., Amsterdam.

Association of Official Agricultural Chemists (1940). "Methods of Analysis," p. 371. AOAC, Washington, D.C.

Association of Official Agricultural Chemists (1960). "Official Methods of Analysis," 5th ed., pp. 650 and 675. AOAC, Washington, D.C.

Association of Official Analytical Chemists (1975). "Official Methods of Analyses," 12th ed., Chapter 43, p. 885. AOAC, Washington, D.C.

Belsey, R., DeLuca, H. F., and Potts, J. T. (1971). *J. Clin. Endocrinol. Metab.* **33,** 554.

Bjorkhem, I., and Holmberg, T. (1976). *Clin. Chim. Acta* **68,** 215.

Brockmann, H. (1936). *Hoppe-Seyler's Z. Physiol. Chem.* **241,** 104.

Brockmann, H., and Chen, Y. (1936). *Hoppe-Seyler's Z. Physiol. Chem.* **241,** 129.

Chen, P. S., and Bosmann, H. B. (1964). *J. Nutr.* **83,** 133.

Chen, P. S., Terepka, R., and Lane, K. (1964). *Anal. Biochem.* **8,** 34.

Christakos, S., and Norman, A. W. (1979). *Endocrinology* **104,** 1495.

Clements, J. A., Forbes, J., Olliff, C. J., and Rogers, A. R. (1967). *J. Pharm. Pharmacol.* **19,** Suppl., 1035.

Coates, M. E., and Holdsworth, E. S. (1961). *Br. J. Nutr.* **15,** 131.

Cruye, A. A. M., and de Leenheer, A. P. (1974). *J. Steroid Biochem.* **5,** 302.

Cruze-Coke, E. (1939). *C. R. Seances Soc. Biol. Ses Fil.* **105,** 238.

DeWitt, J. B., and Sullivan, M. X. (1946). *Ind. Eng. Chem. Anal. Ed.* **18,** 117.

Eisman, J. A., Shephard, R. M., and DeLuca, H. F. (1977). *Anal. Biochem.* **80,** 298.

Evans, J. R. (1972). *Clin. Chim. Acta* **42,** 343.

Fieser, L. F., and Fieser, M. (1959). "The Steroids," pp. 90–168. Van Nostrand-Reinhold, Princeton, New Jersey.

Fuchs, L., and Beck, Z. (1933). *Chem. Zentralbl.* **11,** 1903.

Gharbo, S. A., and Gosser, L. A. (1974). *Analyst* **99,** 222.

Haftman, E., and Mosettig, E. (1960). *In* "Biochemistry of Steroids," p. 63. Academic Press, New York.
Halden, W., and Tzoni, H. (1936). *Nature (London)* **137,** 909.
Harrison, H. E., and Harrison, H. C. (1960). *Am. J. Physiol.* **199,** 265.
Haussler, M. R., Zerwekh, J. E., Helle, J. E., Rizzardo, R. H., and Pechet, M. M. (1973). *Proc. Natl. Acad. Sci. U.S.A.* **70,** 2248.
Hibberd, K. A., and Norman, A. W. (1969). *Biochem. Pharmacol.* **18,** 2342.
Hofsass, H., Grant, A., Alcino, N. J., and Greenbaum, S. (1976). *J. Assoc. Off. Anal. Chem.* **59,** 251.
Johnson, R. L. (1975). Ph.D. Dissertation, University of California, Riverside.
Jones, G., and DeLuca, H. F. (1975). *J. Lipid Res.* **16,** 448.
Kobayashi, T., and Adachi, A. (1973). *J. Nutr. Sci. Vitaminol.* **19,** 311.
Koshy, K. T., and Vanderslik, A. L. (1976). *Anal. Biochem.* **74,** 282.
League of Nations (1931). "Report of Congress on Vitamin Standards," No. C. H. 1055(1). League of Nations, Geneva.
League of Nations (1935). *Bull. Health Organ. League Nations* **4,** No. 3, 540.
McCollum, E. V., Simmonds, N., Shipley, P. G., and Park, E. A. (1922). *J. Biol. Chem.* **54,** 41.
Marcussen, E. (1939). *Dan. Tidsskr. Farm.* **13,** 141.
Martin, D. L., and DeLuca, H. F. (1969a). *Arch. Biochem. Biophys.* **134,** 139.
Martin, D. L., and DeLuca, H. F. (1969b). *Am. J. Physiol.* **216,** 1351.
Mulder, F. J., and deVries, E. J. (1974). *J. Assoc. Off. Anal. Chem.* **57,** 1349.
Mulder, F. J., deVries, E. J., and Keuning, K. J. (1965). *Pharm. Weekbl.* **100,** 1457.
Mulder, F. J., deVries, E. J., and Borsje, B. (1971). *J. Assoc. Off. Anal. Chem.* **54,** 1168.
Murray, T. M., Arnold, B. M., Tam, W. H., and Hitchman, A. J. W. (1974). *Metab., Clin. Exp.* **23,** 829.
Myrtle, J. F., and Norman, A. W. (1971). *Science* **171,** 78.
Nelson, E. M. (1949). *J. Assoc. Off. Agric. Chem.* **32,** 801.
Nield, C. H., Russell, W. C., and Zimmerli, A. (1940). *J. Biol. Chem.* **136,** 73.
Norman, A. W., Mitra, M. N., Okamura, W. H., and Wing, R. M. (1975). *Science* **188,** 1013.
Panalaks, T. (1971). *J. Assoc. Off. Anal. Chem.* **54,** 1299.
Passannante, A. J., and Avioli, L. V. (1966). *Anal. Biochem.* **15,** 287.
Reynolds, J. J. (1974). *Calcif. Tissue Res.* **15,** 333.
Robinson, F. (1937). *Chem. Ind. (Anal.)* **56,** 191.
Rygh, O. (1935). *Nature (London)* **136,** 396.
Sallis, J. D., and Holdsworth, E. S. (1962). *Am. J. Physiol.* **203,** 4972.
Schachter, D., and Rosen, S. M. (1959). *Am. J. Physiol.* **196,** 357.
Shear, M. J. (1925). *Proc. Soc. Exp. Biol. Med.* **23,** 546.
Sheppard, A. J., LaCroix, D. E., and Prosser, A. R. (1965). *J. Assoc. Off. Anal. Chem.* **51,** 839.
Sklan, D., Budowski, P., and Katz, M. (1973). *Anal. Biochem.* **56,** 606.
Steenbock, H., and Herting, D.-C. (1955). *J. Nutr.* **57,** 449.
Stoeltzner, W. (1928). *Muench. Med. Wochenschr.* **75,** 1584.
Tompkins, D. F., and Tscherne, R. J. (1974). *Anal. Chem.* **46,** 1602.
Topelmann, H., and Schuhknecht, W. (1935). *Z. Vitaminforsch.* **4,** 11.
Tsukida, K., and Saiki, K. (1972). *Int. J. Vitam. Nutr. Res.* **42,** 242.
U.S. Pharmacopeia (1934). Xth ed., Interum Suppl. No. 2. Mack Printing Co.
U.S. Pharmacopeia (1950). XIV ed., p. 794. Mack Printing Co.
U.S. Pharmacopeia (1955). XV ed., p. 889. Mack Printing Co.
U.S. Pharmacopeia (1960). XVI ed., p. 910. Mack Printing Co.
U.S. Pharmacopeia (1975). XIX ed., p. 633. Mack Printing Co.
Waddell, J. (1934). *J. Biol. Chem.* **105,** 711.

Wardynska, H., Paczek, K., and Galecka, H. (1973). *Acta Pol. Pharm.* **30,** 587.
Wasserman, R. H., and Taylor, A. N. (1962). *Proc. Soc. Exp. Biol. Med.* **109,** 633.
Wasserman, R. H., Corradino, R. A., Fullmer, C. S., and Taylor, A. N. (1974). *Vitam. Horm. (N.Y.)* **32,** 299.
Wilkie, J. B., Jones, S. W., and Kline, O. L. (1958). *J. Am. Pharm. Assoc.* **47,** 385.
Wilson, T. H., and Wiseman, G. (1954). *J. Physiol.* **123,** 116.
Wolf, L. K. (1938). *Z. Vitaminforsch.* **7,** 277.
World Health Organization (1950). *W.H.O., Tech. Rep. Ser.* **3,** 7.

CHAPTER

5

Vitamin D Metabolites and Analogs

I. INTRODUCTION

A. Metabolism of Vitamin D

A totally new era in the field of vitamin D research has dawned since 1969, with the discovery of the metabolism of vitamin D into eight metabolites (Fig. 5-1.) There had been several attempts to study the metabolism of vitamin D in the period from 1940 to 1960; the usual protocol involved the administration of pharmacological doses of vitamin D with attempts to evaluate its tissue distribution and possible metabolism by measuring the biological activity of the various fractions. These studies were largely unsuccessful because of the unavailability of radioactive vitamin D with a sufficiently high specific activity to permit detection of small amounts of transformed steroid. In 1960, radioactive vitamin D with a specific activity high enough to permit the administration and measurement of truly physiological quantities of the steroid became available (Norman and DeLuca, 1963; Neville and DeLuca, 1966; DeLuca *et al.*, 1968) (see also Table 3-3).[1]

It quickly became apparent that vitamin D was subject to a complex series of transformations into more polar products (Norman *et al.*, 1964; Lund *et al.*, 1967; Lund and DeLuca, 1966; Mori *et al.*, 1967; Callow *et al.*, 1966). Our understanding of the metabolism of vitamin D progressed rapidly and within five years five new metabolites of vitamin D had been isolated and chemically characterized. Then in 1979 DeLuca and Schnoes (1979) reported the structures of three additional metabolites. A logical consequence of these developments was a reawakening of interest on the part of organic chemists in the challenges posed by the structures of the various vitamin D metabolites, particularly those of the biologically active forms, $1,25(OH)_2D_3$ and $24,25(OH)_2D_3$.

B. Opportunity for Structure–Function Studies

With the recognition of the metabolic pathway for the production of the biologically active forms of vitamin D, it was possible for chemists, clinicians, pharmacologists, and biochemists to envision a detailed assessment of the structural features of the vitamin D molecule that were required for the development of biological responses. This objective is important for a number of reasons. For the biochemist it provides insight into the determination of the structural requirements of the molecule necessary to produce specific biological responses, i.e., intestinal calcium transport or bone calcium mobilization. For the chemist such studies permit the development of a topological model or "blueprint," which can

[1]A discussion of physiological doses of vitamin D is given in Chapter 4. In general, for the rat or chick a daily dose of 10 IU (0.65 nmole; 250 ng) is sufficient to permit normal calcium metabolism and growth.

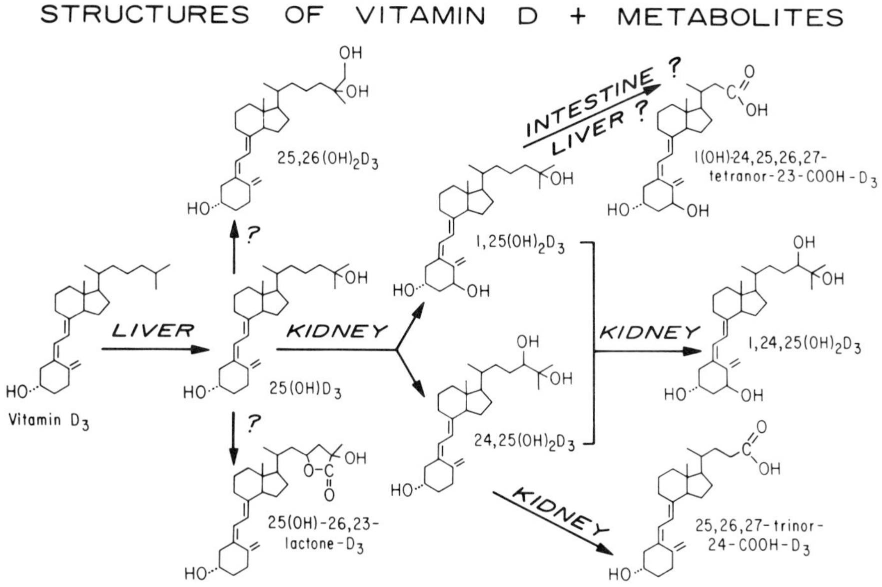

Figure 5-1. Metabolic pathway for vitamin D transformation.

be informative both for the planning of specific syntheses of new analogs and for quantitatively describing or correlating the effect of structural modifications on biological activity. For the clinician there is immense potential in such structure–function studies because new analogs may have a different pattern of biological responses than the natural metabolites. For example, one can envision analogs that exhibit greater biological activity than even 1,25$(OH)_2D_3$ or, alternatively, analogs that selectively are active in the intestine but are relatively less active in bone. Still further, it is possible that the structural requirements for an "antivitamin D" can be pinpointed. A wide battery of techniques are available which permit the biological screening of new analogs, including diverse *in vivo* and *in vitro* procedures. These will be detailed at a later point in this chapter (Section IV,A).

II. ISOLATION, CHARACTERIZATION, AND CHEMICAL SYNTHESIS OF VITAMIN D METABOLITES

A. 25$(OH)D_3$

The first metabolite of vitamin D to be isolated and chemically characterized was 25$(OH)D_3$. This landmark achievement was carried out in the laboratory of Professor H. F. DeLuca at the University of Wisconsin and signaled the start of a

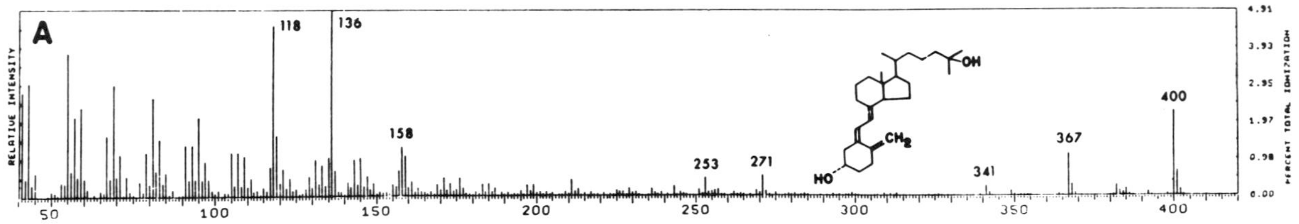

A
RELATIVE INTENSITY
PERCENT TOTAL IONIZATION
118
136
158
253
271
341
367
400
OH
CH2
HO
50
100
150
200
250
300
350
400
4.91
3.93
2.95
1.97
0.98
0.00

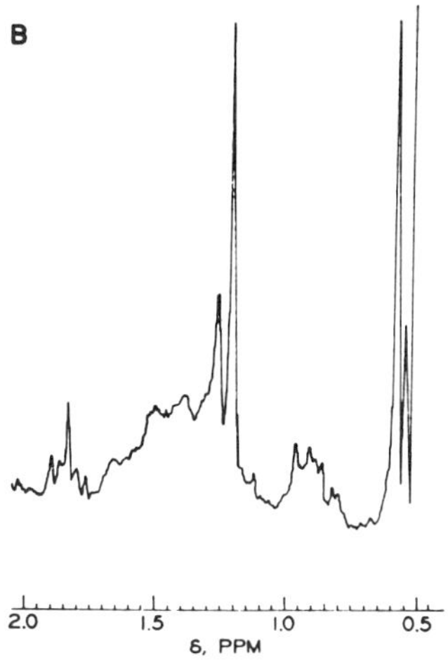

Figure 5-2. Mass spectrum (A) and NMR spectrum (B) of 25(OH)D_3. The NMR spectrum was taken at 100 MH_z. Blunt *et al.* (1968b); reproduced by permission of the publisher. Copyright by the American Chemical Society.

completely new era in vitamin D research. 25(OH)D_3 was obtained from porcine blood after the administration of massive doses of low specific activity [^{3}H]vitamin D (6.25 mg/day for 26 days) (Blunt *et al.*, 1968a,b). Milligram quantities of the polar metabolite of vitamin D were isolated in pure form, and the substance was chemically characterized through a combination of ultraviolet spectroscopy, gas–liquid partition chromatography, mass spectrometry, and nuclear magnetic resonance (NMR) analyses. The ultraviolet spectrum of 25(OH)D_3 is essentially identical to that of vitamin D_3, as shown in Fig. 3-2. Figure 5-2 shows the mass spectrum and the NMR spectrum of 25(OH)D_3.

The mass spectrometer is of inestimable value in terms of the insights provided into the structure of the new metabolites. This was first demonstrated in the determination of the structure of 25(OH)D_3. Of prime importance is the fact that the high-resolution mass spectrometer can provide molecular weights to six or seven significant figures; because the molecular weight can be determined to this degree of accuracy, the empirical formula can be unequivocally established. The molecular weight of the metabolite 25(OH)D_3 was found to be 400.3343, which indicated that the empirical formula was $C_{27}H_{44}O_2$. The presence of the second hydroxyl in the side chain could be deduced by evaluation of the fragment with a peak at *m/e* 271.2053 ($C_{19}H_{27}O$). This peak, containing only one of the two oxygen atoms of the intact molecule, could be produced only by loss of the side chain by cleavage of the bond between C-17 and C-20. Furthermore, the peak at *m/e* 59.0492 (C_3H_7O) in the spectrum of the metabolite but not in that of the parent vitamin could arise only by a cleavage of the C-24–C-25 bond with a hydroxyl group being attached to C-25. The location of the hydroxyl group on

C-25 has been confirmed through study of the 100-MH_z NMR spectrum of the metabolite.

The chemical synthesis of 25(OH)D_3 has been recorded by a number of groups (Campbell *et al.*, 1969; Halkes and van Vliet, 1969; Blunt and DeLuca, 1969; Morisaki *et al.*, 1973a; Partridge *et al.*, 1974). All of these syntheses are relatively simple and depend on the ready availability of the precursor 25-oxy-26-norcholesterol. Through a simple Grignard reaction, followed by introduction of the Δ^7 double bond and subsequent irradiation, 25(OH)D_3 can be isolated in a straightforward fashion. The synthesis of Morisaki *et al.* (1973a) is somewhat more interesting in that they used as starting material the sterol fucosterol, or $\Delta^{5,24(28)}$stigmastadien-3β-o1, which is a naturally occurring sterol found in the marine brown alga *Phaeophyceae*. Trinh-Toan *et al.* (1977) completed an X-ray crystallographic analysis of the stereochemical relationships of the monohydrate of 25(OH)D_3.

B. 25(OH)D_2

25-Hydroxyergocalciferol [25(OH)D_2] was isolated and chemically characterized in 1969 by Suda *et al.* The metabolite was isolated, by a scheme essentially identical to that employed for 25(OH)D_3, from the blood obtained from four pigs given radioactive vitamin D_2 (12.5 mg/day for 26 days). After extensive silicic acid and Sephadex-LH chromatography, 314 μg were isolated in pure form. Once again, the application of ultraviolet spectroscopy, gas–liquid partition chromatography, NMR resonance spectrometry, and mass spectrometry to both the free and trimethylsilyl either derivatives proved to be essential for the structure determination.

The mass spectrum of 25(OH)D_2 is shown in Fig. 5-3. It displays a molecular ion of *m/e* 412, which is an increase of 16 mass units over the molecular weight of vitamin D_2; this again suggests the incorporation of an additional oxygen atom. High-resolution mass spectrometry gave a molecular ion of 412.3341, which is consistent with an empirical formula of $C_{28}H_{44}O_2$. In addition, the metabolite displayed intense peaks at *m/e* 136 ($C_9H_{12}O$) and *m/e* 118 (C_9H_{10}) deriving from ring A of the molecule and including C-6 and C-7. Furthermore, both the metabolite and the parent vitamin D_2 had peaks at *m/e* 271, which reflected a composition of $C_{19}H_{27}O$ resulting from loss of the entire side chain through cleavage of the bond between C-17 and C-20. The biological activity of 25(OH)D_2 was found to be 1.5 times greater than that of vitamin D_2 or D_3 in curing rickets in rats (Suda *et al.*, 1969).

C. 1,25$(OH)_2D_3$

The modern era of vitamin D research was placed on firm footing by the elucidation of the chemical structure of the metabolite of vitamin D that had

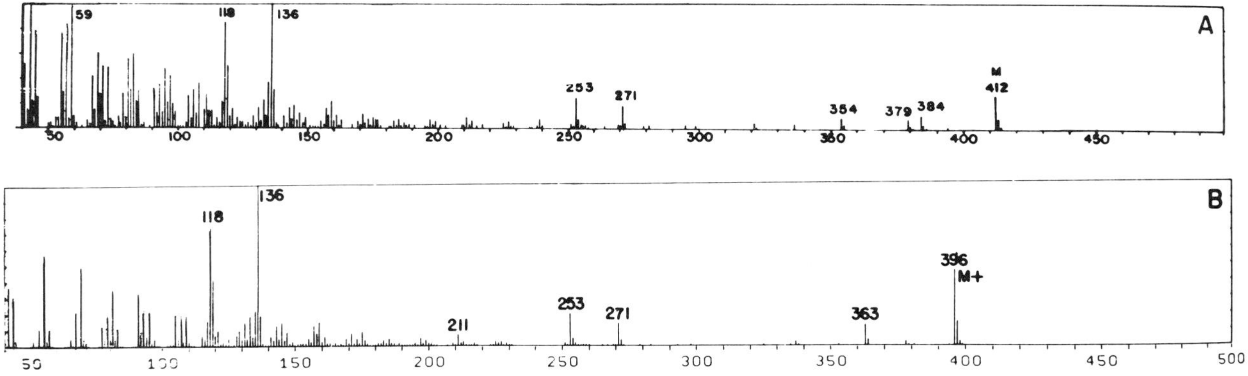

Figure 5-3. Mass spectra of (A) $25(OH)D_2$ and (B) D_2. Taken from Suda *et al.* (1969); reproduced by permission of the authors and publisher. Copyright by the American Chemical Society.

previously been proposed by Norman's and Kodicek's laboratories to be the biologically active form (Haussler *et al.*, 1968; Myrtle *et al.*, 1970; Kodicek *et al.*, 1970; Myrtle, 1971; Myrtle and Norman, 1971a). The chemical characterization of the structure of $1,25(OH)_2D_3$ was reported virtually simultaneously (within 6–8 weeks) by the laboratories of Kodicek (Lawson *et al.*, 1971), Norman (Norman *et al.*, 1971), and DeLuca (Holick *et al.*, 1971).

The mass spectrum and NMR spectrum of crystalline $1,25(OH)_2D_3$ are shown in Fig. 5-4. The high-resolution mass spectrum indicated an *m/e* of 416.32900, which was consistent only with an empirical formula of $C_{27}H_{44}O_3$. Once again, interpretation of the high-resolution mass spectrum played an indispensable role in the elucidation of the structure of a vitamin D metabolite. The α orientation of the hydroxyl on C-1 was deduced from metabolism experiments involving [1α-^{3}H]vitamin D_3. Both Lawson *et al.* (1969a,b) and Myrtle and Norman (1971b) reported the specific loss of tritium in the 1α position as vitamin D was metabolized to $1,25(OH)_2D_3$ (see Table 6-2). This was confirmed by comparing the biological and chemical properties of the chemically synthesized $1,25(OH)_2D_3$ and the biosynthetically produced $1,25(OH)_2D_3$.

The chemical synthesis of $1,25(OH)_2D_3$ has presented unusual challenges to the organic chemist inasmuch as hydroxyl groups must be introduced at completely opposite ends of the secosteroid molecule. This places stringent requirements on appropriate starting materials. The first chemical synthesis of $1,25(OH)_2D_3$ was reported by Semmler *et al.* (1972); unfortunately, their total yield was less than 0.005%. This led for some time to acceptance of the view that $1,25(OH)_2D_3$ was too difficult to synthesize to permit production of large quantities of the product steroid.

The potential clinical and agricultural market for $1,25(OH)_2D_3$ is tabulated in Table 5-1. It can be estimated that, to treat all patients with renal osteodystrophy, some 30 g of $1,25(OH)_2D_3$ would be required annually, whereas to employ $1,25(OH)_2D_3$ for renal osteodystrophy, osteoporosis, anticonvulsant-induced osteomalacia, and milk fever would require 1–4 kg of $1,25(OH)_2D_3$ annually.

In retrospect it can be appreciated that, although the view that $1,25(OH)_2D_3$ was too difficult and expensive to synthesize was erroneous, it was also fortuitous. This view more than any other stimulated the development of analogs of $1,25(OH)_2D_3$. The principal analog that was synthesized lacked the 25-hydroxyl group, i.e., $1\alpha(OH)D_3$ (Harrison *et al.*, 1973, 1974; Kaneko *et al.*, 1973a; Barton *et al.*, 1973; Furst *et al.*, 1973; Holick *et al.*, 1975b; Okamura *et al.*, 1975b).

In 1975, however, a major breakthrough occurred in the laboratory of Dr. Milan Uskoković and co-workers at Hoffmann-La Roche in Nutley, New Jersey. They synthesized, for the first time, significant quantities (i.e., greater than 50 mg) and by 1978 had produced hundreds of grams of $1,25(OH)_2D_3$. As yet no formal details of their synthesis have been published; however, a key inter-

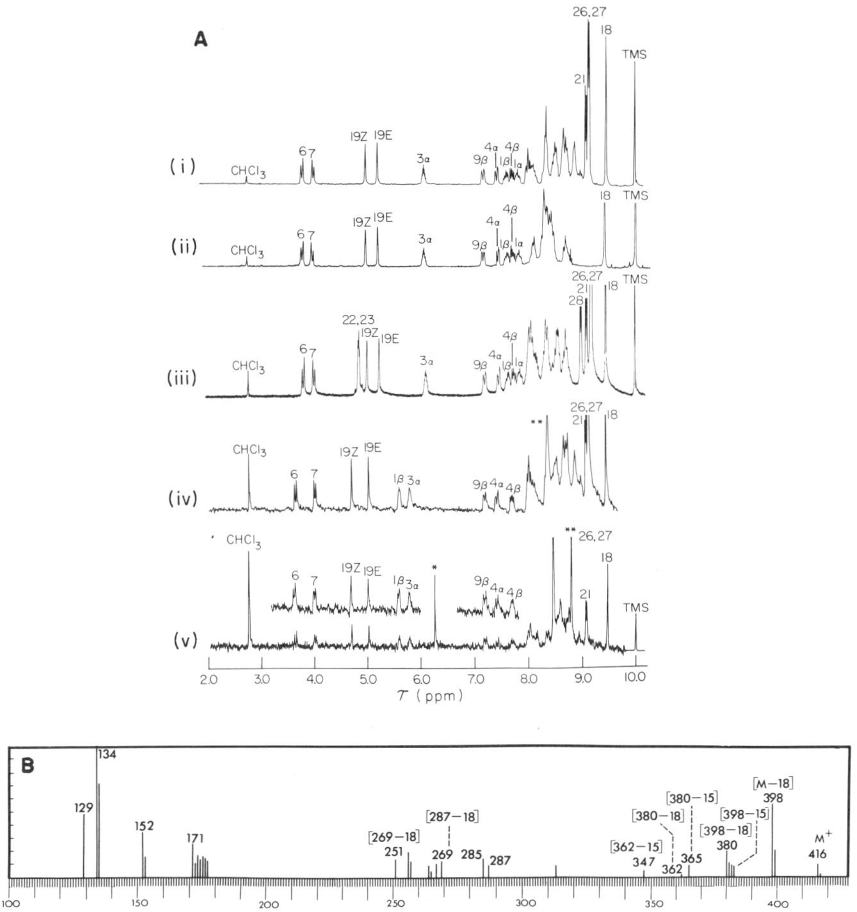

Figure 5-4. (A) High-resolution NMR spectrum at 300 MH_z of (i) D_3, (ii) octanor-D_3, (iii) D_2, (iv) $1\alpha(OH)D_3$, and (v) $1,25(OH)_2D_3$ in deuterochloroform solvent. MeSi (TMS) and chloroform (218O H_z) apart appear as internal standards. Impurities are marked with asterisks. From Wing *et al.* (1975), reproduced by permission of the authors and publisher. (B) Mass spectrum of $1,25(OH)_2D_3$. Taken from unpublished work of Okamura *et al.* 1977).

mediate compound is $1,25(OH)_2$-cholesterol (Narwid *et al.*, 1974b; Rubio-Lightbourn *et al.*, 1973; Morisaki *et al.*, 1973a,b,c).

Paaren *et al.* (1978) have devised a highly efficient procedure that permits direct C-1 hydroxylation of a variety of vitamin D compounds. The method involves conversion of vitamin D tosylates to 3,5-cyclovitamin D derivatives, allylic oxidation with SeO_2, followed by acid-catalyzed solvolysis to $1\alpha(OH)$ derivatives. This procedure was used to synthesize, in 10–15% yields, $1,25(OH)_2D_3$, $1\alpha(OH)D_3$, and $1\alpha(OH)D_2$.

TABLE 5-1
Potential Industrial Market for $1,25(OH)_2D_3$

Proposed application	Number of potential subjects	Proposed daily dosage (μg)	Required yearly amount (g)
Renal failure			
Now on dialysis	20,000	0.5	3.6
Severe CRF with bone disease (not now dialyzed)	40,000	0.5	7.3
Moderate CRF (possible prophylactic treatment)	500,00	0.1	18.2
Anticonvulsant-treated epilepsy[a]	620,000	0.1–0.5	22.6–113.1
Osteoporosis[b]	3,229,000	0.1–0.15	117–589
Milk fever (dairy cows)[c]	6,700,000	100–500	670–3350
Estimated total (g)			840–4080

[a]The frequency of occurrence of epilepsy in the United States is 3.1/1000; 90% of epileptics are treated with some anticonvulsant and may develop anticonvulsant-induced osteomalacia.

[b]Of the female population in the United States, 31.4% is 45 years or older. The total female population in 1977 was 102,858,000; if 10% develop osteoporosis, 3,229,000 might require treatment.

[c]There are 11,909,000 dairy cows in the United States (1976); of these 6,700,000 are bred annually. The incidence rate of milk fever is 4.8%. It might be appropriate to treat all 6,700,000 prophylactically.

D. $1,25(OH)_2D_2$

The isolation and chemical characterization of $1,25(OH)_2D_2$ was carried out in 1975 by Jones *et al*. Through the chemical synthesis of [3α-^{3}H]vitamin D_2 it was possible to detect the existence in the rat of a polar metabolite that was believed to be the active form of vitamin D_2.

In subsequent experiments it was isolated in pure form from an *in vitro* chick kidney mitochondrial incubation and identified unequivocally as $1,25(OH)_2D_2$. Only 4.17 μg of pure metabolite were obtained for chemical determination and bioassay. Mass spectrometry of the metabolite showed a molecular ion at *m*/*e* 428. The presence of three hydroxyl functions was demonstrated by the formation of a tris(trimethylsilyl ether) derivative with a molecular weight of 644.

E. $24,25(OH)_2D_3$

$24,25(OH)_2D_3$ was isolated and chemically characterized by Holick *et al.* (1972c). It was first erroneously reported that the structure of this metabolite was $21,25(OH)_2D_3$ by Suda *et al.* (1970b). Regrettably there is a period in the literature during which a number of investigators referred to what was actually $24,25(OH)_2D_3$ as $21,25(OH)_2D_3$. To date there has been no evidence of the actual existence of $21,25(OH)_2D_3$; accordingly, this terminology is no longer used.

The metabolite $24,25(OH)_2D_3$ was isolated in pure form by incubating radioactive $25(OH)D_3$ with homogenates obtained from the kidneys of rachitic chicks. After extensive column chromatography, 200 μg of the metabolite were recovered in pure form and chemically characterized by a mass spectrometry, ultraviolet absorption spectrophotometry, and specific chemical reactions. Figure 5-5 presents the mass spectrum of $24,25(OH)_2D_3$. It shows the parent molecular ion at *m/e* 416, suggesting the incorporation of an additional oxygen function into the substrate $25(OH)D_3$. In addition, the peaks at *m/e* 271, 253 (271–H_2O), 136, and 118 (136-H_2O) are identical to those for both vitamin D_3 and $25(OH)D_3$, demonstrating that the additional oxygen functionality is located in the side chain.

The location of the additional hydroxyl group on C-24 was eventually determined by the technique of periodate cleavage; this procedure is applicable when there are vicinal hydroxyls on adjacent carbons. Thus, a characteristic feature of $24,25(OH)_2D_3$ is its lability to treatment with periodate.

It should be noted that the introduction of a hydroxyl group on C-24 can occur with one or two stereochemical orientations, either *R* or *S*. The stereochemistry of the biosynthesized $24,25(OH)_2D_3$ could not be determined until 1975, when advances in the chromatographic techniques, i.e., high-pressure liquid chromatography, made it possible to separate the *R* and *S* epimers from one another. It was then shown by means of chromatography of radioactive, biosynthesized $24,25(OH)_2D_3$ with authentic chemically synthesized $24(R),25(OH)_2D_3$ or $24(S),25(OH)_2D_3$ of known configuration that the biosynthesized material migrated exclusively with the *R* epimer (Tanaka *et al.*, 1975a,b).

The chemical synthesis of $24,25(OH)_2D_3$ has been reported by a number of laboratories. The first synthesis was probably that of a racemic mixture of $24(R),25(OH)_2D_3$ and $24(S),25(OH)_2D_3$ by Lam *et al.* (1973) and Seki *et al.* (1973). This was followed by the stereospecific syntheses of the two epimers by Redel *et al.* (1974a, 1975), Ikekawa *et al.* (1975b), as well as Milhaud *et al.* (1974), Seki *et al.* (1975), and Partridge *et al.* (1976).

F. $1,24,25(OH)_3D_3$

The metabolite $1,24,25(OH)_3D_3$ was first isolated by Holick *et al.* (1973b) from incubations of chick kidney homogenates, in which $24,25(OH)_2D_3$ was employed as a substrate. Subsequently, Kleiner-Bossaller and DeLuca (1974) reported that $1,24,25(OH)_3D_3$ could be produced *in vitro* from incubations with

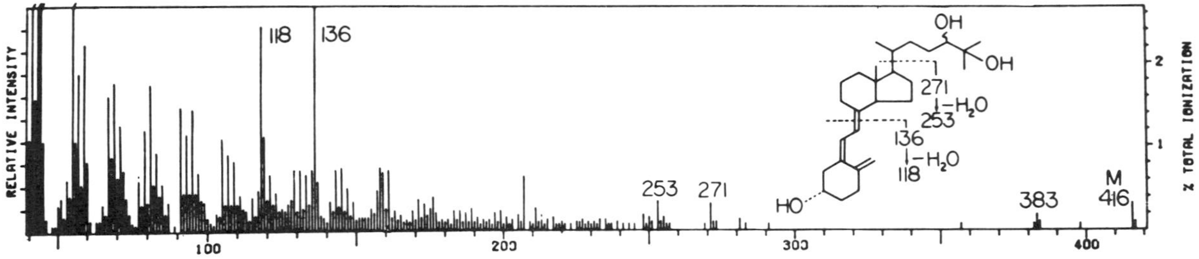

Figure 5-5. Mass spectrum of $24,25(OH)_2D_3$. Taken from Holick *et al.* (1972c); reproduced by permission of the authors and publisher. Copyright by the American Chemical Society.

the appropriate kidney homogenates of either $24,25(OH)_2D_3$ or $1,25(OH)_2D_3$. However, no unequivocal evidence has yet appeared, indicating that $1,24,25(OH)_3D_3$ actually is a metabolite present in significant concentrations *in vivo* (Holick *et al.*, 1973b; Friedlander and Norman, 1975; Tanaka *et al.*, 1977).

The chemical characterization of $1,24,25(OH)_3D_3$ by Holick *et al.* (1973b) again employed extensive column chromatography (yielding only 2–3 μg) followed by ultraviolet and mass spectrometry and treatment with periodate. The mass spectrum of the metabolite (see Fig. 5-6) and its trimethylsilyl ether derivative showed molecular ion peaks at *m/e* 432 and 720, respectively, demonstrating that an additional hydroxyl function had been incorporated into the parent $24,25(OH)_2D_3$. Furthermore, the peaks at *m/e* 287, 269 (287-H_20), and 251 (287-$2H_20$) in the mass spectrum of the metabolite arose from the loss of the entire side chain by cleavage of the bond between C-17 and C-20; this confirmed the lack of an additional hydroxyl functionality in the side chain. Continuing the analysis, the fragments *m/e* 152 and 134 (152-H_20), due to ring A plus C-6 and C-7, had also been previously observed in the mass spectrum of $1,25(OH)_2D_3$ and established that the additional hydroxyl functionality was in ring A.

No information was available on the stereochemistry of the hydroxyls at either the 1 or 24 position; however, it was presumed that the substrate that had been biosynthesized was $24(R),25(OH)_2D_3$ and that the subsequent hydroxyl introduced at the 1 position would be in the α configuration as in $1,25(OH)_2D_3$.

The chemical synthesis of $1,24(R),25(OH)_3D_3$ and $1,24(S),25(OH)_3D_3$ has been carried out by Ikekawa *et al.* (1975a) as well as by the research group led by Uskokovic at Hoffmann-La Roche (Partridge *et al.*, 1977).

G. $25,26(OH)_2D_3$

The isolation and chemical characterization of $25,26(OH)_2D_3$ was carried out by Suda *et al.* (1970c). The $25,26(OH)_2D_3$ was obtained from the same blood samples that had been employed for the isolation of $25(OH)D_3$ namely, that of pigs given pharmacological doses of vitamin D_3. The mass spectrum of $25,26(OH)_2D_3$ is given in Fig. 5-7.

The chemical synthesis of $25,26(OH)_2D_3$ has been reported by Seki *et al.* (1973), Lam *et al.* (1975a), and Redel *et al.* (1973, 1974b). The synthesis by Redel and co-workers produced a mixture of both C-25 epimers. It was ultimately possible to separate these epimers by high-pressure liquid chromatography at the intermediate stage of $25,26(OH)_2D_3 3\beta,26$-diacetate. This led to an X-ray diffraction analysis (Cesario *et al.*, 1978) and determination of the absolute configuration of the epimers at C-25. Recently Redel *et al.* (1978) determined that the biologically occurring epimer was $25R,26(OH)_2D_3$.

The *in vivo* site of production of $25,26(OH)_2D_3$ is unknown, and the steroid has no known or proposed biological functions.

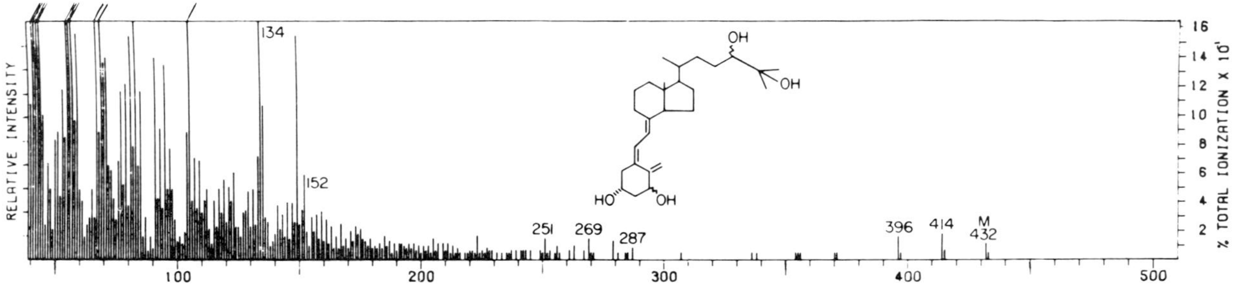

Figure 5-6. Mass spectrum of $1,24,25(OH)_3D_3$. Taken from Lam *et al.* (1975a); reproduced by permission of the authors and publisher.

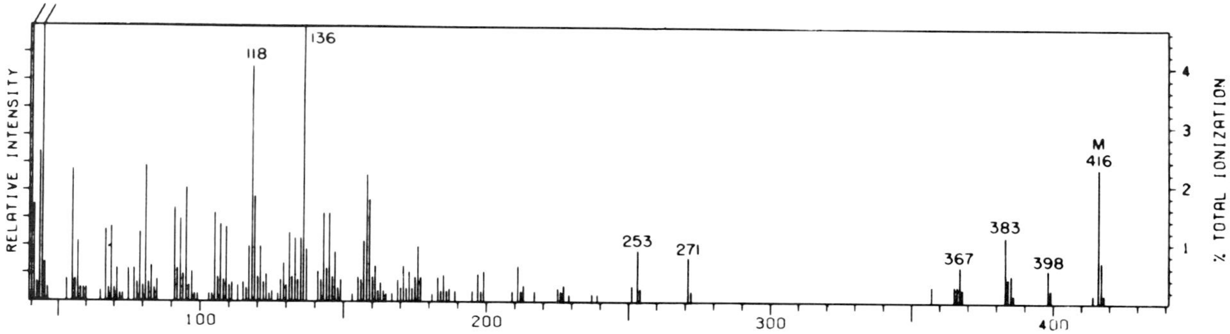

Figure 5-7. Mass spectrum of $25,26(OH)_2D_3$. Taken from Lam *et al.* (1975a); reproduced by permission of the authors and publisher.

H. 1-(OH)-24,25,26,27-Tetranor-23-COOH-D_3

DeLuca and Schnoes (1979) have reported preliminary data concerning the existence and structure of three side-chain metabolites of vitamin D_3. The first of these was detected by the intravenous administration to rats of a mixed dose of [26,27-^{14}C]- and [3α-^{3}H]-1,25$(OH)_2D_3$. At 3 or 6 hours the animals were killed, the livers removed, homogenized, lyophilized, and extracted with methanol–chloroform–water, pH 8.0, to yield a chloroform phase containing 50% of the tissue radioactivity and an aqueous-methanol layer containing 39% of the radioactivity. The ^{3}H/^{14}C ratio of the organic phase was unchanged from that of the administered dose, while the ^{3}H/^{14}C ratio of the polar, water extract was elevated threefold. This suggested that the metabolite was a side-chain cleavage product that had lost C-26 and C-27. The aqueous soluble fraction from the livers was then sequentially (a) chromatographed on a DEAE-Sephadex column, (b) chromatographed on a Sephadex-LH-20 column, (c) methylated in diazomethane, (d) rechromatographed on Sephadex-LH-20, and (e) finally purified by extensive HPLC chromatography.

From 57 rats given a 1 μg dose of 1,25$(OH)_2D_3$, ultimately 1.8 μg of chromatographically homogeneous metabolite was isolated. This metabolite exhibited a typical *cis*-triene uv absorption curve with a λ_{max} of 264 nm and λ_{min} at 228 nm. The mass spectrum of the methylated product gave a parent molecular ion at m/e 388. A detailed analysis of the mass spectra suggested that the likely structure was that of 1,25$(OH)_2D_3$ that had lost four carbons from its side chain, namely C-24, C-25, C-26 and C-27. The side chain was now terminated in a carboxyl functional group on C-23. Thus the structure is proposed to be 1α,3β-dihydroxy-9,10 seco-24,25,26,27-tetranor-5,7,10(19)-cholestatriene-23-oic acid. The structure is included in Fig. 5-1.

The biological activity of this metabolite is not yet known and accordingly, its true significance in the vitamin D endocrine system remains to be elucidated. Although this metabolite was isolated from liver extracts, it is not yet certain whether this is its sole site of synthesis. Some evidence (DeLuca and Schnoes, 1979) exists supporting its production also in the intestine. The cleavage of the side chain between C-23 and C-24 suggests that a 1,25$(OH)_2D_3$-23-hydroxylase must exist to produce the putative metabolite 1,23,24,25$(OH)_4D_3$. This would then permit steroid side-chain cleavage by known enzymatic mechanisms at the C-23, C-24 vicinal hydroxyls.

I. 25(OH)-26,23-Lactone-D_3

In the course of investigating the 24,25$(OH)_2D_3$ region of Sephadex-LH-20 chromatography of plasma extracts from chicks, preliminary evidence was obtained for the existence of a new vitamin D metabolite. This metabolite was ultimately resolved from 24,25$(OH)_2D_3$ via reversed-phase HPLC chromatog-

TABLE 5-2
Synthesis and Biological Activity of Vitamin D Metabolites[a]

Structure no.	Compound	Biological activity[b] ICA	Biological activity[b] BCM	Synthesis	Biological activity
1	$25(OH)D_3$	+++	+++	Okamura *et al.* (1975b), Campbell *et al.* (1969), Halkes and van Vliet (1969), Blunt and DeLuca (1969), Morisaki *et al.* (1973a,b), Partridge *et al.* (1974)	
2	$25(OH)D_2$	+++	+++		Suda *et al.* (1969)
3	$1,25(OH)_2D_3$	+++	+++	Okamura *et al.* (1975a,b), Semmler *et al.* (1972), Paaren *et al.* (1978)	Semmler *et al.* (1972)
4	$1,25(OH)_2D_2$	+++	+++		Jones *et al.* (1975)
5	$24,25(OH)_2D_3$	+++	0	Seki *et al.* (1973, 1975), Redel *et al.* (1974a, 1975), Lam *et al.* (1973), Ikekawa (1975b), Partridge *et al.* (1976)	Lam *et al.* (1973), Boyle *et al.* (1973), Holick *et al.* (1972c), Milhaud *et al.* (1974), Redel *et al.* (1975), Ikekawa *et al.* (1975a,b), Miravet *et al.* (1976), Henry *et al.* (1976)
6	$25,26(OH)_2D_3$	++	ND	Redel *et al.* (1973, 1974b), Lam *et al.* (1975a)	Redel *et al.* (1974b, 1977), Miravet *et al.* (1976)
		+	0	Lam *et al.* (1975a)	
		++	++	Milhaud *et al.* (1974)	
7	$1,24,25(OH)_3D_3$	++	++	Ikekawa *et al.* (1975b)	Holick *et al.* (1975c), Procsal *et al.* (1977)

[a] See Fig. 5-8A for structures.

[b] Relative bone calcium mobilization (BCM) and intestinal calcium transport (ICA) activities are expressed as follows: +++, highly active; ++, moderately active; +, slightly active; 0, inactive; ND, activity not determined.

raphy (DeLuca and Schnoes, 1979). The isolation procedure started with 16 liters of plasma which were heated to 70° for 1 hr and then centrifuged. The protein pellet was extracted with chloroform/methanol and the resulting fraction was extracted and sequentially (a) chromatographed on Sephadex-LH-20, (b) re-chromatographed on Sephadex-LH-20, and (c) then chromatographed on two different regular phase HPLC columns. From the 16 liters of plasma, 8 μg of chromatographically homogeneous metabolite was obtained. In a separate, parallel experiment, 5 μg of pure metabolite was isolated from 1100 ml of plasma obtained from chicks dosed with 10 million IU (153 nmol) of vitamin D_3. This metabolite exhibited a uv spectrum typical of the *cis*-triene vitamin D system. Analysis of the mass spectra suggested that the structure was 3β-25-dihydroxy-9,10 seco-5,7,10(19)-cholestatrieno-26,23-lactone. The structure is included in Fig. 5-1.

As yet, the biological activities of this metabolite have not been determined. Also, no information is available concerning its tissue site of biosynthesis. Again, the presence of an enzyme capable of hydroxylating C-23 of the side chain of vitamin D seco-steroids is suggested.

J. 25,26,27-Trinor-24-COOH-D_3

In separate experiments, DeLuca and Schnoes (1979) studied, under *in vitro* conditions, the further metabolism of $24,25(OH)_2D_3$. They incubated rat kidney homogenates in the presence of NADPH, molecular oxygen, and $24,25(OH)_2$-[3α-^{3}H]D_3 and detected the presence of appreciable amounts of a new water-soluble metabolite. The isolation procedure for this metabolite was then carried out exactly as described above for the C-23 acid of $1,25(OH)_2D_3$.

This metabolite gave the expected uv absorption spectrum of the vitamin D *cis*-triene system. Analysis of the mass spectra suggested that the structure was 3β-hydroxy-9,10-seco-25,26,27-trinor-5,7,10(19)-cholestatriene-24-oic acid.

No information is available describing the biological activity of this metabolite.

A summary of the chemical syntheses and biological activities of the five principal vitamin D metabolites is given in Table 5-2. As yet, the three recently characterized side-chain metabolites (Fig. 5-1) have not been chemically synthesized nor have their biological activities been thoroughly assessed.

III. ANALOGS OF VITAMIN D AND ITS METABOLITES

A. General Considerations

A challenging problem to the organic chemist and biochemist has been to determine the essential structural features of all metabolites of vitamin D in terms of their biological activity. Studies of this type were stimulated greatly by the intriguing observations of the unusual importance of the 1α-hydroxyl group. (a) Neither vitamin D (Wong *et al.*, 1972; Holick *et al.*, 1972b) nor 25(OH)D_3 (Wong *et al.*, 1972; Holick *et al.*, 1972b) was able to stimulate intestinal calcium uptake or bone calcium resorption in nephrectomized rats, whereas the biological response of 1,25$(OH)_2D_3$ was unaffected by nephrectomy; (b) 5,6-*trans*-25(OH)D_3 (Holick *et al.*, 1972a) and 5,6-*trans*D_3 (Holick *et al.*, 1972a) were found to be biologically active in nephrectomized rats; and (c) two other pseudo[2] 1α analogs of 1,25$(OH)_2D_3$, dihydrotachysterol$_3$ (Hibberd and Norman, 1969; Suda *et al.*, 1970a; van de Vliervuet *et al.*, 1959) and isotachysterol$_3$ (Holick *et al.*, 1973c), were claimed to exhibit high biological activity.[3]

Support for structure–function studies was also derived from the observations that shortening the side chain of vitamin D as in octanor-D_3 (vitamin D without any side chain) (A. W. Norman and W. H. Okamura, unpublished observations) or as in 1α(OH)-pregnane-D_3 (Lam *et al.*, 1975b) abolished biological activity.

In the following sections, a summary is presented of many of the analogs of vitamin D that have been chemically synthesized and for which a formal publication exists. These are tabulated in Tables 5-3, 5-4, 5-5, and 5-6. When appropriate some qualitative information on the biological activity of these steroids is also indicated in terms of their ability to stimulate intestinal calcium absorption (ICA) or bone calcium mobilization (BCM). However, it remains for the reader to refer to the actual papers for details concerning the routes and methods of chemical synthesis as well as for a more thorough assessment of the biological activity evaluations.

B. A-Ring Analogs

*1. 5,6-*cis*-Steroids*

Table 5-3 lists the chemical syntheses and reported biological activities of A-ring analogs of vitamin D that belong to the 5,6-*cis* series. Figure 5-8 presents the structure of the A-ring analogs that have been chemically synthesized to date.

*2. 5,6-*trans*-Steroids*

Table 5-4 lists the chemical syntheses and the reported biological activities of A-ring analogs of vitamin D that belong to the 5,6-*trans* series. Figure 5-9 presents the chemical structure of these 5,6-*trans* A-ring analogs.

[2]A pseudo 1α-hydroxyl-containing analog is a compound whose 3β-hydroxyl group occupies a position geometrically equivalent to that of the 1α-hydroxyl group of 1,25$(OH)_2D_3$. This is the case for all 5,6-*trans* compounds that possess the requisite 3β-hydroxyl.

[3]According to Dr. J. Babcock, Upjohn Co. (personal communication), the structure assignments of isotachysterol$_3$ and isovitamin D_3 were reversed in the paper by Holick *et al.* (1973c), and their reportedly biologically active isotachysterol is actually isovitamin D_3.

TABLE 5-3
Synthesis and Biological Activity of A-ring Analogs of Vitamin D (5,6-*cis* Series)[a]

Structure no.	Compound	Biological activity[b] ICA	Biological activity[b] BCM	Synthesis	Biological activity
8	Previtamin D_3	++	++	Velluz and Amiard (1961)	Hanewald *et al.* (1961)
9	$1\alpha(OH)D_3$	+++	+++	Okamura *et al.* (1975a,b), Harrison *et al.* (1973, 1974), Kaneko *et al.* (1973a), Barton *et al.* (1973), Furst *et al.* (1973), Holick *et al.* (1975b,c), Paaren *et al.* (1978), Pelc (1977)	Harrison *et al.* (1973), Holick *et al.* (1973a, 1975c), Haussler *et al.* (1973), Pechet and Hesse (1974), Toffolon *et al.* (1975)
10	3-Deoxy-$1\alpha(OH)D_3$	++	ND	Lam *et al.* (1974), Norman *et al.* (1975b)	Lam *et al.* (1974), Norman *et al.* (1975b)
11	$4\alpha(OH)D_3$	ND	ND	Pelc (1974), Kaneko *et al.* (1975)	
12	$2\alpha(OH)D_3$	0	0	Kaneko *et al.* (1974)	Kaneko *et al.* (1972)
13	$1\alpha(OH)$-epi-D_3	++	0	Semmler *et al.* (1972), Sheres *et al.* (1975), Okamura and Pirio (1975)	Semmler *et al.* (1972), A. W. Norman *et al.* (unpublished results)
14	3-Deoxy-1,25$(OH)_2D_3$	+++	++	Okamura *et al.* (1975a)	Okamura *et al.* (1975a)
15	3-Deoxy-A-homo-D_3	ND	ND	Sine *et al.* (1974)	
16	3-Deoxy-3α-methyl-$1\alpha(OH)D_3$	ND	ND	Okamura *et al.* (1978)	Strating (1952)
17	DHV_3-II[c]	0	0	Okamura *et al.* (1977)	A. W. Norman (unpublished results)
18	DHV_3-III[c]	++	++	Okamura *et al.* (1977)	A. W. Norman (unpublished results)
19	19(OH)DHV_3-II[c]	0	0	Hammond *et al.* (1977)	A. W. Norman (unpublished results)
20	19(OH)DHV_3-III[c]	0	0	Hammond *et al.* (1977)	A. W. Norman (unpublished results)
21	3-Deoxy-3β-chloro-D_3	0	0	Bernstein *et al.* (1948, 1949), Bide *et al.* (1948)	Bernstein *et al.* (1948, 1949), Bide *et al.* (1948)
22	3-Deoxy-3β-bromo-D_3	0	0	Bernstein *et al.* (1948, 1949), Bide *et al.* (1948)	Bernstein *et al.* (1948, 1949), Bide *et al.* (1948)

23	3-Deoxy-3β-sulfhydryl-D_3	0	0	Strating and Backer (1950), King *et al.* (1948)	Bernstein and Sax (1951)
24	3-Oxo-D_3	0	0	Bide *et al.* (1948)	Bide *et al.* (1948)
25	1α,2$\alpha$$(OH)_2D_3$	+++	+++	T. Suda (unpublished results)	T. Suda (unpublished results)
26	2$\beta$$(OH)D_3$	ND	ND	Kaneko *et al.* (1974, 1975)	Kaneko *et al.* (1974, 1975)
27	1$\beta$$(OH)D_3$	ND	ND	Kaneko *et al.* (1974)	Kaneko *et al.* (1974)
28	1,24$(OH)_2D_3$	++	++	Morisaki *et al.* (1975), Koizuma *et al.* (1975)	Kawashima *et al.* (1977)
29	3-Methyl-D_3	ND	ND	Strating (1952)	
30	3-Deoxy-3-hydroxymethyl-D_3	ND	ND	Strating (1952)	
31	3-Deoxy-3-carboxymethyl-D_3	ND	ND	Strating (1952)	
32	17-Nor-17-(2,2-ethylenedioxy)-1$\alpha$$(OH)D_3$	0	0	Sakamoto *et al.* (1975)	
33	17-Nor-17-(2,2-ethylenedioxy)-2$\beta$$(OH)D_3$	ND	ND	Sakamoto *et al.* (1975)	
34	19-Nor-3-deoxy-1$\alpha$$(OH)D_3$	ND	ND	Mazur *et al.*[d]	
35	19-Nor-3-deoxy-1$\beta$$(OH)D_3$	ND	ND	Mazur *et al.*[d]	
36	19-Nor-3-deoxy-D_3	ND	ND	Mazur *et al.*[d]	
37	3α-Methyl-D_3	ND	ND	Mazur *et al.*[d]	
38	19-Nor-4,4-dimethyl-D_3	ND	ND	Mazur *et al.*[d]	
39	19-Nor-4,4-dimethyl-1$\alpha$$(OH)D_3$	ND	ND	Mazur *et al.*[d]	
40	4,4-Dimethyl-1α(OH)-epi-D_3	ND	ND	Mazur *et al.*[d]	
41	4,4-Dimethyl-1α(OH)-3-oxo-D_3	ND	ND	Mazur *et al.*[d]	
	3-Deoxy-3-amino-D	ND	ND	Mazur *et al.*[d]	
	3-Deoxy-3-amino-D_3	ND	ND	Zbiral (1978)	
	3-Deoxy-3-epiamino-D_3	ND	ND	Zbiral (1978)	
	1$\alpha$$(OH)D_2$	+++	+	Paaren *et al.* (1978), Reeve *et al.* (1978)	
	3-Deoxy-3α-methyl-1,25$(OH)_2D_3$	++	++	Okamura *et al.* (1978)	
	1α(OH)-25-F-D_3	++	++	Napoli *et al.* (1978)	

[a]See Fig. 5-8B for structures.

[b]Relative bone calcium mobilization (BCM) and intestinal calcium transport (ICA) activities are expressed as follows: +++, highly active; ++, moderately active, +, slightly active; 0, inactive; ND, activity not determined.

[c]DHV_3, dihydrovitamin$_3$; DHT_3, dihydrotachysterol$_3$.

[d]Personal communication from Dr. Y. Mazur.

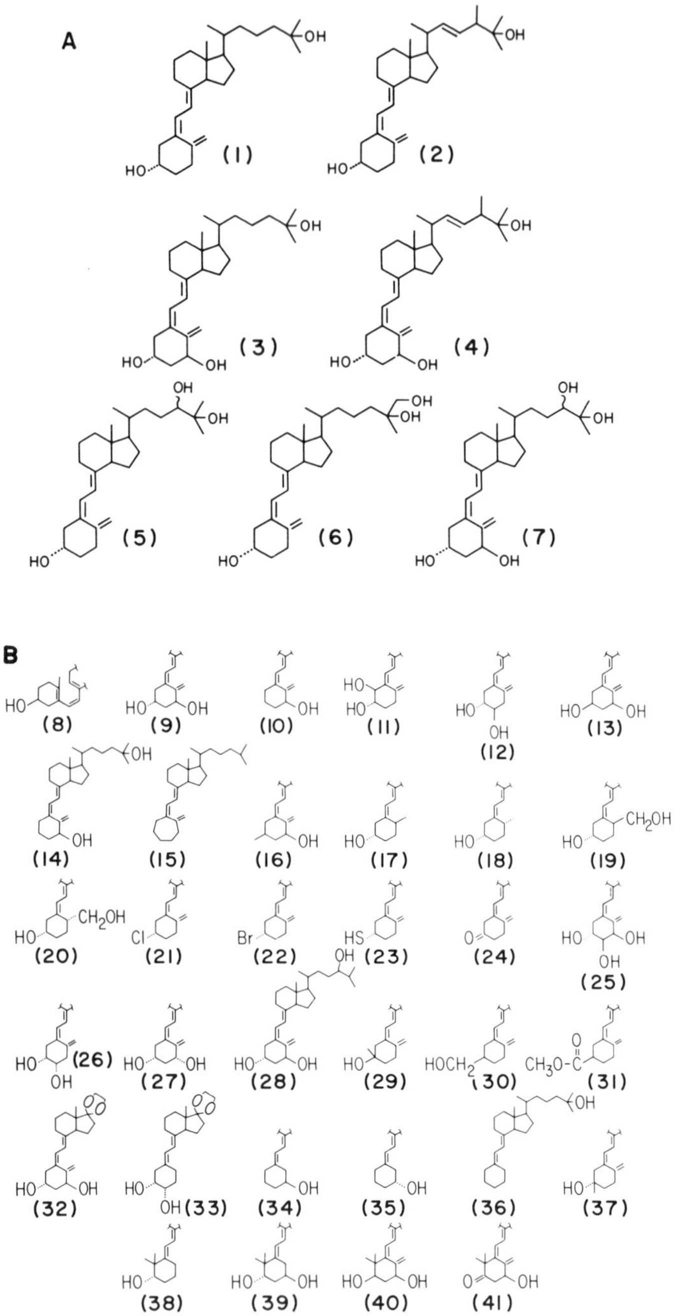

Figure 5-8. (A) Structures of metabolites of vitamin D_3. (B) Structures of A-ring analogs of vitamin D (5,6-*cis* series) (see Tables 5-2 and 5-3). No entries appear in Table 5-3 for structures 34–41; they are discussed in the text.

TABLE 5-4
Synthesis and Biological Activity of A-Ring Analogs of Vitamin D (5,6-*trans* Series)[a]

Structure no.	Compound	Biological activity[b] ICA	Biological activity[b] BCM	Synthesis	Biological activity
42	5,6-*trans*-D_3	++	++	W.H. Okamura (unpublished results)	Strating (1952), Holick *et al.* (1973c)
43	25(OH)-5,6-*trans*-D_3	++	0	Okamura *et al.* (1975), Holick *et al.* (1972a), Strating (1952)	Holick *et al.* (1972a)
44	DHT_3[c]	++	++	Okamura *et al.* (1977)	van de Vliervuet *et al.* (1959)
45	DHT_2	+	+		van de Vliervuet *et al.* (1959)
46	25(OH)DHT_3[c]	++	++		Okamura *et al.* (1974), Halkes and van Vliet (1969), Blunt and DeLuca (1969)
47	DHV_3-IV[c]	++	++	Okamura *et al.* (1977)	A. W. Norman (unpublished results)
48	19-OH-DHT_3[c]	0	0	W.H. Okamura (unpublished results)	A. W. Norman (unpublished results)
49	19-OH-DHV_3-IV[c]	0	0	W.H. Okamura (unpublished results)	A. W. Norman (unpublished results)
50	$Tachysterol_3$	0	0	W.H. Okamura (unpublished results)	A. W. Norman (unpublished results)
51	$Isotachysterol_3$	++	++	von Werder (1957), Sklan and Budowski (1973)	von Werder (1957), Holick *et al.* (1973c)
52	Isovitamin-D_3	++	++	von Werder (1957)	von Werder (1957)
53	25(OH)-Iso-$tachysterol_3$	++	++	von Werder (1957)	von Werder (1957)
54	5,6-*trans*-Preg-D_3	0	0	Holick *et al.* (1975a)	Holick *et al.* (1975a)
55	5,6-*trans*-27-Nor-25(OH)D_3	++	0	Holick *et al.* (1975a)	Holick *et al.* (1975a)
56	5,6-*trans*-26,27-Dinor-25(OH)D_3	++	0	Holick *et al.* (1975a)	Holick *et al.* (1975a)
57	24-Nor-5,6-*trans*-25(OH)D_3	+	+	Holick *et al.* (1972a), Mourino *et al.* (1978)	Holick *et al.* (1972a), Mourino *et al.* (1978)
58	11α(OH)D_3	0	0	Velluz and Amiard (1961)	
	24-Nor-1,25$(OH)_2D_3$	++	++	Mourino *et al.* (1978)	Mourino *et al.* (1978)

[a]See Fig. 5-9 for structures.

[b]Relative bone calcium mobilization (BCM) and intestinal calcium transport (ICA) activities are expressed as follows: +++, highly active; ++, moderately active; +, slightly active; 0, inactive; ND, activity not determined.

[c]DHV_3, $dihydrovitamin_3$; DHT_3, $dihydrotachysterol_3$.

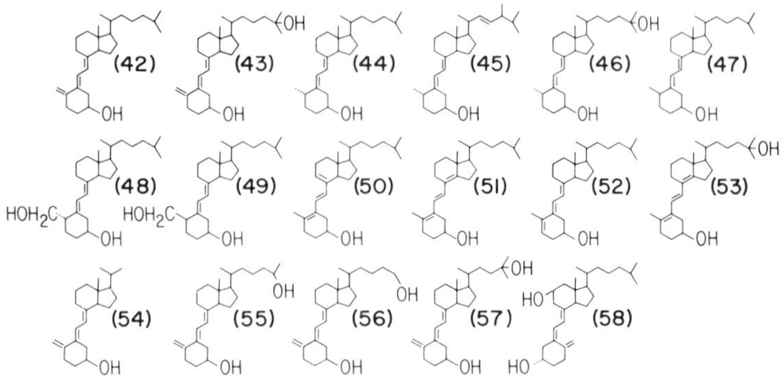

Figure 5-9. Structure of A-ring analogs of vitamin D (5,6-*trans* series) (see Table 5-4).

C. Side-Chain Analogs

Table 5-5 lists the chemical syntheses and reported biological activities of side-chain analogs of vitamin D. The structures of the side-chain analogs that have been synthesized to date are given in Fig. 5-10.

D. Other Analogs Related to Vitamin D

The chemical syntheses and reported biological activities of other relevant steroids whose structures are related to vitamin D are given in Table 5-6. The chemical structures of these relevant steroids are shown in Fig. 5-11.

IV. STRUCTURE–FUNCTION STUDIES

A. Problems of Evaluation

In view of the development of our understanding of the metabolism of vitamin D as well as our recognition of the steroid hormonelike mode of action of $1,25(OH)_2D_3$ in its target organ, the intestine, it is now possible to consider a detailed structure–function analysis of the vitamin D endocrine system. This is an ambitious project, and as yet only preliminary insights have been gained.

Currently there are numerous techniques available for both *in vivo* and *in vitro* biological screening of new analogs. Some of the standardized techniques concerned with the measurement of intestinal calcium absorption and bone calcium mobilization are discussed in Chapter 4; the large number of more recently developed *in vitro* assays are described in detail in other chapters of this book. These include (a) the determination of the enzymatic rate of conversion of $25(OH)D_3$ to $1,25(OH)_2D_3$ using chick kidney homogenates of mitochondrial

TABLE 5-5
Synthesis and Biological Activity of Side-Chain Analogs of Vitamin D[a]

Structure no.	Compound	Biological activity[b] ICA	Biological activity[b] BCM	Synthesis	Biological activity
3	$1,25(OH)_2D_3$	+++	+++	Frolick and DeLuca (1972)	Frolick and DeLuca (1972)
59	Octanor-D_3	0	0	Wing *et al.* (1975)	A. W. Norman (unpublished results)
60	Preg-D_3	0	0	Holick *et al.* (1975a)	Holick *et al.* (1975a)
61	1α(OH)-Preg-D_3	0	0	Lam *et al.* (1975a)	Lam *et al.* (1975b)
62	27-Nor-25(OH)D_3	+	+	Holick *et al.* (1975a), Bontekoe *et al.* (1970)	Holick *et al.* (1975a)
63	26,27-Dinor-25(OH)D_3	+	+	Holick *et al.* (1975a), Bontekoe *et al.* (1970)	Holick *et al.* (1975a)
64	$20,25(OH)_2D_3$	ND	ND	Bontekoe *et al.* (1970)	
65	27-Nor-$20,25(OH)_2D_3$	ND	ND	Bontekoe *et al.* (1970)	
66	25,26,27-Trinor-24(OH)D_3	ND	ND	Bontekoe *et al.* (1970)	
67	22(*S*),22(OH)D_4	ND	ND	Crump *et al.* (1973)	
68	24(*R*),24(OH)D_3	+++	+++	Ikekawa *et al.* (1975a)	Ikekawa *et al.* (1975a), Tanaka *et al.* (1975b)
69	24(*S*),24(OH)D_3	+++	0	Ikekawa *et al.* (1975a)	Ikekawa *et al.* (1975a), Tanaka *et al.* (1975b)
70	24α-Homo-D_3	+	+	Louw *et al.* (1955)	Louw *et al.* (1955)
71	$24\alpha,24\beta$-Dihomo-D_3	0	0	Louw *et al.* (1955)	Louw *et al.* (1955)
72	23,24,25,26,27-Pentanor-22-(*N*,*N*-diethylamido)D_3	0	0	Louw *et al.* (1955)	Louw *et al.* (1955)
73	23,24,25,26,27-Pentanor-22-(*N*,*N*-diethylamino)D_3	0	0	Louw *et al.* (1955)	Louw *et al.* (1955)
74	Vitamin D_4	Activity similar to D_3 in rats		Grab (1936)	

(*continued*)

TABLE 5-5 *(Continued)*

Structure no.	Compound	Biological activity[b] ICA	Biological activity[b] BCM	Synthesis	Biological activity
75	Vitamin D_5	Some antirachitic potency		Wunderlich (1936)	
76	Vitamin D_6	Negligible activity		Haslewood (1939), Wunderlich (1936)	
77	17β(OH)-Octanor-D_3	"Feebly active"		Windaus and Naggatz (1939)	
78	25,26,27-Trinor-24-carboxy-D_3	Inactive		World Health Organization (1950)	
79	Pentanor-25(OH)D_3	0	0	Johnson (1975)	Johnson (1975)
80	22,23,24-Trinor-25(OH)D_3	0	0	Johnson (1975)	Johnson (1975)
81	23,24-Dinor-25(OH)D_3	0	0	Johnson (1975)	Johnson (1975)
82	24-Nor-25(OH)D_3	0	0	Johnson (1975)	Johnson (1975)
		+++	0	Holick *et al.* (1972a)	Holick *et al.* (1972a)
83	Homo-25(OH)D_3	++	+++	Johnson (1975)	Johnson (1975)
84	25,26,27-Trinor-D_3	ND	ND	Vries and Backer (1952)	
85	26,27-Dinor-D_3	ND	ND	Vries and Backer (1952)	
86	27-Nor-D_3	ND	ND	Vries and Backer (1952)	
87	24α-Homo-27-nor-D_3	ND	ND	Vries and Backer (1952)	
88	26,27-Dinor-25-phenyl-D_3	ND	ND	Vries and Backer (1952)	
89	25-Aza-D_3	0	0	Onisko *et al.* (1977)	
90	25-Fluoro-D_3	ND	ND	Onisko *et al.* (1977)	
91	24,25-Dehydro-D_3	ND	ND	Onisko *et al.* (1977)	
92	25,26-Dehydro-D_3	ND	ND	Onisko *et al.* (1977)	
	1,24$(OH)_2D_3$	++	++	Morisaki *et al.* (1975), Koizumi *et al.* (1975)	Kawashima *et al.* (1977)

[a]See Fig. 5-10 for structures 59–92; Fig. 5-8A for structure 3.

[b]Relative bone calcium mobilization (BCM) and intestinal calcium transport (ICA) activities are expressed as follows: +++, highly active; ++, moderately active; +, slightly active; 0, inactive; ND, activity not determined.

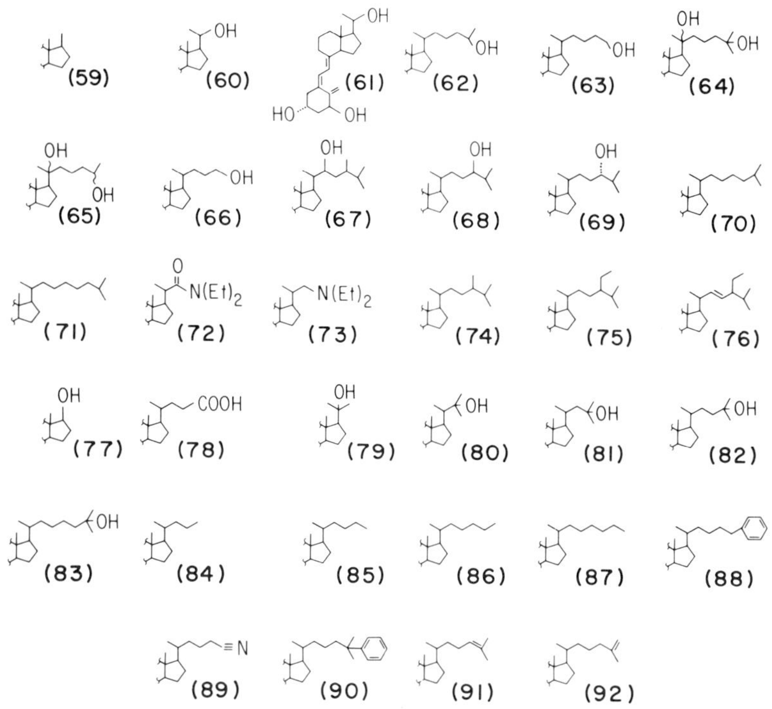

Figure 5-10. Structure of side-chain analogs of vitamin D (see Table 5-5).

TABLE 5-6
Synthesis of Some Steroids Related to Vitamin D[a,b]

Structure no.	Compound	Synthesis
93	1α(OH)-7-Dehydrocholesterol	Freeman *et al.* (1974), Kaneko *et al.* (1974)
94	1α(OH)-cholesterol	Mitra *et al.* (1974), Kaneko *et al.* (1973b), Morisaki *et al.* (1973a)
95	1,25$(OH)_2$-cholesterol	Morisaki *et al.* (1973c), Rubio-Lightbourn *et al.* (1973), Narwid *et al.* (1974b)
96	25(OH)-cholesterol	Partridge *et al.* (1974), Narwid *et al.* (1974a), Morisaki *et al.* (1973b)
97	24,25$(OH)_2$-cholesterol	Seki *et al.* (1973)
98	25,26$(OH)_2$-cholesterol	Seki *et al.* (1973)

[a]See Fig. 5-11 for structures.

[b]None of the steroids listed in this table have any biological activity; none are secosteroids, and thus they do not satisfy the minimal structural requirement for vitamin D biological activity.

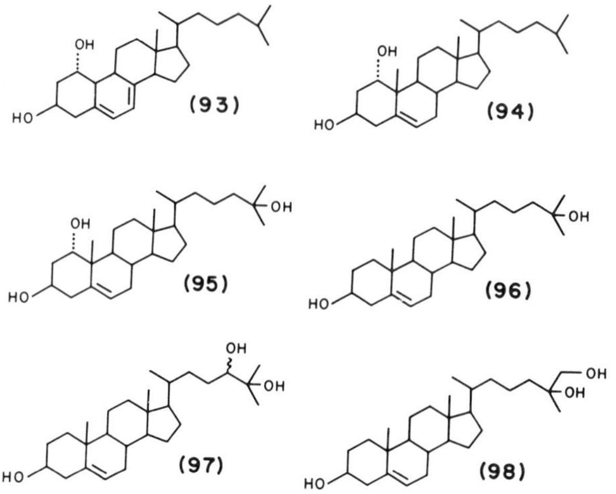

Figure 5-11. Structures of steroids related to vitamin D (See Table 5-6).

preparations (Henry and Norman, 1974, 1975a,b) (see Chapter 6); (b) a steroid radiocompetition assay for 25(OH)D_3 employing its serum binding protein (Haddad and Chyu, 1971; Norman *et al.*, 1976; Osborn, 1976), in which the test compound is allowed to compete with radioactive 25(OH)D_3 for its plasma binding protein (see Chapter 8); (c) a steroid radiocompetition assay in which radioactive 1,25$(OH)_2D_3$ competes with the test steroid in a recombined cytosol–chromatin incubation mixture prepared from the intestinal mucosa of rachitic chicks (Brumbaugh and Haussler, 1974; Procsal *et al.*, 1975 (see Fig. 7-16, Table 7-12, and Chapters 7 and 8); (d) a bone culture assay in which the analog or metabolite is tested for its ability to mediate the release of $^{45}Ca^{2+}$ from prelabeled calvaria obtained from fetal rats (Raisz *et al.*, 1972; Reynolds, 1974) (see Fig. 12-3); and finally (e) a radial immunoassay for the ability of the test compound to induce the synthesis a vitamin D-dependent calcium-binding protein either *in vivo* (Corradino *et al.*, 1968) or by acting on organ culture intestines obtained from embryonic chicks (Corradino, 1972, 1973 (see Fig. 4-5).

Table 5-7 lists some of the obvious problems that confront the chemist or biochemist in initiating any thorough structure–function analysis of analogs. Although it is laborious to conduct all the assays for any one analog, it is essential, in view of the major efforts often required to chemically synthesize a particular steroid, that it be evaluated in as many systems as possible.

Three important bioassay variables must be kept in mind when one is considering any results. These include: (a) the time required for the appearance of the maximal biological response; (b) the size of the dose required to produce the maximal biological response; and (c) the magnitude or intensity of the maximal

TABLE 5-7
Problems of Assay of New Vitamin D Metabolites of Analogs

1. Which bioresponse should be measured (ICA, BCM[b] or other)?
2. Should the assay be *in vivo* or *in vitro*?
3. How should the dose be administered? (orally, ip, or ic)[a]
4. Problems related to physiology and biochemistry of the action of vitamin D
   a. Steroid structural requirements (metabolism–transport–interaction with target tissue receptors)
      i. 25-Hydroxylation and/or 1-hydroxylation
      ii. 5,6-*cis* versus 5,6-*trans* vitamin D compounds
      iii. Equilibrium of A-ring conformers
      iv. Side-chain effects
      v. Effects of missing, altered, or added functional groups
   b. Consequence of catabolism

[a]ip, intraperitoneally; ic, intracardially.
[b]ICA = intestinal Ca^{2+} absorption; BCM = bone calcium mobilization.

response. While points (a) and (b) are obvious, some comment about the intensity of maximal response is appropriate. If one assumes efficient delivery of a steroid to the tissue where the biological response is to be generated, then one must consider the intensity or magnitude of the response that can be produced there. Under simple conditions the natural steroid and related analog will produce the same total magnitude of response, but different concentrations will be required to produce this maximal response. However, in light of the elegant work of Samuels and Tomkins (1970), it is apparent that the situation often may not be as simple as this. In studies employing analogs of the glucocorticoids in which production of the enzyme tyrosine aminotransferase in HTC cells in tissue culture was measured, it was clear that there were at least three different levels of maximal response obtainable. These levels could be related to the structural class of the analog being tested, and these classes were referred to as (a) optimal inducers, or those that gave the expected normal magnitude of response; (b) suboptimal inducers, or those that generated only a fraction of the response of the optimal inducers; and (c) inactive compounds (Baxter *et al.*, 1972; Higgins *et al.*, 1973).

B. Structural Features Required for Optimization of Vitamin D Activity

Any detailed consideration of the structure required for optimization of biological activity of vitamin D soon reduces to a careful analysis and comparison with the structure of the biologically active form of the vitamin $1,25(OH)_2D_3$. The laboratories of Norman and Okamura in Riverside, California (Norman *et al.*, 1975a, b, 1976; Procsal *et al.*, 1975, 1976), as well as those of DeLuca and

Schnoes in Madison, Wisconsin (Schnoes and DeLuca, 1974), have attempted to define the particular attributes of $1,25(OH)_2D_3$ that so exquisitely optimize the biological activity of vitamin D_3.

Procsal *et al.* (1975) focused on the interaction of $1,25(OH)_2D_3$ and related analogs with the intestinal cytosol–chromatin receptor under *in vitro* conditions as well as on the *in vivo* assay of intestinal calcium absorption and bone calcium mobilization. A summary of these data is given in Table 5-8. From these results we have concluded that the hydroxyl groups located at the 1α and 25 positions appear to be of equal importance for the binding of $1,25(OH)_2D_3$ to its receptor. A 3β-OH group does not appear, on the other hand, to be as important as a hydroxyl at the 1α or 25 position since 3-deoxy-$1\alpha(OH)D_3$ and 3-deoxy-$1,25(OH)_2D_3$ were both effective in comparison to $1\alpha(OH)D_3$ or $1,25(OH)_2D_3$, respectively (Norman *et al.*, 1976).

A *cis* configuration for the A ring is preferred over the *trans* configuration. This conslusion was based on a comparison of the results obtained with 25(OH)-5,6-*trans*-D_3 versus 3-deoxy-$1,25(OH)_2D_3$. For 25-hydroxyl analogs of the 5,6-*trans* series, a methyl group at C-10 with an *S* configuration results in a better competitor than does a C-10 methylene group [based on results obtained with 25(OH)DHT_3 versus 25(OH)-5,6-*trans*-D_3]. Furthermore, it became apparent from the results of Johnson *et al.* (1975), who compared the biological activities of a homologous series of 25-hydroxylated side-chain analogs of vitamin D, that there is virtually no toleration by the chick of 25-hydroxylated analogs having shortened or lengthened side chains. As yet, little information is available from structure–function studies concerning structural modifications of either the triene system or, more importantly, rings C and D. A further discussion of these relationships is given in Chapter 7.

C. Possible Relationship of Steroid Conformation to Biological Activity

As discussed in Chapter 3, one of the chemical properties unique to the seco structure of vitamin D is that the A- ring is dynamically equilibrated between two chair–chair conformers. This conclusion is based on the 300-MHz NMR spectroscopic evaluation of vitamin D and related secosteroids in solution (Wing *et al.*, 1974, 1975). There have been some hints of the existence of conformational mobility of vitamin D secosteroids from the X-ray crystallographic analyses of Knobler *et al.* (1972, Hodgkin *et al.*, 1963). The novel structural feature of the calciferols is conformational mobility of the A and seco-B rings. Thus, the substituent groups in the A-ring of vitamin D secosteroids may be either equatorially or axially oriented. Whereas all four rings of such classic steroid hormones as estrogen, hydrocortisone, aldosterone, ecdysterone, and testosterone are held relatively rigidly together, only the C and D rings of the calciferols are as conformationally immobile.

In view of the well-known stereospecificities of enzymes, receptors, and other binding proteins in their biological activities, it seems reasonable to assume that only one of the two vitamin D chair conformations represents the optimally active molecular topology. At the steroid hormone receptor level of intestinal calcium transport, we have suggested that it is the equatorial 1α-hydroxyl conformer of 1,25$(OH)_2D_3$ that is important (Okamura *et al.*, 1974) (see also the discussion in Chapter 7).

The relative proportion of the A-ring conformers at equilibrium can be estimated by the nature of the substituents and their relative stereochemistries (i.e., whether they are oriented α or β). It should be noted that, in cyclohexane and related compounds, equatorial substituents are sterically favored over axial substituents (Eliel *et al.*, 1967).

We have proposed that vitamin D-like molecules should be relatively more active if there is a conformational bias in favor of the 1α-hydroxyl being equatorial rather than axial. As was pointed out by Okamura *et al.* (1974), a thorough test of this proposition can be reasonably accomplished only by comparing 1α-containing analogs that are identical in structure and stereochemistry at rings C and D, at their side chain, and also with regard to the precise orientation of their intercyclic atoms, C-6, C-7, C-8, and C-9. Furthermore, the relative position, but not necessarily the stereochemistry or oxidation state, of the C-19 should be similar. Thus, comparisons between molecules with a C-19 positioned as in D_3 and those with a C-19 located as in 5,6-*trans*-D_3 are not necessarily ideal test comparison cases.

The conformational population ratios for the A- ring of some analogs of 1,25$(OH)_2D_3$ are shown in Table 5-9. It is apparent that changing the substituent groups on the A- ring of these secosteroids mediates dramatic changes in the conformational ratio of the 1α-hydroxyl or pseudo 1α-hydroxyl functional group.

The hypothesis of Okamura *et al.* (1974) was originally based on a comparison of the biological activities of DHT_3 and DHV_3-IV (dihydrovitamin$_3$). These secosteroids are epimeric at C-19 and thus would be anticipated to have greatly differing conformational ratios of their pseudo 1α-hydroxyl functional groups (see Table 5-8). In this respect it was well known that DHT_3 was highly biologically active (Hibberd and Norman, 1969), whereas there were reports in the literature (von Werder, 1957; Norman *et al.*, 1976) (see also Fig. 7-18) that DHV_3-IV possessed little if any biological activity. Thus, since DHT_3 has a bias of 9 : 1 in favor of the equatorial versus axial orientation for its pseudo 1α hydroxyl group, this was consistent with the requirements of our three-dimensional "blueprint."

TABLE 5-8
Summary of Biological Activity of Vitamin D Metabolites and Analogs

Steroid	Assays[a,b] (relative activity): Rat line test	Assays[a,b] (relative activity): Intestinal calcium absorption[e]	Assays[a,b] (relative activity): Bone calcium mobilization[e]	Bone ash[f] (calculated) doubling dose (ng/day)	Steroid competition assay[c] (relative concentration required for 50% competition): Intestine	Steroid competition assay[c] (relative concentration required for 50% competition): Plasma
Metabolites						
D_3	1.0	1.0	1.0	189	10,000	>30
D_2	1.0					40
$25(OH)D_3$	1.4	2.0	2	226	900	1.0
$25(OH)D_2$	1.4					3
$1,25(OH)_2D_3$	1–2[d]	4–10	5	25	1.0	10
$1,25(OH)_2D_2$	1–2					
$24(R),25(OH)_2D_3$		0.5	0.02	445	5,000	
$24(S),25(OH)_2D_3$		0.01	0.02	24,170	5,000	
$1,24(R),25(OH)_3D_3$		1.0	1.0	465	2.5	
$1,24(S),25(OH)_3D_3$				3,194	3.0	
$25,26(OH)_2D_3$		1.0	1.0			
23,24-Dinor-$25(OH)D_3$						60

Analogs					
5,6-*cis* (*Z*) series					
3-Deoxy-1,25$(OH)_2D_3$				8	
3-Deoxy-1α$(OH)D_3$	0.5	1.0		5,000	>1,200
1α$(OH)D_3$			22	900	130
1α(OH)-epi-D_3				5,000	
25$(OH)D_3$					
DHV_3-II					
DHV_3-III					
19(OH)DHV_3-II				>10,000	
19(OH)DHV_3-III				>10,000	
5,6-*trans* (*E*) series					
DHT_3				>10,000	>200
25(OH)DHT_3				90	720
DHV_3-IV				>10,000	
19(OH)DHT_3				>10,000	
19(OH)DHV-IV				>10,000	
5,6-*trans*-D_3			12,730	>10,000	>200
25(OH)-5,6-*trans*-D_3					

[a]This table is a compilation of published data from many laboratories as well as some unpublished observations of Norman and Okamura. Although every effort was made to select data from assays that included appropriate reference controls, this was not possible in every instance. Of necessity some subjective judgment was exercised, for which this author takes responsibility. Literature citations for each steroid are provided in Tables 5-1 to 5-4.

[b]The conduct of these assays is described in Chapters 4 and 10.

[c]Taken from data of Norman *et al.* (1976). That for the intestine is a cytosol–chromatin assay for 1,25$(OH)_2D_3$, and that for the plasma measures competition with 25$(OH)D_3$ for a binding protein.

[d]Since this assay requires 1 week and because of the rapid clearance rates of 1,25$(OH)_2D_3$, it is important to administer the steroid daily.

[e]Measures response to an acute dose of the test steroid in a rachitic chick. See, for example, Norman and Wong (1972) and Henry *et al.* (1976).

[f]This is the daily oral dose required to double the tibia ash weight in chicks fed a rachitogenic diet. Abstracted from Boris *et al.* (1977).

TABLE 5-9
Conformational Population Ratios for the A Ring of Some Analogs of $1,25(OH)_2D_3$[a]

Secosteroid	Hydroxyl group on C-3: % equatorial/% axial	Hydroxyl group on C-1[b]: % equatorial/% axial
5,6-*cis* series		
D_3	55:45	—
$1,25(OH)_2D_3$	45:55	55:45
3-Deoxy-$1,25(OH)_2D_3$	—	70:30
$1\alpha(OH)D_3$	45:55	55:45
DHV_3-II	90:10	—
DHV_3-III	10:90	—
$1\alpha(OH)$-3-epi-D_3	30:70	30:70
5,6-*trans* series		
DHT_3	—	89:11
5,6-*trans*-D_3	—	79:21
DHV-IV	—	42:58

[a] From published studies and unpublished observations of W. H. Okamura, R. M. Wing, and A. W. Norman. (See Norman *et al.*, 191976; Okamura and Pirio, 1975.)

[b] For steroids in the 5,6-*trans* series, data given are for the pseudo 1-hydroxyl group.

Our laboratories are now actively engaging in the synthesis of many additional compounds so that this hypothesis can be more critically tested.

D. Analog Studies

1. Selectively Active Analogs

One intriguing prospect is designing an analog that has selective biological activity. It would be most favorable for clinical purposes and as a probe in biochemical systems to have analogues that would interact only with the intestinal receptor system (i.e., intestinal calcium absorption) or the bone receptor system (i.e., bone calcium mobilization). In spite of the large number of analogs that have been reported (see Tables 5-3 to 5-6) there are only a few reports of those that might have this desired selectivity. To date, the most impressive results have been obtained with the analogs 3-deoxy-$1\alpha(OH)D_3$ and 3-deoxy-$1,25(OH)_2D_3$ (see Fig. 5-12). The former analog can stimulate intestinal calcium absorption in the chick while having a relatively much less effective interaction in terms of bone calcium mobilization (Norman *et al.*, 1976). A similar documentation of the relative lack of activity of 3-deoxy-$1,25(OH)_2D_3$ on bone calcium mobilization has been obtained in the *in vitro* bone calvaria assay system (personal communication Dr. A. Boris, Hoffmann-La Roche, Nutley, New

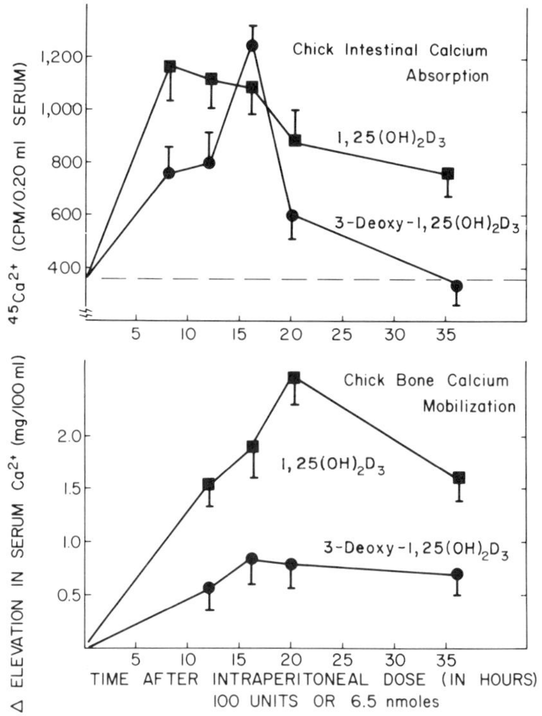

Figure 5-12. Differential biological responses of intestinal calcium absorption and bone calcium mobilization to doses of 3-deoxy-1,25$(OH)_2D_3$ in the chick. Taken from Norman *et al.* (1976); reproduced by permission of the publisher.

Jersey). Apparently, the presence of a 3β-hydroxyl is more essential for interaction with bone receptors than with intestinal receptors in the chick. It will be of interest to learn whether other analogs can be designed with similar differentiation of biological responses.

2. *Analogs That May Function as "Antivitamins"*

The incorporation of another attractive biological activity into a vitamin D analog would involve the synthesis of a steroid that would block in a general or selective way the actions of vitamin D or its biologically active metabolites. The first analog with such properties was discovered in the laboratories of Norman and Okamura. We reported that 24-nor-25$(OH)D_3$ blocked the vitamin D_3 stimulation of intestinal calcium absorption and bone calcium mobilization in the chick (Johnson *et al.*, 1975). It should be recalled that lengthening or shortening the side chain of 25$(OH)D_3$ by as little as one carbon virtually abolished all biological activity. Thus, it was most surprising that the steroid 24-nor-25$(OH)D_3$ when given 2–12 hrs in advance of vitamin D_3 was able to abolish completely any of the biological responses in both intestine and bone. It was also intriguing that the 24-nor analog did not inhibit the biological responses generated by administration of $25(OH)D_3$ or $1,25(OH)_2D_3$. Thus, the prospect exists that this 24-nor analog may be capable of functioning in some way as an "antivitamin" at least in terms of the parent vitamin D_3. Further studies are currently underway to explore this possibility in more detail.

More recently two additional analogs have been reported to have antivitamin D activity. Our laboratories (Hammond *et al.*, 1977) have found that 19-(OH)DHV$_3$II, but not DHV$_3$-II, will block intestinal calcium absorption and bone calcium mobilization in the chick when it is administered slightly prior to vitamin D_3. This is an intriguing result since this antivitamin analog has its apparently critical inhibitory-producing functionality (the 19-hydroxyl) present on the A ring, whereas 24-nor-$25(OH)D_3$ is altered in its side chain. Also, Onisko *et al.* (1977) reported that 25-azavitamin D_3 has some antivitamin properties against vitamin D_3 in the rat.

3. *Summary*

It should be apparent from the foregoing comments that only moderate progress has been made in carrying out a complete "systems analysis" of the structure–function relationships existing between vitamin D_3, its intermediary metabolites, the final biologically active form, $1,25(OH)_2D_3$, and various related analogs. This is a formidable task, and the results that have been described above should be considered to be only preliminary. It is difficult to anticipate which structural parameters in a molecule may prove to be of importance to the biosystem. For example, the fact that 24-nor-$25(OH)D_3$ can block the action of vitamin D_3 but not $25(OH)D_3$, or the fact that the bone calcium mobilization system prefers the presence of a 3β-hydroxyl more than does the intestinal calcium absorption system, could not have been predicted in advance. The exact structural requirements of vitamin D metabolites and analogs pertaining to the architecture of the receptors present in the intestine, kidney, and bone and the plasma carrier proteins are clearly of critical importance in determining the nature and extent of the biological responses and the smooth interfunctioning of the various components of this sophisticated endocrine system.

REFERENCES

Barton, D. H. R., Hesse, R. H., Pechet, M. M., and Rizzardo, E. (1973). *J. Am. Chem. Soc.* **95**, 2748.

Baxter, J. D., Rousseau, G. G., Benson, M. C., Garcea, R. L., Ito, J., and Tomkins, G. M. (1972). *Proc. Natl. Acad. Sci. U.S.A.* **69**, 1892.

Bernstein, S., and Sax, K. J. (1951). *J. Org. Chem.* **16**, 685.

Bernstein, S., Sax, K. J., and Subbarow, Y. (1948). *J. Org. Chem.* **13,** 837.

Bernstein, S., Oleson, J. J., Ritter, H. B., and Sax, K. J. (1949). *J. Am. Chem. Soc.* **71**, 2576.

Bide, A. E., Henbest, H. B., Jones, E. R. H., and Wilkenson, R. A. (1948). *J. Chem. Soc. P.* 1788.

Blunt, J. W., and DeLuca, H. F. (1969). *Biochemistry* **8**, 671.

Blunt, J. W., DeLuca, H. F., and Schnoes, H. (1968a). *Chem. Commun.* p. 801.

Blunt, J. W., DeLuca, H. F., and Schnoes, H. K. (1968b). *Biochemistry* **7**, 3317.

Bontekoe, J. S., Wignall, A., Rappoldt, M. P., and Roborgh, J. R. (1970). *Int. J. Vitam. Res. Nutr.* **40**, 589.

Boris, A., Hurley, J. F., and Trmal, T. (1977). *J. Nutr.* **107**, 194.

Boyle, I. I., Omdahl, J. L., Gray, R. W., and DeLuca, H. F. (1973). *J. Biol. Chem.* **248**, 4174.

Brumbaugh, P. F., and Haussler, M. R. (1974). *J. Biol. Chem.* **249**, 1258.

Callow, R. K., Kodicek, E., and Thompson, G. A. (1966). *Proc. R. Soc. London, Ser. B* **164**, 1–20.

Campbell, J. A., Squires, D. M., and Babcock, J. C. (1969). *Steroids* **13**, 567.

Cesario, M., Guilhern, J., Pascard, C., and Redel, J. (1978). *Tetrahedron Lett.* p. 1097.

Corradino, R. A. (1972). *Science* **179**, 402.

Corradino, R. A. (1973). *Nature (London)* **243**, 41.

Corradino, R. A., Wasserman, R. H., Pubols, M. H., and Chang, S. I. (1968). *Arch. Biochem. Biophys.* **124**, 378.

Crump, D. R., Williams, D. H., and Pelc, B. (1973). *J. Chem. Soc.* p. 2731.

DeLuca, H. F., and Schnoes, H. K. (1979). Recent Developments in the Metabolism of Vitamin D. In "Vitamin D: Recent Basic Advances and their Clinical Application (Proceedings of the Fourth Workshop on Vitamin D)" (A. W. Norman, K. Schaefer, D. von Herrath, H.-G. Grigoleit, E. B. Mawer, T. Suda, H. F. DeLuca, and J. W. Coburn, eds) Walter de Gruyter Publishing Company, Elmsford, New York.

DeLuca, H. F., Weller, M., Blunt, J. W., and Neville, P. E. (1968). *Arch. Biochem. Biophys.* **124**, 122.

Eliel, E. L., Allinger, N. L., Angyal, S. J., and Morrison, G. A. (1967). in *Conform. Anal., Pap. Int. Symp.*, 1966. Chapter 2.

Freeman, D., Acher, A., and Mazur, Y. (1974). *Tetrahedron Lett.* p. 261.

Friedlander, E. J., and Norman, A. W. (1975). *Arch. Biochem. Biophys.* **170**, 731.

Frolick, C. A., and DeLuca, H. F. (1972). *J. Clin. Invest.* **51**, 2900.

Furst, A., Labler, L., Meier, W., and Pfoertner, K. H. (1973). *Helv. Chim. Acta* **56**, 1708.

Grab, W. (1936). *Hoppe-Seyler's Z. Physiol. Chem.* **243**, 63.

Haddad, J. G., Jr., and Chyu, K. J. (1971). *J. Clin. Endocrinol. Metab.* **33**, 992.

Halkes, S. J., and van Vliet, N. P. (1969). *Recl. Trav. Chim. Pays-Bas* **88**, 1080.

Hammond, M. L., Mourino, A., Blair, P., Wecksler, W. R., Johnson, R. L., Norman, A. W., and Okamura, W. H. (1977). *In* "Vitamin D: Biochemical, Chemical and Clinical Aspects Related to Calcium Metabolism" (A. W. Norman *et al.*, eds.), de Gruyter, Berlin.

Hanewald, K. H., Rappoldt, M. P., and Roborgh, J. R. (1961). *Rec. Trav. Chim. Pays-Bas* **80**, 1003–1014.

Harrison, R. G., Lythgoe, B., and Wright, P. W. (1973). *Tetrahedron Lett.* p. 3649.

Harrison, R. G., Lythgoe, B., and Wright, P. W. (1974). *J. Chem. Soc.*, p. 2654.

Haslewood, G. A. D. (1939). *Biochem. J.* **33**, 454.

Haussler, M. R., Myrtle, J. F., and Norman, A. W. (1968). *J. Biol. Chem.* **243**, 4055.

Haussler, M. R., Zerwekh, J. E., Hesse, R. H., Rizzardo, E., and Pechet, M. M. (1973). *Proc. Natl. Acad. Sci. U.S.A.* **70**, 2248.

Havinga, E. (1973). *Experientia* **29**, 1181.

Henry, H. L., and Norman, A. W. (1974). *J. Biol. Chem.* **249**, 7529.

Henry, H. L., and Norman, A. W. (1975a). *Comp. Biochem. Physiol. B* **50**, 431.

Henry, H. L., and Norman, A. W. (1975b). *In* "Proceedings of the Second Workshop on Vitamin D

and Problems Related to Uremic Bone Disease" (A. W. Norman *et al.*, eds.), p. 1. de Gruyter, Berlin.
Henry, H. L., Norman, A. W., Taylor, A. N., Hartenbower, D. L., and Coburn, J. W. (1976). *J. Nutr.* **106**, 724.
Hibberd, K. A., and Norman, A. W. (1969). *Biochem. Pharmacol.* **18**, 2347.
Higgins, S. J., Rousseau, G. G., Baxter, J. D., and Tomkins, G. M. (1973). *J. Biol. Chem.* **248**, 5866.
Hodgkin, D. C., Rimmer, B. M., Dunitz, J. D., and Trueblood, K. N. T. (1963). *J. Chem. Soc.* p. 4945.
Holick, M. F., Schnoes, H. K., DeLuca, H. F., Suda, T., and Cousins, R. J. (1971). *Biochemistry* **10**, 2799.
Holick, M. F., Garabedian, M., and DeLuca, H. F. (1972a). *Biochemistry* **11**, 2715.
Holick, M. F., Garabedian, M., and DeLuca, H. F. (1972b). *Science* **176**, 1146.
Holick, M. F., Schnoes, H. K., DeLuca, H. F., Gray, R. W., Boyle, I. T., and Suda, T. (1972c). *Biochemistry* **11**, 4251.
Holick, M. F., Semmler, E. J., Schnoes, H. K., and DeLuca, H. F. (1973a). *Science* **180**, 190.
Holick, M. F., Kleiner-Bossaller, A., Schnoes, H. K., Kasten, P. M., Boyle, I. T., and DeLuca, H. F. (1973b). *J. Biol. Chem.* **248**, 6691.
Holick, M. F., DeLuca, H. F., Kasten, P. M., and Korycka, M. F. (1973c). *Science* **180**, 964.
Holick, M. F., Garabedian, M., Schnoes, H. K., and DeLuca, H. F. (1975a). *J. Biol. Chem.* **250**, 226.
Holick, M. F., Holick, S. A., Tavela, T., Gallagher, B., Schnoes, H. K., and DeLuca, H. F. (1975b). *Science* **190**, 576.
Holick, M. F., Kasten-Schraufrogel, P., Tavela, T., and DeLuca, H. F. (1975c). *Arch. Biochem. Biophys.* **166**, 63.
Ikekawa, N., Morisaki, M., Koizumi, N., Sawamura, M., Tanaka, Y., and DeLuca H. F. (1975a). *Biochem. Biophys. Res. Commun.* **62**, 485.
Ikekawa, N., Morisaki, M., Koizumi, N., Kato, Y., and Takeshita, T. (1975b). *Chem. Pharm. Bull.* **23**, 695.
Johnson, R. L. (1975). Ph.D. Dissertation, University of California, Riverside.
Johnson, R. L., Okamura, W. H., and Norman, A. W. (1975). *Biochem. Biophys. Res. Commun.* **67**, 797.
Jones, G., Schnoes, H. K., and DeLuca, H. F. (1975). *Biochemistry* **14**, 1250.
Kaneko, C., Yamada, S., Sugimoto, A., Ishikawa, M., Suda, T., Suzuki, M., and Sasaki, S. (1972). *J. Chem. Soc.* p. 1104.
Kaneko, C., Yamada, S., Sugimoto, A., Eguchi, Y., Ishikawa, M., Suda, T., Suzuki, M., Kabuta, S., and Sasaki, S. (1973a). *Steroids* **23**, 75.
Kaneko, C., Yamada, S., Sugimoto, A., Ishikawa, M., Sasaki, S., and Suda, T. (1973b). *Tetrahedron Lett.* p. 2239.
Kaneko, C., Sugimoto, A., Eguchi, Y., Yamada, S., and Ishikawa, M. (1974). *Tetrahedron* **30**, 2701.
Kaneko, C., Yamada, S., Sugimoto, A., and Ishikawa, M. (1975). *Chem. Pharm. Bull.* **23**, 1616.
Kawashima, K., Hoshina, Y., Hashimoto, Y., Takeshita, T., Ishimoto, S., Noquichi, T., Ikekawa, N., and Morisaki, M. (1977). *FEBS Lett.* **76**, 177.
King, L. C., Dodson, R. M., and Subluskey, L. A. (1948). *J. Am. Chem. Soc.* **70**, 1176.
Kleiner-Bossaler, A., and DeLuca, H. F. (1974). *Biochim. Biophys. Acta* **338**, 489.
Knobler, C., Romers, C., Braun, P. B., and Hornstra, J. (1972). *Acta Crystallogr., Sect. B* **28**, 2097.
Kodicek, E., Lawson, D. E. M., and Wilson, P. W. (1970). *Nature (London)* **228**, 763.

Koizumi, N., Morisaki, M., Ikekawa, N., Suzuki, A., and Takeshita, T. (1975). *Tetrahedron Lett.* p. 2203.

Lam, H.-Y., Schnoes, H. K., Deluca, H.F., and Chen, T. C. (1973). *Biochemistry* **12**, 4851.

Lam, H.-Y., Onisko, B. L., Schnoes, H. K., and DeLuca, H. F. (1974). *Biochem. Biophys. Res. Commun.* **59**, 845.

Lam, H.-Y., Schnoes, H. K., and DeLuca, H. F. (1975a). *Steroids* **25**, 247.

Lam, H.-Y., Schnoes, H. K., DeLuca, H. F., Reeve, L., and Stern, P. H. (1975b). *Steroids* **26**, 422.

Lawson, D. E. M., Wilson, P. W., Barker, D. C., and Kodicek, E. (1969a) *Biochem. J.* **115**, 263.

Lawson, D. E. M., Wilson, P. W., and Kodicek, E. (1969b). *Biochem. J.* **115**, 269.

Lawson, D. E. M., Fraser, D. R., Kodicek, E., Morris, H. R., and Williams, D. H. (1971). *Nature (London)* **230**, 228.

Louw, D. F., Strating, J., and Backer, H. J. (1955). *Recl. Trav. Chim. Pays-Bas* **74**, 1540.

Lugtenburg, J., and Havinga, E. (1969). *Tetrahedron Lett.* **28**, 2391.

Lund, J., and DeLuca, H. F. (1966). *J. Lipid Res.* **7**, 739.

Lund, J., DeLuca, H. F., and Horsting, M. (1967). *Arch. Biochim. Biophys.* **120**, 513.

Milhaud, G., Labat, M.-L., Redel, J. (1974). *C. R. Hebd. Seances Acad. Sci.* **279**, 827.

Miravet, L., Redel, J., Carré, M., Queille, M. L., and Bordier, P. (1976). *Calcif. Tissue Res.* **21**, 145.

Mitra, M. N., Norman, A. W., and Okamura, W. H. (1974). *J. Org. Chem.* **39**, 2931.

Mori, H., Lund, J., Neville, P. F., and DeLuca, H. F. (1967). *Arch. Biochem. Biophys.* **120**, 508.

Morisaki, M., Rubio-Lightbourn, J., and Ikekawa, N. (1973a). *Chem. Pharm. Bull.* **21**, 457.

Morisaki, M., Bannai, K., and Ikekawa, N. (1973b). *Chem. Pharm. Bull.* **21**, 1853.

Morisaki, M., Rubio-Lightbourn, J., Ikekawa, N., and Takeshita, T. (1973c). *Chem. Pharm. Bull.* **21**, 2568.

Morisaki, M., Koizumi, N., Ikekawa, N., Takeshita, T., and Ishimoto, S. (1975). *J. Chem. Soc.* p. 1421.

Mourino, A., Blair, P., Wecksler, W., Johnson, R. L., Norman, A. W., and Okamura, W. H. (1978). *J. Med. Chem.* **21**, 1025.

Myrtle, J. F. (1971). Ph.D. Dissertation, University of California, Riverside.

Myrtle, J. F., and Norman, A. W. (1971a). *Science* **171**, 79

Myrtle, J. F., and Norman, A. W. (1971b). *Steroids* **17**, 619.

Myrtle, J. F., Haussler, M. R., and Norman, A. W. (1970). *J. Biol. Chem.* **245**, 1190.

Napoli, J. L., Fivizzani, M. A., Schnoes, H. K., and Deluca, H. F. (1978). *Biochemistry* **17**, 2387.

Narwid, T. A., Cooney, K. E., and Uskokovic, M. R. (1974a). *Helv. Chim. Acta* **57**, 771.

Narwid, T. A., Blount, J. F., Iacobelli, J. A., and Uskokovic, M. R. (1974a). *Helv. Chim. Acta* **57**, 781.

Neville, P. F., and DeLuca, H. F. (1966). *Biochemistry* **5**, 2201.

Norman, A. W., and DeLuca, H. F. (1963). *Biochemistry* **2**, 1160.

Norman, A. W., and Wong, R. G. (1972). *J. Nutrition* **102**, 1709.

Norman, A. W., Lund, J., and DeLuca, H. F. (1964). *Arch. Biochem. Biophys.* **108**, 12.

Norman, A. W., Myrtle, J. F., Midgett, R. J., Nowicki, H. G., Williams, V., and Popjak, G. (1971). *Science* **173**, 51.

Norman, A. W., Procsal, D. A., Okamura, W. H., and Wing, R. M. (1975a). *J. Steroid Biochem.* **6**, 461.

Norman, A. W., Mitra, M. N., Okamura, W. H., and Wing, R. M. (1975b). *Science* **188**, 1013.

Norman, A. W., Johnson, R. L., Osborn, T. W., Procsal, D. A., Carey, S. C., Hammond, M. L., Mitra, M. N., Pirio, M. R., Rego, A., Wing, R. W., and Okamura, W. H. (1976). *Clin. Endocrinol.* (N.Y.) **5**, 121s.

Okamura, W. H., and Pirio, M. R. (1975). *Tetrahedron Lett.* **49**, 4317.
Okamura, W. H., Norman, A. W., and Wing, R. M. (1974). *Proc. Natl. Acad. Sci. U.S.A.* **71**, 4194.
Okamura, W. H., Mitra, M. N., Procsal, D. A., and Norman, A. W. (1975a). *Biochem. Biophys. Res. Commun.* **65**, 24.
Okamura, W. H., Hammond, M. L., Pirio, M. R., Wing, R. M., Rego, A., Mitra, M. N. and Norman, A. W. (1975b). *In* "Proceedings of the Second Workshop on Vitamin D and Problems Related to Uremic Bone Disease" (A. W. Norman *et al.*, eds.), p. 1. de Gruyter, Berlin.
Okamura, W. H., Hammond, M. L., Rego, A., Norman, A. W., and Wing, R. M. (1977). *J. Org. Chem.* **42**, 2284.
Okamura, W. H., Mitra, M. N., Pirio, M. R., Mourino, A., Carey, S. C., and Norman, A. W. (1978). *J. Org. Chem.* **43**, 574.
Onisko, B. L., Schnoes, H. K., and DeLuca, H. F. (1977). *Tetrahedron Lett.* **13,** 1107.
Osborn, T. (1976). Ph.D. Dissertation, University of California, Riverside.
Paaren, H. E., Hamer, D. E., Schnoes, H. K., and DeLuca, H. F. (1978) *Proc. Natl. Acad. Sci. (U.S.A.)* **75**, 2080.
Partridge, J. J., Faber, S., and Uskoković, M. R. (1974). *Helv. Chim. Acta* **57,** 764.
Partridge, J. J., Toome, V., and Uskoković, M. R. (1976). *J. Am. Chem. Soc.* **98,** 3739.
Partridge, J. J., Shivey, S. J., Baggiolini, E. G., Hennessy, B., and Uskoković, M. (1977). *In* "Vitamin D: Biochemical, Chemical and Clinical Aspects Related to Calcium Metabolism" (A. W. Norman *et al.*, eds), p. 47. de Gruyter, Berlin.
Pechet, M. M., and Hesse, R. H. (1974). *Mol. Cell. Endocrinol.* **1**, 305.
Pelc, B. (1974). *J. Chem. Soc.* p. 1436.
Pelc, B. (1977). *Steroids* **30**, 193.
Procsal, D. A., Okamura, W. H., and Norman, A. W. (1975). *J. Biol. Chem.* **250**, 8382.
Procsal, D. A., Okamura, W. H., and Norman, A. W. (1976). *J. Clin. Nutr.* **29**, 1271.
Procsal, D. A., Henry, H. L., Friedlander, E. J., and Norman, A. W. (1977). *Arch. Biochem. Biophys.* **179**, 229.
Raisz, L. G., Trummel, C. L., Holick, M. F., and DeLuca, H. F. (1972). *Science* **175**, 768.
Redel, J., Bell, P., Delbarre, F., and Kodicek, E. (1973). *C. R. Hebd. Seances Acad. Sci.* **276**, 2907.
Redel, J., Bell, P., Delbarre, F., and Kodicek, E. (1974a). *C. R. Hebd. Seances Acad. Sci.* **278**, 529.
Redel, J., Bell, P. A., Bazely, N., Calando, Y., Delbarre, F., and Kodicek, E. (1974b). *Steroids* **24**, 463.
Redel, J., Bazely, N., Calando, Y., Delbarre, F., Bell, P. A., and Kodicek, E. (1975). *J. Steroid Biochemi.* **6**, 117.
Redel, J., Miravet, L., Bazely, N., Calando, Y., Carré, M., and Delbarre, F. (1977). *C. R. Hebd. Seances Acad. Sci.* **285,** 443.
Redel, J., Bazely, N., Tanaka, Y., and DeLuca, H. F. (1978). *FEBS Lettr.* **94,** 228.
Reeve, L. E., Schnqes, H. K., and DeLuca, H. F. (1978). *Arch. Biochem. Biophys.* **186**, 164.
Reynolds, J. J. (1974). *Calcif. Tissue Res.* **15**, 333.
Rubio-Lightbourn, J., Morisaki, M., and Ikekawa, N. (1973). *Chem. Pharm. Bull.* **21**, 1854.
Sakamoto, H., Sugimoto, A., Kaneko, C., Suda, T., and Sasaki, S. (1975). *Chem. Pharm. Bull.* **23**, 1733.
Samuels, H. H., and Tomkins, G. M. (1970). *J. Mol. Biol.* **52**, 57.
Schnoes, H., and DeLuca, H. F. (1974). *Vita. Horm. (N.Y.)* **32**, 385.
Seki, M., Rubio-Lightbourn, J., Morisaki, M., and Ikekawa, N. (1973). *Chem. Pharm. Bull.* **21**, 2783.
Seki. M., Koizumi, N., Morisaki, M., and Ikekawa, N. (1975). *Tetrahedron Lett.* p. 15.

Semmler, E. J., Holick, M. F., Schnoes, H. K., and DeLuca, H. F. (1972). *Tetrahedron Lett.* p. 4147.
Sheres, M., Berman, E., Freeman, D., and Mazur, Y. (1975). *J. Chem. Soc., Chem. Commun.* p. 643.
Sine, S. M., Conklin, T. E., and Okamura, W. H. (1974). *J. Org. Chem.* **39**, 3797.
Sklan, D., and Budowski, P. (1973). *Anal. Biochem.* **52**, 584.
Strating, J. (1952). *Recl. Trav. Chim. Pays-Bas* **71,** 822.
Strating, J., and Backer, H. J. (1950). *Recl. Trav. Chim. Pays-Bas* **69**, 909.
Strating, J., and Backer, H. J. (1951). *Recl. Trav. Chim. Pays-Bas* **70**, 389.
Suda, T., DeLuca, H. F., Schnoes, H. K., and Blunt, J. W. (1969). *Biochemistry* **8**, 3515.
Suda, T., Hallick, R. B., DeLuca, H. F., and Schnoes, H. F. (1970a). *Biochemistry* **9**, 1651.
Suda, T., DeLuca, H. F., Schnoes, H. K., Ponchon, G., Tanaka, Y., and Holick, M. F. (1971b). *Biochemistry* **9**, 2917.
Suda, T., DeLuca, H. F., Schnoes, H. K., Tanaka, Y., and Holick, M. F. (1970c). *Biochemistry* **9**, 4776.
Tanaka, Y., Frank, H., DeLuca, H. F., Koizumi, N., and Ikekawa, N. (1975a). *Biochemistry* **14**, 3293.
Tanaka, Y., DeLuca, H. F., Ikekawa, N., Morisaki, M., and Koizumi, N. (1975b). *Arch. Biochem. Biophys.* **170**, 620.
Tanaka, Y., Castillo, L., and DeLuca, H. F. (1977). *J. Biol. Chem.* **252**, 1421.
Toffolon, E. P., Pechet, M. M., and Isselbacher, K. (1975). *Proc. Natl. Acad. Sci. U.S.A.* **72**, 229.
Trinh-Toan, Ryan, R. C., Simon, G. L., DeLuca, H. F., Calabrese, J. C., and Dahl, L. F. (1977). *Journal Chem. Soc. Perkin Trans.* **I**, 109.
van de Vliervuet, J. L. J., Westerhof, P., Keverling-Buisman, J. A., and Havinga, E. (1959). *Recl. Chim. Trav. Pays-Bas* **75**, 1179.
Velluz, L., and Amiard, G. (1961). *Hebd. Seances Acad. Sci.* **253**, 603.
von Werder, F. (1957). *Justus Leibigs Ann. Chem.* **603**, 15.
Vries, H., and Backer, H. J. (1952). *Recl. Trav. Chim. Pays-Bas* **71**, 719.
Windaus, A., and Naggatz, J. (1939). *Justus Liebigs Ann. Chem.* **542**, 204.
Wing, R. M., Okamura, W. H., Pirio, M. R., Sine, S. M., and Norman, A. W. (1974). *Science* **186**, 939.
Wing, R. M., Okamura, W. H., Rego, A., Pirio, M. R., and Norman, A. W. (1975). *J. Am. Chem. Soc.* **97**, 4980.
Wong, R. G., Norman, A. W., Reddy, C. R., and Coburn, J. W. (1972). *J. Clin. Invest.* **51**, 1287.
World Health Organization (1950). *W.H.O. Tech. Rep. Ser.* **3**.
Wunderlich, W. (1936). *Hoppe-Seyler's Z. Physiol. Chem.* **241**, 116.
Zbiral, E. (1978). *Tetrahedron* **34**, 713.

CHAPTER 6

Metabolism of Vitamin D

I. INTRODUCTION

A. Background

Before the recent advent of radioactive vitamin D with high specific activity (see Chapter 3), it was not possible to determine whether vitamin D was converted to further metabolites. The extreme biological potency of vitamin D, coupled with the lack of physical or chemical means for the direct assay of physiological concentrations (see Chapter 4), meant that investigators had to rely on slow and imprecise biological assays. Early experiments carried out with nonradioactive vitamin D provided some preliminary insight into the tissue distribution and putative metabolism of the vitamin (Heymann, 1937a,b; Morgan and Shimotori, 1943). Heymann (1937a,b) administered 200,000 IU (5 mg) of viosterol (a commercial preparation of vitamin D_3) to rabbits and detected via biological assay the presence of vitamin D activity in blood, liver, and skin. The studies by Morgan and Shimotori (1943) involved the administration of 40,000 IU (1 mg) to dogs; they were able to account for 10% of the administered dose on the basis of activity present in the kidney, heart, large intestine, brain, lung, spleen, muscle, fat, skin, and hair. In the 1950's Cruickshank *et al.* (1953, 1954) studied the fate of a massive dose of vitamin D_2 (1 mg) in a single rat and were able to account for 25% of the administered dose in the bones, intestine, and feces. They concluded that the remainder was probably metabolized to biologically inactive steroids.

The most important question, however, that could not be answered by means of biological assays concerned the potential metabolism of vitamin D to biochemically active as well as inactive forms. By 1955–1960 many laboratories were already cognizant of the possibility that the delay in biological response to vitamin D in terms of initiation of intestinal calcium absorption might be due to the necessity for time-dependent metabolism to an "active" compound. It is interesting that the adrenal glands had been suggested by both Raoul and Gounelle (1958) and Sallis and Holdsworth (1962) as the possible site of this putative vitamin D metabolism. Raoul and Gounelle (1958) claimed that 87% of an intravenously injected dose of 104 nmoles (1600 IU) of nonradioactive vitamin D_2 accumulated in the rat adrenals within 30 min. This conclusion, however, was based only on a uv difference spectrum obtained from total lipid extracts of rat adrenals. Sallis and Holdsworth (1962) implicated the adrenal glands by use of a presumed specific inhibitor of adrenal action. Administration of this compound, 1-(2-chlorophenyl)-1-(4-chlorophenyl)-2,2-dichloroethane (*o,p'*-DDD), for 3 days to rachitic chicks abolished both adrenal function and the ability to respond to a dose of 6.5 nmoles (100 IU) of vitamin D_3.

The adrenal vitamin D metabolism hypothesis, however, can be refuted for the following reasons:

1. Although Quartermann (1965) found, as had Raoul and Gounelle (1958), that there was an increase in the concentration of a component in the rat adrenal shortly after intracardial injection of vitamin D, this compound had chromatographic properties quite different from those of vitamin D and, most importantly, it had no antirachitic activity.

2. Radioactive vitamin D shows no tendency to localize in the adrenals (Norman and DeLuca, 1963; Haussler and Norman, 1967) (see Chapter 7).

3. The compound *o,p'*-DDD is not a specific inhibitor of only adrenal function. It also inhibits the labeling of intestinal mucosal ribonucleic acid by [^{3}H]uridine (Norman, 1966). Furthermore, this compound belongs to the class of polychlorinated hydrocarbons, and it is now known that many of these substances are capable of interfering with the metabolism of vitamin D (see Section VI).

4. Vitamin D-deficient, adrenalectomized rats can still respond to vitamin D administration in terms of increased intestinal calcium absorption and bone calcium mobilization (Czarnowska-Misztal *et al.*, 1966).

Sahashi and co-workers (1962; Tanaka *et al.*, 1963; Higaki *et al.*, 1965a,b) postulated that there is a relationship between vitamin D and sulfate metabolism on the basis of their finding of higher amounts of sulfate in tibia of rachitic chicks that had received vitamin D_3. They proposed that chick liver has the requisite enzymes to form vitamin D sulfate. They further claimed to have isolated such a compound in the urine of rabbits that received 5 mg (200,000 IU) of vitamin D_2. In more recent studies (Sahashi *et al.*, 1967a,b) these investigators detected the presence of vitamin D sulfate in milk, and they stated that it has a biological activity equivalent to that of unesterified vitamin D. The significance of these observations is unknown at present; however, they do not form the basis for our understanding of the metabolism of vitamin D to its steroid/or hormonally active form.

B. Discovery of Vitamin D Metabolism

The modern era of the study of vitamin D, which has provided an opportunity to define the biochemical and physiological basis of its action, became possible because of the availability of radioactive vitamin D with high specific activity (see Chapter 3). It is now possible to trace the fate of physiological doses of this steroid and to determine its preferential sites of localization at the tissue, cellular, and subcellular levels. It is possible with many of the available preparations to detect unequivocally the presence of metabolites after administration of a small physiological dose (0.065–0.65 nmole; 1–10 IU) to vitamin D-deficient rats or chicks. However, the detection of new metabolic forms was also dependent on the development of modern chromatographic techniques for separation of the parent vitamin from other chemical forms that were either less polar or more polar than the parent vitamin (see Chapter 3). An important consideration in evaluating the early literature concerning the metabolism of radioactive vitamin D is the specific molecular site in the steroid of the incorporation of labeled component, whether it be tritium or carbon-14. If the radioactive vitamin D is "labeled" in only one specific position, it is possible that a metabolic conversion will release this radioactivity as water, carbon dioxide, or a small organic molecule. In the process the investigator will have lost his tag on the major steroid nucleus. On the other hand, such a specific labeling also has the potential of providing a clear insight into the metabolic step under study.

Kodicek and co-workers (Kodicek, 1956) were the first to demonstrate the metabolism of vitamin D into more polar substances. They reported the existence of breakdown products in the small and large intestine, bone, liver, and feces and stated that all new polar products present were devoid of biological activity. However, the significance of their work is somewhat clouded by the unphysiological doses that they administered to the rats (1 mg, or 40,000 IU).

The first detailed study of the metabolism of physiological doses of vitamin D was carried out by Norman *et al.* (1964) and then extended in independent studies by Lund and DeLuca (1966) and Haussler and Norman (1967). In the studies of Norman *et al.* (1964) and Lund and DeLuca (1966), the methanol–chloroform extraction of intestinal mucosa, kidney, and blood, followed by careful gradient elution chromatography on long columns of silicic acid, indicated that most tissues contained at least four metabolites of vitamin D. Figure 6-1 is a chromatographic profile of the pattern of metabolites present in intestinal mucosa and plasma after administration to rachitic chicks of an intracardial dose of 0.65 nmole (10 IU) of vitamin D_3 15 hr prior to sacrifice. The major metabolite in the plasma designated at that time as peak IV (or 4) was shown by Norman

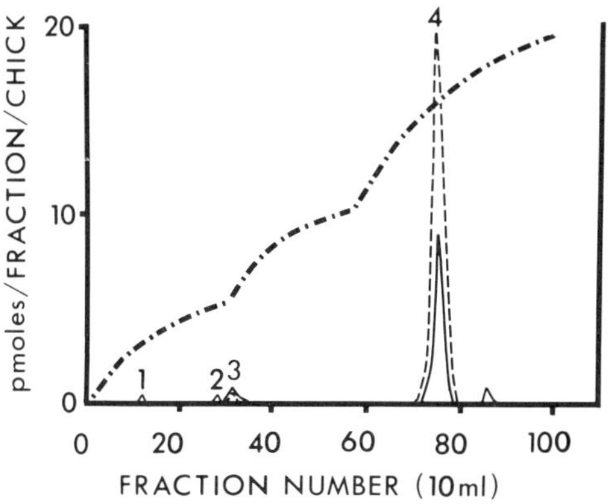

Figure 6-1. Silicic acid chromatography of intestinal and plasma lipids. Separate groups of six chicks each received an intracardial dose of [4-^{14}C]- or [1,2-^{3}H]vitamin D_3 (0.65 nmole; 10 IU) 15 hr before the intestines and plasma from each group were separately extracted for total lipids. The ^{3}H-labeled intestinal lipids were mixed with the ^{14}C-labeled plasma lipids and simultaneously chromatographed on a 30-g (1 × 80 cm) silicic acid column with gradient elution as described by Norman *et al.* (1971c). Peak 3, unmetabolized vitamin D_3; ———, intestine; ---, plasma; –·–·–, gradients.

et al. (1964) and Lund and DeLuca (1966) to have biological activity that ranged from one-half as active to somewhat more active than the parent vitamin D. This was the first clear-cut demonstration of the existence of a biologically active metabolite of vitamin D that was chromatographically distinct from the parent vitamin and that was generated *in vivo*.

Between 1966 and 1971, many papers appeared from the laboratories of DeLuca (in Madison, Wisconsin), Kodicek (in Cambridge, England), Norman (in Riverside, California), and Stanbury (in Manchester, England) concerning the efforts to understand and describe the metabolism of vitamin D. It is difficult to make comparisons of the conclusions proposed by these various research groups since each laboratory used its own characteristic chromatographic separation scheme as well as nomenclature for the as yet uncharacterized metabolites. The Madison group felt that metabolite IV was the most relevant, whereas the Cambridge group felt that peak "P" was deserving of further study. The Riverside group actively supported the actions of metabolite 4B, and the Manchester group of Stanbury supported metabolite V. Figure 6-2 shows a comparison made by Norman *et al.* (1971c) of a lipid sample that was divided into fourths and subjected to the chromatography systems of Madison, Cambridge, Manchester, and Riverside. The lipid sample contained ^{3}H-labeled metabolites from the intestine and ^{14}C-labeled metabolites from the plasma of rachitic chicks administered 0.65 nmole (10 IU) of [^{3}H]vitamin D_3 or [^{14}C]vitamin D_3. Table 6-1 is a summary of the terminology of the separation schemes employed by the four research groups for evaluation of the pattern of metabolites in the intestine. It is apparent that metabolite 4A (Riverside) was synonymous with peak IV (Madison), peak IV (Manchester), and 25-hydroxycholecalciferol (Cambridge); similarly, metabolite 4B (Riverside) was found to be synonymous with peak V (Madison), peak V (Manchester), and peak "P" (Cambridge).

An interesting aspect of the period between 1967 and 1971 concerned the controversy as to whether $25(OH)D_3$ or $1,25(OH)_2D_3$ was the "biologically active form of vitamin D." On the one hand, DeLuca's research group strongly advocated that $25(OH)D_3$, which was the predominant metabolite in the blood, was the active form of vitamin D (DeLuca, 1969a–e), whereas Norman's group in Riverside maintained that the predominant vitamin D metabolite present in the intestine, $1,25(OH)_2D_3$, was the biologically active form of vitamin D (Haussler *et al.*, 1968; Haussler and Norman, 1969; Norman *et al.*, 1969; Myrtle *et al.*, 1970; Myrtle and Norman, 1971a,b). In retrospect, the primary reason for this disagreement related both to the fact that the Madison group focused on blood metabolites and the Riverside group on intestinal metabolites and to the difference in chromatographic techniques employed by the two laboratories (see Fig. 6-2). In 1968 DeLuca's research group (Blunt *et al.*, 1968a,b) isolated and chemically characterized the vitamin D metabolite $25(OH)D_3$; it was isolated in pure form from plasma obtained from pigs that had received massive doses of

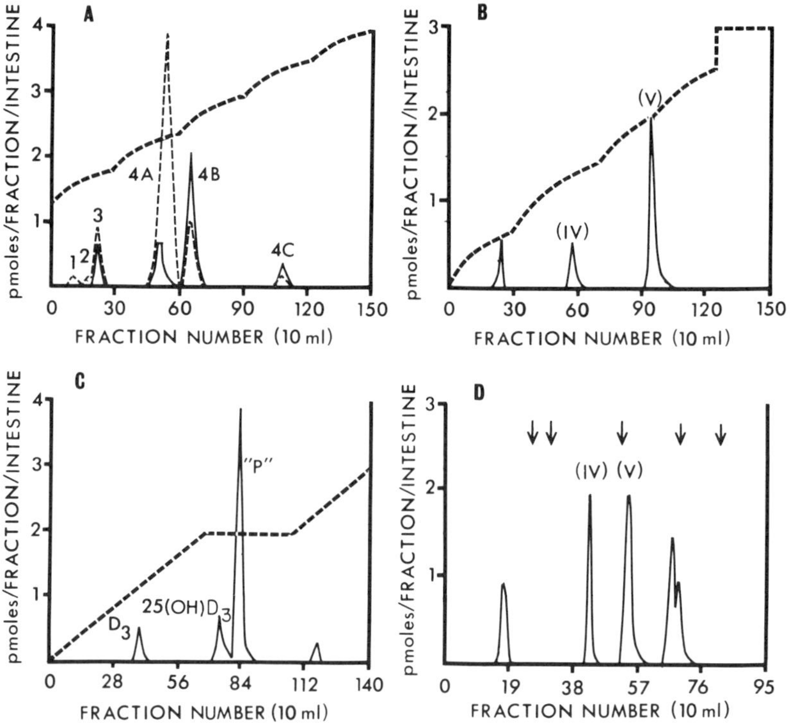

Figure 6-2. Silicic acid chromatography of a standard sample of intestinal lipids in four chromatographic systems. (A) Riverside, elution system III; (B) Madison, elution system IV; (C) Cambridge elution system; and (D) Manchester elution system. A group of 16 rachitic chicks received [4-^{14}C]vitamin D_3 or [1^{3}H]vitamin D_3 (0.65 nmole; 10 IU) 15 hr before sacrifice. After organic solvent extraction of total tissue lipids, the solvent was removed under nitrogen and then replaced with hexane. Equal aliquots were applied to each column. The details of the solvent elution schedule for each elution system are described by Norman *et al.* (1971a). The pattern of intestinal metabolites observed is shown by the solid lines. In (A), plasma lipids, designated by the dashed line, were cochromatographed on the same column (heavy dashed line) gradients. In (D), the successive changes of the solvents used for batch elution are designated by the vertical arrows. All fractions were 10 ml. The results presented here are of historical interest in that in 1968–1969, when these four laboratories were studying the metabolism of vitamin D, there was no consistency of chromatography methodology or terminology; accordingly, there was no agreement concerning the definitive existence of 1,25$(OH)_2D_3$. Taken from Norman *et al.* (1971c).

vitamin D_3 on a regular basis for several weeks. It was quickly shown by Blunt *et al.* (1968b) that the biological activity of 25(OH)D_3 was approximately 1.4 times that of the parent vitamin D in terms of the stimulation of intestinal calcium absorption and bone calcium mobilization. It was not appreciated by the Madison research group that 25(OH)D_3 was not the predominant vitamin D metabolite in the intestine at the time of initiation of biological response (see Fig. 6-3). In part

TABLE 6-1
Terminology of Separation Schemes for Intestinal Metabolites of Vitamin D_3[a]

Gradient system	Laboratory	Reference	Peak		Amount of metabolites (pmoles/g mucosa)	
			4A [25(OH)D_3]	4B [1,25$(OH)_2D_3$]	4A [25(OH)D_3]	4B [1,25$(OH)_2D_3$]
II	Riverside (Norman and associates)	Norman *et al.* (1969), Haussler *et al.* (1968)	4A	4B	3.2	8.4
III	Madison (DeLuca and associates)	DeLuca (1969a,d)	Peak IV	Peak V	2.6	7.8
IV	Cambridge (Kodicek and associates)	Lawson *et al.* (1969c, 1971b)	25(OH)D_3	Peak "P"	3.2	6.5
V	Manchester (Stanbury and associates)	Mawer *et al.* (1969, 1971a)	Peak IV	Peak V	2.6	7.8

[a] All chromatographic systems were set up according to published procedures; aliquots of the same sample of chick intestinal metabolites obtained 15 hr after 10 IU of [^{14}C]vitamin D_3 were chromatographed in each.

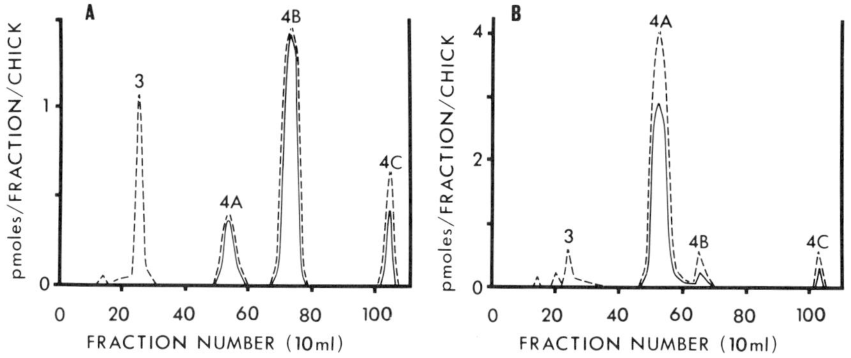

Figure 6-3. Silicic acid chromatography of intestinal (A) and plasma (B) lipids of chicks receiving 25(OH)[4-^{14}C]D_3 and [1,2-^{3}H]vitamin D_3. One group of 4 chicks each received 0.26 nmole of 25(OH)[4-^{14}C]D_3 intracardially 15 hr prior to being killed. A second group of 11 chicks received 0.65 nmole (10 IU) of [1,2-^{3}H]vitamin D_3 16 hr prior to being killed and was utilized as a control. Both intestinal lipid samples (A) and both plasma lipid samples (B) were combined and chromatographed on silicic acid columns as described by Myrtle *et al.* (1970). Peak 3 is unmetabolized vitamin D_3; ---, ^{3}H from vitamin D_3; ———, ^{14}C from metabolite 4A [25(OH)D_3]. Metabolite 4B is now known to be 1,25$(OH)_2D_3$.

this was due to the inability of the chromatographic systems to clearly resolve 25(OH)D_3 and 1,25$(OH)_2D_3$ from one another as well as to the Madison group's enthusiasm for the properties of the first chemically characterized metabolite of vitamin D. However, as is apparent in Fig. 6-3, the pattern of vitamin D metabolites in the intestine differs radically from that in the plasma. In the plasma the major species is peak 4A, or 25(OH)D_3; in the intestine it is metabolite 4B, or 1,25$(OH)_2D_3$. In 1970 (Ponchon *et al.*, 1970) the Madison group acknowledged that 1,25$(OH)_2D_3$ might be the biologically active form of vitamin D in the intestine.

A second interesting aspect in the series of developments during the period from 1967 to 1971, which resulted in the ultimate chemical characterization of 1,25$(OH)_2D_3$, was the discovery of the Cambridge research group that their peak "P" metabolite incurred a loss of tritium in its production. When a mixed dose of [1,2-^{3}H]vitamin D_3 and [4-^{14}C]vitamin D_3 was administered to rachitic rats or chicks, with an initial $^{14}C/^{3}H$ ratio of 1.0, the $^{14}C/^{3}H$ ratio present in their peak "P" metabolite increased to 3.0, a value that was consistent with a 60% loss of tritium. Furthermore, the 25(OH)D_3 in plasma had no measurable tritium loss (Lawson *et al.*, 1969c, 1971b). Most importantly the Cambridge group noted, in agreement with reports of the Riverside group, that the peak "P" metabolite in the intestinal mucosa was associated principally with the intestinal cell nuclei (Lawson *et al.*, 1969a). As could be predicted there was a highly significant loss of tritium in the nuclear localized peak "P" metabolite such that the $^{14}C/^{3}H$ ratio was elevated to 5.5. Similar data obtained by Myrtle and Norman (1971b) are shown in Table 6-2. It is apparent that both the peak "P" metabolite and metabolite 4B undergo an approximate 40% loss of tritium from the starting dose of [1,2-^{3}H]vitamin D_3 that was originally administered. Bell and Kodicek (1970) had evaluated the percent distribution of total tritium in the 1α (47%), 1β (15%), and $2\alpha,2\beta$ (36%) positions of [^{3}H]vitamin D_3, suggesting that the structure of the metabolites in peak "P" and 4B, which were known to be derived from 25(OH)D_3, had an additional oxygen functionality incorporated at C-1; thus, the investigators from Riverside and Cambridge proposed that the structure of their vitamin D polar metabolites was 1,25$(OH)_2D_3$ (Lawson *et al.*, 1971a; Myrtle and Norman, 1971b).

A third important observation made concerning vitamin D metabolism in 1968–1971 by both the Riverside (Haussler *et al.*, 1968; Haussler and Norman, 1969; Myrtle *et al.*, 1970) and Cambridge groups (Lawson *et al.*, 1969a,b,c) was that metabolite 4B and peak "P" metabolite were localized in the nuclear and chromatin fraction of the intestinal mucosa. As discussed in detail in Chapter 7, this observation provides one of the bases for the proposal that the mode of action of 1,25$(OH)_2D_3$ is like that of other steroid hormones. Since it was already known by 1968 that the response to vitamin D could be inhibited by actinomycin D and that vitamin D was capable of stimulating the biosynthesis of RNA in the intestinal mucosa (see Fig. 7-15), it was not unreasonable for the Riverside and

TABLE 6-2
Tritium Loss during the Metabolism of a Mixed Dose of [1,2-^{3}H] and [4-^{14}C]Cholecalciferol[a,b]

Tissue	Dose	$^{3}H/^{14}C$ ratio: D_3	25(OH)D_3	1,25$(OH)_2D_3$	Loss of tritium in 1,25$(OH)_2D_3$
Chick					
Intestine	3.22	3.13	3.07	1.75	46
Skeleton	3.22	3.15	3.13	1.93	40
Blood	3.22	3.10	3.21	3.40	0
Kidney	3.22	2.92	3.02	1.72	47
Rat					
Intestine	3.22	3.19	3.19	1.90	41
Blood	3.22	3.23	3.18	2.57	20

[a]Taken from Myrtle and Norman (1971b).

[b]Rachitic chicks received a mixed dose of 0.065 nmole of [1,2-^{3}H]vitamin D_3 (Amersham/Searle, Inc.) and 0.58 nmole of [4-^{14}C]vitamin D_3. Vitamin D-deficient rats received 0.13 and 1.17 nmole, respectively, of the identical steroids. Silicic acid chromatography resolved the tissue radioactivity into the parent metabolite cholecalciferol (D_3) and 4B [1,25$(OH)_2D_3$]. The ratios in several minor metabolites also resolved are not shown here.

TABLE 6-3
Relative Biological Activities of Vitamin D_3, $25(OH)D_3$, and $1,25(OH)_2D_3$ in Stimulating Intestinal Calcium Transport and Bone Calcium Mobilization *in Vivo*

Steroid tested	Activity relative to an equivalent amount of vitamin D_3	
	Bone calcium mobilization[a] (±S.E.M.)	Intestinal calcium absorption[b] (±S.E.M.)
$1,25(OH)_2D_3$	5.47±1.36 (3)	4.74±1.09 (3)
$25(OH)D_3$	1.53±0.20 (3)	1.78±0.23 (3)
D_3	1.0	1.0

[a]Taken from Wong *et al.* (1972b).
[b]Taken from Myrtle and Norman (1971a).

Cambridge research groups to strongly support the view that their as yet chemically uncharacterized metabolite was the biologically active form of vitamin D in the intestine.

A most important facet of the problem concerned the biological activity of the peak "P" metabolite and metabolite 4B. Norman's laboratory was the first to report that metabolite 4B was "significantly more active" than the parent vitamin D (Haussler *et al.*, 1968). This was followed by the more quantitative study of Myrtle and Norman (1971a), who stated that their metabolite 4B [$1,25(OH)_2D_3$] was a minimum of 4.7 ± 1.1 (S.D.) times more active than the parent vitamin D in stimulating the intestinal absorption of calcium; these data are summarized in Table 6-3. Another important property of metabolite 4B [$1,25(OH)_2D_3$] was that it greatly shortened the lag in time between administration of the dose and development of maximal response of intestinal calcium absorption; for $1,25(OH)_2D_3$ the lag was only 9–12 hr, whereas for the parent vitamin D and intermediate $25(OH)D_3$ the lag was at least 24–48 hr. These important data are summarized in Fig. 6-4. Similar supportive results were forthcoming from the laboratories of both Rasmussen (Haussler *et al.*, 1971) and Kodicek (Kodicek *et al.*, 1970).

On the basis of the data available in 1970, both peak "P" metabolite and metabolite 4B satisfied all identifiable prerequisites of being the "active form" of vitamin D in the target organ, the intestine: (a) It was the most biologically active form of vitamin D known; (b) it was the predominant metabolite of vitamin D in the intestine after administration of a physiological dose of vitamin D; (c) it acted considerably faster than either $25(OH)D_3$ or the parent vitamin D in stimulating intestinal calcium transport; and (d) it localized in the nucleus of the intestine, a location consistent with its proposed steroid hormone mode of action and with the observation that actinomycin D was capable of blocking the biological response to vitamin D.

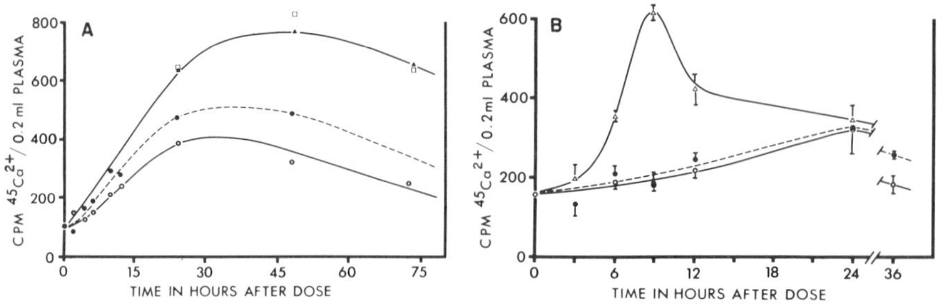

Figure 6-4. Time course of the intestinal calcium transport response after administration of $1,25(OH)_2D_3$. Transport was assayed as described by Myrtle and Norman (1970). In (A), the compounds assayed were dissolved in 1,2-propanediol and administered intracardially: ○, 10 IU (0.65 nmole) of vitamin D_3; ●, 10 IU of $25(OH)D_3$; , 50 IU of vitamin D_3; ▲, 50 IU (325 nmoles) of vitamin D_3. In (B), the compounds were administered orally: ○, 5 IU of vitamin D_3; ●, 5 units (0.325 nmole) of $25(OH)D_3$; △, 1.8 units (0.117 nmole) of metabolite $1,25(OH)_2D_3$. Each point represents the average ± S.E. for $^{45}Ca^{2+}$ absorption of three to five chicks. (Copyright by the American Association for the Advancement of Science.)

Thus, the modern era of vitamin D research came into full bloom with the simultaneous yet independent reports from three laboratories that the chemical structure of metabolites "P", 4B, and V was in fact $1,25(OH)_2D_3$ (Lawson *et al.*, 1971b; Norman *et al.*, 1971a; Holick *et al.*, 1971). Detailed in Chapter 4 are the data supporting the chemical characterization of the five vitamin D metabolites: $25(OH)D_3$, $1,25(OH)_2D_3$, $24,25(OH)_2D_3$, $25,26(OH)_2D_3$, and $1,24,25(OH)_3D_3$.

II. VITAMIN D

A. Photochemical Production

Hess and Weinstock (1922) were the first to show that an antirachitic substance was produced in the skin when it was irradiated with ultraviolet light. Goldblatt and Soames (1923) reported that the antirachitic substance produced in the skin by ultraviolet irradiation could be transported to other parts of the body. Ultimately, Windaus and Bock (1936) were able to isolate and chemically characterize 7-dehydrocholesterol from organic solvent extracts of pigskin. Bunker *et al.* (1940) reported that uv light of wavelength of 297 nm was equally effective in curing rickets in rats and activating 7-dehydrocholesterol under *in vitro* conditions. This result strongly suggests that the natural precursor of vitamin D in mammals is 7-dehydrocholesterol. Recently, Holick *et al.* (1977a,b) reported results of experiments in which 7-[3α,3-^{3}H]dehydrocholesterol was topically applied to the epidermis of shaved rats. These animals then were irradiated with uv light; 24 hr later Holick *et al.* succeeded in isolating and chemically characterizing radioactive previtamin D_3. This important result suggests that the photochemical pathway for conversion of 7-dehydrocholesterol to vitamin D_3 *in vivo* is very similar to that which occurs *in vitro* in the organic chemistry laboratory. One point of speculation concerns the possible physiological advantage of the relatively slow "dark" conversion of previtamin D_3 to vitamin D_3. Table 3-2 documents that at 40°C the equilibrium ratio of vitamin D_3 to previtamin D_3 is 89:11. Furthermore, the time required to achieve equilibrium starting with 100% previtamin D_3 is 8–12 hr at 40°C (Hanewald *et al.*, 1961). Thus, the animal requires only intermittent exposure of his epidermal 7-dehydrocholesterol to ultraviolet light to ensure a continuous delivery of vitamin D_3 to the systemic circulation. These photochemical "facts of life" concerning previtamin D_3-vitamin D_3 interconversions undoubtedly provide advantageous benefits to the animal by ensuring a continuous supply of the vitamin even in the absence of ultraviolet exposure.

There has been some question concerning the exact route of absorption of vitamin D produced in the epidermis. Some investigators have proposed that it is resorbed through the basal layers of the squamous tissue, whereas others have held that it is absorbed only via an animal licking his skin or fur or via birds' preening activities. In an early report Rekling (1927) claimed that rats who were prevented from licking their fur were not protected from rickets by ultraviolet irradiation. Similarly, Hou in a series of papers (1927, 1929, 1930, 1931) reported that chicks who had their preen glands surgically removed were not protected from rickets by ultraviolet light. The claims of these early workers have fallen into disfavor as a consequence of more recent experimentation. Knoles (1935) presented evidence contradictory to that of Hou in that he found that chicks without preen glands were protected from rickets by exposure to ultraviolet light. Also, Koch and Koch (1941) found, via biological activity measurements, significant quantities of vitamin D activity in chick skin, whereas none was present in either the feathers or preen glands of birds that had been irradiated. Ponsold and Pfennigsdorf (1954) showed that antirachitic activity that is produced in the skin as a consequence of external ultraviolet irradiation is absorbed through the basal layers of the skin rather than via oral ingestion.

As yet there are not many quantitative reports concerning the production capability of skin that is exposed to defined energies of light at defined wavelengths. The only papers are those of Bekemeier and co-workers (Bekemeier, 1958, 1959; Bekemeier and Pfennigsdorf, 1959), who reported surprisingly high yields of vitamin D in explants of skin that were exposed to ultraviolet light under defined conditions. As deduced from its antirachitic potency, egg yolk contains significant quantities of vitamin D (see Table 13-2). Fraser and Emtage (1976) presented evidence obtained from radiochemical tracer studies that the specific transport of vitamin D_3 to the egg yolk is mediated by the vitamin D-binding protein, transcalciferin, present in the blood (see Chapter 8).

B. Possible Nonphotochemical Production

As reported in Tables 3-1 and 13-2, there are strikingly large quantities of vitamin D in the oil extracts prepared from the livers of various species of fish. Inasmuch as most of these species have a habitat in seawater well below the penetration level of ultraviolet rays from sunlight, a most interesting question concerns the source of this vitamin D. Steenbock and Black (1925) first suggested that these high levels of vitamin D in fish liver were due to the ingestion of phytoplankton or plankton that had been irradiated at the surface by sunlight. However, biological assays of plankton extracts have failed to show high enough vitamin D activity to support the view that this plant material serves as a source of fish vitamin D.

On the basis of extensive nutritional and biochemical studies (carried out without the availability of radioactive vitamin D preparations), Bills (1954) proposed that fish can biosynthesize vitamin D by a nonphotochemical process. More recently, Nes and co-workers examined the possible enzymatic conversion of radioactive 7-dehydrocholesterol to vitamin D by liver homogenates obtained from various species of fish. They synthesized 7-[4-^{14}C]dehydrocholesterol (Kulkarni *et al.*, 1963) and incubated it with homogenates of liver obtained from Atlantic striped bass, obtaining preliminary evidence that there was a modest nonphotochemical production of vitamin D by this enzyme system (Blondin *et al.*, 1967). In separate studies, Ozumi and Monder (1972) were able to detect neither enzymatic, nonphotochemical production of vitamin D in the goldfish nor further metabolism of radioactive vitamin D or 25(OH)D_3. Still later studies by Sugisaki *et al.* (1974) involving goldfish (*Carassius auratus* L.) that had been injected with DL-[2-^{14}C]mevalonate or with sodium[1,2-^{14}C]acetate also gave no evidence of metabolic conversion and incorporation of radioactivity into vitamin D over a 10-day period while the fish were maintained in the dark.

It is apparent that considerable additional work is required to define the existence of a nonphotochemical pathway for the production of vitamin D (or possibly its metabolites) as well as to identify the biochemical mechanism by which this transformation might occur.

C. Intestinal Absorption

Considerable effort has been exerted to identify the pathway of intestinal absorption of vitamin D that has been orally ingested. An understanding of this process was deemed to be of importance particularly in the era during which vitamin D was believed to be an essential trace dietary constituent, i.e., a legitimate vitamin. However, with the acceptance of the more modern view that vitamin D is in reality a steroid hormone and with particular appreciation of the fact that adequate amounts of vitamin D can be produced by daily exposure of small portions of the skin to ultraviolet light, there is little necessity for presuming that the body has evolved a detailed absorption mechanism for the steroid.

Greaves and Schmidt (1933) were the first to demonstrate the need for bile salts to facilitate the intestinal absorption of vitamin D; Heymann (1937a,b) obtained confirmatory data supporting this view. Somewhat later Schachter *et al.* (1964), using low specific activity radioactive vitamin D that was placed in a solution of ethanol and propylene glycol in a ligated intestinal loop, concluded that vitamin D is absorbed largely from the jejunum of the rat, principally via the lymphatic system, and ultimately carried by the chylomicrons into the bloodstream. Norman and DeLuca (1963) administered physiological doses of high specific activity radioactive vitamin D in vegetable oil to rachitic rats and obtained evidence suggesting that the ileum was the primary site of absorption of vitamin D in the rat.

Rosenstreich *et al.* (1971) reported that vitamin D is absorbed throughout the complete small intestinal tract in the baboon. Hollander and Truscott (1976) studied the site and mechanism of the initial uptake of radioactive vitamin D present in pharmacological concentrations (0.3 m*M*) in everted sacs prepared from rat intestine. Their results indicate that vitamin D is taken up by the intestinal epithelial cells by means of a nonsaturable passive diffusion mechanism; the highest rate of uptake was associated with the duodenum and jejunum.

D. Vitamin D 25-Hydroxylase

1. Localization and Properties of the Enzyme

After the isolation and chemical characterization by Blunt *et al.* (1968a,b) of $25(OH)D_3$ from porcine plasma, attention turned to identification of the site of production of this vitamin D metabolite. It was known from the earlier work of Norman and DeLuca (1963) with rats as well as from the studies of Avioli *et al.* (1967a,b) on human beings that, after intravenous administration of radioactive vitamin D_3, the plasma radioactivity falls rapidly within 20–40 min and then "rebounds" to a high level before assuming a regular decay curve. Particularly on the basis of the rat data, it appeared that uptake of vitamin D by the liver was occurring. These results anticipated the clear demonstration by Ponchon and DeLuca (1969) that the liver was capable of mediating the hydroxylation of vitamin D_3 to form $25(OH)D_3$. Subsequently, Ponchon *et al.* (1969) surgically isolated the liver from the circulatory system and almost completely eliminated the rat's ability to produce $25(OH)D_3$; this technique reduced by 90% the circulating levels of $25(OH)D_3$ produced after administration of an intravenous dose of [^{3}H]vitamin D_3. More recently Olson *et al.* (1976), by utilization of the surgical technique of hepatectomy, obtained confirmatory evidence that in the rat the liver is probably the sole site of production of $25(OH)D_3$. Since it is not possible to carry out a total hepatectomy in vitamin D-deficient rats and keep the animals alive for the duration of a biological assay, it is not possible to definitively test this premise.

Tucker *et al.* (1973), who worked with rachitic chicks, reported that there was evidence of low 25-hydroxylation activity in the intestine and kidney as well as in the liver. In spite of these observations, it is now generally accepted that the liver is the tissue responsible for the production of 25(OH)D.

Some biochemical characteristics of the vitamin D 25-hydroxylase have been described. However, in relation to the current understanding of the biochemistry of renal hydroxylation processes, the present level of understanding of the 25-hydroxylase is minimal. Direct confirmation of the presence of vitamin D 25-hydroxylase enzymatic activity in liver tissue was obtained by Horsting and DeLuca (1969), who incubated homogenates of liver tissue with [^{3}H]vitamin D and detected chromatographically the presence of very small quantities of tritiated 25(OH)D_3. The 25-hydroxylation process was found to be stimulated by molecular oxygen in the presence of NADPH. Horsting (1970) reported that the enzyme activity was associated with the liver mitochondrial fraction, that the Michaelis constant K_m for vitamin D was 3×10^{-8} *M*, that the pH optimum was 6.9 and that the enzyme was not inhibited by the presence of carbon monoxide.

Subsequently, Bhattacharyya and DeLuca (1974a) presented clear evidence that the vitamin D 25-hydroxylase activity was instead associated with the liver microsomal and not the mitochondrial fraction of the cell. The enzyme reaction clearly requires the presence of NADPH and molecular oxygen. Cinti *et al.* (1976) presented spectral evidence that a microsomal NADPH-cytochrome *P*-450 reductase enzyme system is associated with the biotransformation of vitamin D to 25(OH)D_3. This suggests that vitamin D metabolism by the liver occurs via a mixed-function oxidase system, a common means of hydroxylation of many steroids and drugs. An explanation for the conflicting views on the subcellular localization of the vitamin D 25-hydroxylase activity was provided by Bjorkhen and Holmberg (1978). They established that both purified mitochondrial and microsomal fractions from rat liver had the enzymatic capacity to 25-hydroxylate vitamin D_3. However, the greatest proportion of the activity was associated with the mitochondria. To date, however, no isolation or purification of the vitamin D 25-hydroxylase system has been reported.

2. *Regulation of Vitamin D 25-Hydroxylase*

An interesting endocrinological aspect of the conversion of vitamin D to 25(OH)D_3 concerns the possibility that this enzymatic step is subject to physiological regulation. Bhattacharyya and DeLuca (1973, 1974a,b) reported that the 25-hydroxylase is subject to regulation in the rat and the chick. Thus, a rat that has received abundant dietary quantities of vitamin D_3 will not convert the same proportion of D_3 to 25(OH)D_3 as a rat that has not received vitamin D_3. From their studies in the chick, Bhattacharyya and DeLuca (1974a) concluded that regulation of the 25-hydroxylase occurs as a consequence of a direct feedback by vitamin D; however, the biochemical basis of this effect was not elucidated. In contrast, Tucker *et al.* (1973) were not able to demonstrate any regulation of $25(OH)D_3$ production in the chick by variations in the dietary intake of vitamin D_3.

More recently, Rojanasathit and Haddad (1976) in studies in the rat found that serum $25(OH)D_3$ levels did not influence any "feedback" regulation of the 25-hydroxylase but, rather, only reflected the activity of this enzyme.

Sulimovici and Roginsky (1976) found that the liver 25-hydroxylase of vitamin D-deficient rats was enhanced 24 hr after the injection of N^6-2-*O*-dibutyryladenosine 3′, 5′-monophosphate (an analogue of cyclic AMP). These provocative results, which suggest the capacity for regulation of the vitamin D 25-hydroxylase, have not yet been confirmed in other laboratories.

Sulimovici and Roginsky (1977) also reported that chronic administration of the anticonvulsants phenobarbital or diphenylhydantoin *in vivo* inhibits rat liver 25-hydroxylase. These results may be relevant to anticonvulsant-induced osteomalacia (see Chapter 13), which occurs in man.

One interesting system, which has been the subject of only minimal study, is the metabolism of vitamin D by avian embryos. Fraser and Emtage (1976) injected [^{3}H]vitamin D_3 into fertile chick eggs and found that the bulk of the steroid remained unchanged although there was limited metabolism to $25(OH)D_3$.

Available observations in man concerning the regulated production of $25(OH)D_3$ are less certain, largely because it is impossible to be absolutely sure of the levels of vitamin D_3 ingested or produced in the skin. Mawer and coworkers (1971b) reported that a greater fraction of vitamin D is converted to a more polar metabolite, which they believe to be $25(OH)D_3$, in vitamin D-deficient subjects than in patients who have received substantial quantities of vitamin D. Hahn *et al.* (1972) found increased plasma levels of 25(OH)D, as measured by a steroid displacement binding assay, in subjects receiving larger quantities of vitamin D. These data imply that a certain fraction of added vitamin D was converted to $25(OH)D_3$ and are consistent with the view that this metabolic step is not particularly stringently regulated. Similar results were reported by Haddad and Stamp (1974).

III. 25-HYDROXYVITAMIN D

A. 25-Hydroxyvitamin D 1-Hydroxylase

1. Localization and Properties of the Enzyme

Aside from the extensive efforts required to chemically characterize the eight known metabolites of vitamin D, clearly the most outstanding discovery made in the modern era of vitamin D research was the identification of the kidney as the site of production of 1,25$(OH)_2D_3$. Fraser and Kodicek (1970) were the first to report the unique biosynthesis by the kidney of their biologically active vitamin D metabolite known as peak "P." In a nephrectomized rat, there was no conversion of [^{3}H]vitamin D_3 to metabolite peak "P." These investigators were able to detect the production of this substance by incubation of homogenates of chick kidney with their preparation of [4-^{14}C,1-^{3}H]vitamin D_3 and to observe the characteristic "tritium loss" that had been previously reported to be associated with the intestinal polar metabolite. They did not, however, demonstrate that this kidney-produced metabolite that was "deficient in tritium" had the biological activity characteristic of the intestinal metabolite "P." Virtually simultaneously, Norman *et al.* (1971b) reported the results of incubations of 25(OH)[26,27-^{3}H]D_3 with homogenates of intestine, kidney, bone, and liver (see Fig. 6-5A). Only the kidney homogenate produced a ^{3}H-labeled metabolite that exactly comigrated in silicic acid chromatography with their intestinal metabolite 4B produced *in vivo*. As shown in Fig. 6-5B the intestinal metabolite 4B and the kidney-derived metabolite 4B exactly comigrated in two separate chromatographic systems. The kidney is now considered to be the sole source of this important vitamin D metabolite. Most significantly, Norman *et al.* (1971b) were the first to demonstrate that this metabolite produced from kidney homogenate

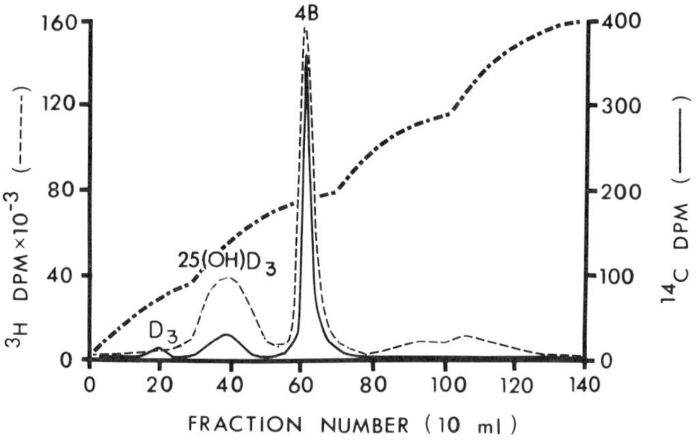

Figure 6-5A. Silicic acid chromatography of ^{3}H-labeled metabolites produced *in vitro* from a kidney homogenate and ^{14}C-labeled metabolites obtained from chick intestines *in vivo*. A kidney homogenate was incubated with 25(OH)[26,27-^{3}H]D_3 as described by Norman *et al.* (1971b). The homogenate lipids were extracted and cochromatographed on a 30-g silicic acid column with intestinal lipids obtained from rachitic chicks that had received 0.65 nmole (10 IU) of [4-^{14}C]vitamin D_3 intracardially 17 hr prior to sacrifice. Metabolites were eluted with successive exponential gradients of diethyl ether, 50% (v/v) 1,2-dichloroethane, acetone, and methanol. (———) ^{14}C; (---) ^{3}H; (—-—-—) gradients.

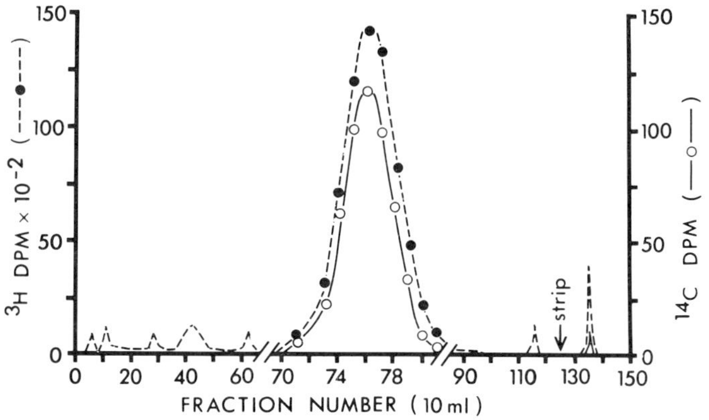

Figure 6-5B. Cochromatography of ^{3}H-labeled metabolite 4B [$1,25(OH)_2D_3$] (*in vitro*) and ^{14}C-labeled metabolite 4B [$1,25(OH)_2D_3$] (*in vivo*). The metabolites produced *in vitro* and *in vivo* were obtained from a silicic acid column exactly as described in Fig. 6-5A and applied to a 20-g celite liquid-liquid partition column, as described by Norman *et al.* (1971b). Stripping of the column with 100% 1,2-dichloroethane was started with the collection of fraction 125.

incubations *in vitro* had biological activity in terms of stimulating intestinal calcium absorption. More specifically, this metabolite 4B [$1,25(OH)_2D_3$] produced *in vitro* was over four times as active as the parent vitamin D_3 (Myrtle and Norman, 1971a; Norman *et al.*, 1971b). Also, during this period of time, similar reports were emanating from the Madison and Manchester research groups. Gray *et al.* (1971) reported that the kidney was the principal locus of production of their metabolite V. They also demonstrated that in an anephric animal it was not the associated uremia that resulted in the inability to produce the new polar metabolite, but rather it was the absence of the kidney. Also, Mawer *et al.* (1971b) found that their metabolite peak "P" had no "tritium loss" when it was obtained from the plasma of nephrectomized rats.

There have been few instances in calcium- and phosphorus-related research as dramatic as those surrounding the discovery that the biologically active form of vitamin D is produced by the kidney. The most important concept to emerge is that there is, in reality, an endocrine system for processing vitamin D and that the kidney is the crucial endocrine gland charged with the responsibility of producing and secreting the biologically active form, $1,25(OH)_2D_3$. The classic method of demonstrating that an organ has an endocrine role in the economy of the organism is to create a deficit of its hormone by surgical removal or chemical inactivation of the organ in question. With regard to vitamin D and its highly biologically active $1,25(OH)_2D_3$, this criterion was satisfied by the observations of Fraser and Kodicek (1970), Gray *et al.* (1971), and Wong *et al.* (1972a). The results from the last-named group are shown in Fig. 6-6. These workers administered physiological doses of vitamin D_3, $25(OH)D_3$, or $1,25(OH)_2D_3$ to vitamin

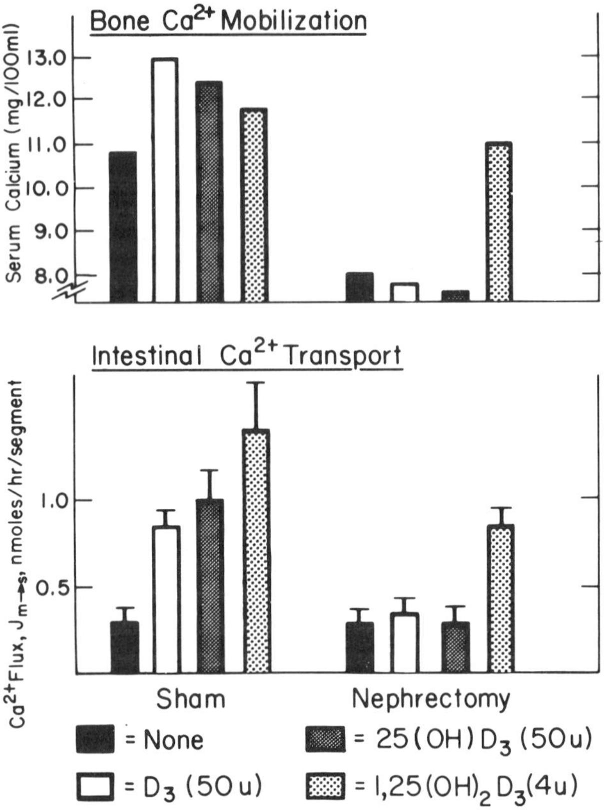

Figure 6-6. Inhibition of biological responses to vitamin D_3 and 25(OH)D_3 but not 1,25(OH)$_2$$D_3$ by nephrectomy in the rat. Groups of vitamin D-deficient rats were subjected to either sham or bilateral nephrectomy. Then the indicated dose of vitamin D steroid was administered, and the biological response of intestinal calcium absorption or bone calcium mobilization was measured 24 hr later. From Wong *et al.* (1972a).

D-deficient rats that had undergone either a sham operation or total nephrectomy. In the absence of the kidneys only 1,25(OH)$_2$$D_3$ was capable of initiating the classic biological responses of vitamin D: stimulation of intestinal calcium absorption and mobilization of bone calcium (measured by elevation of serum calcium). In the absence of the kidney, vitamin D_3 and 25(OH)D_3 in moderate doses were both completely devoid of biological activity. These observations demonstrate that a deficit of the biologically active (hormonally active) form of vitamin D can be created by surgical removal of the kidneys and that this deficit can be overcome by administration of the steroid hormone 1,25(OH)$_2$$D_3$, and they support the concept that the kidney is the endocrine organ for the production of this hormonally active form of vitamin D. When these results were coupled with the further critical evaluation of the biological activity properties of $1,25(OH)_2D_3$, there was full support for this view. Myrtle and Norman (1971a) and Norman and Wong (1972) reported that $1,25(OH)_2D_3$ is 13–15 times as effective as vitamin D in stimulating the intestinal absorption of calcium and 5–6 times as effective as the parent vitamin in stimulating serum calcium elevation. When $1,25(OH)_2D_3$ was administered on a daily basis for 3 weeks, it was at least as active if not more active than the parent vitamin D in terms of every parameter tested (bone ash, serum calcium, and rate of growth) (Norman and Wong, 1972).

In view of the foregoing developments it has been appropriate to invest a considerable effort to understand the biochemical properties of the 25-hydroxyvitamin D_3 1-hydroxylase. Because of the exquisitely complicated anatomical and morphological relationships in the kidney, an intriguing problem was the determination of the precise localization of this enzyme. The initial report of Fraser and Kodicek (1970) suggested that the enzyme activity was associated with either the crude nuclear or heavy mitochondrial fraction of the cell. It has now been clearly shown by Gray *et al.* (1972) as well as Midgett *et al.* (1973) that the $25(OH)D_3$ 1-hydroxylase is exclusively associated with the mitochondrial fraction of the kidney. Furthermore, Midgett *et al.* (1973) reported that the enzymatic production of $1,25(OH)_2D_3$ was found only in the renal cortex of rat, man, and dog but was absent from the renal medulla. There are many other precedents for steroid hydroxylation reactions being localized subcellularly in the mitochondria, such as the side-chain cleavage of cholesterol to form pregnenolone and 11β-hydroxylation of 11-deoxycortisol to form cortisol in the adrenal cortex (Cooper *et al.*, 1968).

Ghazarian *et al.* (1973), through the use of ^{18}O, demonstrated that the source of the oxygen introduced into the 1α position of $25(OH)D_3$ was molecular oxygen rather than water. This observation clearly demonstrated that the $25(OH)D_3$ 1-hydroxylase was a "mixed-function oxidase." Mixed-function oxidases catalyze the consumption of one molecule of oxygen (O_2) per molecule of substrate; one atom of the oxygen molecule appears in the product, and the other is reduced to water by a hydrogen donor other than the substrate, usually NADPH. In an important study, Henry and Norman (1974) described the development of an enzyme assay that was capable of detecting initial reaction velocities of the 1-hydroxylase as low as 0.2 pmole/min. The level of the 1-hydroxylase enzyme activity was found to vary over a 6- to 10-fold range, depending on whether the kidney mitochondria were isolated from vitamin D-deficient or vitamin D-replete chicks; the K_m for $25(OH)D_3$ was $1–2 \times 10^{-7}$ M in both mitochondrial preparations (see Fig. 6-7). Malate and succinate were the most effective electron donors for the hydroxylation process. The pattern of inhibition of 1-hydroxylase activity seen in the presence of antimycin, rotenone, oligomycin, and cyanide,

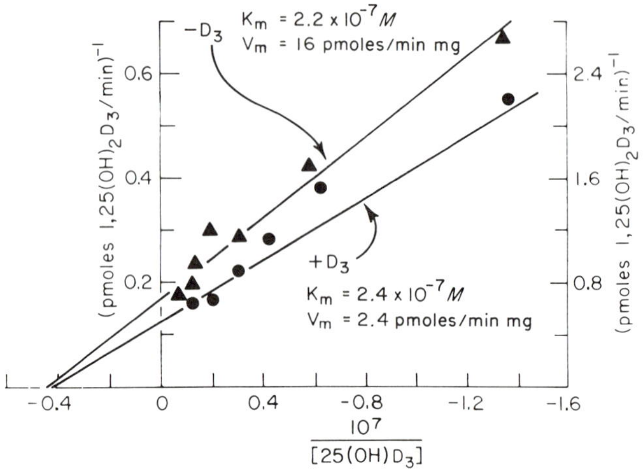

Figure 6-7. Determination of Michaelis constant for $25(OH)D_3$ for chick kidney $25(OH)D_3$ 1-hydroxylase. The determination was carried out separately in kidney mitochondria obtained from vitamin D-deficient or vitamin D-replete chicks, as described by Henry and Norman (1974).

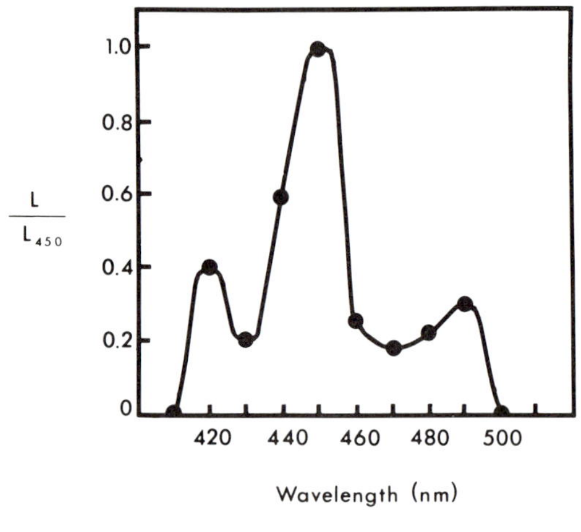

Figure 6-8A. Photochemical action spectrum of $25(OH)D_3$ 1-hydroxylase. Initial rates of mitochondrial 1-hydroxylase activity were determined as described by Henry and Norman (1976) under an atmosphere of 20% O_2, 40% CO, and 40% N_2 in the absence or presence of light of the indicated wavelength. A noninhibited control, 20% O_2 and 80% N_2, was run in each experiment. The light sensitivity factor L at each wavelength was determined from the equation

$$L = [(K_1 - K_d)/K_1](1/I)$$

where K_1 and K_D are the partition constants in the presence and absence of light, respectively, and I is the relative light intensity at the given wavelength. Results are expressed as the value of L at each wavelength relative to that at 450 nm.

when malate or succinate and intact mitochondria were employed, was consistent with the concept that the 1-hydroxylase is similar to many other steroid mixed-function oxidases.

Although previous workers (Fraser and Kodicek, 1970; Gray *et al.*, 1972) had suggested that the 1-hydroxylase activity was sensitive to inhibition by carbon monoxide, no detailed data supporting this interaction were presented. Henry and Norman (1974) determined unequivocally that the partition coefficient (K), a measure of the sensitivity of the enzyme to carbon monoxide, for CO inhibition of the 1-hydroxylase was 1.0, a value quite comparable to that of other steroidogenic hydroxylases (see Fig. 6-8B). Furthermore, and most importantly, the wavelength of light most effective in reversing CO inhibition was 450 nm. This was the first direct, unequivocal evidence for the involvement of cytochrome P-450 with the renal 1-hydroxylase (Fig. 6-8A). The minor peaks in the photochemical action spectra given in Fig. 6-8A at 420 and 490 nm have also been reported for the adrenal cholesterol side-chain cleavage system (Simpson and Boyd, 1967) and for liver microsomal taurodeoxycholic acid 7α-hydroxylase (Trulzsch *et al.*, 1973). Ultimately, Ghazarian *et al.* (1974) and Pedersen *et al.*

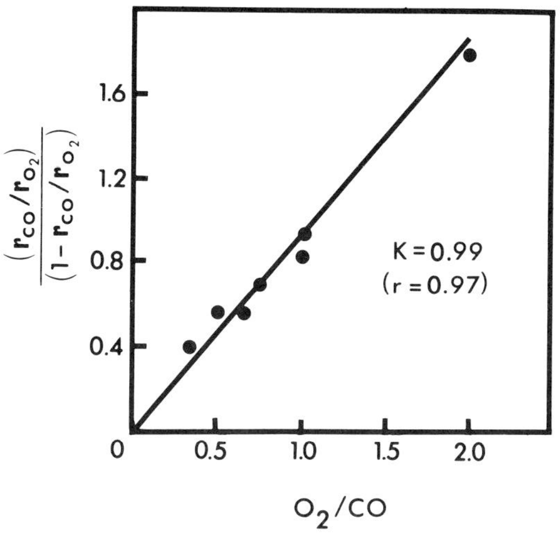

Figure 6-8B. Effect of CO/O_2 ratio on $25(OH)D_3$ 1-hydroxylase activity. The value of r_{CO} was obtained by measuring initial reaction rates of chick kidney mitochondrial $25(OH)D_3$ 1-hydroxylase as described by Henry and Norman (1976) in a closed system under atmospheres of the following CO and O_2 composition, the balance being nitrogen. At 10% O_2, CO was 10, 20, or 30%; at 15% O_2, CO was 20%; at 20% O_2, CO was 10, 20, or 30%. The rate in the absence of CO, r_{O_2}, was measured separately at 10, 15, and 20% O_2. The slope K was determined by a linear regression analysis of the data and is the partition constant from the equation

$$(r_{CO}/r_{O_2})/(1 - r_{CO}/r_{O_2}) = K(O_2/CO)$$

(1976) were able to develop a solubilized preparation of chick kidney mitochondria that was enriched in cytochrome *P*-450 and also contained an iron–sulfur ferridoxin-like protein (similar to adrenodoxin in adrenal cortex mitochondria), which was capable of functioning as an intermediate in the transport of electrons from NADPH to the cytochrome *P*-450 moiety. These results strongly support the suggestion of these workers that the kidney mitochondrial $25(OH)D_3$ 1-hydroxylase system consists of a renal ferredoxin reductase (presumably a flavoprotein), renal ferredoxin, and cytochrome *P*-450.

With the emergence of the concept that the renal $25(OH)D_3$ 1-hydroxylase is a critical enzyme both as a possible control point in the regulation of vitamin D metabolism (see below) and as an integral part of the overall endocrine regulation of normal calcium and phosphorus homeostasis, it became pertinent to evaluate the presence of this enzyme activity in the kidneys of various species and classes of vertebrates. The presence of the 1-hydroxylase in renal tissues of a species would be strong presumptive evidence that the species in question had a requirement for vitamin D metabolism for normal calcium and phosphorus homeostasis. Little information is actually available concerning the general requirement for vitamin D among all the classes of vertebrates. Henry and Norman (1975a) surveyed 28 species of vertebrate classes and detected in 26 of them evidence for the existence of the renal $25(OH)D_3$ 1-hydroxylase (Table 6-4). The level of 1-hydroxylase activity in most normal adult animals ranged from 2 to 10 pmoles/min per gram of kidney. As expected, the highest enzyme activity occurred in birds (chicks and ducks) that were severely rachitic at the time of analysis. The detection of the 1-hydroxylase activity in both fresh- and saltwater fish is the first demonstration of the further metabolism of vitamin D in this vertebrate class. The presence of 1-hydroxylase in primates was also demonstrated. These results concerning the phylogenetic distribution of the 1-hydroxylase are in excellent agreement with the separate studies of Hay and Watson (1976a,b), who carried out a phylogenetic study of the presence of plasma binding protein for $25(OH)D_3$ (see Chapter 8).

Another interesting aspect of the comparative biochemistry of the $25(OH)D_3$ 1-hydroxylase concerns its ontogenetic appearance in the kidney: When in the embryological development of the kidney does the 1-hydroxylase appear? Certainly there is an immediate need for $1,25(OH)_2D_3$ at birth, particularly in the chick, to facilitate the intestinal absorption of calcium and normal bone development. However, the report of Taylor and Wasserman (1972) indicating that calcium-binding protein (CaBP) could not be found in the intestinal mucosa of chick embryos or of newly hatched chicks raised the question as to when developmentally the ability to produce $1,25(OH)_2D_3$ appeared. Both Moriuchi and DeLuca (1974) and Bishop and Norman (1975) studied the metabolism of $25(OH)D_3$ in the chick embryo. They found that the renal 1-hydroxylase enzyme system was present as early as day 9 of chick embryo life (12 days before hatch).

TABLE 6-4
25-Hydroxycholecalciferol 1-Hydroxylase Activity in Vertebrate Kidneys[a]

Scientific name	Common name	Activity (pmoles/min per g kidney)
Carassius auratus	Goldfish	3
Salmo gairdneri	Rainbow trout	1
Cyprinus carpio	Carp	78
Sebastus carnatus	Rockfish	5
Epinephelus labrifornus	Sea bass	7
Scorpaena guttata	Sculpin	2
Sarda chiliensis	Bonito	4
Paralabrax clathratus	Kelp bass	4
Rana pipiens	Green frog	8
Rana macroglossa	Thick-tongued frog	13
Iguana iguana	Green iguana	6
Terrapene carolina bauri	Box turtle	56
Caiman fucus	Caiman	7
Thamnophis elegans vagrans	Garter snake	1
Gallus domesticus	Chick (rachitic)	520
	Chick (+D)[b]	140
	Chicken	8
Anas platyrhynchus	Duck (rachitic)	390
Meleagris gallopavo	Turkey	9
Columba livia	Pigeon	2
Oryctolagus cuniculus	Rabbit (−D)[b]	90
Mus musculus	Mouse	1
Rattus norvegicus	Rat (−D)[d]	90
Cavia porcellus	Guinea pig (−D)[b]	10
Bos taurus	Cow	2
Ovis aries	Sheep	3
Bison bison	Bison	13
Saimiri sciurea	Squirrel monkey (−D)[b]	
	No. 1	435
	No. 2	22

[a] Taken from Henry and Norman (1975a). (Copyright by Pergamon Press, Ltd.)

[b] Tissues were obtained from animals raised on a diet without vitamin D_3 (−D) or supplemented with vitamin D_3 (+D).

Furthermore, the enzyme activity increased sixfold to a maximal level precisely on the day of hatching, day 21. Thus, it is quite apparent that embryonic chick kidneys have the capacity to support the production of $1,25(OH)_2D_3$. These results suggest that the reason for the absence of CaBP in embryonic chick intestine is not a lack of $1,25(OH)_2D_3$ but perhaps an absence of intestinal cytosol receptors for this steroid.

It has long been known that, in the chick, vitamin D_2 is only approximately one-tenth as active as vitamin D_3 (see Chapter 4). Various theories have been put forth to explain this discrimination against the side chain of vitamin D_2. A distinct possibility was that either the liver vitamin D 25-hydroxylase or the kidney 25(OH)D 1-hydroxylase had a reduced affinity for the vitamin D_2 metabolites, which would then result in a reduced output of $1,25(OH)_2D_3$. Jones *et al.* (1976) carried out an *in vitro* study of the liver 25-hydroxylation of vitamin D_2 and the kidney 1α- and 24(*R*)-hydroxylations of $25(OH)D_3$ in order to determine whether the discrimination against vitamin D_2 seen in chicks *in vivo* is a result of a block of one or more of the steps in the metabolic pathway required to produce the biologically active form. Vitamin D_2 hydroxylation reactions in the chick were reported to be virtually identical with those observed with the vitamin D_3 series, with regard to both the Michaelis constant K_m for the substrates and the maximal velocity rates obtainable. It was known from the previous work of Imrie *et al.* (1967) and Drescher *et al.* (1969) that vitamin D_2 was much more rapidly metabolized and excreted in the chick than vitamin D_3; thus, the report of Jones *et al.* (1976) does not really explain the discrimination by the chick against vitamin D_2.

Botham *et al.* (1976) isolated and highly purified an iron-containing protein from rat serum, which when added *in vitro* to isolated chick kidney mitochondria was a potent inhibitor of the $25(OH)D_3$ 1-hydroxylase. The physiological significance of the protein inhibitor is not known. However, its presence in rat tissues may explain the inability of many investigators to demonstrate significant activities *in vitro* of the renal 1-hydroxylase in mammalian renal homogenate or mitochondrial preparations.

2. *Regulation of 25(OH)D_3 1-Hydroxylase*

a. Background. A most significant development in our understanding of the mechanism of action of vitamin D concerns the fact that the renal production of $1,25(OH)_2D_3$ may be regulated in some fashion in response to changing endocrinological or physiological "signals." An important practical aspect of the possible regulation of the renal 25(OH)D 1-hydroxylase is that the organism can regulate the amount of the exceedingly potent $1,25(OH)_2D_3$ in accordance with its calcium needs. In the period between 1971 and 1975 it was variously suggested that the enzymatic activity of the $25(OH)D_3$ 1-hydroxylase is affected by changes in serum calcium, serum phosphorus, parathyroid hormone, calcitonin, cyclic AMP, vitamin D metabolites, and other associated factors including diphosphonates, pH, and steroid hormones. On the one hand, these are extremely stimulating and provocative suggestions because they propose a relationship with other known regulators of calcium homeostasis (PTH and calcitonin), but, on the other hand, these putative interrelationships pose immense problems to the experimentalist who would like to delineate the biochemical details of these proposed regulatory effects.

The problem of the regulation of the 1-hydroxylase can be divided into four major areas: (a) the chemical nature of possible signals to the kidney; (b) possible responses of kidney cells to these signals, which may result in changed intracellular concentrations and/or mitochondrial concentrations of calcium, phosphate, or cyclic AMP; (c) possible subsequent effects on the activity of the mitochondrially localized renal 1-hydroxylase system; and (d) an increased or decreased rate of production of $1,25(OH)_2D_3$. However, any change in the production of $1,25(OH)_2D_3$ must be explainable in biochemical terms. It could be due to (a) alterations in the balance between the biosynthesis and biodegradation of the 1-hydroxylase enzyme itself, (b) activation or inactivation of a steady-state quantity of this enzyme, or (c) an indirect effect on enzyme activity because of the change in substrate or cofactor availability. The fact that the enzyme $25(OH)D_3$ 1-hydroxylase is localized within the mitochondria imposes severe restrictions on the procedures that can be employed to study possible mechanisms of enzyme regulation. Shown in Fig. 6-9 is an example of how dietary vitamin D alters the specific activity of the renal $25(OH)D_3$ 1-hydroxylase. It is apparent that in the presence of dietary vitamin D the level of the 1-hydroxylase activity is quite low but, as soon as the dietary D_3 is withdrawn, there is a marked four-to fivefold rise in the activity of the enzyme, which can occur within 15–35 hr. If the same enzyme data are calculated on a per bird basis (i.e., per pair of kidneys) rather than on a concentration basis (specific activity or picomoles per minute per milligram of protein), the same difference in enzyme activity is apparent. This is consistent with the hypothesis that in the absence of D_3 there is a marked increase in the concentration of active enzyme molecules. These data are presented simply to emphasize the dynamic, short time scale aspects of regulation of the $25(OH)D_3$ 1-hydroxylase.

b. Minerals. *i. Calcium.* As indicated above, modulation of the renal production of $1,25(OH)_2D_3$ by the prevailing mineral status has been suggested as a functional regulatory mechanism. Experiments evaluating the effects of calcium on the 1-hydroxylase have been carried out in intact animals as well as in isolated kidney tubules or kidney mitochondrial preparations. Boyle *et al.* (1971) studied the effect of variations in dietary calcium on the metabolism *in vivo* of administered doses of tritiated $25(OH)D_3$. It should be appreciated that these investigators could not directly measure the changes in enzyme activity of the 1-hydroxylase since an enzyme assay was not carried out, but simply measured the alterations in vitamin D metabolism that occurred *in vivo* as a consequence of changing mineral availability. They reported that vitamin D-deficient rats fed a diet containing a high calcium content (3%) had a lower intestinal content of $1,25(OH)_2D_3$ than rats receiving a diet with 0.47% calcium. Most interestingly,

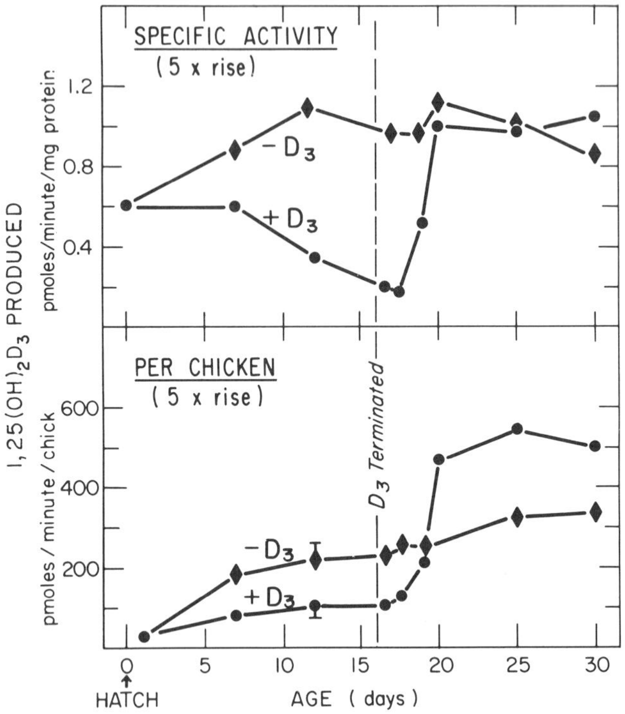

Figure 6-9. Effect of dietary vitamin D_3 on the renal level of $25(OH)D_3$ 1-hydroxylase. Groups of chicks were raised from the day of hatching on a diet of 0.6% calcium, 0.4% phosphate and received either 15 IU (975 pmoles) of vitamin D_3 orally per day or only vehicle (1,2-propanediol). On day 16, the dietary vitamin D_3 was terminated. Triplicate $25(OH)D_3$ 1-hydroxylase assays were conducted on kidney homogenates at the indicated points. The same enzyme data are calculated in two ways: top panel gives the specific activity per milligram of protein; bottom panel gives enzyme activity on a per bird basis (Henry *et al.*, 1974).

these workers reported an apparent reciprocal relationship between the production by the kidney of $1,25(OH)_2D_3$ and $24,25(OH)_2D_3$ [see below for discussion of $25(OH)D_3$ 24-hydroxylase]. This intriguing possibility has been extensively supported by work from the Madison group; particularly, Omdahl *et al.* (1972) found an inverse relationship between dietary calcium and the percentage of radioactivity recovered as $1,25(OH)_2D_3$ following the administration of radioactive $25(OH)D_3$.

Henry *et al.* (1974) and Friedlander *et al.* (1977a,b) carried out extensive studies that attempted to correlate the steady-state level of the renal $25(OH)D_3$ 1-hydroxylase measured *in vitro* with the dietary intake of calcium and phosphorus. The amount of enzyme present was inversely related to dietary and serum calcium but was unrelated to dietary, serum, or renal tissue phosphorus levels. It is important to note that these studies concerned direct measurement of the 1-hydroxylase activity under defined conditions rather than the indirect assessment that occurs during *in vivo* measurements.

Any assessment of potential effects of changing serum calcium or dietary calcium levels on the 1-hydroxylase activity must include consideration of effects of parathyroid hormone (PTH). The regulatory actions of PTH are discussed below. Larkins *et al.* (1973, 1974a) and MacIntyre *et al.* (1974) claimed that the low-calcium diet favored the production of $1,25(OH)_2D_3$ from $25(OH)D_3$, even in animals that had been parathyroidectomized. This suggests that changes in the activity of the $25(OH)D_3$ 1-hydroxylase could be produced by variations of the calcium intake independent of alterations in the circulating levels of PTH. However, the results of Hughes *et al.* (1975), who measured plasma levels of $1,25(OH)_2D_3$ (via a steroid competition assay) in vitamin D-replete rats, either with or without their parathyroid glands, found no evidence for the ability of low dietary calcium levels to increase circulating levels of $1,25(OH)_2D_3$ in the absence of the parathyroid gland. Interestingly, Hughes *et al.* (1975) did report that, in the absence of the parathyroid glands, low dietary phosphate conditions were capable of elevating circulating levels of $1,25(OH)_2D_3$. This important observation suggests that perturbations in serum calcium levels as compared to serum phosphorus levels manifest their effects on the production of $1,25(OH)_2D_3$ by distinctly different mechanisms.

As a result of the foregoing considerations concerning the modulation of the renal production of $1,25(OH)_2D_3$ by altering the prevailing dietary mineral levels, many investigators have explored the metabolism of $25(OH)D_3$ *in vitro* by employing either isolated preparations of kidney tubules or, more frequently, highly purified preparations of isolated mitochondria. Henry and Norman (1974, 1976) reported inhibition of the 1-hydroxylase by low calcium concentrations (10^{-5} to 10^{-4} *M*) in isolated chick kidney mitochondrial preparations obtained from either vitamin D-deficient or vitamin D-replete birds (see Fig. 6-10). Other investigators have also observed inhibitory effects of calcium at higher (10^{-4} to 10^{-3} *M*) concentrations (Fraser and Kodicek, 1973; Galante *et al.*, 1973; Colston *et al.*, 1973). It has also been reported, however, that calcium has no effect on the *in vitro* metabolism of $25(OH)D_3$ to $1,25(OH)_2D_3$ (Ghazarian and DeLuca, 1974). Still other investigators employing mitochondria previously depleted of calcium by extensive washing with EGTA (a highly efficient chelator of calcium) have observed that the addition of increasing concentrations of calcium first activates and then inhibits 1-hydroxylation (at 10^{-6} *M*) (Suda *et al.*, 1973) or is without effect (Bikle *et al.*, 1975). It would seem that extensive washing of mitochondrial membranes with EGTA might remove the vestigial levels of calcium that are associated with and are important for membrane structure; thus, one could

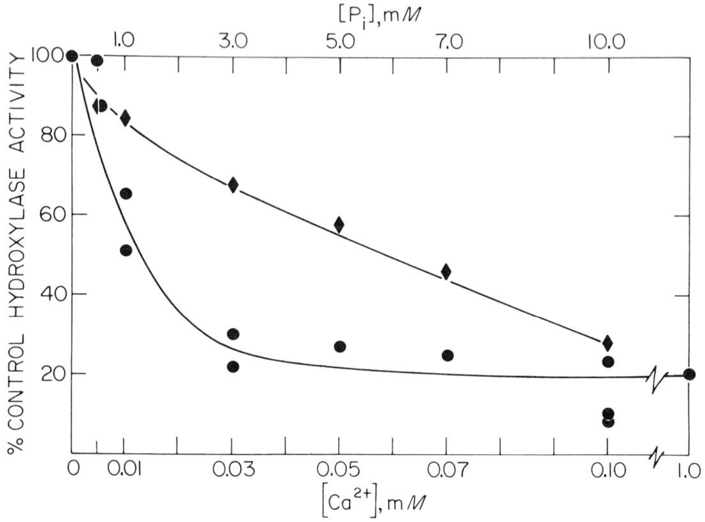

Figure 6-10. Effects of calcium or phosphate on the activity of chick renal $25(OH)D_3$ 1-hydroxylase (●—●, Ca^{2+}; ◆—◆, P_i). From Henry and Norman (1976).

rationalize the apparent activating effect of very low calcium concentrations with subsequent inhibitory effects at higher calcium concentrations.

Horiuchi *et al.* (1974) reported that the production of $1,25(OH)_2D_3$ by mitochondria from chick kidneys increased as the calcium concentration was elevated from 0 to 0.2 m*M* and then fell off as the concentration was increased to 0.7 m*M*. Henry and Norman (1976) studied both the effects of a hypotonic medium, and the effects of freezing and thawing of the mitochondria, and found that there was a significant inhibition of the 1-hydroxylase by as little as 0.02 m*M* calcium in mitochondria obtained from both vitamin D-deficient and vitamin D-treated chicks. These observations supported the hypothesis that the inhibition of the $25(OH)D_3$ 1-hydroxylase by calcium was specific and not due to a nonspecific effect of calcium on mitochondrial metabolism. A partial reversal of calcium inhibition of 1-hydroxylase activity by employing the calcium ionophore A-23187 was also noted, suggesting that it is intramitochondrial calcium which is responsible for the inhibition of the 1-hydroxylase.

ii. Phosphorus. The effects of phosphate on 1-hydroxylation have been less widely investigated than those of calcium but with no more agreement in results and interpretation. Again the effects of phosphate have been studied both *in vivo* and *in vitro*. Interest in the possible role of phosphate in vitamin D metabolism undoubtedly first arose because of the striking similarities between the skeletal lesions of osteomalacia and those present in a condition of phosphate depletion (Day and McCollum, 1939; Lotz *et al.*, 1964). Haddad *et al.* (1971) were the first to study the effects of phosphate depletion on vitamin D metabolism in the rat. However, despite their reports of poor growth, hypercalcemia, florid rickets, and hypophosphatemia in the phosphate-depleted animals, the metabolism of radioactive vitamin D was not different from that in rats that had received adequate dietary levels of inorganic phosphate. An interesting observation made in the chick by both Haddad *et al.* (1971) and Morrissey and Wasserman (1971) was that dietary phosphate depletion stimulated the intestinal absorption of calcium virtually as much as did dietary calcium depletion. More recently, Edelstein *et al.* (1978) made the puzzling observation that phosphate depletion in the rat, unlike the chick, does not stimulate the absorption of intestinal calcium or the level of intestinal calcium-binding protein. The significance of these observations will be discussed below.

Tanaka and DeLuca (1973), in studies involving phosphate-depleted rats given radioactive $25(OH)D_3$, found larger quantities of $1,25(OH)_2D_3$ in the plasma than they did in rats fed normal levels of dietary phosphate. Most provocatively, the quantity of $1,25(OH)_2D_3$ in the serum appeared to vary inversely with the level of serum phosphorus, whereas the amount of $24,25(OH)_2D_3$ was found to vary directly with serum phosphorus. Tanaka and DeLuca suggested that a reduced renal content of phosphate was an important factor in stimulating the activity of the $25(OH)D_3$ 1-hydroxylase and that the effects of phosphate occurred independently of the parathyroid glands. This interesting suggestion concerning the effect of phosphate depletion in stimulating metabolic conversion of $25(OH)D_3$ to $1,25(OH)_2D_3$ received much attention, principally in the clinical fields, since phosphate depletion was suggested to be a means of activating by diet the production of $1,25(OH)_2D_3$ in individuals with chronic renal failure. However, it should once again be appreciated that the data of Tanaka and DeLuca (1973) were obtained *in vivo* and cannot be considered to be indicative of "activating effects" of low phosphate levels directly on renal 1-hydroxylase. In fact, in repeated investigations by Henry and Norman (1974) as well as by Friedlander *et al.* (1977a,b) and Montecuccoli *et al.* (1977a), no basis to support this contention has been found. Instead, it appears that the major effects of low dietary phosphate levels do not occur directly on the renal 1-hydroxylase system per se but through other independent biological mechanisms (see discussion below).

Several laboratories have explored the effects of phosphate added *in vitro* to incubations of either kidney tubule preparations or isolated mitochondria. Bikle and Rasmussen (1975) reduced dietary phosphate intake in vitamin D-deficient chicks and noted that the activity of the renal $25(OH)D_3$ 1-hydroxylase as measured *in vitro* in mitochondria was not enhanced by phosphate restriction above the already high levels due to a vitamin D deficiency. Furthermore, Bikle and Rasmussen (1975) found that varying the phosphate concentration *in vitro* in the presence of 1 to 2 m*M* calcium had a biphasic effect on the activity of the 1-hydroxylase measured in tubule preparations. As the phosphate concentration was increased from 0 to 0.6 m*M*, there was a reduced production of $1,25(OH)_2D_3$ by the enzyme. However, as the concentration of phosphate was elevated above 1.2 m*M*, the enzyme activity increased. In other experiments carried out *in vitro* with chick kidney mitochondrial preparations, Henry and Norman (1974) found that phosphate at a concentration of 5×10^{-3} *M* produced a 50% inhibition of the 1-hydroxylase activity (see Fig. 6-10).

It is to be anticipated that the pioneering efforts of Henry (1977a) to develop a primary cell culture system capable of metabolizing $25(OH)D_3$ to both $1,25(OH)_2D_3$ and $24,25(OH)_2D_3$ will provide informative biochemical results in the future. Similarly, the monkey kidney cell culture system of David and DeLuca (1977), which converts $25(OH)D_3$ to only $24,25(OH)D_3$, may prove to be of value.

A further discussion of the integrated interactions of changing calcium and phosphorus status on vitamin D metabolism can be found in Section III,D.

iii. Magnesium and Potassium. Since magnesium depletion is believed to affect parathyroid secretion (Suh *et al.*, 1973; Reddy *et al.*, 1973), it might be postulated that magnesium depletion would affect the metabolism of $25(OH)D_3$ to $1,25(OH)_2D_3$. Evaluation of this possibility by Hartenbower *et al.* (1975) provided no evidence that magnesium depletion of either chicks or rats affected $25(OH)D_3$ metabolism when measured both *in vivo* and *in vitro*.

Bikle *et al.* (1976) presented evidence that the mitochondrial concentration of potassium may be crucial in determining the activity of the $25(OH)D_3$ 1-hydroxylase. They found in *in vitro* studies with isolated chick renal mitochondria that increasing the medium concentration of K^+ from 1 to 50 m*M* led to a sixfold increase in the production of $1,25(OH)_2D_3$.

c. Peptide Hormones. *i. Parathyroid Hormone.* One potential, important modulator of $25(OH)D_3$ metabolism by the kidney is the peptide hormone PTH. Although the various experimental observations pertaining to PTH are difficult to relate, it now appears that this peptide hormone should be considered a potential trophic factor capable of stimulating the biosynthesis of $1,25(OH)_2D_3$.

In 1972 there were simultaneous reports by Garabedian *et al.* (1972), Rasmussen *et al.* (1972), and Galante *et al.* (1972b) which implicated PTH involvement in the metabolism of $25(OH)D_3$ to $1,25(OH)_2D_3$. Garabedian *et al.* (1972) evaluated the production of $1,25(OH)_2D_3$ from radioactive $25(OH)D_3$ *in vivo* in vitamin D-deficient rats that had been subjected to thyroparathyroidectomy (TPTX) and found significantly reduced quantities of an apparent $1,25(OH)_2D_3$ in the plasma. However, it is difficult to interpret their results because in order to ensure survival of their TPTX rats they administered small quantities of nonradioactive $1,25(OH)_2D_3$ to prevent fatal hypocalcemia. Galante *et al.* (1972b) reported the consequences of administering PTH extract in large doses to vitamin D-deficient, nonrachitic rats; these workers noted that the administration of PTH resulted in a reduction in the apparent plasma levels of radioactive $1,25(OH)_2D_3$.

The report of Rasmussen *et al.* (1972) was based on an *in vitro* study of the conversion of radioactive $25(OH)D_3$ to $1,25(OH)_2D_3$ via a preparation of isolated renal tubules obtained from vitamin D-deficient chicks. They, too, found that the rate of conversion was enhanced by low concentrations of PTH (5 or 50 ng/ml). However, a puzzling aspect of this observation was the report of Shain (1972), who was working in the Rasmussen laboratory at the same time; he found no effect of added purified PTH (10 μg/ml) on the metabolism of radioactive $25(OH)D_3$ in kidney tubules obtained from vitamin D-deficient chicks.

Shortly thereafter, Fraser and Kodicek (1973) measured *in vitro* the activity of 1-hydroxylase in homogenates of whole kidneys obtained from vitamin D-deficient chicks and found a modest effect of the *in vivo* administration of bovine PTH in doses of 30 units per 100 g body weight every 6 hr for 48 hr. However, this important observation had not been duplicated until the report by Henry (1977a,b), who found a dose–response relationship between the amount of purified PTH administered over a 7-hr period to vitamin D-replete chicks and the resulting steady-state level of the $25(OH)D_3$ 1-hydroxylase. The more PTH administered, the higher was the specific activity of the 1-hydroxylase (see Fig. 6-11).

One important approach to this problem is to surgically remove the parathyroid glands and evaluate the effects on 1-hydroxylase specific activity. Fraser and Kodicek (1973) and Henry *et al.* (1974) carried out parathyroidectomy of vitamin D-deficient chicks, and Garabedian *et al.* (1972), Tanaka and DeLuca (1973), Seymour and DeLuca (1974), and Favus *et al.* (1974) evaluated the consequences of parathyroidectomy in the rat. In general, in each experimental circumstance there was a marked fall in the specific activity of the 1-hydroxylase associated with removal of the parathyroid gland; however, Galante *et al.* (1973)

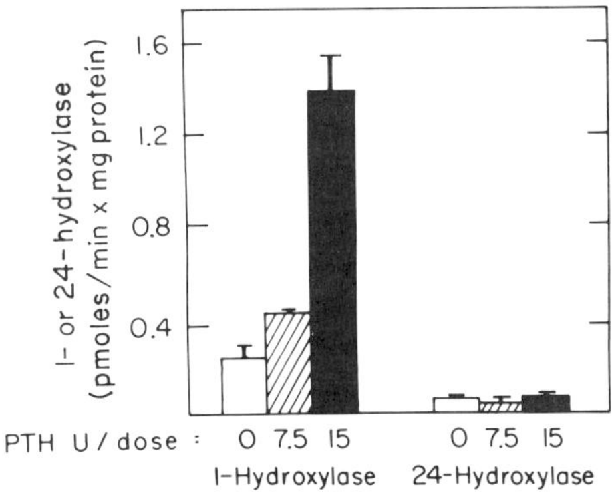

Figure 6-11. Effects of repeated doses of bovine PTH on the specific activity of chick kidney $25(OH)D_3$ 1-hydroxylase. Reproduced by permission from Henry (1977a).

could obtain this effect only in animals that had been given a dietary source of vitamin D_3 (see Fig. 6-12).

Favus *et al.* (1974) reported the results of an interesting experiment in which adaptation of intestinal calcium absorption to differing levels of dietary calcium was evaluated in TPTX rats as well as sham-operated controls. They found, surprisingly, that in spite of the reduced plasma levels of 1,25$(OH)_2D_3$, which presumably occurred due to the absence of the trophic actions of PTH on renal 1-hydroxylase, there were normal levels of the 1,25$(OH)_2D_3$ localized in the intestine in both the sham-operated and TPTX animals. Somewhat in contrast to these results, Seymour and DeLuca (1974) concluded that hypoparathyroid animals cannot synthesize appreciable quantities of 1,25$(OH)_2D_3$. However, Hughes *et al.* (1975) found, on the basis of a steroid competition assay, that phosphate depletion is capable of elevating circulating levels of 1,25$(OH)_2D_3$ in animals devoid of parathyroid glands. Thus, the absence of parathyroid glands and PTH does not abolish completely the renal capability of producing 1,25$(OH)_2D_3$.

ii. Calcitonin. At approximately the same time that MacIntyre's research group (Galante *et al.*, 1972b) was reporting effects of PTH in depressing the metabolism of 25(OH)D_3, the same laboratory was also reporting stimulatory effects of calcitonin on the production of 1,25$(OH)_2D_3$ *in vivo* (Galante *et al.*, 1972a). However, there have been no follow-up reports which describe in detail the putative actions of calcitonin or amplify the original observations. Also, no

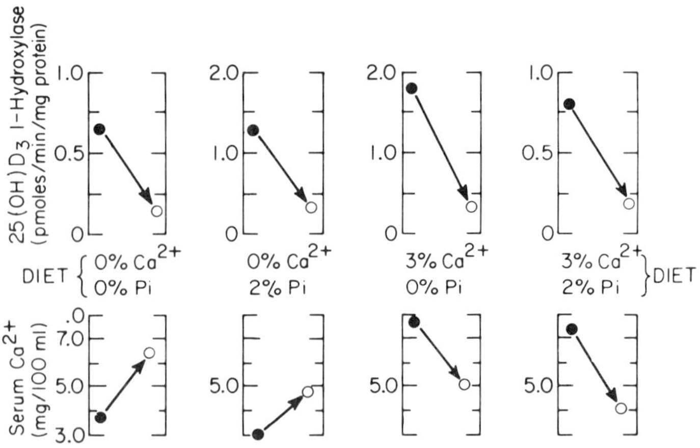

Figure 6-12. Effects of parathyroidectomy on the specific activity of renal 25(OH)D_3 1-hydroxylase. Chicks were raised on a rachitogenic diet containing the indicated levels of dietary Ca and P. After 3 weeks they were subjected to total parathyroidectomy; 15 hr later the enzyme assay for 25(OH)D_3 1-hydroxylase was carried out as described by Henry and Norman (1974). Taken from Henry *et al.* (1974).

other laboratories have been able to repeat these results. One must postulate only with reservation that calcitonin may be a regulatory agent in the metabolism of vitamin D.

iii. Prolactin. Spanos *et al.* (1976a) reported that administration of ovine prolactin daily for a period of 7 days to either vitamin D-deficient or vitamin D-supplemented chicks resulted in a doubling of the specific activity of the $25(OH)D_3$ 1-hydroxylase as measured *in vitro*. However, this effect could be observed only when the enzyme was assayed within 2–3 hr after the final subcutaneous injection of the prolactin. A single subcutaneous injection of prolactin was also found to provide a maximal elevation of the 1-hydroxylase within 1 hr. The effect abated 3 hr after the prolactin dose. This observation was confirmed via measurement of the increased levels of plasma $1,25(OH)_2D_3$ that occurred after prolactin administration to the chick (Spanos *et al.*, 1976b). Clearly, some care must be taken in the evaluation of these results since one would not necessarily anticipate action by a mammalian prolactin in an avian species. However, in the event that this is a valid observation, extrapolation of these results to mammals may well explain the known marked increases in calcium and phosphorus absorption that occur in late phases of pregnancy and lactation, both times when plasma prolactin levels are high (Horrobin, 1974).

iv. Cyclic AMP. An extremely challenging problem to the biochemist concerned with the molecular basis for regulation of the renal $25(OH)D_3$ 1-hydroxylase is to elucidate the specific means whereby PTH and possibly prolactin are able to stimulate the production of $1,25(OH)_2D_3$. Inasmuch as peptide hormones are not believed to enter cells but rather are thought to exert their actions via a "second messenger" such as cyclic AMP, it would seem that the actions of PTH must occur through the intervention of this nucleotide. However, to date no consistent effects have been observed with the addition of cyclic AMP to mitochondrial preparations obtained from vitamin D-replete or vitamin D-deficient chicks (Rasmussen *et al.*, 1972; Shain, 1972; Larkins *et al.*, 1974a). An intriguing possibility, however, is that cyclic AMP may well activate a protein kinase present in the cell containing the 1-hydroxylase which phosphorylates some component(s) of the $25(OH)D_3$ 1-hydroxylase so as to convert it from an inactive to an active species. There is precedent for this proposed model. Reed and co-workers (Linn *et al.*, 1969) reported that the mitochondrial enzyme α-ketoglutarate dehydrogenase is converted from an inactive to an active form by the action of a cAMP-activated kinase; conversely, a specific phosphatase has been found to inactivate this enzyme. It might well be possible that such a system also mediates the effects of the changing circulating concentrations of PTH so that the output of $1,25(OH)_2D_3$ can be carefully regulated to meet the calcium demands of the organism.

d. Vitamin D Status. There is agreement among all laboratories that dietary vitamin D_3 or $1,25(OH)_2D_3$ is capable of diminishing the specific activity of the

$25(OH)D_3$ 1-hydroxylase. It was shown by Henry and Norman (1974) that this effect was not due to any technical errors caused by the presence of nonradioactive pools of vitamin D metabolites during the enzyme assay; the lowered enzyme specific activity apparently reflects a genuine reduction in the net number of catalytic centers concerned with the production of $1,25(OH)_2D_3$ (see Fig. 6-9).

Garbedian *et al.* (1972) first noted effects of dietary vitamin D on the production of $1,25(OH)_2D_3$. However, a detailed interpretation of their results is complicated since they were measuring metabolism of vitamin D *in vivo* in animals that had been thyroparathyroidectomized. Subsequently, Henry and Norman (1974) and Henry *et al.* (1974) reported dramatic differences in the specific activity of the renal 1-hydroxylase, which were dependent on the vitamin D status of the birds from which the mitochondria had been isolated. These results are shown in Fig. 6-9; the levels of the renal 1-hydroxylase were studied as a function of withdrawal of dietary vitamin D_3. From the initiation of the experiment on the day of hatching of the chicks to day 26, it is apparent that in the presence of dietary vitamin D_3 the level of $25(OH)D_3$ 1-hydroxylase was quite low, but as soon as dietary vitamin D was withdrawn there was a marked four- to fivefold rise in the activity of the enzyme. Similar results were obtained by administration and withdrawal of $1,25(OH)_2D_3$ (Henry *et al.*, 1974). These results are consistent with the hypothesis that in the absence of vitamin D there is a marked increase in the concentration of active enzyme molecules capable of catalyzing this reaction. This could be due to either changes in the rate of biosynthesis or biodegradation of the 1-hydroxylase activity.

A study of the turnover time, $t_{\frac{1}{2}}$, of the $25(OH)D_3$ 1-hydroxylase is reported in Fig. 6-13. Advantage was taken of the fact that administration of the inhibitor of protein synthesis, cycloheximide, prevents translation of existing messenger RNA for the 1-hydroxylase. Thus, the fall in enzyme activity that occurs is a measure of the degradation rate of the $25(OH)D_3$ 1-hydroxylase. It is apparent that the 1-hydroxylase has a $t_{\frac{1}{2}}$ of 4 to 5 hr in both the vitamin D-deficient and vitamin D-replete birds. Thus, it can be proposed that the change in 1-hydroxylase specific activity which occurs as a consequence of the administration of vitamin D is due to a reduction in the rate of biosynthesis of the 1-hydroxylase enzyme. In a vitamin D-deficient bird, the rate of synthesis of the enzyme is 7.5 hr^{-1}, or some 4.7 times greater than that of a vitamin D-replete bird.

Larkins *et al.* (1974b) found that the conversion of $25(OH)D_3$ to $1,25(OH)_2D_3$ in suspensions of kidney tubules decreased following preincubation with $1,25(OH)_2D_3$ itself. They proposed that this effect was due to a "feeding back" of $1,25(OH)_2D_3$ to the nucleus of the appropriate kidney cells to effect a reduction in the rate of biosynthesis of the 1-hydroxylase. This is an extremely interesting suggestion in light of the proposed steroid hormone mechanism of action for $1,25(OH)_2D_3$ in the target intestinal mucosa. As yet no additional data have been forthcoming from the laboratory of MacIntyre to support the nuclear localization

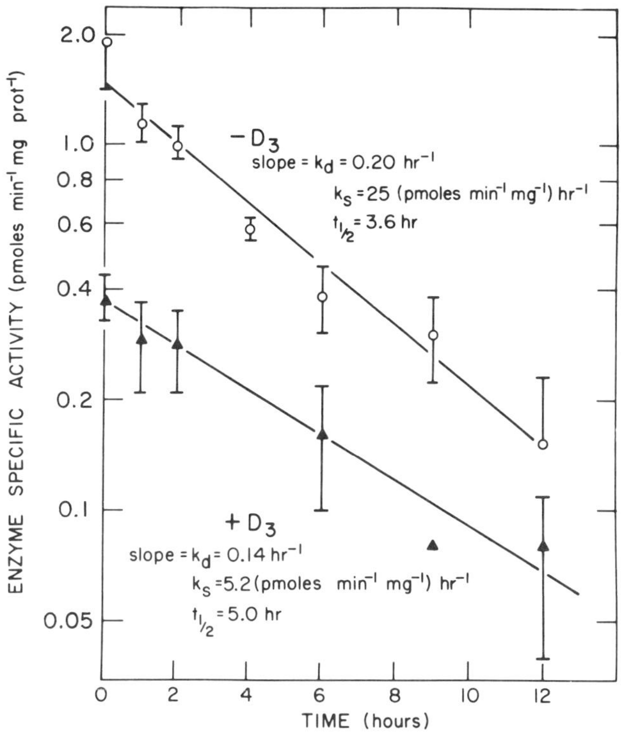

Figure 6-13. Effect of cycloheximide on $25(OH)D_3$ 1-hydroxylase activity in vitamin D-replete or vitamin D-deficient chicks. Cycloheximide was given (80 μg per 100 g) at 0, 4, and 8 hr. Enzyme assays were conducted in triplicate on pooled homogenates from four to five birds. The slopes of each line were determined by a least-squares analysis. From Berlin and Schimke (1965), the slope k_d is equal to the rate of enzyme degradation, and the half-life $t_{\frac{1}{2}}$ and rate of synthesis could be determined from the following equations:

$$t_{\frac{1}{2}} = \frac{\ln 2}{k_d} \quad \text{and} \quad E_o = \frac{k_s}{k_o}$$

Here, E_0 is the steady-state concentration of the enzyme prior to administration of the cycloheximide; k_s is the zero-order rate constant describing the rate of synthesis of the enzyme; k_d is the first-order rate constant describing the rate of decay of the enzyme. Key: ▲—▲, $t_{\frac{1}{2}} = 5.0$ hrs; $k_d = 0.139$ hr^{-1}; $k_s = 2.66$ e.u. (enzyme units) mg^{-1} hr^{-1}. ○—○, $t_{\frac{1}{2}} = 3.6$ hr; k_d, 0.195 hr^{-1}; $k_s = 7.54$ e.u. mg^{-1} hr^{-1}. Taken from Henry *et al.* (1974).

and perturbation of the rate of biosynthesis of the renal 1-hydroxylase system. However, the results do suggest a teleological explanation for the localization of the $25(OH)D_3$ 1-hydroxylase enzyme system in the kidney tubule. In this location it is uniquely capable of sensing and responding to fluctuations in calcium concentration in the tubule. In the face of high plasma and urinary calcium levels, the intracellular calcium concentration could rise and directly inhibit the

1-hydroxylase (see above); also, $1,25(OH)_2D_3$ could feed back to the nucleus of that cell to reduce the further biosynthesis of 1-hydroxylase enzyme molecules.

e. Other Factors. *i. Diphosphonates.* Some studies on the regulation of the metabolism of vitamin D have focused on the involvement of ethane-1-hydroxy-1,1-diphosphonate (EHDP) in this process. As a class, diphosphonates are compounds that contain phosphorus–carbon bonds in place of the usual phosphorus–oxygen–carbon bonds; accordingly, they are analogues of phosphoesters, which are resistant to hydrolysis because of the lack of the oxygen moiety. Diphosphonates are known to interfere with bone mineral metabolism (King *et al.*, 1970) as well as intestinal calcium absorption (Bonjour *et al.*, 1972a). It has been suggested that these effects may be partially attributable to inhibition of the production of $1,25(OH)_2D_3$ by the kidney. Particularly, Bonjour and Fleisch and associates (Bonjour *et al.*, 1972a) proposed that the EHDP impairment of intestinal calcium absorption is due to specific perturbations of the metabolism of vitamin D by the kidney. Similar views were expressed by Bar and Hurwitz (1973), who found that EHDP treatment reduced the intestinal levels of the vitamin D-dependent calcium-binding protein.

It was reported (Hill *et al.*, 1973; Baxter *et al.*, 1974) that treatment of vitamin D-deficient animals with EHDP *in vivo* reduced the enzymatic production of $1,25(OH)_2D_3$ under both *in vivo* and *in vitro* conditions. Support for this view was also obtained by Bonjour *et al.* (1972b). Thus, there is a distinct possibility that EHDP was selectively interfering with the normal metabolism of $25(OH)D_3$ to its biologically active form. However, it was quite evident from the data of Hill *et al.* (1973) and further elaborated in detail by Taylor *et al.* (1973, 1975) that, although EHDP could block the response to vitamin D given chronically, a single acute dose of vitamin D given to vitamin D-deficient animals treated with EHDP resulted in a normal amount of $1,25(OH)_2D_3$ and a normal intestinal biological response. This normal response to the acute dose of vitamin D was followed within several days by an apparent inhibition of metabolism of vitamin D administered chronically. Thus, the view was expressed by these investigators that inhibition of the biosynthesis of $1,25(OH)_2D_3$ could not be attributed to a direct action of EHDP on the renal $25(OH)D_3$ 1-hydroxylase but appeared to be the result of action of the drug on the normal response to vitamin D. In confirmation of this suggestion are the results of Baxter *et al.* (1974) and Henry and Norman (1975a), who reported that direct addition of EHDP to renal mitochondrial preparations *in vitro* resulted in inhibition only when the drug was present at unreasonably high concentrations, i.e., greater than 1.0 mM. Possibly over a prolonged period of time the EHDP concentrations might build up in the kidney tissue and produce morphological damage, which would result in impaired metabolism of vitamin D. An equally attractive possibility is that there may be an end organ inhibition of the biological response to $1,25(OH)_2D_3$ at the target organ, the intestine (Krawitt *et al.*, 1973; Bonjour *et al.*, 1975).

ii. Nonvitamin D—Steroid Hormone Effects. There is abundant clinical evidence that sex hormones play an important role in calcium metabolism (Frame *et al.*, 1973; Rasmussen and Bordier, 1974). The widespread occurrence of postmenopausal osteoporosis could in some way be related to perturbations in circulating levels of estrogens and androgens. It is known that in birds there are marked increases in serum calcium levels at the time of initiation of ovulation prior to the formation of the eggshell. To date there are only a few brief reports commenting on the possible intervention of sex steroid hormones in vitamin D metabolism. Nicholson *et al.* (1976) observed that estradiol stimulated the production of 25(OH)D_3 from the parent vitamin D in the Japanese quail. In homogenates made from the livers of immature quail of either sex, very little 25(OH)D_3 was formed; however, after administration of exogenous estradiol, the situation was reversed. Kenny *et al.* (1976) and Tanaka *et al.* (1976) presented evidence consistent with the view that there is a strong regulation by the sex hormones estradiol and testosterone of the renal 25(OH)D_3 1-hydroxylase. They, too, employed Japanese quail for their experimental studies. A single injection of 5 mg of estradiol-17β-OH into a male bird completely suppressed the normal endogenous level of the 25(OH)D_3 24-hydroxylase (see below) and greatly elevated the 25(OH)D_3 1-hydroxylase activities. Castrated male chicks exhibited an estradiol response only when they had been pretreated with testosterone. Montecuccoli *et al.* (1977b) found highly correlated levels of intestinal calcium-binding protcin with the specific activity of the renal 25(OH)D_3 1-hydroxylase during the egg-laying cycle of Japanese quail.

The results obtained with the sex steroids estradiol and testosterone, when studied in conjunction with the reports described above concerning the effects of the peptide hormone prolactin, strongly suggest that there may be an integrated endocrine interaction between calcium and phosphorus homeostasis, the regulated metabolism of vitamin D, and reproductive hormones.

Spanos *et al.* (1977) found that a single injection of 2 mg of cortisol to vitamin D-replete chicks resulted 16 hr later in an inhibition of the renal 25(OH)D_3 24-hydroxylase and a marked stimulation of the 25(OH)D_3 1-hydroxylase. Surprisingly, this effect could be duplicated under *in vitro* conditions. Thus, the presence of cortisol (50 ng/ml) stimulated the 1-hydroxylase activity of chick kidney tubule preparations obtained from vitamin-D deficient chicks. The possible physiological significance of enhanced production of 1,25$(OH)_2D_3$ before and during the well-documented inhibition of intestinal calcium transport by glucocorticoids remains to be established (see Chapter 13). In contrast Edelstein and Noff (1977) found that hydrocortisone administration to rats that had received chronic doses of radioactive vitamin D_3 significantly reduced the intestinal and renal levels of 1,25$(OH)_2D_3$.

iii. Metabolic Acidosis. Lee *et al.* (1977) demonstrated from *in vivo* studies in rats given dietary ammonium chloride that the resulting systemic acidosis led to a reduced rate of production of 1,25$(OH)_2D_3$. Similarly, Booth *et al.* (1977) found in studies in the chick that the development of a vitamin D-deficient state was accompanied by the onset of metabolic acidosis. Thus, the possibility must be considered that metabolic acidosis in man, which is often associated with hypercalciuria and hyperphosphaturia, might in part be due to perturbations of vitamin D metabolism in general and the 25$(OH)D_3$ 1-hydroxylase in particular. In that regard it may be useful to apply the six-compartment computer-generated model of 25$(OH)D_3$ metabolism developed by Omdahl *et al.* (1977) to the problem of vitamin D metabolism in acidosis.

B. 25-Hydroxyvitamin D 24-Hydroxylase

1. Localization and Properties of the Enzyme

The metabolite 24,25$(OH)_2D_3$ is also produced by the kidney. At present there is an emerging picture concerning the biological functions of 24,25$(OH)_2D_3$; there is some recent evidence suggesting its interaction at the parathyroid gland (Henry *et al.*, 1977) as well as at the bone (see Chapters 12 and 13). The only report on the subcellular localization and biochemical properties of the 25$(OH)D_3$ 24-hydroxylases is that by Knutson and DeLuca (1974). A fact that is crucial to the manipulation and study of the 24-hydroxylase is that its specific activity is elevated in animals raised on a high-calcium (3%), vitamin D-supplemented diet. Knutson and DeLuca (1974) reported that the 25$(OH)D_3$ 24-hydroxylase activity was exclusively localized in the kidney mitochondria obtained from these vitamin D-replete animals. The only cofactors required for the enzymatic reaction were NADPH and molecular oxygen. The NADPH could be generated through the oxidation of succinate and malate in a fashion reminiscent of that reported for the 25$(OH)D_3$ 1-hydroxylase. The mitochondrial electron transport inhibitors antimycin and cyanide also inhibit the 24-hydroxylase. Magnesium was not a required cofactor. It is rather puzzling that carbon monoxide was claimed not to inhibit the 24-hydroxylase. In view of the clear demonstration that CO inhibits the 1-hydroxylase, one might anticipate that a similar inhibitory action would be noted with the 25$(OH)D_3$ 24-hydroxylase. Madhok *et al.* (1977) showed that the oxygen inserted in the 24 position is derived exclusively from $^{18}O_2$. Therefore, like the 25$(OH)D_3$ 1-hydroxylase, the 25$(OH)D_3$ 24-hydroxylase system is also a mixed-function oxidase.

2. Regulation of 25$(OH)D_3$ 24-Hydroxylase

Data obtained in several laboratories suggest that the activity of the renal 25$(OH)D_3$ 24-hydroxylase may be subject to regulation. Garbedian *et al.* (1972) first showed that, following thyroparathyroidectomy, rats fed a low-calcium diet suffered a loss in their ability to synthesize 1,25$(OH)_2D_3$ and a concomitant increase in their ability to biosynthesize $24,25(OH)_2D_3$. Furthermore, they demonstrated that the ability of a TPTX rat to produce $1,25(OH)_2D_3$ could be restored by the administration of PTH. This observation suggested to these investigators that there was a reciprocal relationship between the biological production of $1,25(OH)_2D_3$ and $24,25(OH)_2D_3$. Thus, under circumstances that stimulated the production of $1,25(OH)_2D_3$ there would be a repression of the ability to produce $24,25(OH)_2D_3$; conversely, under endocrinological conditions that stimulated the production of $24,25(OH)_2D_3$ there would be a repression of the biosynthesis of $1,25(OH)_2D_3$.

In an apparent confirmation of this observation, Tanaka and DeLuca (1974) reported that production of $24,25(OH)_2D_3$ could be stimulated in vitamin D-deficient rats by the dietary administration of $1,25(OH)_2D_3$. However, the dietary administration of $24,25(OH)_2D_3$ was without effect on the pattern of 1-hydroxylase and 24-hydroxylase activities. Tanaka *et al.* (1975) followed the sequence of events that occurred after the administration of $1,25(OH)_2D_3$ in terms of the measurable levels of the $25(OH)D_3$ 24-hydroxylase. They reported that alterations in the 24-hydroxylase by PTH or $1,25(OH)_2D_3$ are not related to changes in circulating levels of serum calcium or phosphorus. They further found that actinomycin D or cycloheximide given *in vivo* reduced the 24-hydroxylase specific activity very rapidly. This is consistent with the view that the regulation of this enzyme might be of physiological importance in calcium and phosphorus homeostasis. Unfortunately, this interesting concept has not received experimental support from other laboratories (see Section III,D below).

Henry (1979) presented convincing evidence, using primary cell culture of chick kidney cells, that the 1-hydroxylase and 24-hydroxylase activities are reciprocally related. Cells grown in the absence of $1,25(OH)_2D_3$ have a high $25(OH)D_3$ 1-hydroxylase activity and no $25(OH)D_3$ 24-hydroxylase activity, whereas cells grown in the presence of as little as 5×10^{-9} *M* $1,25(OH)_2D_3$ have a lowered 1-hydroxylase and a modestly elevated 24-hydroxylase activity. From this system Henry presented clear evidence of the ability of $1,25(OH)_2D_3$ to direct the production of $24,25(OH)_2D_3$.

C. Production of $1,24,25(OH)_3D_3$

With the demonstration that the kidney had the enzymatic capacity to not only 1-hydroxylate but also 24-hydroxylate $25(OH)D_3$, it was not unexpected to find that both enzymatic hydroxylation processes could occur on the same substrate to produce $1,24,25(OH)_3D_3$. Boyle *et al.* (1973) were the first to show that $24,25(OH)_2D_3$ could be metabolized by rat kidney homogenates to yield a more polar vitamin D metabolite. This steroid was subsequently isolated by Holick *et al.* (1973) from incubations of chick kidney homogenates and chemically characterized as $1,24,25(OH)_3D_3$. Shortly thereafter, Kleiner and DeLuca (1974) reported the production *in vitro* of the new trihydroxy steroid from 1,25$(OH)_2D_3$ by rat kidney homogenates. It should be emphasized that the chemical characterization of this trihydroxy metabolite, 1,24,25$(OH)_3D_3$, has been effected only on material that was produced under *in vitro* conditions in homogenates from either rat kidney or chick kidney. Tanaka *et al.* (1977) showed that 1,25$(OH)_2D_3$ and 25$(OH)D_3$ can be 24-hydroxylated to yield 1,24,25$(OH)_3D_3$ or 24,25$(OH)_2D_3$ by chick kidney homogenates *in vitro* as well as in anephric rats *in vivo*. They further noted that the 24-hydroxyl was in the *R* configuration. These results describing the extrarenal production of 1,24(*R*),25$(OH)_2D_3$ led to the report by Kumar *et al.* (1978) of the presence in the rat intestine (but not chick intestine) of a 25$(OH)D_3$ 24-hydroxylase and 1,25$(OH)_2D_3$ 24-hydroxylase. The physiological significance of this observation is not yet known.

A major question, however, remains as to whether 1,24,25$(OH)_3D_3$ actually occurs *in vivo* under physiological circumstances. Holick *et al.* (1973) claimed to observe the presence of a metabolite peak on Sephadex LH-20 chromatography which was more polar than 1,25$(OH)_2D_3$ and which was sensitive to periodate; this would be consistent with the identification of this peak as 1,24,25$(OH)_3D_3$, but it does not constitute conclusive proof. In contrast, Friedlander and Norman (1975) definitely demonstrated that chick kidney homogenates have the capability of converting both 24,25$(OH)_2D_3$ and 1,25$(OH)_2D_3$ to a more polar metabolite, which was tentatively identified as 1,24,25$(OH)_3D_3$ on the basis of its chromatographic mobility and susceptibility to periodate cleavage. However, it was not possible to demonstrate the presence of this steroid *in vivo* in lipid extracts obtained from intestine, liver, kidney, or blood of chickens raised on either high (3%) or low (0.05%) dietary calcium levels and given chronic physiological doses of high specific activity radioactive vitamin D for 8 days. The crucial issue here is whether 1,24,25$(OH)_3D_3$ is produced from vitamin D_3; *in vivo* experiments that employ 25$(OH)D_3$, 1,25$(OH)_2D_3$, or 24,25$(OH)_2D_3$ as substrate can never provide an unequivocal answer (see also DeLuca, 1978). Thus, the role, if any, of 1,24,25$(OH)_3D_3$ in calcium and phosphorus homeostasis remains to be determined.

D. Integrated Regulation of the Renal Metabolism of 25$(OH)D_3$

Hay and Watson (1976a,b) carried out a remarkably thorough study of the presence of plasma transport proteins for 25$(OH)D_3$ in 22 species of fish, 12 species of amphibians, 5 species of reptiles, 19 species of birds, and 72 species from 14 orders of mammals: this is consistent with a universal presence in vertebrates of the vitamin D endocrine system.

In view of the proposed steroid hormone mode of action for 1,25$(OH)_2D_3$ and identification of the endocrine system for its production, a pertinent problem is to identify and describe in detail the integrated operation of this endocrine system.

This problem is all the more challenging since, although the kidney is the site of production of $1,25(OH)_2D_3$, it is also clearly capable of producing $24,25(OH)_2D_3$ and possibly $1,24,25(OH)_3D_3$. In this regard, the proposal of DeLuca and coworkers (Tanaka and DeLuca, 1973, 1974) that there is a reciprocal relationship between the enzymatic production of $1,25(OH)_2D_3$ and $24,25(OH)_2D_3$ by the kidneys is quite intriguing. Another important challenge is to quantitatively determine the relationship between stimulation of intestinal calcium transport and regulation of the renal 1-hydroxylase and 24-hydroxylase.

It is known that intestinal calcium absorption is adaptively regulated by the organism so that there is an increased efficiency of calcium absorption under conditions in which the calcium demand of the organism is high (e.g., conditions of low dietary calcium levels) (Nicolaysen, 1938) (see Fig. 6-14). However, it is also known that augmentation of intestinal calcium absorption may occur under conditions of adequate or normal dietary calcium levels if the dietary phosphorus

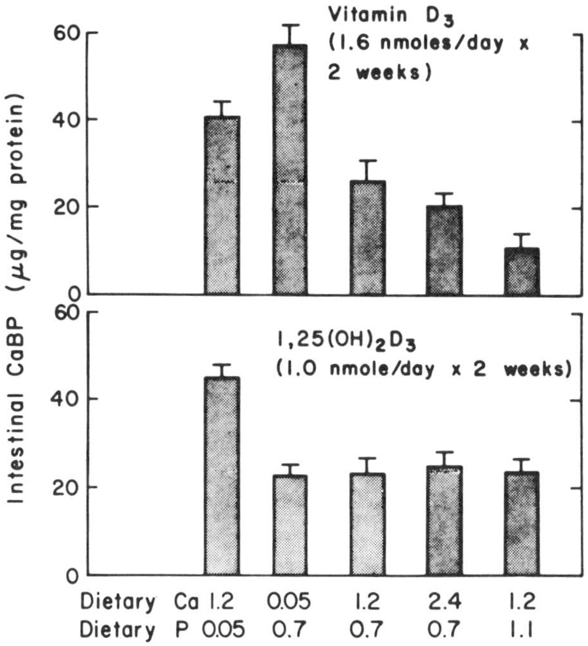

Figure 6-14. Differential production of intestinal CaBP following daily administration of vitamin D_3 or $1,25(OH)_2D_3$. Groups of six to eight chicks, 14 days old, were raised on the indicated experimental diets for an additional 2 weeks, during which time they received 1.6 nmoles/day of vitamin D_3 (upper panel) or 1.0 nmoles/day of $1,25(OH)_2D_3$ (lower panel). Analysis of the diets indicated that the percent calcium was low, 0.05%; normal, 1.2%; high, 2.4%. Dietary phosphorus was low, 0.05%; normal, 0.7%, high, 1.1%. The standard error of the mean is indicated. From Friedlander *et al.* (1977a,b).

level is very low (Carlsson, 1953) (see also Chapter 10). Much evidence has accumulated to suggest that adaptation to the varying calcium demands of an organism involves the endocrine-mediated regulation of production of $1,25(OH)_2D_3$. This steroid then localizes in the nuclear fraction of the intestinal mucosa and initiates the *de novo* biosynthesis of a new protein, a calcium-binding protein (CaBP). Morrissey and Wasserman (1971) clearly documented the direct relationship between elevation of CaBP levels and enhanced intestinal absorption capability for calcium in the chick. Since it is known that $1,25(OH)_2D_3$ stimulates the intestinal biosynthesis of CaBP, an important mode of regulation of the appearance of CaBP may occur via regulation by the kidney of the biosynthesis of $1,25(OH)_2D_3$. As described in preceding sections of this chapter, the process of regulation of the 1-hydroxylase is exceedingly complicated; however, an important point agreed on by all laboratories is that there is a highly significant inverse correlation between the $25(OH)D_3$ 1-hydroxylase activity and serum calcium levels (Henry *et al.*, 1974). This may simply be a manifestation of the trophic actions of PTH. Under conditions of hypocalcemia there would be an elevated circulating concentration of PTH, which would result in an enhanced production of $1,25(OH)_2D_3$ by the kidney. Associated with this would be a concomitant stimulation of the biosynthesis of CaBP in the intestine and a resulting stimulation of intestinal calcium absorption.

Possible mechanisms involved in the enhanced calcium absorption produced by phosphorus deficiency are not yet clear. The role of the $25(OH)D_3$ 1-hydroxylase in this phenomenon is certainly not obvious, although Tanaka and DeLuca (1973, 1974) as well as Baxter and DeLuca (1976) reported that phosphate deprivation results in a modest stimulation of the $25(OH)D_3$ 1-hydroxylase measured under defined *in vitro* conditions. Another interesting aspect of this problem relates to the observation by Bar and Wasserman (1973), Ribovich and DeLuca (1975), as well as Friedlander *et al.* (1977a,b) that administration of pseudo 1α-steroids (such as dihydrotachysterol) or $1,25(OH)_2D_3$ eliminates the adaptation of intestinal calcium transport by chicks or rats raised on low-calcium diets but does not eliminate the stimulation of intestinal calcium transport by low-phosphorus diets. These results clearly suggest that dietary phosphate deprivation may stimulate calcium transport by an as yet unrecognized mechanism.

The laboratories of Norman (Friedlander *et al.*, 1977a,b; Norman *et al.*, 1977) and Bar (Montecuccoli *et al.*, 1977a,b; Edelstein *et al.*, 1978) have carried out extensive studies to probe the steady-state relationships existing under various dietary calcium and phosphorus conditions between the $25(OH)D_3$ 1-hydroxylase and the $25(OH)D_3$ 24-hydroxylase activity, the circulating levels of $1,25(OH)_2D_3$ in the plasma and intestinal mucosa, and the precise level of chick intestinal CaBP. Since the levels of CaBP parallel very closely those of intestinal calcium absorption (Morrissey and Wasserman, 1971), quantitation of this protein represents a good measure of the level of intestinal calcium absorption activity. Figure 6-14 shows the comparative effects of either daily dietary vitamin D or $1,25(OH)_2D_3$ administration on the steady-state level of intestinal CaBP in chicks raised under various dietary calcium and phosphorus conditions. Clearly, in the presence of dietary vitamin D, levels of CaBP and, by inference, intestinal calcium absorption were significantly elevated under both low-calcium and low-phosphorus dietary conditions. However, when $1,25(OH)_2D_3$ was present under identical dietary conditions, the adaptive response to the low calcium content of the diet was totally eliminated, whereas that due to low phosphorus content was still clearly present. Since the level of CaBP can be significantly elevated by low dietary phosphorus conditions, even in the presence of high levels of exogenous $1,25(OH)_2D_3$, a pertinent question was, What role, if any, does the renal $25(OH)D_3$ 1-hydroxylase play in adapting to changing phosphorus levels? Figure 6-15 shows the highly significant inverse correlation between serum calcium levels (4–11.5 mg per 100 ml) and the specific activity of the 1-hydroxylase. Excluding serum calcium values above 11.5 mg per 100 ml is

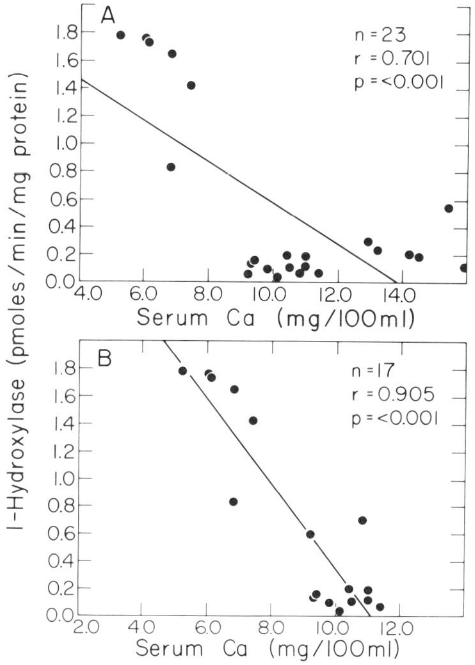

Figure 6-15. Relationship between specific activity of $25(OH)D_3$ 1-hydroxylase and serum calcium levels. Groups of six to eight chicks, 14 days old, were fed one of four diets described in Fig. 6-14. (A) includes all $25(OH)D_3$ 1-hydroxylase values for all serum calcium determinations; (B) excludes $25(OH)D_3$ 1-hydroxylase values for serum calcium levels above 11.5 mg per 100 ml or phosphorus levels below 4 mg per 100 ml. From Friedlander *et al.* 1977a,b).

equivalent to excluding chicks that had a serum phosphorus concentration below 4 mg per 100 ml. For chicks receiving adequate vitamin D and balanced mineral diets, a normal serum calcium level is 9–11 mg per 100 ml and a normal serum phosphorus level is 5–7 mg per 100 ml.

When the same type of analysis is repeated with the serum phosphorus concentrations, two significant trends can be observed in the relation of the 1-hydroxylase to serum phosphorus levels. Figure 6-16A shows the positive relationship for the 25(OH)D_3 1-hydroxylase for all levels of serum phosphorus, whereas Figs. 6-16B and C demonstrate the relationships obtained upon subdividing the population according to appropriate levels of serum phosphorus. Excluding serum phosphorus levels below 4 mg per 100 ml (Fig. 6-16B) yields a highly significant positive correlation between the steady-state level of the 1-hydroxylase and serum phosphorus levels. When serum phosphorus concentrations above 8 mg per 100 ml are excluded (Fig. 6-16C), a different relationship emerges. Now there is a modest inverse correlation between the 1-hydroxylase level and the corresponding serum phosphorus level. Thus, under the appropriate conditions, phosphorus depletion is capable of effecting a small, twofold increase in the steady-state level of the renal 25(OH)D_3 1-hydroxylase.

In view of the results of Boyle *et al.* (1971) suggesting an inverse relationship between circulating levels of 1,25$(OH)_2D_3$ and 24,25$(OH)_2D_3$ depending on the dietary calcium and phosphorus conditions, and also because of their more recent reports (Baxter and DeLuca, 1976), it was important to evaluate the steady-state level of the renal 25(OH)D_3 24-hydroxylase activity. Figures 6-17A and B show the relationship between 24-hydroxylase activity and serum calcium and serum phosphorus levels, respectively. It should be noted that the highest achieved steady-state levels of the 25(OH)D_3 24-hydroxylase are markedly lower than those of the 25(OH)D_3 1-hydroxylase—at best only 10% of the activity of the 1-hydroxylase. Furthermore, there is no apparent correlation between the 24-hydroxylase and serum calcium levels.

Since CaBP is specifically induced by the steroid hormone 1,25$(OH)_2D_3$ and since production of 1,25$(OH)_2D_3$ by the renal 1-hydroxylase can be modulated over a wide range, one would expect a positive relationship between the 25(OH)D_3 1-hydroxylase activity of the kidney and the levels of CaBP in the intestine. This possibility is confirmed by the data presented in Fig. 6-18. The results appear to follow a hyperbolic relationship similar to that of classic Michaelis–Menten enzyme kinetics. A double reciprocal plot of the data, shown in the inset of Fig. 6-18, yields a linear relationship. The intercept of the line on the ordinate indicates that the maximal amount of CaBP that could be produced is around 60 μg per milligram protein. The specific activity of the 25(OH)D_3 1-hydroxylase, which is capable of producing the half-maximal value of CaBP, is approximately 0.2 pmole/min per milligram protein. It is interesting that the corresponding serum calcium value that will yield this specific activity is the normal value, 10 mg per 100 ml (Fig. 6-13).

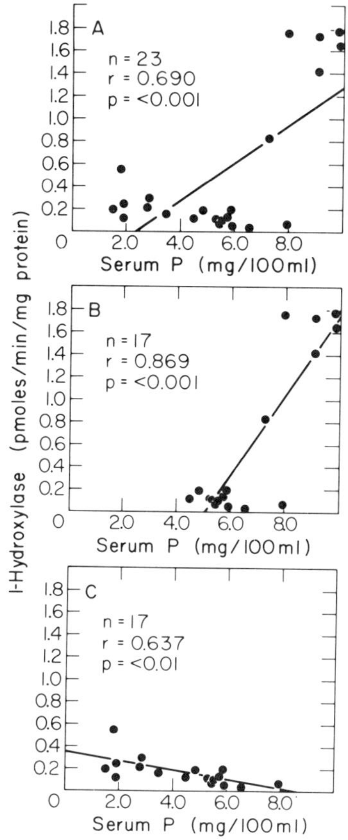

Figure 6-16. Relationship between specific activity of $25(OH)D_3$ 1-hydroxylase and serum phosphorus levels. Groups of six to eight chicks, 14 days old, were fed diets varying in calcium and phosphorus as described in Fig. 6-14 and received vitamin D_3 daily for 2 weeks. (A) includes $25(OH)D_3$ 1-hydroxylase for all serum phosphorus determinations; (B) excludes $25(OH)D_3$ 1-hydroxylase values for serum phosphorus levels below 4 mg 100 ml; (C) excludes $25(OH)D_3$ 1-hydroxylase values for serum phosphorus levels above 8 mg per 100 ml. From Friedlander *et al.* (1977a,b).

Figure 6-19 depicts the close relationship between the amount of radioactive $1,25(OH)_2D_3$ isolated from the intestinal mucosa and the amount of intestinal CaBP present there. The serum levels of calcium and phosphorus are indicated at the bottom of the figure. Both moderate hypocalcemia (6.4 mg per 100 ml) and severe hypophosphatemia (2.1 mg per 100 ml) result in a two- to threefold increase in the amount of radioactive $1,25(OH)_2D_3$ localized in the intestinal mucosa as well as in the steady-state amount of CaBP present there. These results substantiate the cause and effect relationship between these two processes under steady-state conditions.

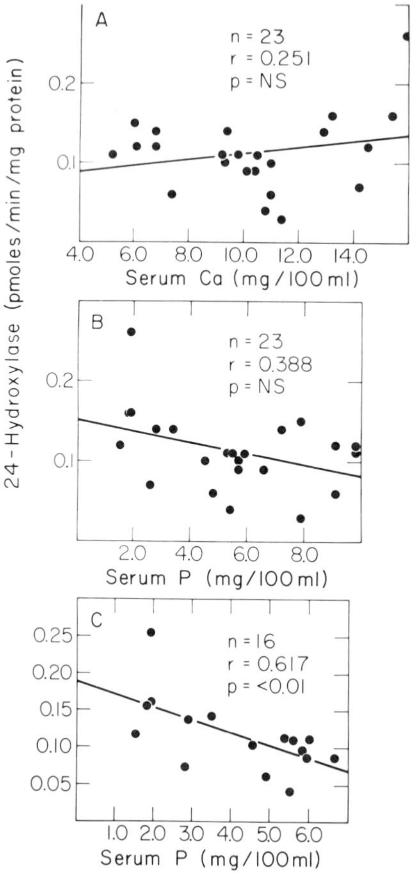

Figure 6-17. Relationship between specific activity of 25(OH)D_3 24-hydroxylase and circulating levels of serum calcium and phosphorus. The experimental protocol is the same as in Fig. 6-14 to 6-16. (A) 25(OH)D_3 24-hydroxylase values for all serum calcium levels; (B) 25(OH)D_3 24-hydroxylase values for all serum phosphorus levels; (C) excludes 25(OH)D_3 24-hydroxylase values for serum phosphorus levels above 7 mg/100 ml. From Friedlander *et al.* (1977a,b).

Figure 6-20 is a model presented by Norman *et al.* (1977) of our current understanding of calcium and phosphorus homeostasis as it pertains to regulation of the kidney levels of 25(OH)D_3 1-hydroxylase and 25(OH)D_3 24-hydroxylase (Fig. 6-20A) and the steady-state relationships between intestinal levels of CaBP which are endocrinologically linked to the circulating levels of serum calcium and serum phosphorus (Fig. 6-20B). In terms of the renal 1-hydroxylase, the dominant factor in its regulation is the circulating serum calcium level; under circumstances of lowered serum calcium levels, there is a sharp rise in the enzymatic capacity for production of 1,25$(OH)_2D_3$. As the animal becomes

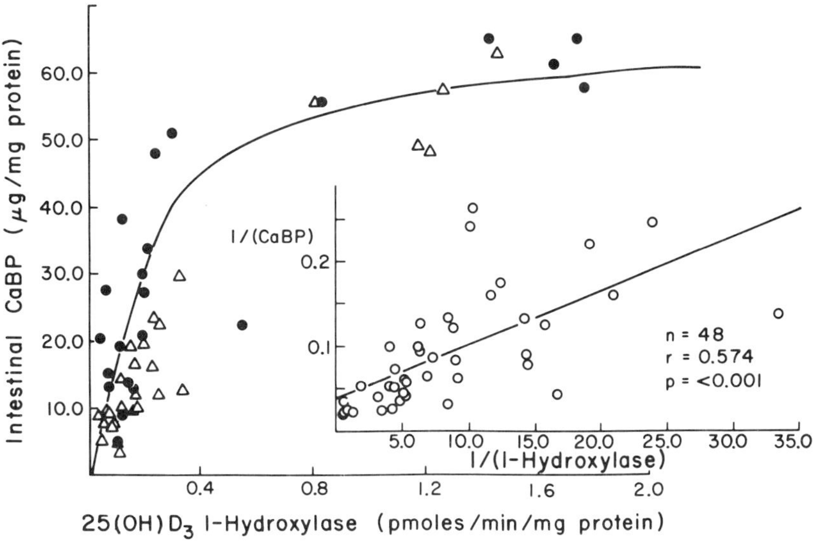

Figure 6-18. Relationship between intestinal CaBP and steady-state level of 25(OH)D_3 1-hydroxylase levels. Groups of six to eight chicks, 14 days old, were fed diets of varying calcium and phosphorus content and were administered daily doses of 1.6 nmoles/day vitamin D_3. Data in main panel are plotted as a function for a rectangular hyperbola, and the inset panel presents the same data plotted in a double reciprocal fashion (●—● and △—△ are data points from two separate experiments; ○—○ all the same data points plotted in a double reciprocal fashion). From Friedlander *et al.* (1977a).

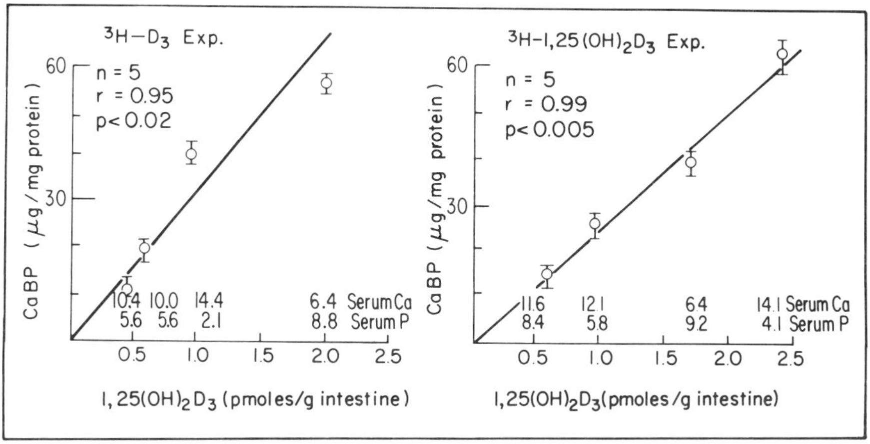

Figure 6-19. Relationship between the amount of tritiated 1,25$(OH)_2D_3$ isolated from the intestinal mucosa and the corresponding levels of intestinal CaBP under hypocalcemic, hypophosphatemic, and normal conditions. Groups of five chicks, 14 days old, were given nonradioactive vitamin D_3 for 1 week and [$1\alpha,2\alpha$-^{3}H]vitamin D_3 for the second week. Dietary calcium and phosphorus levels are the same as those described for Figs. 6-14 to 6-19. For intestinal CaBP the standard error of the mean is shown. From Friedlander *et al.* (1977a,b).

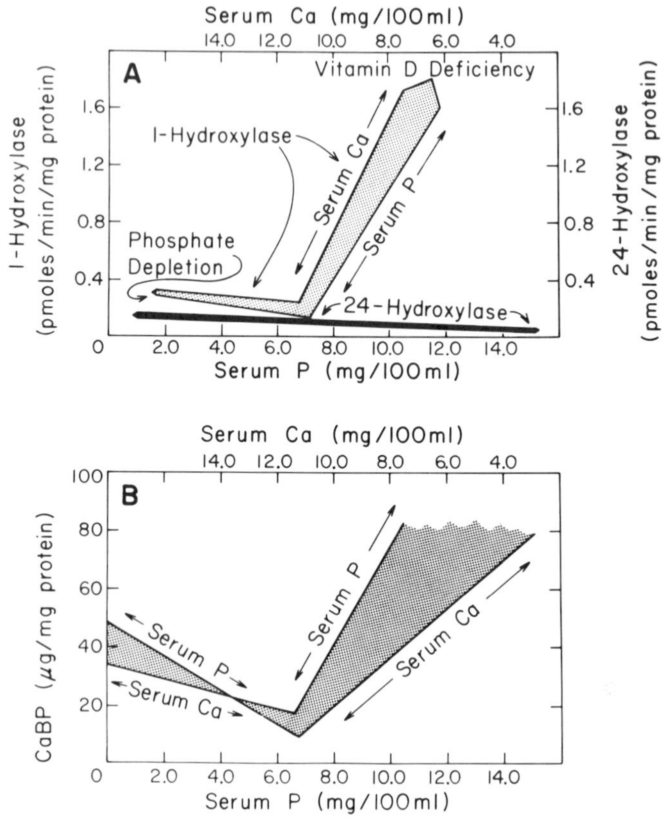

Figure 6-20. Summary of steady-state relationships between 25(OH)D_3 1-hydroxylase and 25(OH)D_3 24-hydroxylase specific activities (A) and level of intestinal calcium-binding protein (CaBP) (B) and serum Ca or serum P levels.

increasingly vitamin D-deficient, a 10- to 20- fold increase can occur in the enzymatic capacity for the production of the steroid hormone 1,25$(OH)_2D_3$. There is also a modest yet quite significant increase in the 1-hydroxylase activity under circumstances of dietary phosphate depletion; however, this response, in comparison to the dominant effects of serum calcium, seems of questionable physiological significance. It should be recalled from Fig. 6-16 that phosphate depletion may play a more important role in the actual binding of 1,25$(OH)_2D_3$ to the intestinal mucosa tissue. This fact is also apparent in Fig. 6-20B, which summarizes the relationships between changing serum calcium and serum phosphorus levels and steady-state levels of CaBP. Once again, it would appear that the downward perturbation of serum calcium levels is capable of inducing a more dramatic elevation of intestinal CaBP levels than is a downward perturbation of serum phosphorus levels. However, it should also be apparent by comparison of Figs. 6-20A and B that phosphate depletion is capable of exerting a relatively greater effect on the intestinal level of CaBP than on the specific gravity of the renal 25$(OH)D_3$ 1-hydroxylase.

E. Production of 25,26$(OH)_2D_3$

One of the eight chemically characterized metabolites of vitamin D is 25,26$(OH)_2D_3$. However, at present there is no information describing where this steroid is biologically produced, although it is generally agreed that it is not a renal metabolite. The naturally occurring epimer is 25R,26$(OH)_2D_3$ (Redel *et al.*, 1978).

IV. 1,25$(OH)_2D_3$ METABOLISM: UNRESOLVED PROBLEMS

Although an extensive amount of information has been collected concerning the metabolism of vitamin D to its hormonally active form, 1,25$(OH)_2D_3$, until recently no information was available concerning the breakdown or clearance of the hormonally active form. In 1975, DeLuca and co-workers initiated a study of

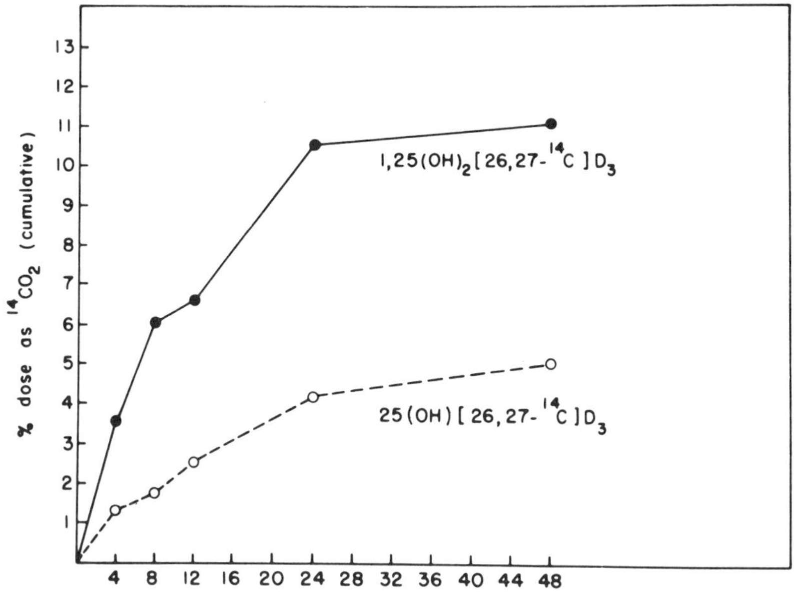

Figure 6-21. Time course of $^{14}CO_2$ in expired air of rachitic chicks given either 650 pmoles (10 U) of 25(OH)[26,27-^{14}C]D_3 or 325 pmoles (5 U) of 1,25$(OH)_2$[26,27-^{14}C]D_3 intravenously. Reproduced from Kumar and DeLuca (1976b) by permission of the authors and publisher.

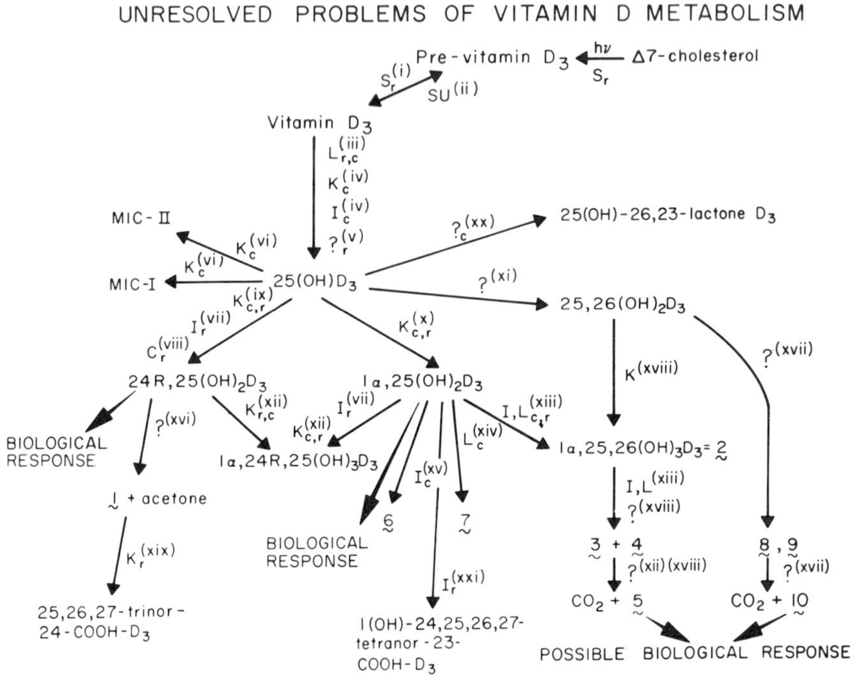

Figure 6-22. Unresolved problems of vitamin D metabolism. This figure summarizes the metabolic interconversions of vitamin D to known steroids as well as several postulated metabolites that have not yet been characterized but whose existence appears likely. Capital letters indicate tissues that have the indicated vitamin D metabolism capability: SU, sea urchin; L, liver; K, kidney; I, intestine; C, cartilage. Superscript numbers in parentheses refer to notes below; subscripts indicate that the tissues with the indicated vitamin D metabolic capability were derived from either the chicken (c) or rat (r). The numbers **1–10** represent postulated vitamin D metabolites whose structures are discussed in the following notes. (i) Hobbs and Pennock (1978) demonstrated *in vivo* an isomerizing enzyme in the sea urchin *Psammechinus miliaris* capable of intraconverting D_3 and pre-D_3. (ii) Bjorkhem and Holmberg (1978) unequivocally showed that the vitamin D_3 25-hydroxylase is found in both rat liver mitochondria and microsomal fractions. (iii) Tucker *et al.* (1973) showed that both intestinal and kidney homogenates from chick but not rat can convert D_3 to 25(OH)D_3. Krawitt (1978) stated that there is no detectable 25-hydroxylase in human intestinal mucosa. (iv) Ribovich and DeLuca (1978a,b) carried out experiments in which rats raised on a variety of Ca and P dietary regimens received daily 250-ng (10-IU) doses for 2 weeks of high specific activity (19 Ci/mmole) [1,2-^{3}H]vitamin D_3. They reported the existence in the blood and/or intestine of at least 13 unidentified vitamin D metabolites designated A, A_T, A′, E, II, V_{t_1}, V_{t_2}, V_b, V'_c, VI, VII, VIII, IX. The structural relationships of these metabolites to the proposed structures discussed in this figure are not known. (v) Ghazarian and DeLuca (1977) demonstrated chick kidney microsomal metabolism *in vitro* of 25(OH)D_3 to two more polar metabolites, MIC-I and MIC-II. See also Bikle and Rasmussen (1974). (vi) Kumar *et al.* (1978) showed that rat intestinal but not chick intestinal homogenates can 24(*R*)-hydroxylate both 25(OH)D_3 and 1,25(OH)$_2D_3$. (vii) Garabedian *et al.* (1974) showed extra renal production *in vivo* in nephrectomized rats of 24,25(OH)$_2D_3$ from 25(OH)D_3; Garabedian *et al.* (1978) found that cartilage tissue has a low specific activity 25(OH)D_3 24(*R*)-hydroxylase. (viii) Boyle *et al.* (1971) reported that mitochondria from chicks or rat kidneys could 24-hydroxylate 25(OH)D_3.

the metabolism of $25(OH)[26,27\text{-}^{14}C]D_3$ as well as $1,25(OH)_2[26,27\text{-}^{14}C]D_3$. Thus Harnden *et al.* (1976) and Kumar *et al.* (1976b) reported on the metabolism of these steroids in rats and Kumar and DeLuca (1976) reported on the metabolism of these steroids in chicks. In both systems there was a rapid evolution of $[^{14}C]$carbon dioxide within 4 hr after administration of the radioactive $1,25(OH)_2D_3$. Some of the data are presented in Fig. 6-21. The exceedingly

---

(ix) Henry *et al.* (1974) showed that the renal $25(OH)D_3$ 1-hydroxylase is a mixed-function steroid hydroxylase located in the mitochondrial fraction. (x) The enzymatic site of production of $25,26(OH)_2D_3$ is not known. (xi) Knutson and DeLuca (1974), Friedlander and Norman (1975), and Tanaka *et al.* (1977) demonstrated that $1,24,25(OH)_3D_3$ can be produced *in vitro* by rat and/or chick mitochondrial preparations using as substrates either $1,25(OH)_2D_3$ or $24(R),25(OH)_2D_3$. (xii) Kumar *et al.* (1976), Harnden *et al.* (1976), and Kumar and DeLuca (1976) showed that after giving physiological doses of $1,25(OH)_2[26,27\text{-}^{14}C]D_3$ to chicks or intact or nephrectomized rats, up to 25–35% of the administered ^{14}C is evolved as $^{14}CO_2$ within 6–9 hr; presumably at least one new steroid, **5**, is formed as a coproduct. It is possible to postulate at least three other metabolites, **2, 3, 4,** representing the C-26 (or C-27) hydroxyl **2**, aldehyde **3**, and carboxyl **4** metabolites, respectively, of $1,25(OH)_2D_3$, which would be formed to ultimately permit release of the C-26 (or C-27) as carbon dioxide by conventional steroid metabolic conversions. Thus, **5** might be 26- or 27-nor-1α(OH)-25-ketovitamin D_3, and **2** would be the $1,25,26(OH)_3D_3$. See also the report of Ribovich and DeLuca (1978c). (xiii) E. J. Friedlander (1978) reported the presence in liver of a less polar metabolite, 7, of $1,25(OH)_2D_3$ that was not an ester. (xiv) Norman and Henry (1979) studied the enzymatic conversion by chick intestinal homogenates of $1,25(OH)_2D_3$ to a H_2O-soluble unknown metabolite, **6.** (xv) If $24(R),25(OH)_2D_3$ undergoes further metabolism by vicinal cleavage of the C-24–C-25 bonds, the products would be acetone plus **1**, the 25,26,27-trinor,-C-24-aldehyde-vitamin D_3. (xvi) If $25,26(OH)_2D_3$ undergoes the same pathway of further metabolism as $1,25(OH)_2D_3$ discussed above under note (12), three similar steroids, **8, 9,** and **10,** would be produced. They might be the C-26 (or C-27) aldehyde **8** and carboxyl **9** metabolites of $25,26(OH)_2D_3$, which could ultimately lead to CO_2 evolution and 26- or 27-nor-25-ketovitamin D_3 **10.** (xvii) Ribovich and DeLuca (1978b) presented some evidence that $25,26(OH)_2D_3$ may be 1α-hydroxylated to yield $1,25,26,(OH)_3D_3$. If $1,25,26(OH)_3D_3$ undergoes the same pathway of further metabolism as **2** discussed above under note (xii), the same three steroids, **3, 4** and **5**, would be produced. They might be the C-26 (or C-27) aldehyde **3** and carboxyl **4** metabolites of $1,25,26(OH)D_3$, which could ultimately lead to CO_2 evolution and 26- or 27-nor-1α,25-ketovitamin D_3, **5.** (xviii) If the aldehyde-containing metabolite **1**, the keto-containing metabolites **5** and **10**, or the carboxyl-containing metabolites **4** and **9** are actually formed, there is then the possibility of ring formation via a hemiacetal, hemiketal, or lactone, respectively, with either the 3β- or 1α-hydroxyl groups on ring A. Such a cyclic structure would have a remarkable resemblance to the polyene antibiotic Filipin (see Fig. 10-8) and might explain the potent effects of Filipin (see Chapter 10) on stimulating calcium uptake by intestinal cells. (xix) DeLuca and Schnoes (1979) have reported the chemical characterization of a side-chain cleavage product of $24,25\text{-}(OH)_2D_3$ that has a C-24 carboxyl group. Its structure was determined to be 25,26,27-trinor-24-COOH-D_3. It was produced in an *in vitro* incubation of a rat kidney homgenate using $24,25(OH)_2$-$[3\alpha\text{-}^3H]D_3$ as a substrate. (xx) DeLuca and Schnoes (1979) have reported the isolation from chick plasma of 25(OH)-26,23-lactone-D_3. (xxi) DeLuca and Schnoes (1979) have studied the further metabolism of $1,25(OH)_2D_3$ and have isolated and characterized from extracts of rat livers the metabolite 1-(OH)-24,25,26,27-tetranor-23-COOH-D_3. It remains to be determined whether the four-carbon side chain fragment which must concomitantly be produced can be further metabolized in a manner to yield CO_2 from C-26 and C-27 as would be predicted from the studies of Kumar and DeLuca (1977).

rapid evolution of the radioactive carbon dioxide suggests that this metabolic pathway may be of some importance to either the functioning of $1,25(OH)_2D_3$ or its clearance from the plasma. Furthermore, Kumar *et al.* (1976a) found that nephrectomy of rats prevented the evolution of $^{14}CO_2$ from radioactive $25(OH)D_3$ but not from $1,25(OH)_2D_3$.

It is apparent from studies of this type that there is much to be learned about the metabolism of vitamin D and particularly the subsequent metabolism of its various metabolites. Figure 6-22 gives a summary of many of the unresolved problems concerning the further metabolism of vitamin D metabolites. As discussed in the notes to this figure there are certainly a number of additional metabolites of vitamin D that will eventually be chemically characterized.

V. VITAMIN D METABOLISM IN MAN

Although the symptoms of a vitamin D deficiency were first recognized in man, studies in man concerning the formation and metabolism of vitamin D have been relatively few. Naturally such studies had to await the development of radioactive preparations of vitamin D with high specific activity. The first well-documented account of the production of more polar metabolites in human subjects from radioactive doses of vitamin D_3 was provided by Avioli *et al.* (1967a,b). Since that time, however, the bulk of the work concerning the metabolism of vitamin D in man has been carried out by Mawer, Stanbury, and co-workers (Mawer *et al.*, 1972, 1975b; Mawer, 1974). Two excellent reviews of their work have appeared (Mawer *et al.*, 1975a; Mawer and Taylor, 1978).

Their principal approach was to administer either [^{3}H]vitamin D_3, ^{3}H-labeled $25(OH)D_3$, or mixed doses of [1,2-^{3}H]vitamin D_3 plus [4-^{14}C]vitamin D_3 and to chromatographically evaluate at subsequent time periods the relative proportions of unaltered vitamin D_3 or $25(OH)D_3$ and dihydroxylated metabolites $1,25(OH)_2D_3$, $24,25(OH)_2D_3$ or $25,26(OH)_2D_3$ that were present in plasma samples. Until the availability of Sephadex LH-20 and high-pressure liquid chromatographic techniques it was impossible to separate the three dihydroxylated metabolites from one another. However, the amount of $1,25(OH)_2D_3$ could be quantitated by either (a) subjecting the dihydroxy metabolite region of the chromatogram to sodium periodate and rechromatographing [both $24,25(OH)_2D_3$ and $25,26(OH)_2D_3$ contain vicinal hydroxyls and would be altered by periodate treatment] or (b) employing mixed doses of [1,2-^{3}H,4-^{14}C]vitamin D_3 so that a "tritium loss" would occur in the peak representing $1,25(OH)_2D_3$. An additional complication in studies of this type is that the tracer dose of vitamin D and its metabolites are subject to dilution by various pools of unlabeled parent vitamin and metabolites.

Mawer and colleagues identified in man several metabolites more polar than vitamin D_3 (Mawer and Stanbury, 1968; Mawer and Schaefer, 1969; Mawer *et al.*, 1969) at exactly the same time that Kodicek, Norman, DeLuca, and co-workers were making similar observations in experimental animals. It was ultimately determined (Mawer *et al.*, 1971b) that the principal metabolite of vitamin D present in human plasma was $25(OH)D_3$, with much smaller quantities of the dihydroxylated metabolites. The most important observation of Mawer and colleagues was that in any given individual the metabolic disposal of vitamin D entering the body appears to be determined by the state of vitamin D nutrition of that individual. This is a reflection, undoubtedly, of the different circulating levels of vitamin D_3 and $25(OH)D_3$, which would be related to the vitamin D intake and ultraviolet exposure of the subject. This observation has the important consequence that a comparison of the kinetics and turnover of vitamin D or metabolites between healthy control or diseased subjects is valid only if the subjects have a comparable vitamin D nutrition.

Mawer *et al.* (1971a, 1973; Stanbury *et al.*, 1971) were the first to show that patients with chronic renal failure could not produce $1,25(OH)_2D_3$. They arrived at this conclusion by assessing the "tritium loss" present in the dihydroxy metabolite region of chromatograms obtained from the plasma of normal subjects or those with severe chronic renal failure or who were anephric (see also Hartenbower *et al.*, 1977).

A landmark study reporting the relationship between vitamin D metabolism and parathyroid function in man (Mawer *et al.*, 1975a) was in excellent agreement with the observations of Henry *et al.* (1974; Norman *et al.*, 1977; Friedlander *et al.*, 1977a,b) obtained in experimental animals (see Fig. 6-23). Considering the limitations of sample size and accessibility, their observations and conclusions are all the more remarkable. Mawer *et al.* (1975a) made several important observations.

1. No normal subjects produced $1,25(OH)_2D_3$ and $24,25(OH)_2D_3$ simultaneously. This is consistent with the suggestion of Boyle *et al.* (1971) and Henry (1979) concerning the reciprocal relationship between the 1-hydroxylase and 24-hydroxylase.
2. In normal subjects with a relative vitamin D deficiency, serum $1,25(OH)_2D_3$ levels were related inversely to both serum $25(OH)D_3$ levels and serum calcium levels but were positively related to serum immunoreactive PTH levels (see Fig. 6-19). No correlation was found between plasma $1,25(OH)_2D_3$ level and serum phosphorus level.
3. All subjects with primary hyperparathyroidism produced simultaneously $1,25(OH)_2D_3$ and $24,25(OH)_2D_3$.
4. In normal individuals the plasma concentration of $1,25(OH)_2D_3$ varied over only a fourfold range (18–75 pg/ml). This is quite compatible with the model of a regulated production of this steroid hormone. Also, their calculated

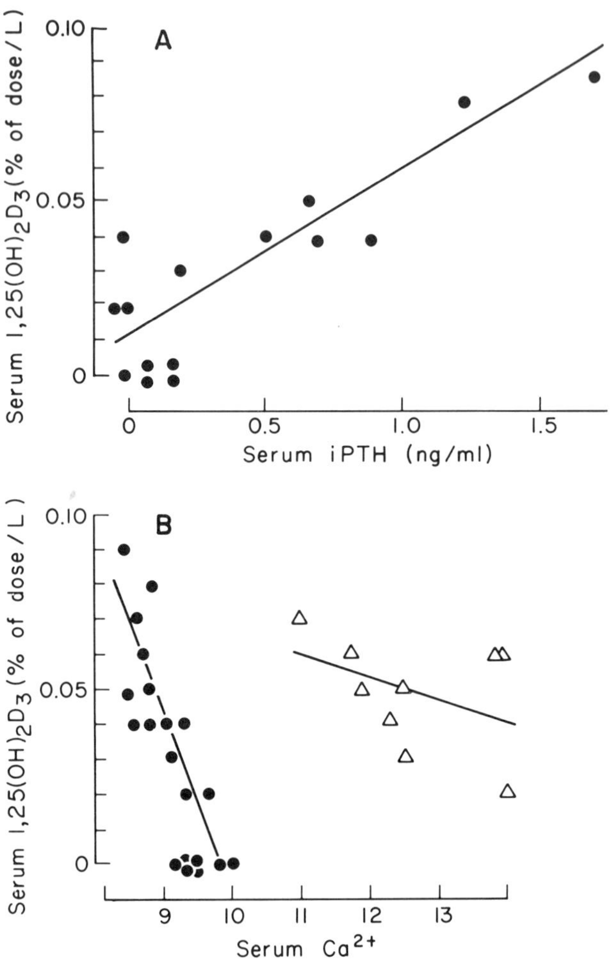

Figure 6-23. (A) Relationship between serum immunoreactive PTH (iPTH) and the serum concentrations of tritiated $1,25(OH)_2D_3$ in normal individuals. (B) Relationships between serum $1,25(OH)_2D_3$ and serum Ca^{2+} (mg/dl) in control subjects (●—●) and patients with primary hyperparathyroidism (△—△). Taken from Mawer *et al.* (1975a) by permission of the authors and publisher.

values for the plasma concentration of $1,25(OH)_2D_3$ are in excellent agreement with those obtained by steroid competition assay, as tabulated in Table 8-7.

5. The production of $1,25(OH)_2D_3$ is regulated directly or indirectly by parathyroid hormone.

Gray *et al.* (1974) studied the fate of labeled vitamin D in normal subjects and anephric patients undergoing maintenance hemodialysis. They found that, although the total pools of plasma $25(OH)D_3$ were equivalent in both groups, the turnover rate of $25(OH)D_3$ in the anephric patients was 1.6 ± 0.1 (S.E.M.) μg/day whereas in the normal subjects it was 2.8 ± 0.3 (S.E.M.) μg/day. Thus, the absence of the kidneys clearly retards the turnover rate of $25(OH)D_3$.

Mawer *et al.* (1975b) and Gray *et al.* (1977) studied the metabolism of tritiated $1,25(OH)_2D_3$ in man. Mawer *et al.* (1975b) found the plasma disappearance of $1,25(OH)_2D_3$ to have a $t_{\frac{1}{2}}$ of 18 to 26 hr. Gray *et al.* (1977) reported that the plasma disappearance curves of tritiated $1,25(OH)_2D_3$ could be resolved into three exponential phases. The average half-lives of the three phases were similar irrespective of the dose (30 pmoles, two subjects; 300–600 pmoles, four subjects): phase I, 4.8 ± 0.2 mins; phase II, 74 ± 46 mins; phase III, 24 ± 5 hr.

Assuming that the phase II rate constant approximates the disappearance of $1,25(OH)_2D_3$ from the plasma compartment, it can be estimated that the plasma pool of $1,25(OH)_2D_3$ is renewed six to eight times daily, whereas the daily plasma turnover is approximately 1.4 nmoles or 0.5 μg/day. This is in excellent agreement with the earlier calculations of Norman and Henry (1974). Also, these experimental results are entirely consistent with the observations that the renal output of $1,25(OH)_2D_3$ in man can be regulated in accordance with his calcium needs.

Krawitt *et al.* (1977) evaluated the absorption, hydroxylation, and excretion of vitamin D_3 in subjects with primary biliary cirrhosis. They found no difference between the 25-hydroxylation of vitamin D_3 in these subjects and that in normal control subjects; however, there was an increased urinary excretion of radioactivity derived from the parent vitamin D_3.

VI. METABOLISM OF VITAMIN D ANALOGS

A. 1α-Hydroxyvitamin D_3

1α-Hydroxyvitamin D_3 [$1\alpha(OH)D_3$] is a highly biologically active analog of $1,25(OH)_2D_3$ in animal systems (Haussler *et al.*, 1973) as well as in man (Chan *et al.*, 1975; Russell *et al.*, 1974; Brickman *et al.*, 1976). The question has been raised as to whether $1\alpha(OH)D_3$ is biologically active in its own right, or whether there is a requirement for its metabolism, i.e., 25-hydroxylation by the liver to give $1,25(OH)_2D_3$, which is the steroid form that elicits the biological responses. This question was pursued indirectly by Haussler and colleagues (Brumbaugh *et al.*, 1974; Zerwekh *et al.*, 1974) using an intestinal cytosol–chromatin assay (see Chapter 8). Also, Holick and co-workers prepared tritiated $1\alpha(OH)D_3$ and studied its metabolism in the rat (Holick *et al.*, 1976a) and in the chick (Holick *et al.*, 1976b). A similar study employing perfused rat livers was carried out by Fukushima *et al.* (1975). All results obtained in the foregoing studies support the view that $1\alpha(OH)D_3$ is obligatorily metabolized to $1,25(OH)_2D_3$ before the initiation of any biological responses. Holick *et al.* (1977a,c) demonstrated the conversion of $1\alpha(OH)[6\alpha\text{-}^3H]D_3$ to $1,25(OH)_2[6\alpha\text{-}^3H]D_3$ in a patient with severe renal failure.

B. Pseudo 1α Analogs

A number of radioactive analogs of $1,25(OH)_2D_3$ have been prepared which belong to the category of pseudo 1α-hydroxysteroids (see Chapter 5). Lawson and Bell (1974) studied the metabolism of tritiated dihydrotachysterol and 5,6-*trans*-vitamin D_3. They reported that both of these steroids were very rapidly metabolized to more polar products in the chick in comparison to the rate of disappearance of control tritiated vitamin D_3. For dihydrotachysterol 20% of the administered dose was excreted in the bile in the first 24 hr, with about 50% of this fraction as a carboxylic acid derivative.

It was previously established by Hallick and DeLuca (1972) that radioactive dihydrotachysterol, and by Holick *et al.* (1972a) that radioactive 5,6-*trans*-D_3 and 25(OH)-5,6-*trans*-D_3, do not undergo hydroxylation at C-1 *in vivo*. Similar results were reported by Lawson and Bell (1974) and Schaefer *et al.* (1975). Holick *et al.* (1972b) found that, although 25(OH)-5,6-*trans*-D_3 stimulated intestinal calcium absorption in the rat, it had little activity for bone calcium mobilization.

A most interesting advance in our understanding of the metabolism of vitamin D and its analogs will occur in the future if radioactive preparations of many of the analogs of $1,25(OH)_2D_3$ and $25(OH)D_3$ listed in Chapter 5 become available.

VII. EFFECTS OF CHLORINATED HYDROCARBONS ON VITAMIN D METABOLISM

There have been many reports in the technical literature that have focused on some of the ecological hazards that result from the widespread occurrence of chlorinated hydrocarbons such as DDT, its major metabolite, DDE, and polychlorinated biphenyls (PCB) in the biosphere (Hickey and Anderson, 1968; Porter and Wiemeyer, 1969; Wiemeyer and Porter, 1970; Peakall, 1969; Switzer *et al.*, 1970; Rehfeld *et al.*, 1972; Scott *et al.*, 1975). These compounds have been suggested as possible causative agents of an altered calcium metabolism that may result in avian reproductive failures. Raptors in Britain, including the peregrine (*Falco peregrinus*), sparrow hawk (*Accipiter nisus*), and golden eagle (*Aquila chrysaetos*), have reproduced less successfully with the increased use of chlorinated hydrocarbons (Ratcliffe, 1967), and egg breakage in the nest seems to be a major part of the phenomenon. In the United States, declining populations of bald eagles (*Haliaetus leucocephalus*) and ospreys (*Pandion haliaetus*) and extirpated populations of peregrines have been related to decreases in eggshell weight (Hickey and Anderson, 1968).

The incorporation of calcium into an eggshell is the end result of an exceedingly complex pathway of calcium metabolism. Dietary calcium is absorbed from the intestine into the blood and then is deposited in the medullary bone, which is comprised primarily of the femur, tibia, and fibula. The medullary bone functions as a temporary depot for the calcium. When the female is not producing an egg, the serum calcium level is 9 mg per 100 ml; during egg production it can approach 30 mg per 100 ml. The final step in the process involves transport of calcium across the eggshell gland and deposition in the shell as calcium carbonate.

In view of this multistep process, it is apparent that there are many potential sites and steps for the deleterious intervention of the chlorinated hydrocarbons. Since the formation and resorption of medullary bone are largely under the control of estrogens and androgens, it has been hypothesized (Kuntzman *et al.*, 1966) that DDT treatment produces a sex hormone imbalance. This hypothesis has been experimentally documented (Nowicki and Norman, 1972); however, to date, a direct link between this finding and the calcification process has not been firmly established.

With the unraveling of the elaborate metabolic pathway for the conversion of vitamin D to its hormonally active forms, and with the identification of the intervention of $1,25(OH)_2D_3$ in the eggshell gland to generate a calcium-binding protein, an alternative attractive hypothesis for the "thin eggshell syndrome" is that chlorinated hydrocarbons may interfere with the function and/or metabolism of vitamin D. Thus, Norman's laboratory (Nowicki *et al.*, 1972a,b; Wong *et al.*, 1973) reported that chronic feeding of low levels of DDT to vitamin D-deficient chicks inhibits the generation of biological response to subsequent administration of physiological doses of vitamin D as measured by stimulation of intestinal calcium absorption and bone calcium mobilization. Also, Wong *et al.* (1974) observed that chronic administration of PCB's to rachitic chicks blocked these same biological responses to physiological doses of vitamin D. These results, considered in conjunction with a report of Peakall (1969) on the effects of DDT on vitamin D metabolism in liver homogenate preparations incubated with radioactive vitamin D, may provide some insight into the basis for the "thin eggshell syndrome." It is apparent from studies of this type that the metabolic pathway for the conversion of vitamin D to its biologically active form is exceedingly vulnerable and may be affected by a surprisingly wide variety of substances.

REFERENCES

Avioli, L. V., Lee, S. W., McDonald, J. E., Lund, J., and DeLuca, H. F. (1967a). *J. Clin. Invest.* **46,** 983.

Avioli, L. V., Williams, F., Lund, J., and DeLuca, H. F. (1967b). *J. Clin. Invest.* **46,** 1907.

Bar, A., and Hurwitz, S. (1973). *Poult. Sci.* **52,** 2338.
Bar, A., and Wasserman, R. H. (1973). *Biochem. Biophys. Res. Commun.* **54,** 191.
Baxter, L. A., and DeLuca, H. F. (1976). *J. Biol. Chem.* **251,** 3158.
Baxter, L. A., DeLuca, H. F., Bonjour, S. D., and Fleisch, H. A. (1974). *Arch. Biochem. Biophys.* **164,** 665.
Bekemeier, H. (1958). *Acta Biol. Med. Ger.* **1,** 756.
Bekemeier, H. (1959). *Hoppe-Seyler's Z. Physiol. Chem.* **314,** 125.
Bekemeier, H., and Pfenningsdorf, G. (1959). *Hoppe-Seyler's Z. Physiol. Chem.* **314,** 120.
Bell, P. A., and Kodicek, E. (1970). *Biochem. J.* **116,** 755.
Berlin, C. M., and Schimke, R. T. (1965). *Mol. Pharmacol.* **1,** 149.
Bhattacharyya, M. H., and DeLuca, H. F. (1973). *J. Biol. Chem.* **248,** 2969.
Bhattacharyya, M. H., and DeLuca, H. F. (1974a). *Arch. Biochem. Biophys.* **160,** 58.
Bhattacharyya, M. H., and DeLuca, H. F. (1974b). *Biochem. Biophys. Res. Commun.* **59,** 734.
Bikle, D. D., and Rasmussen, H. (1974). *Biochim. Biophys. Acta* **362,** 425.
Bikle, D. D., and Rasmussen, H. (1975). *J. Clin. Invest.* **55,** 292.
Bikle, D. D., Murphy, E. W., and Rasmussen, H. (1975). *J. Clin. Invest.* **55,** 299.
Bikle, D. D., Murphy, E. W., and Rasmussen, H. (1976). *Biochim. Biophys. Acta* **437,** 394.
Bills, C. E. (1954). *In* "The Vitamins" (W. H. Sebrell, Jr. and R. S. Harris, eds.), 1st ed., Vol. 2, p. 164. Academic Press, New York.
Bishop, J. E., and Norman, A. W. (1975). *Arch. Biochem. Biophys.* **167,** 769.
Bjorkhem, I., and Holmberg, I. (1978). *J. Biol. Chem.* **253,** 842.
Blondin, G. A., Kulkarni, B. D., and Nes, W. R. (1967). *Comp. Biochem. Physiol.* **20,** 369.
Blunt, J. F., DeLuca, H. F., and Schnoes, H. K. (1968a). *Chem. Commun.* p. 801.
Blunt, J. F., DeLuca, H. F., and Schnoes, H. K. (1968b). *Biochemistry* **7,** 3317.
Bonjour, J.-P., Russell, R. G. G., Morgan, D. B., and Fleisch, H. A. (1972a). *Am. J. Physiol.* **224,** 1011.
Bonjour, J.-P., Herrath, D. V., Schaefer, K., and Fleisch, H. (1972b). *Experientia* **28,** 726.
Bonjour, J.-P., Trechsel, U., Fleisch, H., Schenk, R., DeLuca, H. F., and Baxter, L. A. (1975). *Am. J. Physiol.* **229,** 402.
Booth, B. E., Tsai, H. C., and Morris, R. C., Jr. (1977). *Meta. Clin. Exp.* **26,** 1099.
Botham, K. M., Ghazarian, J. G., Kream, B. E., and DeLuca, H. F. (1976). *Biochemistry* **15,** 2130.
Boyle, I. T., Gray, R. W., and DeLuca, H. F. (1971). *Proc. Natl. Acad. Sci. U.S.A.* **68,** 2131.
Boyle, I. T., Omdahl, J. L., Gray, R. W., and DeLuca, H. F. (1973). *J. Biol. Chem.* **248,** 4174.
Brickman, A. S., Coburn, J. W., Friedman, G. R., Okamura, W. H., Massry, S. G., and Norman, A. W. (1976). *J. Clin. Invest.* **57,** 1540.
Brumbaugh, P. F., Haussler, D. H., Bressler, R., and Haussler, M. R. (1974). *Science* **183,** 1089.
Bunker, J. W. M., Harris, R. S., and Mosher, L. M. (1940). *J. Am. Chem. Soc.* **62,** 508.
Carlsson, A. (1953). *Acta Pharmacol. Toxicol.* **9,** 32.
Chan, J. C., Oldham, S. B., Holick, M. F., and DeLuca, H. F. (1975). *J. Am. Med. Assoc.* **234,** 47.
Cinti, D. L., Golub, E. E., and Bronner, F. (1976). *Biochem. Biophys. Res. Commun.* **72,** 546.
Colston, K. W., Evans, I. M. A., Galante, L., MacIntyre, I., and Moss, D. W. (1973). *Biochem. J.* **134,** 817.
Cooper, D. Y., Narasimhulu, S., Rosenthal, O., and Estabrook, R. W. (1968). *In* "Functions of the Adrenal Cortex" (K. W. McKerns, ed.), Vol. II, p. 897. Appleton, New York.
Cruickshank, E. M., Kodicek, E., and Armitage, P. (1953). *Biochem. J.* **54,** 337.
Cruickshank, E. M., Kodicek, E., and Armitage, P. (1954). *Biochem. J.* **58,** 172.
Czarnowska-Misztal, E., Zull, J. E., and DeLuca, H. F. (1966). *Nature (London)* **210,** 96.
David, J., and DeLuca, H. F. (1977). *Endocrinology* **101,** 1184.
Day, H. G., and McCollum, E. V. (1939). *J. Biol. Chem.* **130,** 269.
DeLuca, H. F. (1969a). *Am. J. Clin. Nutr.* **22,** 412.
DeLuca, H. F. (1969b). *J. Agric. Food Chem.* **17,** 778.

DeLuca, H. F. (1969c). *Arch. Intern. Med.* **124,** 442.
DeLuca, H. F. (1969d). *Fed. Proc., Fed. Am. Soc. Exp. Biol.* **28,** 1678.
DeLuca, H. F. (1969e). *Calcif. Tissue Res.* **4,** 283.
DeLuca, H. F. (1978). *Proc. Int. Congr. Nephrol., 7th, 1978,* p. 447.
DeLuca, H. F., and Schnoes, H. K. (1979). Recent Developments in the Metabolism of Vitamin D. *In* "Vitamin D: Recent Basic Advances and their Clinical Application (Proceedings of the Fourth Workshop on Vitamin D)" (A. W. Norman, K. Schaefer, D. von Herrath, H.-G. Grigoleit, E. B. Mawer, T. Suda, H. F. DeLuca, and J. W. Coburn, eds.) Walter de Gruyter Publishing Company, Elmsford, New York.
Doboszynska, B, and Datsenko, Z. M. (1966). *Bull. Acad. Pol. Sci., Ser. Sci. Biol.* **14,** 199.
Drescher, D., DeLuca, H. F., and Imrie, M. H. (1969). *Arch. Biochem. Biophys.* **130,** 657.
Edelstein, S., and Noff, D. (1977). *FEBS Lett.* **82,** 115.
Edelstein, S., Noff, D., Sinai, L., Harell, A., Puschett, J. B., Golub, E. E., and Bronner, F. (1978). *Biochem. J.* **170,** 227.
Ezawa, I., Sano, Y., and Ogata, E. (1974). *FEBS Lett.* **43,** 353.
Favus, M. J., Walling, M. W., and Kimberg, D. V. (1974). *J. Clin. Invest.* **53,** 1139.
Frame, B., Parfitt, A. M., and Duncan, H., eds. (1973). "Clinical Aspects of Metabolic Bone Disease," pp. 291–345. Exerpta Med. Found. Amsterdam.
Fraser, D. R., and Emtage, J. S. (1976). *Biochem. J.* **160,** 671.
Fraser, D. R., and Kodicek, E. (1970). *Nature (London)* **228,** 764.
Fraser, D. R., and Kodicek, E. (1973). *Nature (London), New Biol.* **241,** 163.
Friedlander, E. J. (1978). Ph.D. Dissertation, Univ. California, Riverside.
Friedlander, E. J., and Norman, A. W. (1975). *Arch. Biochem. Biophys.* **170,** 731.
Friedlander, E. J., Henry, H., and Norman, A. W. (1977a). *J. Biol. Chem.* **252,** 8677.
Friedlander, E. J., Henry, H., and Norman, A. W. (1977b). *In* "Vitamin D: Biochemical, Chemical and Clinical Aspects Related to Calcium Metabolism" (A. W. Norman *et al.,* eds.), p. 289. de Gruyter, Berlin.
Fukushima, M., Suzuki, Y., Tohira, Y., Matsunaga, I., Ochi, K., Nagano, H., Nishii, Y., and Suda, T. (1975). *Biochem. Biophys. Res. Commun.* **66,** 632.
Galante, L. S., Colston, K. W., MacAuley, S. J., and MacIntyre, I. (1972a). *Nature (London)* **238,** 271.
Galante, L. S., MacAuley, S. J., Colston, K. W., and MacIntyre, I. (1972b). *Lancet* **1,** 985.
Galante, L. S., Colston, K. W., Evans, I. M. A., Byfield, P. G. H., Matthews, E. W., and MacIntyre, I. (1973). *Nature (London)* **244,** 438.
Garabedian, M., Holick, M. F., DeLuca, H. F., and Boyle, I. T. (1972). *Proc. Natl. Acad. Sci. U.S.A.* **69,** 1673.
Garabedian, M., Pavlovitch, M., Fellot, C., and Balsan, S. (1974). *Proc. Natl. Acad. Sci. U.S.A.* **71,** 554.
Garabedian, M., Bailly-Du-Bois, M., Corvol, M. T., Pezant, E., and Balsan, S. (1978). *Endocrinology* **102,** 1262.
Ghazarian, J. G., and DeLuca, H. F. (1974). *Arch. Biochem. Biophys.* **160,** 63.
Ghazarian, J. G., Schnoes, H. K., and DeLuca, H. F. (1973). *Biochemistry* **12,** 2555.
Ghazarian, J. G., and DeLuca, H. F. (1977). *Biochem. Biophys. Res. Commun.* **75,** 550.
Ghazarian, J. G., Jefcoate, C. R., Knutson, J. C., Orme-Johnson, W. H., and DeLuca, H. F. (1974). *J. Biol. Chem.* **249,** 3926.
Goldblatt, H., and Soames, K. M. (1923). *Biochem. J.* **17,** 446.
Gray, R. W., Boyle, I., and DeLuca, H. F. (1971). *Science* **172,** 1232.
Gray, R. W., Omdahl, J. L., Ghazarian, J., and DeLuca, H. F. (1972). *J. Biol. Chem.* **247,** 7528.
Gray, R. W., Weber, H. P., Dominguez, J. H., and Leman, J. (1974). *J. Clin. Endocrinol. Metab.* **39,** 1045.
Gray, R. W., Wilz, D. R., Caldas, A., Leman, J., and DeLuca, H. F. (1977). *In* "Vitamin D:

Biochemical, Chemical and Clinical Aspects Related to Calcium Metabolism'' (A. W. Norman *et al.*, eds.), p. 123. de Gruyter, Berlin.
Greaves, J. D., and Schmidt, C. L. A. (1933). *J. Biol. Chem.* **102,** 101.
Haddad, J. G., and Stamp, T. C. B. (1974). *Am. J. Med.* **57,** 57.
Haddad, J. G., Boisseau, V., and Avioli, L. V. (1971). *J. Nutr.* **102,** 269.
Hahn, T. B., Hindin, B. A., Sharp, C., and Haddad, J. G. (1972). *N. Engl. J. Med.* **287,** 900.
Hallick, R. B., and DeLuca, H. F. (1972). *J. Biol. Chem.* **247,** 91.
Hanewald, K. H., Rappoldt, M. P., and Roborgh, J. R. (1961). *Recl. Trav. Chim. Pays-Bas* **80,** 1003.
Harnden, D., Kumar, R., Holick, M. F., and DeLuca, H. F. (1976). *Science* **193,** 493.
Hartenbower, D. L., Henry, H. L., Norman, A. W., and Coburn, J. W. (1975). *Clin. Sci.* **23,** 322A.
Hartenbower, D. L., Stella, F. J., Norman, A. W., Friedler, R. M., and Coburn, J. W. (1977). *J. Lab. Clin. Med.* **20,** 760.
Haussler, M. R., and Norman, A. W. (1967). *Arch. Biochem. Biophys.* **118,** 145.
Haussler, M. R., and Norman, A. W. (1969). *Proc. Natl. Acad. Sci. U.S.A.* **62,** 155.
Haussler, M. R., Myrtle, J. F., and Norman, A. W. (1968). *J. Biol. Chem.* **243,** 4055.
Haussler, M. R., Thomson, W. W., and Norman, A. W. (1969). *Exp. Cell Res.* **58,** 234.
Haussler, M. R., Boyce, D. W., Littledike, E. T., and Rasmussen, H. (1971). *Proc. Natl. Acad. Sci. U.S.A.* **68,** 177.
Haussler, M. R., Zerwekh, J. E., Hesse, R. H., Rizzardo, E., and Pechet, M. M. (1973). *Proc. Natl. Acad. Sci. U.S.A.* **70,** 2248.
Hay, A. W. M., and Watson, G. (1976a). *Comp. Biochem. Physiol. B* **53,** 163.
Hay, A. W. M., and Watson, G. (1976b). *Comp. Biochem. Physiol. B* **53,** 167.
Henry, H. L. (1977a). *In* ''Vitamin D: Biochemical, Chemical and Clinical Aspects Related to Calcium Metabolism'' (A. W. Norman *et al.*, eds.), p. 125. de Gruyter, Berlin.
Henry, H. L. (1977b). *Biochem. Biophys. Res. Commun.* **74,** 768.
Henry, H. L. (1979). *J. Biol. Chem.* **254,** 2722.
Henry, H. L., and Norman, A. W. (1974). *J. Biol. Chem.* **249,** 7529.
Henry, H. L., and Norman, A. W. (1975a). *Comp. Biochem. Physiol. B* **50,** 431.
Henry, H. L., and Norman, A. W. (1975b). *In* ''Proceedings of the Second Workshop on Vitamin D and Problems Related to Uremic Bone Disease'' (A. W. Norman *et al.*, eds.), p. 1. de Gruyter, Berlin.
Henry, H. L., and Norman, A. W. (1976). *Arch. Biochem. Biophys.* **172,** 582.
Henry, H. L., Midgett, R. J., and Norman, A. W. (1974). *J. Biol. Chem.* **249,** 7584.
Henry, H. L., Taylor, A. N., and Norman, A. W. (1977). *J. Nutr.* **107,** 1918.
Hess, A. F., and Weinstock, M. (1922). *J. Am. Med. Assoc.* **80,** 687.
Heymann, W. (1937a). *J. Biol. Chem.* **118,** 371.
Heymann, W. (1937b). *J. Biol. Chem.* **122,** 256.
Hickey, J. J., and Anderson, D. W. (1968). *Science* **162,** 271.
Higaki, M., Takahashi, M., Suzuki, T., and Sahashi, Y. (1965a). *J. Vitaminol.* **11,** 261.
Higaki, M., Takahashi, M., Suzuki, T., and Sahashi, Y. (1965b). *J. Vitaminol.* **11,** 266.
Hill, L. F., Lumb, G. A., Mawer, E. B., and Stanbury, S. W. (1973). *Clin. Sci.* **44,** 335.
Hobbs, R. N., and Pennock, J. F. (1978). *Biochem. Soc. Trans.* **5,** 1713.
Holick, M. F., Schnoes, H. K., DeLuca, H. F., Suda, T., and Cousins, R. J. (1971). *Biochemistry* **10,** 2799.
Holick, M. F., Garabedian, M., and DeLuca, H. F. (1972a). *Biochemistry* **11,** 2715.
Holick, M. F., Garabedian, M., and DeLuca, H. F. (1972b). *Science* **176,** 1247.
Holick, M. F., Kleiner, A., Schnoes, H. K., Kasten, P. M., Boyle, I. T., and DeLuca, H. F. (1973). *J. Biol. Chem.* **248,** 6691.
Holick, M. F., Tavela, T. E., Holick, S. A., Schnoes, H. K., DeLuca, H. F., and Gallagher, B. M. (1976a). *J. Biol. Chem.* **251,** 1020.

Holick, S. A., Holick, M. F., Tavela, T. E., Schnoes, H. K., and DeLuca, H. F. (1976b). *J. Biol. Chem.* **251,** 1025.

Holick, M. F. Frommer, J., McNeill, S., Richtand, N., Henley, J., and Potts, J. T. (1977a). *In* "Vitamin D: Biochemical, Chemical, and Clinical Aspects Related to Calcium Metabolism" (A. W. Norman *et al.*, eds.), p. 135. de Gruyter, Berlin.

Holick, M. F., Frommer, J. E., McNeil, S. C., Richtand, N. M., Henley, J. W., and Potts, J. T. (1977b). *Biochem. Biophys. Res. Commun.* **76,** 107.

Holick, M. F., deBlanco, M. C., Clark, M. B., Henley, J. W., Neer, R. M., DeLuca, H. F., and Potts, J. T. (1977c). *J. Clin. Endocrinol. Metab.* **44,** 595.

Hollander, D., and Truscott, T. C. (1976). *Am. J. Clin. Nutr.* **29,** 970.

Horiuchi, N., Suda, T., and Sasaki, S. (1974). *FEBS Lett.* **43,** 353.

Horrobin, D. F. (1974). "Prolactin." Med. Tech. Publ. Co. Ltd., Lancaster.

Horsting, M. (1970). Ph.D. Dissertation, University of Wisconsin, Madison.

Horsting, M., and DeLuca, H. F. (1969). *Biochem. Biophys. Res. Commun.* **36,** 251.

Hou, H. C. (1927). *Chin. J. Physiol.* **2,** 568.

Hou, H. C. (1929). *Chin. J. Physiol.* **3,** 171.

Hou, H. C. (1930). *Chin. J. Physiol.* **4,** 79.

Hou, H. C. (1931). *Chin. J. Physiol.* **5,** 11.

Hughes, M. R., Brumbaugh, P. F., Haussler, M. R., Wergedal, J. E., and Baylink, D. J. (1975). *Science* **190,** 578.

Imrie, M. H., Neville, P. F., Snellgrove, A. W., and DeLuca, H. F. (1967). *Arch. Biochem. Biophys.* **120,** 525.

Jones, G., Schnoes, H. K., and DeLuca, H. F. (1976). *J. Biol. Chem.* **251,** 24.

Kenny, A. D., Baksi, S. N., and Pang, P. K. (1976). *Am. J. Physiol.* **230,** 1609.

King, W. R., Francis, M. D., and Michael, W. R. (1970). *Clin. Orthop. Relat. Res.* **78,** 251.

Kleiner, A., and DeLuca, H. F. (1974). *Biochim. Biophys. Acta* **338,** 489.

Knoles, H. R. (1935). *J. Poult. Sci.* **14,** 33.

Knutson, J. C., and DeLuca, H. F. (1974). *Biochemistry* **13,** 1543.

Koch, E. M., and Koch, F. C. (1941). *J. Poult. Sci.* **20,** 33.

Kodicek, E. (1956). *Bone Struct. Metab., Ciba Found. Symp., 1955* pp. 161–171.

Kodicek, E., Lawson, D. E. M., and Wilson, P. W. (1970). *Nature (London)* **228,** 763.

Krawitt, E. L. (1978). *Gastroenterology* **74,** 105.

Krawitt, E. L., Sampson, H. W., Kunin, A. S., and Matthews, J. L. (1973). *Calcif. Tissue Res.* **15,** 21.

Krawitt, E. L., Grundman, M. J., and Mawer, E. B. (1977). *Lancet* **2,** 1246.

Kulkarni, B. D., Blondin, G., and Nes, W. R. (1963). *Steroids* **1,** 21.

Kumar, R., and DeLuca, H. F. (1976). *Biochem. Biophys. Res. Commun.* **69,** 197.

Kumar, R., Harnden, D., and DeLuca, H. F. (1976). *Biochemistry* **15,** 2420.

Kumar, R., Schnoes, H. K., and DeLuca, H. F. (1978). *J. Biol. Chem.* **253,** 3804.

Kuntzman, R., Welch, R., and Conney, A. H. (1966). *Adv. Enzyme Regul.* **4,** 149.

Larkins, R. G., Colston, K. W., Galante, L. S., MacAuley, S. J., Evans, I. M. A., and MacIntyre, I. (1973). *Lancet* **2,** 289.

Larkins, R. G., MacAuley, S. J., Rapoport, A., Martin, T. S., Tulloch, B. R., Byfield, P. G. H., Matthews, E. W., and MacIntyre, I. (1974a). *Clin. Sci. Mol. Med.* **46,** 569.

Larkins, R. G., MacAuley, S. J., and MacIntyre, I. (1974b). *Nature (London)* **252,** 412.

Lawson, D. E. M., and Bell, P. A. (1974). *Biochem. J.* **142,** 37.

Lawson, D. E. M., Wilson, P. W., Barker, D. C., and Kodicek, E. (1969a). *Biochem. J.* **115,** 263.

Lawson, D. E. M., Wilson, P. W., and Kodicek, E. (1969b). *Biochem. J.* **115,** 269.

Lawson, D. E. M., Wilson, P. W., and Kodicek, E. (1969c). *Nature (London)* **222,** 171.

Lawson, D. E. M., Pelc, B., Bell, P. A., Wilson, P. W., and Kodicek, E. (1971a). *Biochem. J.* **121,** 673.

Lawson, D. E. M., Fraser, D. R., Kodicek, E., Morris, H. R., and Williams, D. H. (1971b). *Nature (London)* **230**, 228.
Lee, S. W., Russell, J., and Avioli, L. V. (1977). *Science* **195**, 994.
Linn, T. C., PeHit, F. H., and Reed, L. J. (1969). *Proc. Natl. Acad. Sci. U.S.A.* **62**, 234.
Lotz, M., Ney, R., and Bartter, F. C. (1964). *Trans. Assoc. Am. Physicians* **77**, 281.
Lund, J., and DeLuca, H. F. (1966). *J. Lipid Res.* **7**, 739.
MacIntyre, I., Galante, L. S., Evans, I. M. A., Colston, K. W., Moss, D. W., Matthews, E. W., Byfield, P. G. H., MacAuley, S. J., Larkins, R. G., Hi-lyard, C. J., and Greenberg, P. B. (1974). *Endocrinol., Proc. Int. Symp., 4th, 1973* p. 26.
Madhok, T. C., Schnoes, H. K., and DeLuca, H. F. (1977). *Biochemistry* **16**, 2142.
Mawer, E. B. (1974). *Biochem. Soc. Spec. Publ.* **3**, 27.
Mawer, E. B., and Schaefer, K. (1969). *Biochem. J.* **114**, 74 p.
Mawer, E. B., and Stanbury, S. W. (1968). *Biochem. J.* **110**, 53p.
Mawer, E. B., and Taylor, C. M. (1978). *Proc. Int. Congr. Nephrol., 7th, 1978* p. 469.
Mawer, E. B., Lumb, G. A., and Stanbury, S. W. (1969). *Nature (London)* **222**, 482.
Mawer, E. B., Backhouse, J., Lumb, G. A., and Stanbury, S. W. (1971a). *Nature (London), New Biol.* **232**, 188.
Mawer, E. B., Lumb, G. A., Schaefer, K., and Stanbury, S. W. (1971b). *Clin. Sci.* **40**, 39.
Mawer, E. B., Backhouse, J., Holman, C. A., Lumb, G. A., and Stanbury, S. W. (1972). *Clin. Sci.* **43**, 413.
Mawer, E. B., Taylor, C. M., Backhouse, J., Lumb, G. A., and Stanbury, S. W. (1973). *Lancet* **1**, 626.
Mawer, E. B., Backhouse, J., Hill, L. F., Lumb, G. A., DeSilva, P., Taylor, C. M., and Stanbury, S. W. (1975a). *Clin. Sci. Mol. Med.* **48**, 349.
Mawer, E. B., Backhouse, J., Hughes, S., and Taylor, C. M. (1975b). *Biochem. Soc. Trans.* p. 886.
Midgett, R. J., Spielvogel, A. M., Coburn, J. W., and Norman, A. W. (1973). *J. Clin. Endocrinol. Metab.* **36**, 1153.
Montecuccoli, G., Bar, A., Risenfeld, G., and Hurwitz, S. (1977a). *Comp. Biochem. Physiol. A* **57**, 331.
Montecuccoli, G., Hurwitz, S., Cohen, A., and Bar, A. (1977b). *Comp. Biochem. Physiol. A* **57**, 335.
Morgan, A. F., and Shimotori, N. (1943). *J. Biol. Chem.* **147**, 189.
Moriuchi, S., and DeLuca, H. F. (1974). *Arch. Biochem. Biophys.* **164**, 165.
Morrissey, R. L., and Wasserman, R. H. (1971). *Am. J. Physiol.* **220**, 1509.
Myrtle, J. F., and Norman, A. W. (1971a). *Science* **171**, 78.
Myrtle, J. F., and Norman, A. W. (1971b). *Steroids* **17**, 619.
Myrtle, J. F., Haussler, M. R., and Norman, A. W. (1970). *J. Biol. Chem.* **245**, 1190.
Nicholson, R., Akhtar, M., and Taylor, T. G. (1976). *J. Endocrinol.* **68**, 16.
Nicolaysen, R. (1938). *Acta Physiol. Scand.* **6**, 201.
Norman, A. W. (1966). *Biochem. Biophys. Res. Commun.* **23**, 335.
Norman, A. W., and DeLuca, H. F. (1963). *Biochemistry* **2**, 1160.
Norman, A. W., and Henry, H. L. (1974). *Clin. Orthop. Relat. Res.* **98**, 258.
Norman, A. W., and Henry, H. L. (1979). "Proceedings Fourth Workshop on Vitamin D." (abstract book).
Norman, A. W., and Wong, R. G. (1972). *J. Nutr.* **102**, 1709.
Norman, A. W., Lund, J., and DeLuca, H. F. (1964). *Arch. Biochem. Biophys.* **108**, 12.
Norman, A. W., Haussler, M. R., Adams, T. N., Myrtle, J. R., Roberts, P., and Hubberd, K. H. (1969). *Am. J. Clin. Nutr.* **22**, 2367.
Norman, A. W., Myrtle, J. F., Midgett, R. J., Nowicki, H. G., Williams, V., and Popjak, G. (1971a). *Science* **173**, 51.

Norman, A. W., Midgett, R. J., Myrtle, J. F., and Nowicki, H. G. (1971b). *Biochem. Biophys. Res. Commun.* **42,** 1082.

Norman, A. W., Midgett, R. J., and Myrtle, J. F. (1971c). *J. Lab. Clin. Med.* **78,** 561.

Norman, A. W., Friedlander, E. J., and Henry, H. L. (1977). *Adv. Exp. Med. Biol.* **81,** 211.

Nowicki, H. G., and Norman, A. W. (1972). *Steroids* **19,** 85.

Nowicki, H. G., Wong, R. G., Myrtle, J. F., and Norman, A. W. (1972a). *J. Agric. Food Chem.* **20,** 376.

Nowicki, H. G., Myrtle, J. F., and Norman, A. W. (1972b). *J. Agric. Food Chem.* **20,** 380.

Ogata, E., Ezawa, I., and Sano, Y. (1975). *Arch. Biochem. Biophys.* **171,** 540.

Olson, E. B., Jr., Knutson, J. C., Bhattacharyya, M. H., and DeLuca, H. F. (1976). *J. Clin. Invest.* **57,** 1213.

Omdahl, J. L., Gray, R. W., Boyle, I. T., Knutson, J., and DeLuca, H. F. (1972). *Nature (London), New Biol.* **237,** 63.

Omdahl, J. L., Helinek, G., and Eaton, R. P. (1977). *J. Clin. Invest.* **60,** 1202.

Ozumi, K., and Monder, C. (1972). *Comp. Biochem. Physiol. B* **42,** 523.

Peakall, D. B. (1969). *Nature (London)* **224,** 1219.

Pedersen, J. I., Ghazarian, J. G., Orme-Johnson, N. R., and DeLuca, H. F. (1976). *J. Biol. Chem.* **251,** 3933.

Ponchon, G., and DeLuca, H. F. (1969). *J. Clin. Invest.* **48,** 1273.

Ponchon, G., Keenan, A. L., and DeLuca, H. F. (1969). *J. Clin. Invest.* **48,** 2032.

Ponchon, G., DeLuca, H. F., and Suda, T. (1970). *Arch. Biochem. Biophys.* **141,** 397.

Ponsold, W., and Pfenningsdorf, G. (1954). *Strahlentherapie* **95,** 468.

Porter, R. D., and Wiemeyer, S. N. (1969). *Science* **165,** 199.

Quartermann, J. (1965). *Biochim. Biophys. Acta* **97,** 128.

Raoul, Y., and Gounelle, J. (1958). *C. R. Hebd. Seances Acad. Sci.* **247,** 161.

Rasmussen, H., and Bordier, P. (1974). "Physiological and Cellular Basis of Metabolic Bone Disease." Williams & Wilkins, Baltimore, Maryland.

Rasmussen, H., Wong, M., Bikle, D., and Goodman, D. P. P. (1972). *J. Clin. Invest.* **51,** 2502.

Ratcliffe, D. A. (1967). *Nature (London)* **215,** 208.

Reddy, C. R., Coburn, J. W., Hartenbower, D. L., Friedler, R. M., Brickman, A. S., Massry, S. G., and Jowsey, J. (1973). *J. Clin. Invest.* **52,** 3000.

Rehfeld, B. M., Bradley, R. L., Jr., and Sunde, M. L. (1972). *Poult. Sci.* **51,** 488.

Rekling, E. (1927). *Strahlentherapie* **25,** 568.

Ribovich, M. L., and DeLuca, H. F. (1975). *Arch. Biochem. Biophys.* **170,** 529.

Ribovich, M. L., and DeLuca, H. F. (1978a). *Arch. Biochem. Biophys.* **188,** 145.

Ribovich, M. L., and DeLuca, H. F. (1978b). *Arch. Biochem. Biophys.* **188,** 157.

Ribovich, M. L., and DeLuca, H. F. (1978c). *Arch. Biochem. Biophys.* **188,** 164.

Rojanasathit, S., and Haddad, J. G. (1976). *Biochim. Biophys. Acta* **421,** 12.

Rosenstreich, S. J., Vorwiler, W., and Rich, C. (1971). *J. Clin. Invest.* **24,** 897.

Russell, R. G. G., Smith, R., Walton, R. J., Preston, C., Basson, R., Henderson, R. G., and Norman, A. W. (1974). *Lancet* **2,** 14.

Sahashi, Y., Suzuki, T., Nishikawa, T., Tanaka, T., Takahashi, M., Inaba, S., and Miyazawa, E. (1962). *J. Vitaminol.* **8,** 121.

Sashashi, Y., Suzuki, T., Higaki, M., and Asano, T. (1967a). *J. Vitaminol.* **13,** 33.

Sahashi, Y., Suzuki, T., Higaki, M., Takahashi, M., Asano, T., Hasegawa, T., and Miyazawa, E. (1967b). *J. Vitaminol.* **13,** 37.

Sallis, J. D., and Holdsworth, E. (1962). *Am. J. Physiol.* **203,** 506.

Schachter, D., Finkelstein, J. D., and Kowarski, S. (1964). *J. Clin. Invest.* **43,** 787.

Schaefer, K., Kraft, D., von Herrath, D., and Grigoleit, H.-G. (1975). *Res. Exp. Med.* **165,** 49.

Scott, M. L., Zimmermann, J. R., Marinsky, S., Mullenhoff, P. A., Rumsey, G. L., and Rice, R. W. (1975). *Poult. Sci.* **54,** 350.

Seymour, J. L., and DeLuca, H. F. (1974). *Endocrinology* **94,** 1009.
Shain, S. J. (1972). *J. Biol. Chem.* **247,** 4404.
Simpson, E. R., and Boyd, G. S. (1967). *Eur. J. Biochem.* **2,** 275.
Spanos, E., Colston, K. W., Evans, I. M. S., Galante, L. S., MacAuley, S. J., and MacIntyre, I. (1976a). *Mol. Cell. Endocrinol.* **5,** 163.
Spanos, E., Pike, J. W., Haussler, M. R., Colston, K. W., Evans, I. M. A., Goldner, A. M., McCain, T. A., and MacIntyre, I. (1976b). *Life Sci.* **19,** 1751.
Spanos, E., Colston, K. W., and MacIntyre, I. (1977). *FEBS Lett.* **75,** 73.
Stanbury, S. W., Mawer, E. B., Lumb, G. A., Hill, L. F., Holman, C. A., Jones, M., and Van Den Berg, C. J. (1971). *Endocrinol. Proc. Int. Symp., 3rd, 1971* p. 487.
Steenbock, H., and Black, A., (1925). *J. Biol. Chem.* **64,** 263.
Suda, T., Horiuchi, N., Sasaki, S., Ogata, E., Izawa, I., Nagata, N., and Kimura, S. (1973). *Biochem. Biophys. Res. Commun.* **54,** 512.
Sugisaki, N., Welcher, M., and Monder, C. (1974). *Comp. Biochem. Physiol. B* **49,** 647.
Suh, S. M., Tashjian, A. H., Matsuo, N., Parkinson, D. K., and Fraser, D. (1973). *J. Clin. Invest.* **52,** 153.
Sulimovici, S., and Roginsky, M. S. (1976). *Biochem. Biophys. Res. Commun.* **71,** 1078.
Sulimovici, S., and Roginsky, M. S. (1977). *Life Sci.* **21,** 1317.
Switzer, B., Lewin, V., and Wolfe, F. H. (1970). *Can. J. Zool.* **49,** 69.
Tanaka, Y., Takahashi, M., Miyazawa, E., Higaki, M., Inaba, S., Nishikawa, T., Suzuki, T., and Sahashi, Y. (1963). *J. Vitaminol.* **9,** 62.
Tanaka, Y., and DeLuca, H. F. (1973). *Arch. Biochem. Biophys.* **154,** 566.
Tanaka, Y., and DeLuca, H. F. (1974). *Science* **183,** 1198.
Tanaka, Y., Lorenc, R. S., and DeLuca, H. F. (1975). *Arch. Biochem. Biophys.* **171,** 521.
Tanaka, Y., Castillo, L., and DeLuca, H. F. (1976). *Proc. Natl. Acad. Sci. U.S.A.* **73,** 2701.
Tanaka, Y., Castillo, L., and DeLuca, H. F. (1977). *J. Biol. Chem.* **252,** 142.
Taylor, A. N., and Wasserman, R. H. (1972). *Am. J. Physiol.* **233,** 110.
Taylor, C. M., Mawer, E. B., and Reeve, A. (1973). *Biochem. Soc. Trans.* **1,** 596.
Taylor, C. M., Mawer, E. B., and Reeve, A. (1975). *Clin. Sci. Mol. Med.* **49,** 391.
Trulsch, D., Greem, H., Czygan, P., Hutterer, F., Schaffner, F., Popper, H., Cooper, D. Y., and Rosenthal, H. (1973). *Biochemistry* **12,** 76.
Tucker, G., III, Gagnon, R. E., and Haussler, M. R. (1973). *Arch. Biochem. Biophys.* **155,** 47.
Wiemeyer, S. N., and Porter, R. D. (1970). *Nature (London)* **227,** 737.
Windaus, A., and Bock, F. Z. (1936). *Hoppe-Seyler's Z. Physiol. Chem.* **245,** 168.
Wong, R. G., Norman, A. W., Reddy, C. R., and Coburn, J. W. (1972a). *J. Clin. Invest.* **51,** 1287.
Wong, R. G., Myrtle, J. F., Tsai, H. C., and Norman, A. W. (1972b). *J. Biol. Chem.* **247,** 5728.
Wong, R. G., Nowicki, H. G., and Norman, A. W. (1973). *Pestic. Biochem. Physiol.* **4,** 170.
Wong, R. G., Nowicki, H. G., and Norman, A. W. (1974). *Pesticide Biochem. Biophys.* **4,** 170.
Zerwekh, J. E., Brumbaugh, P. F., Haussler, D. H., Cork, D. S., and Haussler, M. R. (1974). *Biochemistry* **13,** 4097.

CHAPTER

7

The Tissue and Subcellular Localization of Vitamin D and Its Metabolites: A Basis for Their Hormonal Mode of Action

I. TISSUE DISTRIBUTION STUDIES

A. Early Studies (Prior to 1960)

Early efforts to elucidate the tissue distribution of vitamin D were hampered due to the lack of radioactive preparations of the secosteroid. Investigators, of necessity, had to rely on slow and imprecise biological assays. These assays do not indicate the amount of vitamin D steroid present, and more importantly they cannot detect nonbiologically active metabolites that might be produced. Due to the relative insensitivity of the available bioassays, particularly the rat line test (see Chapter 4), it was still necessary to administer massive, unphysiological levels of vitamin D to carry out any experiments.

The first published report concerning the tissue distribution of vitamin D was by Heymann (1937a). He administered 5 mg (200,000 IU) of the viosterol[1] preparation to rabbits and followed the vitamin D activity in various tissues by biological assay; some vitamin D activity was found in blood, liver, and skin. However, it was not possible to calculate the recovery of the administered dose, and thus no quantitative information could be obtained for the fraction of administered dose recovered. The major contribution of Heymann was the identification of the important role of bile in mediating the intestinal absorption of orally administered vitamin D (Heymann, 1936, 1937b,c). This provided direct support for the earlier studies of Greaves and Schmidt (1933), who had first suggested the importance of bile for the intestinal absorption of vitamin D.

Biological assays by Morgan and Shimotori (1943) provided evidence for vitamin D activity in the kidney, heart, large intestine, brain, lung, spleen, muscle, fat, skin, and hair of dogs. No more than 10% of the administered dose of 1 mg (40,000 IU) was accounted for. Warkany *et al.* (1945) also evaluated the concentration of vitamin D activity in human serum during and after periods of ingestion of large doses of vitamin D. Their results suggested the hypothesis that vitamin D was sequestered or ''stored'' in tissues and subsequently released quite slowly into the general circulation, where it was utilized to produce vitamin D-related biological responses. Rosenstreich *et al.* (1971) obtained definitive evidence that the primary storage site for vitamin D in man is not the liver, but the fat depot or adipose tissue.

It was not until the advent of radioactive vitamin D that significant progress was made on the tissue distribution, subcellular localization, and most importantly the metabolism of the vitamin. The presence of the radioactive label increased by many orders of magnitude the ability to detect vitamin D itself and provided for the first time a straightforward means of identifying the presence of metabolites, both biologically active and inactive compounds. Initially, several syntheses of radioactive vitamin D were carried out (Havinga and Botts, 1954; Kodicek, 1955, 1956; Schaltegger, 1960) (see Table 3-3), but the specific activities of these preparations were too low to allow adequate detection of steroid in the tissues following physiological doses of the vitamin (Kodicek, 1956; Blumberg *et al.*, 1959, 1960). [See Norman (1967, 1968) for a review of this work.]

[1]Viosterol was a trade name for a crude preparation of vitamin D.

B. Modern Studies (After 1960)

The first syntheses of radioactive vitamin D that were of high enough specific activity so that the presence of small physiological doses could readily be detected were those of Norman and DeLuca (1963, 1964), Neville and DeLuca (1966), and Imrie *et al.* (1967). These preparations had, respectively, specific activities of 1000 or 26,000 dpm/IU. The laboratory of DeLuca and co-workers as well as those of Norman and co-workers and Kodicek and co-workers independently pursued a study of the tissue distribution and subcellular localization of radioactivity resulting after administration of physiological quantities of the radioactive parent steroid.

Figure 7-1 shows typical data concerning the tissue distribution of radioactivity with time in the rachitic chick after an intracardial dose of 3.25 nmoles (50 IU) of [1,2-^{3}H]vitamin D_3. Within 1 hr after the administration of radioactive vitamin D, all tissues examined had significant amounts of radioactivity. Similar results have been obtained following oral or intraperitoneal administration of tritiated vitamin D_2 or D_3. This testifies to the existence of a rapid and efficient mechanism for systemically transporting vitamin D steroids in the body. One of the hallmarks of vitamin D action in terms of initiation of stimulation of intestinal calcium absorption is the time delay between administration of the vitamin and the onset of biological response. One logical explanation for this lag was that there was a slow transportation of the vitamin to the target tissue, the intestinal mucosa. On the basis of the data presented in Fig. 7-1 this is not a major contribution to the time delay. One interesting aspect of these data is the rapid accumulation of vitamin D by the liver. This was the first clue of the major involvement of this organ in vitamin D metabolism. The major uptake of vitamin D steroid by the liver most likely reflects not only metabolism to 25(OH)D_3 but also binding of both vitamin D and its metabolites to plasma binding proteins specifically designed for the transport of these steroids.

A summary of the distribution of radioactivity in the various organs of rats 24 hr after a dose of 3.25 nmoles (50 IU) of [^{3}H]vitamin D is presented in Table 7-1. It is of interest that well over 90% of the administered dose of the vitamin was accounted for. All the tissues normally associated with the action of vitamin D, i.e., the kidneys, liver, skeleton, and intestine, accumulated a significant amount of the administered dose that was retained in the animal. This was in general agreement with the earlier data of Kodicek (1956) as well as the work of Blumberg *et al.* (1960), who obtained distribution data from *Macacus rhesus* monkeys and rats given large doses of vitamin D (975 nmoles, or 15,000 IU). It is apparent that there is a generalized distribution of radioactivity in virtually all tissues of the body, particularly the muscle and adipose tissue. Another interesting aspect of the data presented in Table 7-1 is the large fraction of radioactivity in bone. Also, a small portion of radioactivity was excreted in the urine; attempts

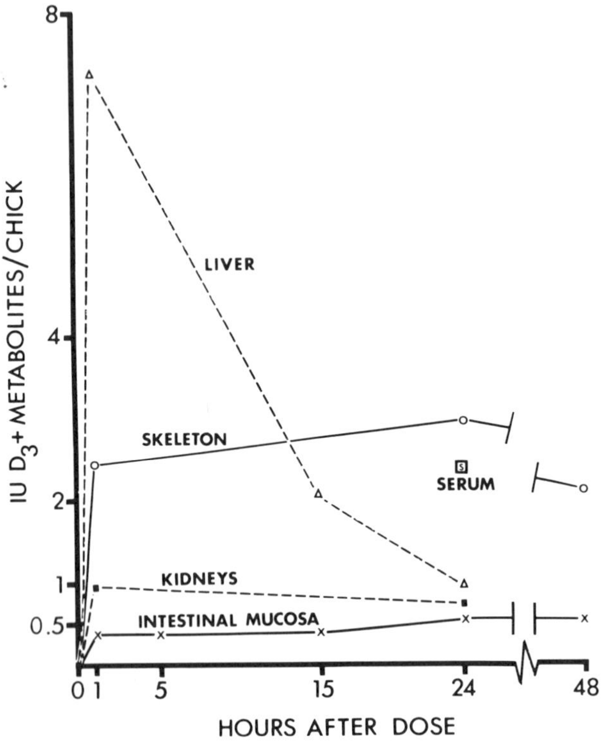

Figure 7-1. Tissue distribution of radioactivity with time in the rachitic chick after an intracardial dose of 50 IU (3.25 nmoles) of [^{3}H]vitamin D_3. The [1,2-^{3}H]vitamin D_3 in 0.20 ml 1,2-propanediol was injected intracardially into rachitic chicks. At the indicated times the chicks were killed and the tissue radioactivity determined by the procedures of Haussler and Norman (1969). The data for the skeleton were obtained by analyzing tibia–fibulas and assuming that the skeleton was 15% of the body weight. Each point is the average of six to eight chicks.

to trap tritiated water from lyophilization of frozen urine failed, suggesting that the tritium present in that fluid was organically bound. Lund *et al.* (1967) reported the presence of esters of vitamin D.

Mawer and colleagues (1972) carried out the only definitive study concerning the distribution and storage of vitamin D and its metabolites in human tissues. A summary of their results is given in Table 7-2. As can be noted, adipose tissue and skeletal muscle are the principal sites of storage of vitamin D and its metabolites in man. Chromatographic evaluation of the radioactivity present in the fat indicated that it was present largely as the parent vitamin; in contrast, the chief form of the steroid present in muscle was 25(OH)D_3.

With the advent of preparations of radioactive 25(OH)D_3 as well as 1,25(OH)$_2D_3$ it has been possible to study the biodynamics of these vitamin D steroids as well. Figure 7-2 presents a comparative study of the tissue distribution of radioactive $1,25(OH)_2D_3$ and vitamin D in both vitamin D-deficient and vitamin D-replete chicks. The result illustrates the transport of the hormonally active form of vitamin D, $1,25(OH)_2D_3$, as it moves from its secretory organ, the kidney, to distal regions of the system and particularly the target organs, the intestine and bone. It is apparent that $1,25(OH)_2D_3$ rapidly equilibrates with all major tissues, including the intestine and bone and also the kidney, liver, and muscle; however, the kinetics of distribution differs markedly when this metabolite is given to vitamin D-replete birds. It is also apparent that there are different

TABLE 7-1
Tissue Localization of Radioactivity in Rats after an Intrajugular Dose of [1,2-^{3}H]Vitamin D_3[a,b]

Tissue	At 4 hr after dose: Percent of dose	Relative incorporation[c]
Blood[d]	12.92±1.96	2472±413
Bone[e]	26.78±3.8	501±73
Bone cells[f]	—	12,525
Heart	0.71±0.20	1409±353
Intestine (small)	1.73±0.07	2305±502
Intestine (large)	0.35±0.03	813±80
Intestinal mucosa[g]	—	7113
Kidney	2.35±0.19	2201±441
Liver	28.50±2.04	5958±893
Lung	1.72±0.49	2739±732
Muscle[h]	8.61±2.75	244±70
Spleen	1.04±0.17	3620±292
Small intestinal contents	5.62±1.05	2831±545
Large intestinal contents plus feces	3.17±0.38	1010±277
Total (%)	96.6	—

[a]Reproduced from Neville and DeLuca (1966) with the kind permission of the American Chemical Society. (Copyright by the American Chemical Society.)

[b]Rats were fed a vitamin D-deficient diet for 3 weeks before being used. Each deficient rat received an intrajugular injection of 10.7 IU of [1,2-^{3}H]vitamin D_3 in 0.2 ml of Tween–NaCl solution. Values plus or minus the standard deviation are averages of three rats at 4 hr.

[c]Relative incorporation expresed as disintegrations per minute per 100 mg dry weight.

[d]This assumes that blood is 6% of body weight.

[e]This assumes that skeleton is 15% of body weight.

[f]This assumes that bone is 4% cells on a dry weight basis and all vitamin D is located in these cells. Activity expressed as per 100 mg dry weight of bone cells.

[g]Calculated on the assumption that small intestine is made up of 30% mucosa and 70% muscle, connective tissue, etc. (on a dry weight basis), and that smooth muscle has the same relative incorporation as skeletal muscle.

[h]This assumes that muscle is 30% of body weight.

TABLE 7-2
Distribution of Vitamin D and Metabolites in Human Tissues[a]

Tissue analyzed	Distribution of Administered Dose among Tissues (%)				
	A (4)[b]	B (16)[b]	C (22)[b]	D (40)[b]	E (59)[b]
Bone	1.8	1.1	0.6	0.8	0.8
Fat	5.4	6.4	8.6	6.2	10.1
Kidney	—	0.1	0.2	0.1	—
Liver	—	1.0	1.3	1.6	0.3
Lung	—	—	0.7	0.6	0.1
Marrow	1.8	2.1	5.5	1.3	3.3
Myocardium	—	0.1	0.1	0.1	0.1
Skeletal muscle	29.5	5.5	8.6	4.1	5.5
Skin	10.8	1.8	2.4	0.9	1.6
Spleen	—	—	0.1	0.2	0.3
Serum	3.3	5.4	3.6	3.0	1.5
Tendon	0.9	—	—	—	0.5
Total recovery	43.5	23.8	31.7	17.5	25.3

[a]Abstracted by permission from Mawer *et al.* (1972). Subjects (A–E) received [^{3}H]vitamin D_3, and data are expressed as a percentage of administered dose recovered via organic solvent extraction of the tissues. Samples were obtained either at autopsy or via amputation or laparotomy.
[b]Number in parentheses indicates time after administration, in days.

kinetics of handling the metabolite 1,25$(OH)_2D_3$ as compared with that of the parent vitamin D. Of significance is the fact that the plasma concentration of 1,25$(OH)_2D_3$ very rapidly reaches a plateau value of 2×10^{-10} *M*, which is then maintained for a prolonged period of time. The amounts of vitamin D, 25$(OH)D_3$, and 1,25$(OH)_2D_3$ present in various tissues 18 hr after the administration of 0.65 nmole (10 IU) of [^{3}H]vitamin D_3 are shown in Table 7-3. Clearly, the intestine contains the highest level of 1,25$(OH)_2D_3$, but the skeleton and blood also contain appreciable amounts of this hormonally active form of vitamin D. In comparison, 25$(OH)D_3$ is present in highest concentrations in the blood; it was because of this observation that DeLuca and co-workers (Ponchon and DeLuca, 1969; DeLuca, 1969) coined the term "circulating hormonally active form" of vitamin D for 25$(OH)D_3$.

It is apparent from the foregoing discussion that both vitamin D and its metabolites are widely distributed in many tissues of the body. However, it is difficult on the basis of these data to more than generally identify which may be target tissues, and certainly no insight can be obtained into proposed biochemical modes of action of vitamin D and its metabolites on the basis of tissue distribution studies.

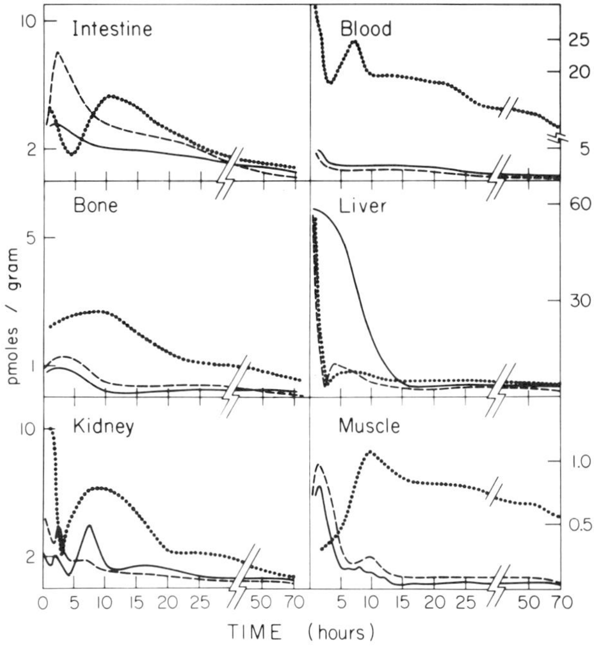

Figure 7-2. Tissue distribution of $1,25(OH)_2D_3$ and vitamin D_3 in vitamin D-deficient or vitamin D-replete chicks. A single oral dose of [4-^{14}C]vitamin D_3 (10 IU; 650 pmoles) was given to groups of rachitic chicks, while a single oral dose of tritiated $1,25(OH)_2D_3$ (5 U; 325 pmoles) was given to groups of rachitic or vitamin D-replete birds. Birds were killed at 20, 40, 60 min and 2, 4, 8, 12, 18, 24, 36, 48, 60, 72 hr, and the radioactivity content of the indicated tissues was determined. Key: ———, $1,25(OH)_2D_3$ in +D chick; - - -, $1,25(OH)_2D_3$ in −D chick; · · ·, ^{14}C in −D chick given ^{14}C-labeled D_3.

TABLE 7-3
Amounts of Vitamin D Metabolites in Various Tissues after Administration of Radioactive Vitamin D[a,b]

Tissue	D_3 (pmoles/chick)	$25(OH)D_3$ (pmoles/chick)	$1,25(OH)_2D_3$ (pmoles/chick)
Intestine	0.47	2.12	8.2
Blood[c]	0.94	37.4	3.8
Skeleton[d]	1.97	7.8	3.5
Kidney	0.25	1.2	0.85
Liver	2.53	2.3	1.0

[a]From Haussler and Norman (1967).

[b]Thirty rachitic chicks received 0.65 nmole (10 IU) of [4-^{14}C]vitamin D_3 intracardially 18 hr before being killed.

[c]Blood values are corrected to the indicated values by assuming a one-third yield of total blood volume.

[d]Results from tibias, fibulas, and femurs were converted to complete chick skeleton values by assuming that the skeleton is 15% of the total body weight.

II. SUBCELLULAR DISTRIBUTION STUDIES

A. Intestinal Mucosa

1. Studies in Vivo

The original approach to the study of the biochemical actions of vitamin D pioneered in the author's laboratory and extensively supplemented by Kodicek, Lawson, and colleagues was to administer *small physiological doses* of radioactive vitamin D, to trace the appearance of the radioactive label in the target tissue, and to ascertain its subcellular localization. In the course of these studies (Haussler and Norman, 1967, 1969; Haussler *et al.*, 1968; Lawson *et al.*, 1969a,b,c, 1971a,b; Myrtle *et al.*, 1970) it became apparent not only that there was a specialized localization of radioactivity within the target intestinal nuclear and chromatin fraction, but also that this radioactivity was not chemically identical to that of the parent vitamin D. Further extensive studies eventually resulted in the demonstration that this substance, which was selectively localized in the target intestine, and its nuclear fraction were chemically distinct from both vitamin D and the intermediate $25(OH)D_3$ (Myrtle *et al.*, 1970). With the concomitant demonstration that this polar metabolite was highly biologically active in terms of stimulating the intestinal transport of calcium (Haussler *et al.*, 1968; Kodicek *et al.*, 1970; Myrtle and Norman, 1971; Haussler *et al.*, 1971), the extensive effort necessary to chemically characterize the compound was undertaken. This resulted in the simultaneous yet independent reports from three laboratories that the chemical structure of this vitamin D metabolite was $1,25(OH)_2D_3$ (Lawson *et al.*, 1971a; Norman *et al.*, 1971; Holick *et al.*, 1971). It should be appreciated that a detailed study of the subcellular distribution of radioactivity in the intestinal mucosa resulting from administration of physiological doses of vitamin D provided a major breakthrough in terms of identifying the presence of the most biologically active or hormonally active form of the parent vitamin, $1,25(OH)_2D_3$.

Figure 7-3 summarizes a large amount of data obtained in the laboratory of the author which are consistent with the view that the biological action of $1,25(OH)_2D_3$ in the intestine is due to the presence of the steroid in the nucleus and its chromatin fraction of this target cell. Shown here are the results of experiments designed to study the localization of radioactivity in the intestine. Irrespective of whether radioactive vitamin D, $25(OH)D_3$, or $1,25(OH)_2D_3$ is given to a rachitic chick, 20, 8, or 4 hr later, respectively, a maximal localization of radioactivity in the intestinal nuclear fraction results (Haussler and Norman, 1967, 1969; Haussler *et al.*, 1968; Lawson *et al.*, 1969a, 1969b). In each instance the nuclear fraction has associated with it approximately 70–80% of the total radioactivity present within the target tissue. Extraction and chromato-

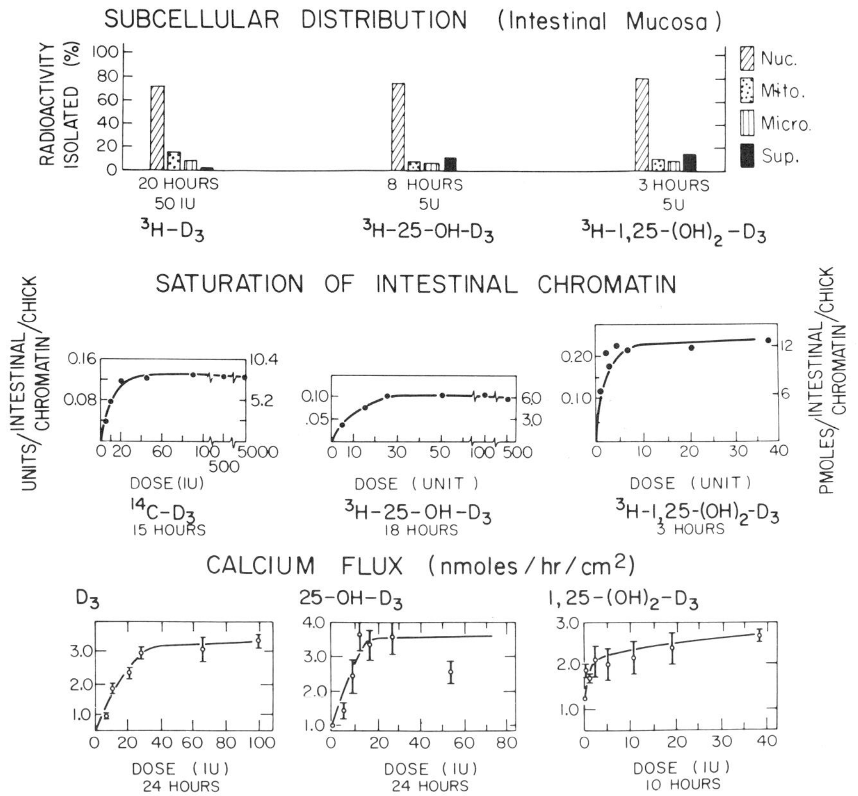

Figure 7-3. Summary of subcellular localization of vitamin D_3 and metabolites (top), saturation of intestinal chromatin receptor with $1,25(OH)_2D_3$ (middle), and stimulation of intestinal calcium transport (bottom) after administration of vitamin D_3 (left), $25(OH)D_3$ (middle), and $1,25(OH)_2D_3$ (right). The plateau values of $1,25(OH)_2D_3$ in the chromatin and the stimulation of calcium transport were measured simultaneously at 24, 15, or 9 hr after vitamin D, $25(OH)D_3$, or $1,25(OH)_2D_3$, respectively. At the time of maximal accumulation (3 hr), a value of 11 to 12 pmoles of $1,25(OH)_2D_3$ per chick intestinal chromatin is found. Taken from Norman (1975).

graphic evaluation of the radioactivity that resulted from the separate administration of the three steroids indicated that in each instance it was exclusively in the chemical form of $1,25(OH)_2D_3$. Further evaluation of the localization of the radioactivity of the crude nuclear fraction of the intestine revealed that it was also present when purified nuclei were prepared (Haussler *et al.,* 1969) or when the subnuclear chromatin fraction was prepared (Haussler *et al.,* 1968; Tsai *et al.,* 1972).

As a consequence of the development of our isolation techniques for chromatin (Haussler *et al.,* 1968), it was possible to carry out dose–response type of studies in which increasing quantities of the three vitamin D steroids were separately administered to groups of rachitic chicks. This was followed by preparation according to our standard procedures of an intestinal chromatin fraction, which was briefly washed with a 1% solution of Triton X-100. When such a procedure was employed, evidence for a finite number of binding sites for $1,25(OH)_2D_3$ in the chromatin fraction was obtained (see middle panel of Fig. 7-3). It was then possible to correlate the dose of vitamin D steroid necessary to saturate the intestinal chromatin fraction with the dose of vitamin D steroid required to give a maximal stimulation of intestinal calcium transport (bottom panels of Fig. 7-3).

A major effort in the course of these experiments was to demonstrate specificity of association of the $1,25(OH)_2D_3$ with the intestinal chromatin fraction. The experiment we devised to test the specificity of localization involved the simultaneous administration of tritiated vitamin D steroid with an equivalent amount of ^{14}C-labeled cholesterol (or vice versa). A receptor molecule or binding site for vitamin D or its metabolites should have little affinity for cholesterol or its metabolites. In addition, the ^{14}C-labeled cholesterol that was found in the intestinal mucosa after injection was probably associated with the membrane components of cells by a nonspecific lipid–lipid interaction. Thus, the ^{14}C-labeled cholesterol present in a given fraction is a means of roughly estimating the amount of steroid that is nonspecifically associated with that subcellular organelle. The ratio of tritium-bound steroid to ^{14}C-bound steroid (or vice versa) will increase when the nuclear fraction is further purified, and an infinite ratio will be obtained when a pure receptor molecule for vitamin D or its metabolites is isolated. Table 7-4 shows the results of such an experiment when [^{14}C]vitamin D_3 and [^3H]cholesterol were simultaneously administered to rachitic chicks, and Table 7-5 shows a similar set of experiments carried out several years later when either $25(OH)[^3H]D_3$ or $1,25(OH)_2[^3H]D_3$ and [^{14}C]cholesterol were simultaneously administered to rachitic chicks. As shown in Table 7-4, the ^{14}C radioactivity resulting from a dose of [^{14}C]vitamin D_3 was very tightly bound to the nuclei and chromatin fractions, for it was stable to repeated washings with 1% Triton X-100. There was a remarkable increase in the ratio of ^{14}C to ^3H, from 0.6 in the homogenate to 10.0 in the Triton-washed chromatin fraction. Furthermore, it can be seen that pretreatment of the rachitic chicks with nonradioactive vitamin D several hours before administration of the ^{14}C-labeled vitamin D_3 prevented subsequent localization of any ^{14}C-labeled steroids in the intestinal mucosa. Apparently, any receptor sites specific for vitamin D or its metabolites, i.e., $1,25(OH)_2D_3$, were previously saturated by the prior administration of the nonradioactive vitamin D. Collectively these results strongly support the contention that there is a specific binding site in the nuclear portion of the intestinal mucosa cell, and more specifically in the chromatin fraction, which accounts for a significant proportion of the $1,25(OH)_2D_3$ steroid present in the intestinal mucosa.

TABLE 7-4

Recovery of Radioactivity from a Dose of [^{14}C]Vitamin D_3 and [^{3}H]Cholesterol in Subcellular Fractions of the Intestinal Mucosa from Rachitic and Normal Chicks[a]

Fraction	Rachitic (−D) chicks: % of ^{14}C (vitamin D_3 + metabolites)	Rachitic (−D) chicks: % of ^{3}H (cholesterol + metabolites)	Rachitic (−D) chicks: $^{14}C/^{3}H$	Normal (+D) chicks: % of ^{14}C (vitamin D_3 + metabolites)	Normal (+D) chicks: $^{14}C/^{3}H$	Normal (+D) chicks: % competition of ^{14}C binding
Homogenate	100	100	0.62	100	0.40	35
Mitochondria	8	17	0.30	17	0.39	0
Microsomes	6	17	0.20	15	0.32	0
Supernatant	12	4	1.67	7	0.51	65
Crude nuclei	75	65	0.71	68	0.39	41
Purified nuclei	47	30	0.95	21	0.38	70
Membrane fractions (from nuclei)	9	14	0.38	21	0.53	0
Chromatin	51	16	2.0	19	0.40	76
Triton-washed chromatin	50	3	10.0	1	0.10	99

[a] Normal (+D) chicks and rachitic (−D) chicks received 10 IU of [4-^{14}C]vitamin D_3 and an equivalent amount of [1,2-^{3}H]cholesterol in 0.2 ml of 1,2-propanediol via intracardial injection 15 hr prior to being killed. In addition, the normal chicks received 5000 IU of nonradioactive vitamin D_3 8 hr prior to the radioactive vitamin. Cellular subfractions were prepared by the procedures of Haussler *et al.* (1968). All purified or subnuclear fractions were prepared from the crude nuclear fraction, not necessarily from the fraction listed above it in this table. All calculations of percent yield were based on the absolute amount present in the homogenate, which was arbitrarily set at 100%. Because the percentage of [^{3}H]cholesterol plus metabolites in the normal chicks was virtually identical to that in the rachitic chicks, only the results from the latter are reported. Percent competition of ^{14}C binding is calculated by comparing the amount (international units) of [^{14}C]vitamin D_3 plus metabolites of the rachitic chicks with that found in a similar fraction of the normal chicks. Triton-washed chromatin was obtained by washing chromatin three times in a 0.01 *M* Tris-buffered solution containing 1% Triton X-100 (a nonionic detergent) followed by centrifugation at 27,000 *g* for 45 min. Each number shown represents an analysis on a single, entire intestinal mucosa and is the average of four determinations. From Norman (1975).

TABLE 7-5

Amounts of 25(OH)[^{3}H]D_3 and Metabolites or 1,25$(OH)_2$[^{3}H]D_3 and Metabolites Relative to [4-^{14}C]Cholesterol and Metabolites in Subcellular Fraction Obtained from Rachitic Chick Intestinal Mucosa[a]

Cell fraction	Ratio of 25(OH)[^{3}H]D_3 and metabolites to [4-^{14}C]cholesterol and metabolites	Ratio of 1,25$(OH)_2$[^{3}H]D_3 and metabolites to [4-^{14}C]cholesterol and metabolites
Homogenate	0.91	8.53
Crude nuclear fraction	1.43	9.58
Mitochondrial fraction	0.48	5.36
Microsomal fraction	0.49	5.66
Supernatant fraction	4.50	11.7
Chromatin fraction	2.00	12.5
Purified chromatin[b]	17.7	36.4

[a] Vitamin D-deficient chicks received 5 units (0.325 nmole) of 25(OH)[^{3}H]D_3 or 1,25$(OH)_2$[^{3}H]D_3 and an equivalent amount of [4-^{14}C]cholesterol in 0.2 ml of 1,2-propanediol via intracardial injection 16 or 8 hr, respectively, prior to death. All purified subnuclear fractions were prepared from the crude nuclear fraction, not necessarily from the fraction listed above it in the table. Each number represents an average of four to eight separate determinations. The ratio of absolute amount of 25(OH)[^{3}H]D_3 and its metabolites or 1,25$(OH)_2$[^{3}H]D_3 and its metabolites to [4-^{14}C]cholesterol and its metabolites in the fraction is computed from the ratio of ^{3}H to ^{14}C and the specific activities of the parent molecules that were administered.

[b] Each chromatin fraction was washed three times with 1.0% Triton X-100 in 0.01 *M* Tris, pH 7.5, before the radioactivity content was determined.

As shown in Table 7-5, similar results were obtained several years later when radioactive preparations of 25(OH)[^{3}H]D_3 and 1,25$(OH)_2$[^{3}H]D_3 were available. Again, there was a remarkable increase in the ratio of vitamin D steroids to cholesterol steroids as the homogenate was fractionated to ultimately yield a purified chromatin fraction. Also, the chromatin-localized radioactivity [exclusively in the chemical form of 1,25$(OH)_2D_3$] was stable to washing three times with a solution of 1% Triton X-100.

It was also possible to further purify the chromatin binding sites for 1,25$(OH)_2D_3$ via selective solubilization of the specific "receptor fraction," which has such a high affinity for this metabolite. This was done by increasing the ionic strength of the incubation media. Extraction of this binding protein from the chromatin resulted in a 170-fold purification over the mucosal homogenate. Characterization of this receptor fraction indicated that it contained a significant amount of RNA in addition to protein and that it might exist in multiple forms, i.e., a species of 50,000–70,000 daltons and a species of a molecular weight greater than 200,000 daltons (Haussler and Norman, 1969).

A summary of many of these complex relationships is given in Table 7-6. Here an attempt has been made to correlate the magnitude of the dose required for saturation of the chromatin binding sites with that required for the development of the maximal biological response. There is an excellent agreement among results obtained from administering separately the three vitamin D steroids. In each instance, the dose required to produce the maximal stimulation of intestinal calcium transport also produced a saturation of chromatin binding sites with equivalent amounts of $1,25(OH)_2D_3$. It should be recalled that the metabolism of $25(OH)D_3$ by the kidney is stringently regulated, and thus under conditions of D_3 or $25(OH)D_3$ administration not all intestinal receptor binding sites for $1,25(OH)_2D_3$ may be filled. In contrast, when $1,25(OH)_2D_3$ is administered directly to the bird, the total binding capacity of the intestinal receptor sites can be quantitated. Furthermore, the time delay required to saturate the chromatin receptor sites is in good agreement with the time necessary to produce maximal calcium transport. The lag was longest for both responses with vitamin D, was intermediate in length with $25(OH)D_3$, and was shortest with the steroid $1,25(OH)_2D_3$. Thus, we have attempted to establish the validity of the concept that there is a strong cause and effect relationship between the appearance of $1,25(OH)_2D_3$ in the intestinal mucosa and the subsequent development of the biological response, an increased intestinal calcium transport.

It is now generally accepted that the prime site of localization of $1,25(OH)_2D_3$ in the intestinal mucosa is the nuclear fraction. However, there have been over the past 10 years various reports disputing this fact (Cousins *et al.*, 1970a,b). Stohs and DeLuca (1967) found that after administration of a physiological dose of 0.65 nmole (10 IU) of vitamin D_3 to rachitic rats the bulk of the radioactivity

TABLE 7-6
Studies on the Mechanism of Action of Vitamin D_3 and Its Metabolites in Stimulating the Intestinal Transport of Calcium[a]

Parameter measured	D_3	$25(OH)D_3$	$1,25(OH)_2D_3$
Dose (pmoles) to produce a maximal Ca^{2+} response	1950	1400	26
Dose (pmoles) necessary to saturate chromatin binding sites	1950	1400	26
Lag time (hr) for maximal Ca^{2+} response	36–48	20–30	8–10
Lag time (hr) before chromatin binding sites are saturated	15–20	12–16	3–4
Maximal amount of $1,25(OH)_2D_3$ (pmoles) bound to chromatin fraction from one chick mucosa[b]	7.8	6.5	11–12
Evidence for specificity of chromatin binding of $1,25(OH)_2D_3$	Yes	Yes	Yes

[a]Taken from Tsai and Norman (1973b).

[b]Determined at the time of maximal $1,25(OH)_2D_3$ uptake by the intestinal mucosa.

in the intestinal mucosa was present in the "crude nuclear debris" fraction. When this fraction was further purified via utilization of 1% citric acid by the procedure of Mirsky and Pollister (1964) to yield a "purified nuclear fraction," less than 10% of the total tissue radioactivity was present. Chen *et al.* (1970) have taken strong exception to the suggestions of Norman's laboratory that $1,25(OH)_2D_3$ is localized in the intestinal chromatin fraction. Although they agree that the steroid is localized in the nuclear fraction, they state that, when highly purified chromatin prepared according to the procedure of Marushige and Bonner (1966) is employed, the $1,25(OH)_2D_3$ remains with a nuclear membrane fraction that is separated from the chromatin during the isolation procedure. Thus, the investigators in DeLuca's laboratory maintain (Chen *et al.*, 1970) that when chromatin is prepared by the method of Haussler *et al.* (1968) as much as 40–60% of the intestinal radioactivity appears in the chromatin fraction but that when chromatin is prepared by the procedure of Marushige and Bonner (1966) less than 10% of the cellular radioactivity of $1,25(OH)_2D_3$ is associated with the "purified chromatin." What seems to be unappreciated by Chen *et al.* (1970) is that there is no one formally correct procedure for the isolation of chromatin, and furthermore the term "chromatin" is only an operational one utilized to designate a fraction that is obtained after a certain specified set of isolation manipulations. The term "chromatin" as employed by the laboratory of Norman and co-workers has always been used to designate an operational procedure for preparation of a subfraction of crude nuclei. Purity of chromatin fractions may be assessed by measurement of overall DNA yield, determination of the DNA/RNA ratio, or electron microscopic evaluation. Both groups (Chen *et al.*, 1970; Haussler *et al.*, 1969) have evaluated their chromatin fractions by the technique of electron microscopy, and no overt differences in the purity of the various fractions are apparent. What is important is that both groups do agree that $1,25(OH)_2D_3$ is localized in the nucleus of the cell.

More recently Chen and DeLuca (1973a) reported the subcellular distribution of tritiated $1,25(OH)_2D_3$ in the intestinal mucosa of vitamin D-deficient rats. They found that 80% of the tritium was located in the crude nuclear debris fraction and that, of the radioactivity associated with this crude nuclear debris fraction, 30–45% was associated with pure chromatin whereas more than 50% of the radioactivity was either extranuclear or loosely bound to the nuclei. This result was followed by a report from the same laboratory (Zile *et al.*, 1978) indicating that autoradiography of frozen sections of intestinal tissue from rachitic chicks given high specific activity (78 Ci/mmole) $1,25(OH)_2[23,24\text{-}^3H]D_3$ demonstrated nuclear localization of the secosteroid.

The experiments discussed above concerning the subcellular localization of vitamin D metabolites after *in vivo* administration of any of the vitamin D steroids represent an important beginning in the understanding of the mode of action of $1,25(OH)_2D_3$. From these observations one may obtain certain clues from which it may ultimately be possible to deduce biochemical details concerning the mode of action of vitamin D in the intestine.

2. *Studies in Vitro*

In view of the results reported above, and particularly in consideration of the current status of investigations underway in other laboratories concerned with the subcellular localization of classic steroid hormones, attempts were initiated to duplicate under *in vitro* conditions the subcellular localization of $1,25(OH)_2D_3$ in the intestinal chromatin fraction. The specificity with which steroid hormones are able to initiate their characteristic physiological responses apparently is dependent on the presence of specific receptor proteins in their target tissue(s). Studies on the mechanism of action of hormones such as estradiol, progesterone, testosterone, aldosterone, and glucocorticoids (Buller and O'Malley, 1976) have established that these steroids participate in a two-step mechanism prior to the initiation of nuclear events required for manifestation of the biological activity. A steroid hormone first must bind to a specific extranuclear receptor protein to form a steroid hormone–receptor complex; this then undergoes an obligatory "activation process" prior to entry of the complex into the nucleus, where it becomes selectively associated with the chromatin fraction. It is proposed that following this sequence of events an enhancement of genetic expression ensues, which ultimately leads to an increased synthesis of key proteins responsible for the development of the characteristic physiological response.

A summary of our more current results obtained in this respect is given in Table 7-7 and Fig. 7-4. Similar studies have been performed by Lawson *et al.*

TABLE 7-7
Incubation *in Vitro* of Tritiated $1,25(OH)_2D_3$ with Different Intestinal Mucosal Fractions[a,b]

Fraction incubated *in vitro*	$1,25(OH)_2D_3$ bound to chromatin fraction (pmole/mg DNA)	Fraction steroid bound (%)
Homogenate	0.50	100
Crude nuclei	0.37	74
Crude nuclei, washed 3×	0.24	48
Chromatin	0.12	24
Cytosol with $1,25(OH)_2D_3$ + crude nuclei	0.62	124

[a] From Tsai and Norman (1973b).

[b] $1,25(OH)_2D_3$ (130 pmoles) was added to each incubation (15 ml) containing the indicated intestinal subcellular fraction. The incubations were carried at 0°–4°C for 30 min. The Triton-washed chromatin fraction was prepared, and the associated radioactivity was determined. Each number is an average of four separate determinations. The cytosol fraction with bound $1,25(OH)_2D_3$ was prepared by incubating cytosol with 130 pmoles of tritiated $1,25(OH)_2D_3$ at 0°–4°C for 30 min and then adding the crude nuclear fraction for a second incubation.

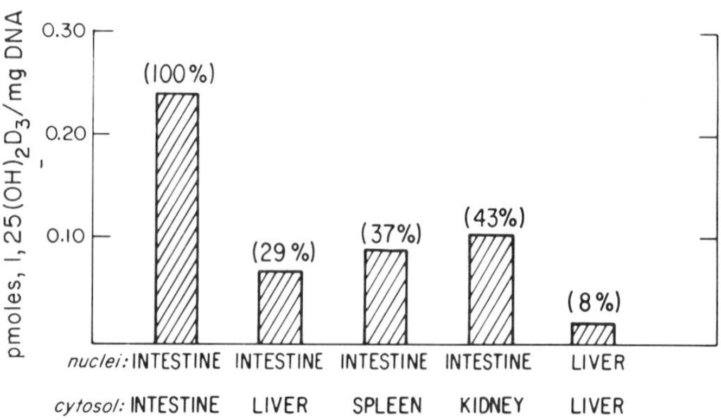

Figure 7-4. Tissue specificity of cytoplasmic and chromatin binding of 1,25$(OH)_2D_3$. Cytosol protein, 60 mg, obtained from different chick tissues was suspended in 10 ml of 0.25 *M* sucrose–TKM (0.05 *M* Tris · HCl, pH 7.5; 0.02 *M* KCl; 0.05 *M* $MgCl_2$) and preincubated with 65 pmoles of 1,25$(OH)_2[^3H]D_3$ at 0°–4°C for 30 min. An intestinal crude nuclear fraction was then added to the "labeled cytosol" and incubated for an additional 30 min at 0°–4°C. Next, the Triton X-100-washed chromatin fraction was prepared according to Tsai and Norman (1973a), and the bound radioactivity was determined.

(1969a,b,c), Lawson and Wilson (1974), Chen and DeLuca (1973b), Brumbaugh and Haussler (1973, 1974), and Bachelet *et al.* (1977). We have attempted to identify the properties, the specificity, and requirements of an intestinal homogenate system that is capable of effecting the localization of 1,25$(OH)_2D_3$ in the intestinal chromatin fraction. As emphasized in Table 7-7, evidence was obtained for the mandatory binding of 1,25$(OH)_2D_3$ to a cytoplasmic receptor required for the association of the steroid with the intestinal chromatin fraction. There is apparently a nuclear receptor or binding site in the intestinal mucosa that will receive either the 1,25$(OH)_2D_3$ or the steroid protein–receptor complex. When 1,25$(OH)_2D_3$ was incubated with the 3× washed crude nuclei or directly with the chromatin fraction, much less 1,25$(OH)_2D_3$ was tightly bound to the subsequently isolated chromatin than when incubations were carried out with whole mucosa homogenates (Tsai and Norman, 1973b). Only when 1,25$(OH)_2D_3$ was preincubated with the cytosol fraction followed by isolation of the chromatin fraction was there a maximal chromatin localization of the steroid.

As shown in Fig. 7-4, the tissue specificity of the cytoplasmic receptor for 1,25$(OH)_2D_3$ was also evaluated. The results indicate that the cytosol of the target tissue, the intestine, is the best mediator of the transfer of 1,25$(OH)_2D_3$ to the nucleus of the intestinal mucosa. There was some localization of 1,25$(OH)_2D_3$ in intestinal chromatin, which was isolated from crude nuclear fractions that had been previously incubated with cytoplasm fractions obtained from the liver, kidney, or spleen. This was possibly due to the presence of a small amount of intestinal cytosol in the crude nuclear fraction of the mucosa. These results, describing *in vitro* conditions that permit the sequential binding of 1,25$(OH)_2D_3$ first to cytoplasmic and then to nuclear receptor, are exactly analogous to those reported to have occurred under both *in vivo* and *in vitro* conditions for many other steroid hormones (Buller and O'Malley, 1976).

Figure 7-5 shows the results of an experiment concerning the temperature dependence of the saturable binding of 1,25$(OH)_2D_3$ to its intestinal cytosol plus chromatin receptor under *in vitro* conditions. These data demonstrate that maximal binding of 1,25$(OH)_2D_3$ at a level of about 21 to 24 pmoles per chick intestinal chromatin (15 mg of DNA) occurs at a concentration of 2.0×10^{-8} *M* at 25°C. When rigorous efforts are made to maintain all incubation components at 0°C, only a greatly reduced amount of 1,25$(OH)_2D_3$ localizes in the reisolated chromatin pellet. This result may be due to either a temperature-dependent "activation" process of the steroid–receptor complex or the slower kinetics of association of steroid ligand with the receptor, which is known to occur at low temperatures (Wecksler, 1978).

The value of 21 to 24 pmoles is approximately two times higher than that obtained *in vivo* when radioactive vitamin D is administered. However, it should be recalled that the renal metabolism of 25$(OH)D_3$ to 1,25$(OH)_2D_3$ is stringently

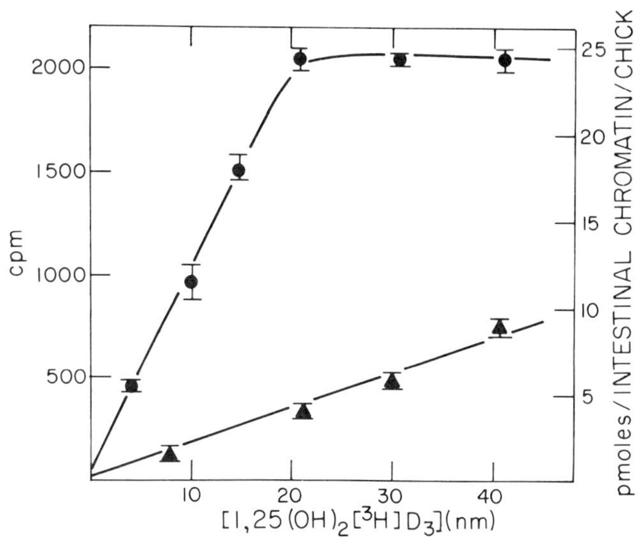

Figure 7-5. Temperature dependence of the saturable binding of 1,25$(OH)_2D_3$ to chick intestinal mucosa chromatin. Increasing amounts of tritiated 1,25$(OH)_2D_3$ (specific activity 2.9 Ci/mmole) were incubated with 0.5 ml of the reconstituted cytosol–chromatin receptor system at 0°C (▲—▲) or 25°C (●—●) for 45 min. The radioactivity bound to chromatin was then determined. Each point represents the average of triplicate measurements ± S.D.

regulated (Henry *et al.*, 1974). This may account for the lower value observed under *in vivo* conditions (see, for example, Fig. 7-3) when vitamin D is administered. When radioactive 1,25$(OH)_2D_3$ is given *in vivo* to rachitic chicks, within 3–4 hr 20–24 pmoles of hormone per chick intestinal chromatin are maximally localized, which compares favorably with the value reported here.

The time course for the binding of 1,25$(OH)_2D_3$ to the intestinal chromatin under *in vitro* conditions is shown in Fig. 7-6. We have observed that the saturation occurs 30 min after initiation of incubation at 25°C and can remain at this level for at least 30 min longer. The results in Figs. 7-5 and 7-6 define a concentration of steroid (2.0×10^{-8} *M*), temperature (25°C), and time (45 mins) required for maximal binding of 1,25$(OH)_2D_3$ to chick intestinal chromatin under the *in vitro* conditions described here.

It has been possible to selectively solubilize the putative steroid–receptor complex that is bound to the intestinal chromatin fraction (Haussler and Norman, 1969). As shown in Fig. 7-7, increasing concentrations of KCl over a narrow range (approximately 0.3 *M*) effect a complete extraction of the ^{14}C-labeled steroid bound to a macromolecule. We have termed the resulting supernatant fraction, after removal of the residual chromatin, the crude receptor fraction.

Figure 7-8 shows the results of sucrose gradients of the intestinal cytosol receptor (Fig. 7-8A) and KCl-extracted protein fraction obtained from the intestinal chromatin (Fig. 7-8B). The cytosol receptor (presumably unactivated) and the receptor retrieved from the intestinal chromatin (which may have been "activated") have identical sedimentation values of 3.5 to 3.7 S. Similar results have

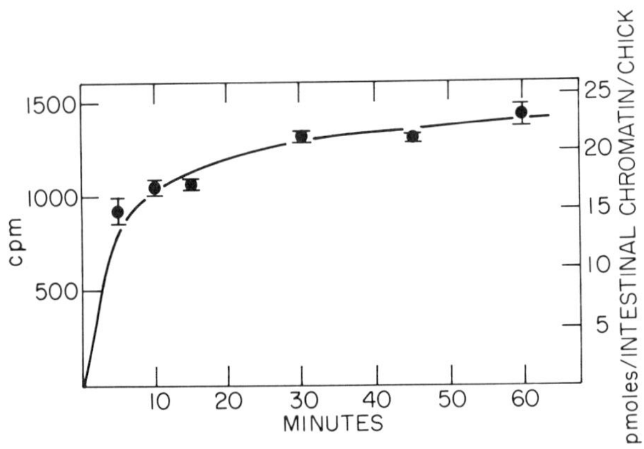

Figure 7-6. Time course for the saturation of chick intestinal mucosa chromatin binding sites with 1,25$(OH)_2D_3$. Reconstituted cytosol-chromatin fractions (1.0 ml) were incubated with 2.0×10^{-8} *M* tritiated 1,25$(OH)_2D_3$ (specific activity 1.1 Ci/mmole) at 25°C for the indicated amount of time. The amount of radioactivity bound to the chromatin following the incubation was determined as described by Tsai and Norman (1973a). Each point represents the average of triplicate measurements ± S.D.

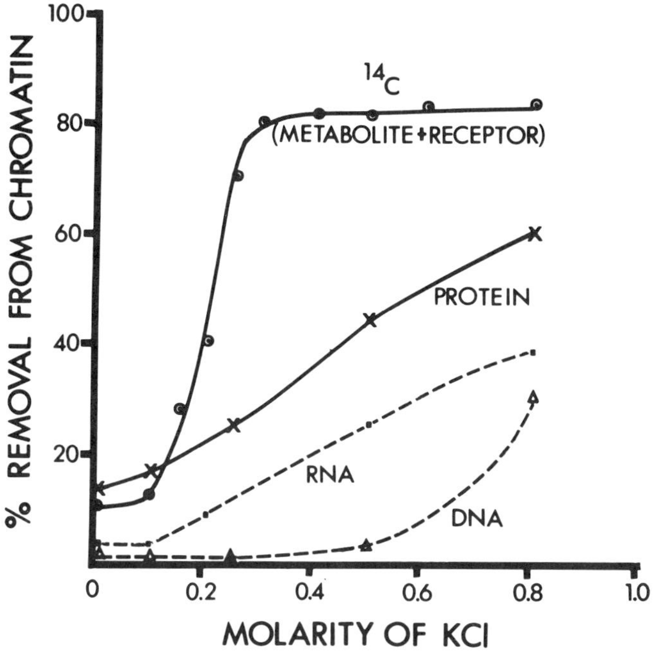

Figure 7-7. Selective solubilization of the chromatin-associated $1,25(OH)_2D_3$ receptor with KCl. Chromatin, which had been prelabeled with $1,25(OH)_2[^{14}C]D_3$ *in vivo,* was homogenized with various concentrations of KCl in 0.01 *M* Tris, pH 7.5 (25 ml). The residual chromatin was recovered by sedimentation at 27,000 g for 1 hr in the RC-2 centrifuge. It was then assayed for ^{14}C radioactivity, and the supernatant was assayed for DNA, RNA, and protein (Haussler and Norman, 1969).

been reported extensively by Haussler and collaborators (Brumbaugh and Haussler, 1974, 1975a,b). On the basis of experiments of this type it can be tentatively concluded that "activation" of intestinal receptors for $1,25(OH)_2D_3$, if it occurs, does not involve major modification in either the size or the shape of the receptor protein. This seems to be a somewhat simpler situation than that observed in other steroid hormone-receptor systems in which receptors of many different sizes may be isolated depending on salt concentration, temperature, or other factors (Buller and O'Malley, 1976).

Other observations consistent with the view that the $1,25(OH)_2D_3$ cytoplasmic receptor is a macromolecule are its elution pattern in Sephadex G-200 chromatography, its sensitivity to treatment with Pronase but insensitivity to RNase and DNase, its heat lability, and its precipitability by ammonium sulfate (Tsai and Norman, 1973b; Wecksler, 1978; and Frolick and DeLuca, 1975).

Recently the laboratories of both DeLuca (Kream *et al.*, 1977a,b) and Norman (Wecksler, 1978) reported the presence of a 3.2–3.5 S cytoplasmic protein in the cytosol of rat intestine which has a high affinity for $1,25(OH)_2D_3$ (see Fig.

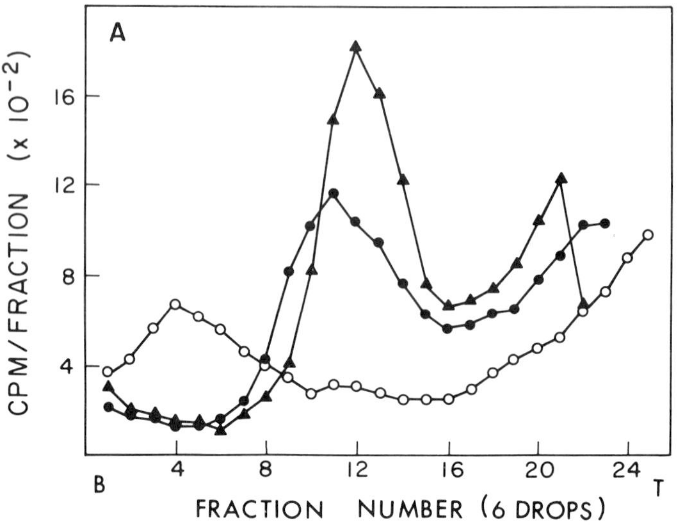

Figure 7-8. Sucrose gradient analysis of intestinal cytosol and KCl-extracted intestinal mucosal chromatin after incubation with 1,25$(OH)_2D_3$. (A) Cytosol was incubated with 0.9 n*M* ^{3}H-labeled steroid for 90 min at 4°C and sedimented through 5–20% sucrose gradients containing 0.3 *M* KCl (▲—▲), 0.15 *M* KCl (●—●), or no KCl (○—○). The receptor appears to aggregate to a larger complex (about 7 S) in the absence of KCl in the sucrose gradients. (B) Reconstituted chromatin and cytosol (2.0 ml) prepared from chick intestinal mucosa was incubated with 1.4×10^{-8} *M* ^{3}H-labeled ligand for 30 min at 23°C. Chromatin was harvested, washed, and extracted with 0.3 *M* KCl. The extract was then sedimented through a high-salt sucrose density gradient. The complex migrates as a 3.7 S species under these conditions.

7-9). Also, Norman's group (Wecksler and Norman, 1979; Wecksler *et al.*, 1979; Wecksler, 1978) presented the first evidence of the existence of an intestinal receptor for 1,25$(OH)_2D_3$ in man (see Fig. 7-10). This human intestinal cytosol receptor for 1,25$(OH)_2D_3$ also has a mobility of 3.5 S on 5–20% sucrose gradients. Thus, it is now firmly established that both avian and mammalian intestinal tissues have a cytosol receptor for 1,25$(OH)_2D_3$. This fact argues strongly that the fundamental mode of action of 1,25$(OH)_2D_3$ is similar in both phylogenic classes.

Figure 7-11 depicts the Scatchard analysis of 1,25$(OH)_2D_3$ binding to the human intestinal receptor; the $K_d = 2.2 \times 10^{-10}$ *M* is in good agreement with the 1,25$(OH)_2D_3$ K_d for chick and rat intestinal receptors (see Table 7-10). As is documented in Table 8-7, the concentration of 1,25$(OH)_2D_3$ in human plasma is 35–50 pg/ml, or approximately 1×10^{-10} *M*. This concentration of ligand would support an approximately 30–50% saturation of the human intestinal 1,25$(OH)_2D_3$ cytosol receptor. Thus, in normal human beings, the extent of saturation of the intestinal receptor is poised midpoint so that a maximal degree

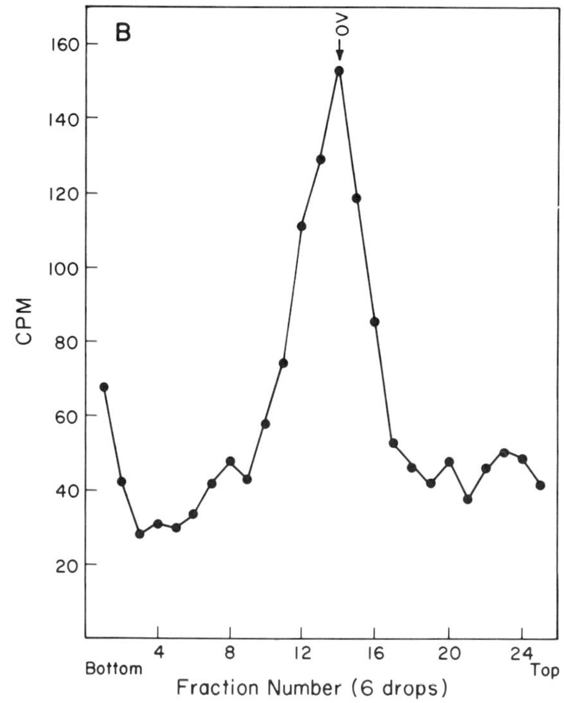

of latitude is available to accommodate either an increased or decreased rate of production of $1,25(OH)_2D_3$ by the kidney. A comparable situation was noted in the chick by Friedlander *et al.* (1977) (see also Fig. 6-18).

B. Bone

A very limited amount of information is available concerning the subcellular localization of vitamin D and its metabolites in bone tissue. Kodicek and Thompson (1965) and Wezeman (1976) reported results concerning the tissue and subcellular localization of tritiated 25 $(OH)D_3$ in bone as determined autoradiographically; regrettably, no definitive conclusions can be drawn due to the lack of consideration of metabolism of the administered steroid. The most definitive studies have been carried out by Weber *et al.* (1971), who developed a simple technique to obtain subcellular fractions from the epiphysis, metaphysis, and diaphysis of chick proximal tibia. Their technique employed the conventional approach of differential centrifugation and isolation of crude nuclear, mitochondrial, and microsomal pellets; the crude nuclear fraction was then further purified by sedimentation through 2.4 *M* sucrose. This methodology enabled

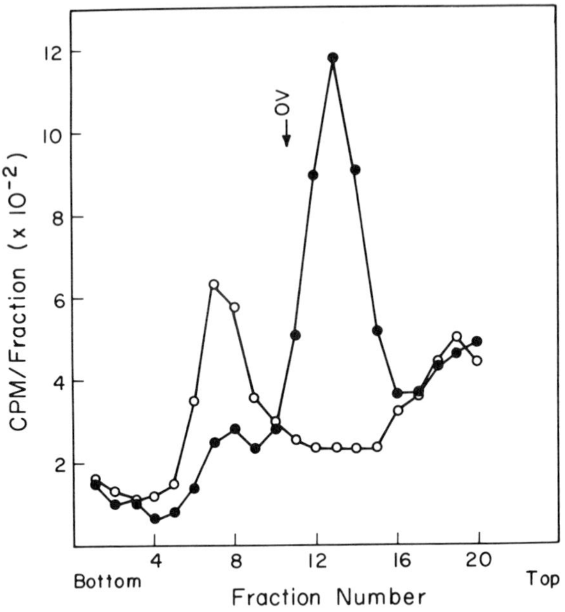

Figure 7-9. Sucrose gradient sedimentation analysis of the rat intestinal mucosa 1,25$(OH)_2D_3$ cytosol receptor. Cytosol was incubated with 1 n*M* tritiated 1,25$(OH)_2D_3$ for 30 min at 23° C in the absence (●—●) or presence (○—○) of 1.4 μ*M* nonradioactive steroid, layed on a sucrose density gradient, and centrifuged as described in Fig. 7-8. The receptor migrates with a 3.2 S sedimentation coefficient on these high-salt gradients.

them to consistently isolate 60–70% of the total bone DNA in the nuclear fraction ultimately obtained. Their experimental protocol involved the administration of [^{14}C]vitamin D_3 to rachitic chicks and at various time intervals assessing the uptake of radioactivity by bone tissue as well as its subcellular localization pattern. They found that 24 hr after administration of [^{14}C]vitamin D, the nuclear fraction contained 27% and the supernatant or soluble portion of the cell had 67% of the total ^{14}C radioactivity recovered. Most importantly, 77% of the radioactivity present in the nuclear fraction could be accounted for by 1,25$(OH)_2D_3$, whereas approximately 10% of the soluble cytoplasmic radioactivity was 1,25$(OH)_2D_3$. Kream *et al.* (1977c) presented preliminary sucrose gradient-derived evidence supporting the existence of a specific high affinity binding protein for 1,25$(OH)_2D_3$ in the cytosol of fetal rat bone. The preferential nuclear localization of 1,25$(OH)_2D_3$ in bone tissue and possible existence of a cytosol receptor for this secosteroid strongly suggest that the mode of action of the steroid in this organ is similar to that postulated above for the intestinal columnar epithelial cells. This will be an area of intensive investigation in the near future.

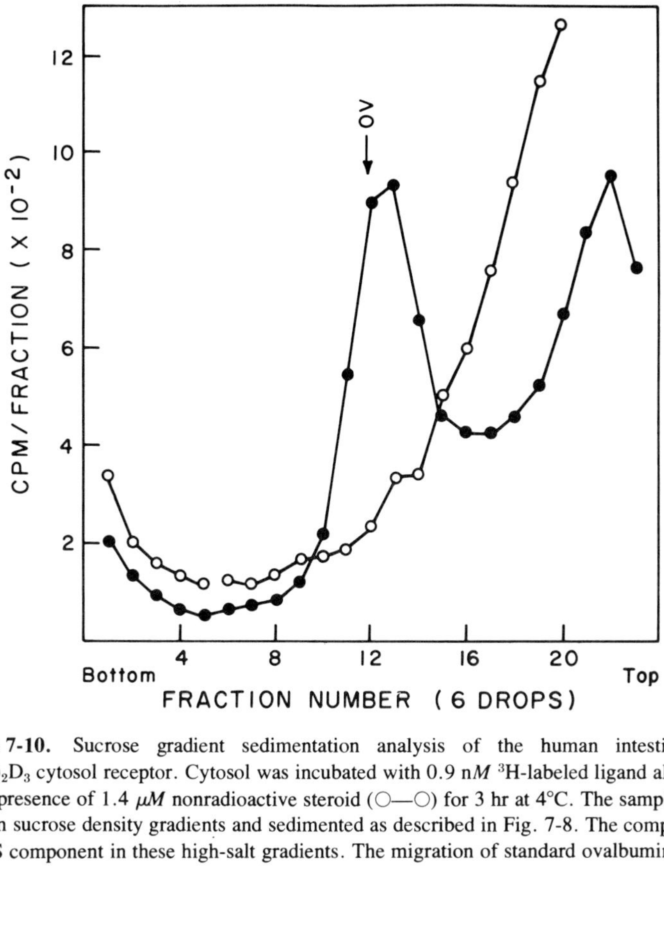

Figure 7-10. Sucrose gradient sedimentation analysis of the human intestinal mucosa $1,25(OH)_2D_3$ cytosol receptor. Cytosol was incubated with 0.9 nM ^{3}H-labeled ligand alone (●—●) or in the presence of 1.4 μM nonradioactive steroid (○—○) for 3 hr at 4°C. The samples were then layered on sucrose density gradients and sedimented as described in Fig. 7-8. The complex migrates as a 3.5 S component in these high-salt gradients. The migration of standard ovalbumin is indicated by OV.

C. Parathyroid Gland

The identification of $1,25(OH)_2D_3$ as the biologically active form of vitamin D and as a part of the endocrine system that regulates calcium metabolism has led to speculation as to the possible interaction of this steroid with another major component of the calcium homeostatic system, namely, the parathyroid hormone (PTH). Much evidence has accumulated which suggests that PTH is capable of maintaining and increasing the renal production of $1,25(OH)_2D_3$ (see Chapter 6); this would suggest that PTH is a trophic factor for the production of $1,25(OH)_2D_3$.

More recently, vitamin D metabolites have been implicated in the regulation of serum PTH levels (Lumb and Stanbury, 1974; Oldham *et al.*, 1973). It has been demonstrated that $1,25(OH)_2D_3$ both decreases immunoreactive PTH *in vivo* and

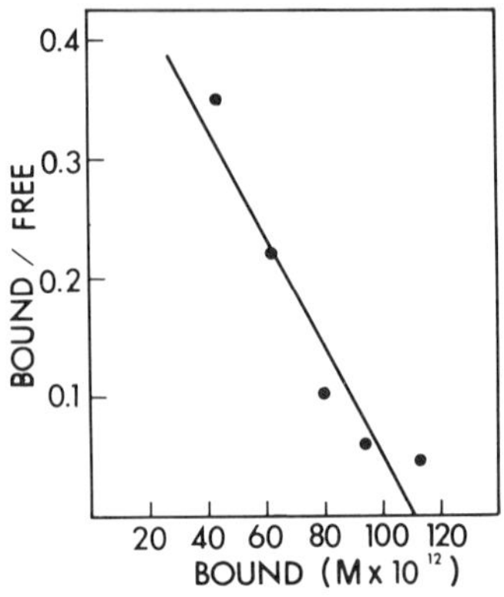

Figure 7-11. Scatchard analysis of the binding of 1,25$(OH)_2D_3$ to its human intestinal cytosol receptor. Various concentrations of ^{3}H-labeled ligand were incubated in the presence or absence of 320-fold excess nonradioactive steroid with human intestinal cytosol for 24 hr at 4°C. Specific binding was determined using the hydroxylapatite assay, and a plot of [bound]/[free] versus [bound] was constructed. The K_d was found to be 2.2×10^{-10} *M*.

inhibits its secretion *in vitro* in organ culture (Chertow *et al.*, 1975; Canterbury *et al.*, 1978). In addition, 1,25$(OH)_2D_3$ alone and in combination with 24,25$(OH)_2D_3$ causes a regression of hyperplastic parathyroid glands *in vivo* (Henry *et al.*, 1977). Observations of this type are suggestive of possible interactions of the steroid at the parathyroid gland level. It is intriguing to wonder whether 24,25$(OH)_2D_3$ may also be involved in regulation of parathyroid gland activities.

Table 7-8 presents the results of an experiment carried out by Henry and Norman (1975) designed to evaluate the localization of 1,25$(OH)_2D_3$ in parathyroid glands. When 1,25$(OH)_2D_3$ was administered to vitamin D-deficient chicks, within 2 hr the concentration of this steroid in the parathyroid glands was four times higher than that in blood and equivalent to levels observed in the

TABLE 7-8
Localization of 1,25$(OH)_2D_3$ in Parathyroid Glands and Other Tissues[a,b]

	Blood	Kidney	Intestine	Parathyroid
dpm/g tissue	520	870	2300	2200
pmoles/g tissue	0.33	0.56	1.5	1.4
Concentration ($\times 10^{-9}$ *M*)	0.44	0.75	2.0	1.9
Concentration ratio to blood	1.0	1.7	4.5	4.3

[a] From Henry and Norman (1975).
[b] Chicks were injected intracardially with 320 pmoles tritiated 1,25$(OH)_2D_3$, and 2 hr later the tissues were removed, lipids extracted, and radioactivity determined.

intestine. Similarly, when $25(OH)D_3$ was administered, the concentration of the metabolite $1,25(OH)_2D_3$ in the parathyroid glands was 2.4 times that in the blood and 60% of that in the intestine. These results were consistent with a concept that the hormonally active form of vitamin D, $1,25(OH)_2D_3$, might interact with the parathyroid glands in a way that might be capable of modulating parathyroid hormone secretion.

Because of these results, it was thought appropriate to initiate studies to determine the subcellular localization of $1,25(OH)_2D_3$ in the parathyroid gland. Wecksler *et al.* (1977) carried out a detailed study of the subcellular localization of tritiated $1,25(OH)_2D_3$ in the parathyroid glands obtained from vitamin D-deficient chicks. We showed that parathyroid glands specifically localize $1,25(OH)_2D_3$ under both *in vivo* and *in vitro* conditions in the nuclear chromatin fraction. As shown in Fig. 7-12 both the parathyroid cytosol and nuclear receptors for $1,25(OH)_2D_3$ have identical *s* values of 3.1–3.5 S. As in the intestine, no major change in sedimentation properties occurs as a consequence of a possible "activation process" which must occur before translocation of the steroid from the cytosol to the nuclear chromatin fraction. Similar results on the sedimentation properties of the parathyroid gland cytosol receptor for $1,25(OH)_2D_3$ in the chick and human adenoma have been reported by Brumbaugh *et al.* (1975) and Hughes and Haussler (1978). It is of further interest that the sedimentation rate for the cytosol receptor obtained from the parathyroid tissue (3.1–3.5 S) is somewhat different from that reported in Fig. 7-8 for the intestinal $1,25(OH)_2D_3$ cytosol receptor (3.5–3.7 S). This suggests that these $1,25(OH)_2D_3$ receptor proteins are not identical. One way of pursuing this question was to carry out "crossover experiments" in which the relative abilities of the parathyroid gland cytosol and intestinal cytosol were compared with regard to their abilities to translocate $1,25(OH)_2D_3$ to chromatin fractions (see Table 7-9). Wecksler *et al.* (1977) reported that, although intestinal mucosa chromatin has a greater capacity to bind $1,25(OH)_2D_3$ than all other tissues evaluated, the parathyroid gland chromatin is clearly a superior concentrator of $1,25(OH)_2D_3$ than either the liver or kidney.

It has also been possible to document the presence of a cytosol receptor for $1,25(OH)_2D_3$ in parathyroid tissue obtained from a human adenoma; Fig. 7-13 depicts a peak in a 5–20% sucrose gradient with a mobility of 3.55 S (Wecksler, 1978). These results appear to substantiate the view that the parathyroid gland of both chicks and man contain receptors for $1,25(OH)_2D_3$. As yet no results are available describing the definite existence of parathyroid receptors for $24,25(OH)_2D_3$.

The biochemical basis of the interaction of $1,25(OH)_2D_3$ in the parathyroid gland is not known. Inasmuch as the steroid is localized in the nuclear chromatin fraction, one would assume that it is concerned with activation of genetic information. This then could be the biochemical means of effecting "feedback" of the trophic actions of PTH on the renal 1-hydroxylase. There is precedent for

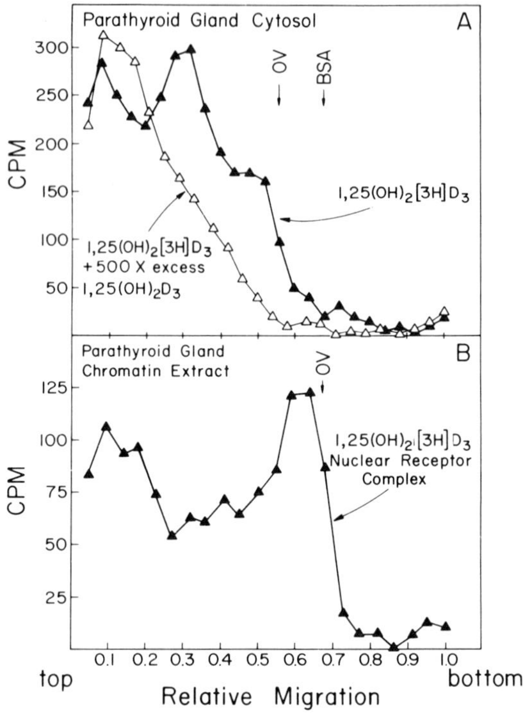

Figure 7-12. Sucrose gradient analysis of cytosol and KCl-extracted chromatin fractions obtained from chick parathyroid glands after incubation with 1,25$(OH)_2D_3$. (A) Parathyroid gland cytosol was incubated with 5.5 n*M* tritiated 1,25$(OH)_2D_3$ in the presence (△—△) or absence (▲—▲) of 500-fold excess nonradioactive 1,25$(OH)_2D_3$. Aliquots of 0.15 ml were layered on 5–20% sucrose gradients and centrifuged for 20 hr at 50,000 rpm. (B) Reconstituted chromatin and cytosol from a 20% parathyroid gland homogenate were incubated with 14 n*M* tritiated 1,25$(OH)_2D_3$, chromatin was isolated and extracted with 0.3 *M* KCl, and 0.15 ml of this KCl extract was applied to a 5–20% sucrose gradient and centrifuged as described above. [^{14}C]Ovalbumin (3.7 S) was included as a sedimentation marker on a parallel gradient. All gradients contained 0.3 *M* KCl. From Wecksler *et al.* (1977).

such "feedback" localization of steroid hormones in endocrine organs that secrete their trophic hormone. It is well known that other steroid hormones under the trophic influence of anterior pituitary hormones may "feed back" in the pituitary or hypothalamus (McEwen *et al.*, 1970). There are specific cytoplasmic receptors (Wise and Payne, 1975; Notides, 1970) for these steroids, and subsequent nuclear localization for some of them has been demonstrated (McEwen *et al.*, 1976; DeKloet *et al.*, 1975). These results suggest that there may be similar modes of action for steroid hormones in both target organ and "feed-

TABLE 7-9
Crossover Experiment to Evaluate Effectiveness of Intestinal Mucosa and Parathyroid Gland Cytosol Fractions in $1,25(OH)_2D_3$ Transfer to Chromatin Fractions[a,b]

	Chromatin source			
Cytosol source	Mucosa	Parathyroid glands	Kidney	Liver
Mucosa	0.72	0.033	0.12	0.13
Parathyroid glands	0.11	0.23	—	—
Kidney	0.11	—	0.02	—
Liver	0.012	—	—	0.006
20 mg/ml bovine serum albumin	0.018			
50 m*M* Tris	0.028			

[a]Experiments were carried out as described by Wecksler *et al.* (1977).
[b]Picomoles tritiated $1,25(OH)_2D_3$ specifically bound to chromatin.

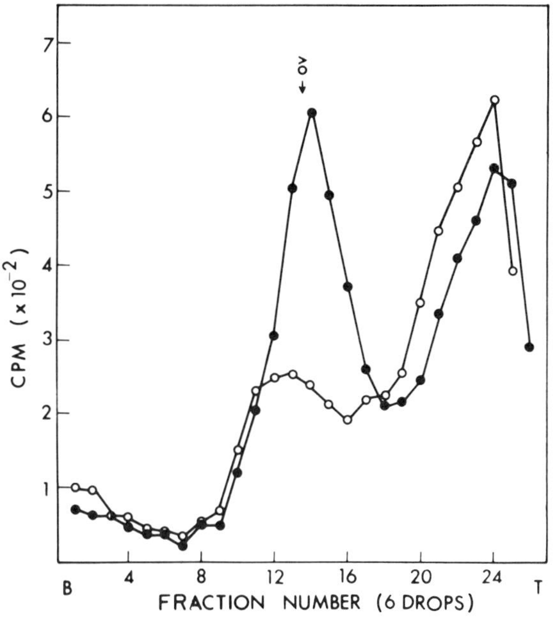

Figure 7-13. Sucrose gradient sedimentation profile of the human parathyroid gland $1,25(OH)_2D_3$ receptor. Cytosol was incubated with tritiated ligand in the absence (●—●) or presence (○—○) of excess nonradiolabeled steroid. The samples were then sedimented through high-salt sucrose density gradients. The peak of tritium representing the receptor migrated at 3.6 S on these gradients.

back" glands. Clearly, however, further work must be undertaken to validate in detail these general suggestions.

Wecksler and Norman (1979; Wecksler, 1978) have completed a detailed comparative study of both the biochemical properties and kinetics and equilibrium binding of $1,25(OH)_2D_3$ to its receptors in chick intestine and parathyroid, rat intestine, and human intestine and parathyroid. The kinetic results are summarized in Table 7-10. The equilibrium dissociation constant K_d was quite similar in all five tissues, with only a threefold variation, e.g., $2.3–7.4 \times 10^{-10}$ *M*, in the three species. Similarly, the second-order kinetic association constants of $1,25(OH)_2D_3$ plus receptor were highly similar, e.g., $0.9–2.5 \times 10^7\ m^{-1}\ min^{-1}$. The principal differences were the first-order dissociation constants, with the $t_{\frac{1}{2}}$ ranging from 18–22 hr for human receptor to 300–900 hr for chick receptor. It is apparent that the cytosol receptor for $1,25(OH)_2D_3$ in these five tissues has a very similar affinity for its ligand.

D. Other Organs (Kidneys, Liver, Brain)

Little specific information is available concerning the subcellular localization of vitamin D and its metabolites in other tissues. Nair and Bucana (1966) examined by gas-liquid chromatography the vitamin D content of liver subcellular fractions prepared by differential centrifugation. Unfortunately, due to the analytical technique that they employed (gas chromatography) and the associated detector sensitivity (see Table 4-2), they were forced to administer unusually large doses of vitamin D, i.e., 0.52–5.20 μmoles (8000–80,000 IU) of vitamin D_2 or D_3 either interperitoneally, intravenously, or orally. They reported that there was

TABLE 7-10
Summary of Kinetic and Equilibrium Binding Studies of $1,25(OH)_2D_3$ Receptors[a,b]

Tissue	K_d ($M \times 10^{10}$)	*n*	k_{on} ($M^{-1}\ min^{-1} \times 10^{-7}$)	*n*	k_{off} ($min^{-1} \times 10^4$)	*n*	$t_{\frac{1}{2}}$ (hr)
Chick intestine	2.3±0.6	5	0.92±0.12[c]	3	0.41±0.15	3	280
			0.55±0.10[d]	3			
Chick parathyroids	2.1	1	1.0	1	0.13	1	890
Rat intestine	7.4±4.1	3	1.7±0.7	2	7.2±0.6	2	16
Human intestine	1.8±0.5	3	2.5	1	6.4±.20	3	18
Human parathyroids	5.4	1	1.2	1	5.3	1	22

[a]Taken from Wecksler (1978), by permission.

[b]Numbers equal the mean ± S.D. of *n* determination; K_d determined at 4°C, k_{on} determined at 0°C, and k_{off} determined at 4°C.

[c]This value was obtained under conditions in which $R_o \neq S_o$ (R = initial concentration of receptor protein and S_o = initial concentration of free $1,25(OH)_2D_3$).

[d]This value was obtained under conditions in which $R_o = S_o$.

essentially a uniform distribution of vitamin D among the nuclear debris fraction, the mitochondrial fraction, and the supernatant cytosol fraction. These results have little physiological meaning in view of the large doses employed.

There are inherent problems in defining the subcellular localization of vitamin D in the liver and, particularly, the kidney since both tissues are sites of vitamin D metabolic transformation. Although specific physiological actions for D metabolites in the kidney (see Chapter 11) that might necessitate nuclear localization have been proposed, the situation is complicated because of the presence of the cytosol receptor for $25(OH)D_3$ as well as the mitochondrially localized $25(OH)D_3$ 1-hydroxylase and $25(OH)D_3$ 24-hydroxylase (Tsai *et al.*, 1973). Thus the unusual success that has been enjoyed with regard to elucidation of the subcellular localization of vitamin D and its metabolites in the intestinal mucosa and parathyroid is perhaps largely due to the fact that these organs are relatively homogenous in terms of cell type and only one major biological activity is resident therein. In contrast, in the kidney, which in the mammal is composed of the cortex and medulla, there is a plethora of cell types, which may tend to "average out" any specialized subcellular localization occurring in only one of the cell types.

Inasmuch as vitamin D-dependent calcium-binding proteins have been detected in the kidney, brain tissue, avian eggshell gland, bone, and pancreas (see Table 10-10), it might be anticipated that one should be capable ultimately of demonstrating a nuclear localization of $1,25(OH)_2D_3$ in these tissues.

III. INTESTINAL NUCLEAR LOCALIZATION OF $1,25(OH)_2D_3$ AS A BASIS FOR ITS STEROID HORMONE MODE OF ACTION

A. Lag in Action of Vitamin D and $1,25(OH)_2D_3$

As discussed in Chapter 1, one of the puzzling aspects of the mechanism of action of vitamin D is the marked time lag that occurs after administration of the steroid before the stimulation of intestinal calcium transport. This time lag was first formally described by Irving (1944); the observation has since been documented by virtually every investigator in the vitamin D field. There are several possible explanations for this time lag. There could be a necessity for (a) a slow transport of the unaltered vitamin to the target organ, (b) a metabolic process by which the vitamin is altered to a biologically active metabolite(s), or (c) mediation of its activity by an inductive mechanism perhaps requiring new RNA and protein synthesis. As described earlier in this chapter, after intercardial administration of vitamin D to rachitic animals, there is a prompt delivery (within 15–30 min) of the steroid to the target organ, the intestine (Fig. 7-1), so that the time delay is not due to slow delivery of either the steroid or metabolites. In view of the comprehensive scheme of vitamin D metabolism, it appears that the time required for metabolism of the parent steroid to $1,25(OH)_2D_3$ is an important factor in the determination of the overall time required for stimulation of intestinal calcium transport.

Figure 7-2 shows the kinetics for appearance of $1,25(OH)_2D_3$ in the intestinal mucosa and its chromatin fraction while figure 10-5 presents the time-course for the appearance of a specific calcium-binding protein in the intestinal mucosa (A) and also the time course of onset of increased intestinal calcium absorption (C). Clearly, the lag time before the appearance of biological response in the intestine is not reduced to zero when the biologically active form of vitamin D, $1,25(OH)_2D_3$, is administered to vitamin D-deficient chicks. (See also figure 6-4B.) There is a finite lag of at least 4 hr before any slight increase in intestinal calcium can be measured. As discussed below, this is most likely due to time-dependent activation of genome information, followed by a concomitant increase in messenger RNA synthesis and specific protein synthesis.

An additional potential contribution to the time lag might be the process of turnover and renewal of the intestinal columnar epithelial cells (see Chapter 10). It is known that these cells undergo progressive maturation and differentiation as they proceed up the intestinal villus. Originally there was concern (Spielvogel *et al.*, 1972) that a portion of the time lag in response to vitamin D might be due to some complex time-dependent requirement for differentiation of the columnar epithelial cells to a state where they would be "receptive" to the presence of $1,25(OH)_2D_3$ or other vitamin D metabolites. It is now known that the $t_{\frac{1}{2}}$ for appearance or decay of all the known intestinal vitamin D-related responses is shorter than the 90–100 hr necessary for complete turnover of intestinal cells.

B. Effects of Actinomycin D and Other Antibiotics on Intestinal Calcium Absorption

It is possible that the further lag in onset of biological response, even after the appearance of the biologically active metabolite, $1,25(OH)_2D_3$, in the intestine is due to a requirement for an increase in synthesis of RNA and subsequent protein synthesis. Perhaps one or several proteins necessary for the mediation of calcium absorption are synthesized by the mucosal cells only under the stimulus of the nuclear-localized $1,25(OH)_2D_3$.

In order to determine whether vitamin D or one of its metabolites was acting analogously to other steroid hormones to initiate the synthesis of new proteins by utilization of stored genetic information, it was essential to establish that certain actions of the vitamin could be blocked by appropriate inhibitors of gene replication, gene transcription, and translation processes.

Eisenstein and Passavoy (1964) first noted that actinomycin D could block the hypercalcemic consequences of the administration of pharmacological doses of vitamin D. However, these workers did not postulate that actinomycin D (an inhibitor of DNA-directed RNA synthesis) would block the actions of physiological levels of the vitamin in the target organ, the intestine. Their results were nonetheless important because they established that the osseous effects of vitamin D are actinomycin D sensitive and, in view of later observations showing that the intestinal actions of vitamin D were also actinomycin D sensitive, they reflected for the first time a fundamental similarity in mode of action of the vitamin in the two target organs.

Norman (1975) and Zull *et al.* (1965) both reported that actinomycin D inhibits the actions of vitamin D in terms of mediating intestinal calcium absorption and elevating serum calcium levels. Typical data are presented in Fig. 7-14.

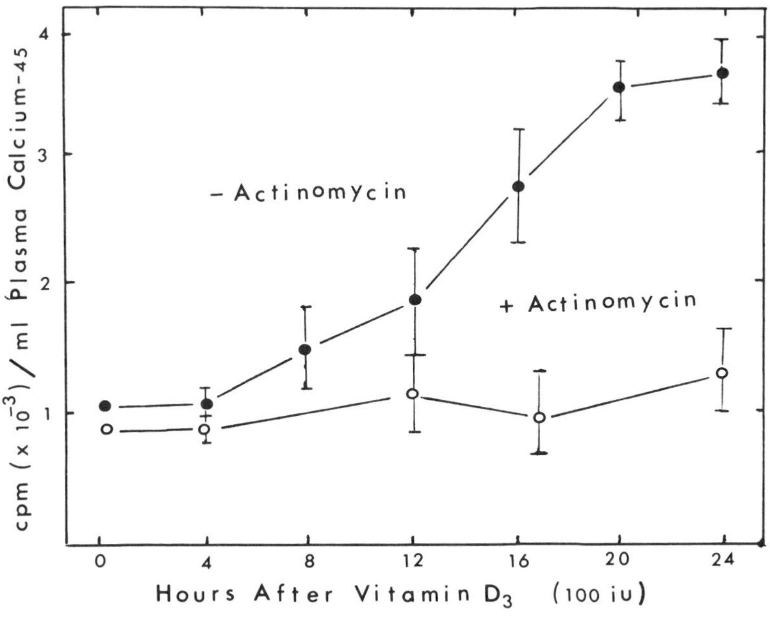

Figure 7-14. The intestinal calcium absorption response of vitamin D-deficient chicks to an oral dose of 100 IU (6.5 nmoles) of vitamin D_3 in the absence (closed circles) and presence (open circles) of actinomycin D. The rachitic chicks received 10 μg actinomycin D per 100 g body weight in 0.20 ml of 0.9% NaCl intraperitoneally 2 hr before the dose of vitamin D_3 (in Wesson oil) was administered orally. At various times after the vitamin D_3 treatment, 2.0 mg of ^{40}Ca + ^{45}Ca (1–3 × 10^6 counts/min) in 0.20 ml was fed orally. Blood from wing veins was drawn with syringes containing heparin 30 and 60 min later. Each point represents the mean of the values obtained on the plasmas of three to five chicks (± S.D.) (Norman, 1965).

These results indicate the effect of an oral dose of 6.5 nmoles (100 IU) of vitamin D_3 on the stimulation of intestinal absorption of calcium in rachitic chicks at various time intervals after administration of the vitamin. No significant enhancement of calcium absorption was observed before 12–16 hr, but, if actinomycin D (10 μg per 110 g of body weight of chick) was injected intraperitoneally 2 hr before the oral administration of the vitamin steroid, the characteristic response of the increased calcium absorption was totally abolished.

A number of laboratories have reported that puromycin (Kunin and Krane, 1965) or actinomycin D treatment *in vivo* inhibits the subsequent action of parathyroid hormone on parathyroidectomized rats, as measured by serum calcium elevation, without altering the hormone's stimulatory effect on renal phosphate excretion (Tashjian *et al.*, 1964; Milhaud *et al.*, 1964; Rasmussen *et al.*, 1964; Tashjian, 1965). However, with the reports that actinomycin D could inhibit the action of vitamin D on mediating intestinal calcium absorption in elevating serum calcium levels, the precise interpretation of the earlier work is subject to question and reinterpretation. The former workers may, in reality,

TABLE 7-11
Effects of Inhibitors of Transcription and Translation on Vitamin D Action

System studied	Inhibitor[a]	Reference
A. Vitamin D-stimulated intestinal	A	Zull *et al.* (1965, 1966)
calcium absorption	A	Norman (1965, 1966a,b)
Measured *in vivo*	A	Harrison and Harrison (1966)
	A	Moriuchi *et al.* (1970)
Measured *in vitro*	A	Bosmann and Chen (1966)
		Ziporin *et al.* (1973)
B. 1,25$(OH)_2D_3$-stimulated intestinal	A	Tanaka *et al.* (1971)
calcium absorption	A	Tsai *et al.* (1973)
Appearance of calcium-binding protein	A, α	Corradino (1973)
C. Metabolism of 25$(OH)D_3$ by kidney	A, C	Gray and DeLuca (1971)
	A, C	Tanaka and DeLuca (1971)
Studies *in vivo*	A	Tanaka *et al.* (1971)
	A	Tsai *et al.* (1973)
Kidney tubules	A, C, P	Shain (1972)
Kidney homogenates	A, C	Tanaka *et al.* (1972)
D. Parathyroid hormone-mediated effects		
Hypercalcemia	P	Kunin and Krane (1965)
	A	Milhaud *et al.* (1964)
	A	Eisenstein and Passavoy (1964)
	A	Tashjian *et al.* (1964)
	A	Tashjian (1965)

[a] Abbreviations for inhibitors: A, actinomycin D; α, α-amanitin; P, puromycin; C, cycloheximide.

have been observing an actinomycin D inhibition of vitamin D action. It should be recalled that Harrison and Harrison (1964) and Rasmussen *et al.* (1963) purported to have shown that vitamin D is required for the hypercalcemic action of parathyroid hormone. Thus, if actinomycin D can inhibit the action of vitamin D, then it could possibly inhibit the permissive effect of the vitamin for parathyroid hormone action.

As documented in Table 7-11, inhibitors of transcription and translation have been widely used to study various aspects of the mode of action of vitamin D and its metabolites. This work is divided principally into three phases: (a) assessment of the effects of actinomycin D on vitamin D- or 1,25(OH)$_2$D$_3$-stimulated intestinal calcium transport as measured either by translocation of the cation or by appearance of the calcium-binding protein (Corradino, 1973); (b) effects of actinomycin D on the hypercalcemic actions of parathyroid hormone; and (c) effects of actinomycin D and cycloheximide on the metabolism of 25(OH)D$_3$ to 1,25(OH)$_2$D$_3$ *in vivo* as well as *in vitro*. There were reports by Gray and DeLuca (1971) and Tanaka and DeLuca (1971) that administration of actinomycin D blocked the metabolic conversion of 25(OH)D$_3$ to the biologically active form. The inference from this suggestion was that actinomycin D blocked the biological response to vitamin D not via inhibition of gene transcription at the intestinal level but simply by blockage of the appearance of the biologically active hormone. However, later studies by this group (Tanaka *et al.*, 1972) and Norman's laboratory (Tsai *et al.*, 1973) (see Fig. 7-15) clearly indicate that actinomycin D

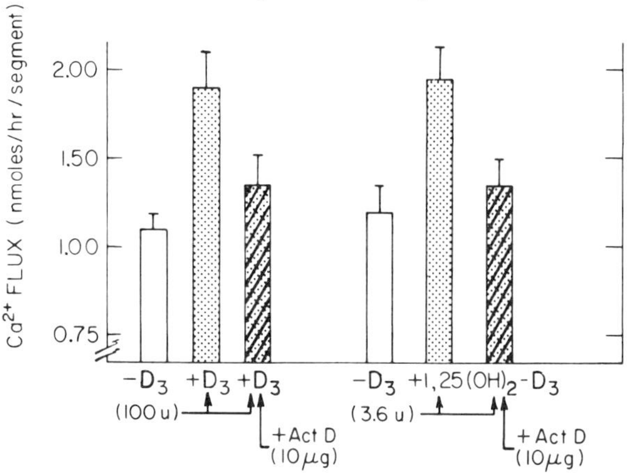

Figure 7-15. Effect of actinomycin D on vitamin D or 1,25(OH)$_2$D$_3$ stimulation of intestinal calcium transport. The indicated doses of vitamin D or 1,25(OH)$_2$D$_3$ were given intracardially either 24 or 10 hr, respectively, before measurement of intestinal calcium transport *in vitro*, according to the procedures of Adams and Norman (1970). Where indicated, a total of 19 μg actinomycin D (Act D) were administered intraperitoneally at intervals prior to the administration of calciferol steroid. (From Tsai *et al.*, 1973, and reproduced by permission of the publisher. Copyright by the American Association for the Advancement of Science.)

blocks the generation of the biological response after administration of $1,25(OH)_2D_3$. As reported in detail by Tsai *et al.* (1973), this is not due to an inhibition by actinomycin D of the localization of $1,25(OH)_2D_3$ in the intestine; normal quantities of the steroid were found in the nucleus and chromatin fractions of that tissue in the presence of the antibiotic.

The appropriate application of antibiotics that block transcriptional events has the consequence of totally inhibiting the normal biological response of both vitamin D and its most active metabolite, $1,25(OH)_2D_3$. Similar results have been obtained for many other steroid hormones; that is, inhibitors of gene transcription events block the generation of biological responses produced by all steroid hormones (Tomkins *et al.*, 1969). Thus, there is a strong analogy between the phenomenological observations concerning the action of vitamin D and its metabolites and that of other classic steroid hormones.

C. Molecular Basis of Steroid Hormone Mode of Action of $1,25(OH)_2D_3$

On the basis of the preceding studies of the chick intestinal mucosal chromatin and cytosol receptor system and by taking advantage of the brilliant advances made in the chemical synthesis of analogs of $1,25(OH)_2D_3$ (see Chapter 5), it has been possible to devise a competitive binding assay for $1,25(OH)_2D_3$ (Procsal *et al.*, 1975, 1976; Brumbaugh and Haussler, 1975a,b). As shown in Fig. 7-16, a linear standard curve is obtained when increasing amounts of nonradioactive $1,25(OH)_2D_3$ are added to the tritiated $1,25(OH)_2D_3$ employed in the assay. The decrease in radioactive steroid bound is due to a dilution of the pool of $1,25(OH)_2D_3$ such that at a ratio of nonradioactive to radioactive steroid equal to 1.0, 50% of the maximal radioactivity bound is measured. One important use of this assay has been to assess the structural requirements of the ligand steroid, $1,25(OH)_2D_3$, for its cytosol and chromatin receptor system. Table 7-12 gives the relative concentrations of steroid required to produce half-maximal competition (defined as relative competitive index, RCI) under these assay conditions.

Several interesting relationships can be deduced from the data given in Fig. 7-16 and Table 7-12. A basic requirement is that any interactive steroid for the intestinal receptor system must be a 9,10-seco compound. This conclusion is supported by the observation that $1,25(OH)_2$-cholesterol did not compete even at a concentration 10,000-fold greater than that of $1,25(OH)_2D_3$. The dramatically decreased ability of either $25(OH)D_3$ or $1\alpha(OH)D_3$ to compete with $1,25(OH)_2D_3$ emphasizes the great importance that must be attributed to the simultaneous presence of both the 25-OH and the 3β-OH group. The 100-fold greater ability of 3-deoxy-$1\alpha,25(OH)_2D_3$ (a steroid that does not contain a 3β-hydroxyl group) to compete than either $1\alpha(OH)D_3$ or $25(OH)D_3$ argues strongly that the requirement for the 3β-OH group is relatively less stringent than that for either the 25-OH or

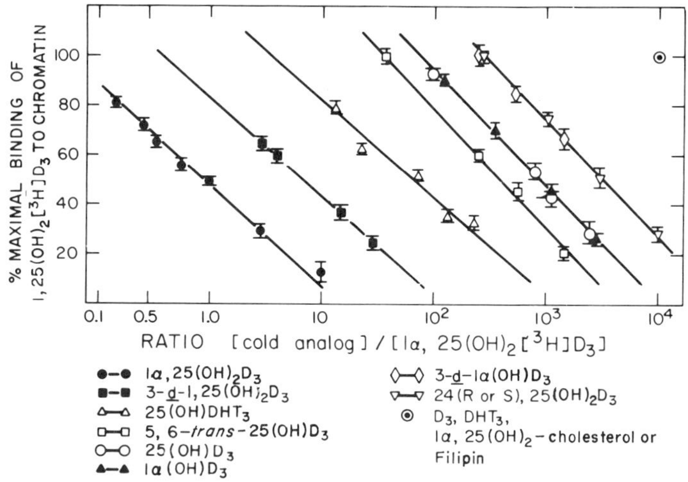

Figure 7-16. Competition of vitamin D_3 analogs with $1,25(OH)_2D_3$ for the chick intestinal receptor system. Increasing concentrations of nonradioactive analogs were incubated for 45 min at 25°C with a reconstituted cytosol-chromatin receptor system in the presence of 2.0×10^{-8} *M* tritiated $1,25(OH)_2D_3$. The percentage of maximal radioactivity tightly bound to the chromatin (radioactivity bound in the absence of analog equals 100%) is plotted as a function of the relative concentration of analog and tritiated $1,25(OH)_2D_3$. Each point represents the average of duplicate of triplicate determinations ± S.D. (From Procsal *et al.*, 1975.)

1α-OH functional group (Procsal *et al.*, 1975, 1976). The relatively greater importance of the 1α-hydroxyl group over that of the 3β-hydroxyl is further emphasized by the observation that vitamin D_3, which lacks both a 25-hydroxyl and 1α-hydroxyl group but does possess the 3β-hydroxyl, is an ineffective competitor, whereas 3-deoxy-$1\alpha(OH)D_3$, which lacks the 3β-hydroxyl and 25-hydroxyl groups but does not have a 1α-hydroxyl, will compete effectively.

The effect of a 180° rotation of the A ring about the 5,6 double bond to produce analogs of the 5,6-*trans* series has also been evaluated. A primary consequence of the 5,6-*trans* isomerization is a change in the orientation of the C-19 methylene group. The isomerization also moves the 3β-hydroxyl to a position sterically equivalent to the 1α-hydroxyl of steroids of the 5,6-*cis* series. This is apparently not sufficient to permit either 25(OH)-5,6-*trans*-D_3 or 5,6-*trans*-D_3 to compete as effectively as their 5,6-*cis* counterparts, 3-deoxy-$1\alpha,25(OH)_2D_3$ and 3-deoxy-$1\alpha(OH)D_3$, respectively. Presumably this difference is a consequence of the change in orientation of the C-19 methylene group. The structures of these analogs are presented in Figs. 5-8 to 5-11.

The critical importance of the length of the side chain is also evident. Johnson *et al.* (1975) reported that 24-nor-$25(OH)D_3$, an analog of $25(OH)D_3$ with one less carbon atom in the side chain, was devoid of biological activity in the chick.

TABLE 7-12
Relative Effectiveness of Structural Analogs of Vitamin D in the $1,25(OH)_2D_3$ Chick Intestinal Receptor Assay

Compound[a]	Series[b]	Relative competitive index[c]
$1,25(OH)_2D_3$	*Z*	100.0
$1,24(R)(OH)_2D_3$	*Z*	98.0
24-Nor-$1,25(OH)_2D_3$	*Z*	44.0
$1,24(R),25(OH)_3D_3$	*Z*	41.0
$1,24(S),25(OH)_3D_3$	*Z*	33.0
3-Deoxy-$1\alpha,25(OH)_2D_3$	*Z*	5.7
$1,24(S)(OH)_2D_3$	*Z*	4.9
$25(OH)DHT_3$	*E*	0.64
25(OH)-5,6-*trans*-D_3	*E*	0.51
$1\alpha(OH)D_3$	*Z*	0.17
$25(OH)D_3$	*Z*	0.17
24-Nor-25(OH)-5,6-*trans*-D_3	*E*	0.10
$19,25(OH)_2DHV_3$-II	*E*	0.09
$19,25(OH)_2DHV_3$-III	*E*	0.09
24-Homo-25(OH)-5,6-*trans*-D_3	*E*	0.06
$24(R),25(OH)_2D_3$	*E*	0.03
$24(S),25(OH)_2D_3$	*E*	0.03
3-Deoxy-$1\alpha(OH)D_3$	*E*	0.03
24-Nor-$25(OH)D_3$	*E*	0.01
24-Homo-$25(OH)D_3$	*E*	0.01
1α(OH)-Epi-D_3	*E*	0.008
DHV_3-IV		0
5,6-*trans*-D_3	*Z*	0
$19(OH)DHT_3$	*Z*	0
$19(OH)DHV_3$-IV	*Z*	0
D_3	*E*	0
3-Deoxy-3α-Me-$1\alpha(OH)D_3$	*E*	0
$19(OH)DHV_3$-II	*E*	0
$19(OH)DHV_3$-III	*E*	0
23,24-Dinor-$25(OH)D_3$	*E*	0
22,23,24-Trinor-$25(OH)D_3$	*E*	0
20,21,22,23,24-Pentanor-$25(OH)D_3$	*E*	0
$1,25(OH)_2$-Cholesterol	—	0

[a] The structures of these steroids are given in Figs. 5-8 to 5-11.

[b] Series: *Z* is 5,6-*cis* series; *E* is 5,6-*trans* series (A ring rotated 180°).

[c] Relative competitive index, or RCI, was calculated from the equation $[\alpha \text{ (competitor)}] \times 100/[1,25(OH)_2D_3]$, where α equals the slope of the line of a plot of 1/percent maximal binding versus nonradioactive analog/[tritiated $1,25(OH)_2D_3$] (see Fig. 7-16). Taken from Procsal *et al.* (1975), Wecksler and Norman (1978); and unpublished observations of P. Siebert and A. W. Norman; see also Eisman and DeLuca (1977).

Recently, Okamura, Norman, and co-workers (Wecksler *et al.*, 1978) completed the synthesis of 24-nor-$1,25(OH)_2D_3$. As reported in Table 7-12 this analog was only 44% as effective as $1,25(OH)_2D_3$ in competing for the intestinal cytosol-chromatin receptor system. Thus, even a slight shortening of the side chain in an analog that possesses the key 1α,25-hydroxyl and even 3β-hydroxyl groups has deleterious effects on optimal ligand binding. A similar result was observed in an analog with its side chain lengthened by one carbon, such as 24-homo-25(OH)-5,6-*trans*-D_3. This analog has a pseudo 1α-OH and a 25-OH and should be compared with 25(OH)-5,6-*trans*-D_3. Clearly, lengthening the side chain also perturbs the optimal structure for tight ligand binding (see Figs. 5-8 to 5-11 for structures).

Our laboratory (Okamura *et al.*, 1977) succeeded in introducing a hydroxyl into the 19 position of the 5,6-*cis* analogs to give 19(OH)DHV_3-II and 19(OH)DHV_3-III. It was reasoned that the presence of the hydroxyl group at the 19 position might, to some limited degree, satisfy the requirements for a 3β-OH group in the 5,6-*trans* series or 1α-OH in the 5,6-*cis* series. However, no significant competition was observed for any of these compounds in our competitive binding assay. Even when the 25-OH group is present in these analogs, as in $19,25(OH)_2DHV_3$-II and $19,25(OH)_2DHV_3$-III, there is no significant enhancement of ligand interaction.

The insertion of a hydroxyl group into the 24 position of $25(OH)D_3$ to give either thc *R* or *S* epimer of $24,25(OH)_2D_3$ significantly reduced the ability of the steroid to compete with $1,25(OH)_2D_3$. Under our assay conditions, it was not possible to discern any significant difference between the two epimers. It should be recalled that the naturally occurring epimer of $24,25(OH)_2D_3$ has its 24-hydroxyl in the *R* configuration (Tanaka *et al.*, 1975).

In general, there is a remarkable correlation between the relative binding of analogs in the chick intestinal receptors system and their relative ability to stimulate intestinal calcium absorption. The following conclusions can be drawn with respect to the structural features required for vitamin D-like biological activity in the intestinal cell:

1. All biologically active compounds must have a 1α-hydroxyl or its geometric equivalent and also a 25-hydroxyl group.
2. The presence of a hydroxyl group at a position geometrically equivalent to the 3β-hydroxyl of $1,25(OH)_2D_3$ is not an absolute requirement.
3. A 5,6-*cis* geometry of the A ring is preferred to 5,6-*trans* geometry. Also, comparison of the binding activities of $25(OH)DHT_3$ with those of 25(OH)-5,6-*trans*-D_3 suggest that, in a steroid of the 5,6-*trans* series, a C-19 methyl group is preferable over a C-19 methylene group.
4. Modifying the side chain by the insertion of a hydroxyl group as in $24,25(OH)_2D_3$ significantly decreases the binding activity of the steroid.

5. Shortening or lengthening the side chain by as little as one carbon as in 24-nor- (one carbon shorter) or 24-homo-5,6-*trans*-25(OH)D_3 (one carbon longer) dramatically reduces the relative competitive effectiveness of the steroid.

Another structural requirement for biological activity was proposed by Okamura, Norman, and co-workers (Okamura *et al.*, 1974; Norman *et al.*, 1976). This model takes into account the chairlike nature of the A ring and proposes that the chair conformer in which the 1α-OH is equatorial as opposed to the axial orientation is the preferred biologically active form. The evidence to support this model is largely derived by comparison of the significant biological activity of DHT_3 (equatorial/axial ratio of 9 : 1) with the inactivity of its structural congener DHV_3-IV (equatorial/axial ratio of 50 : 50) (Knobler *et al.*, 1972; Okamura *et al.*, 1974; Wing *et al.*, 1974, 1975). As shown in Fig. 7-17, the analog in which the pseudo 1α-OH is equatorially oriented (DHT_3) is much more biologically active than the analog with the axially oriented pseudo 1α-OH. Although this observation certainly does not prove our vitamin D steroid blueprint for optimal biological activity (Okamura *et al.*, 1974), it has provided a stimulating basis for much further experimentation.

A challenging problem to the organic chemist and biochemist studying the structure–function relationships between vitamin D secosteroids and the intestinal receptor system is to deduce the advantages and disadvantages of the rapid, chair–chair equilibration of the A ring, which is characteristic of vitamin D steroids. The conformational flexibility of the A ring of 1,25$(OH)_2D_3$ is unique among steroid hormones (see Norman and Henry, 1978).

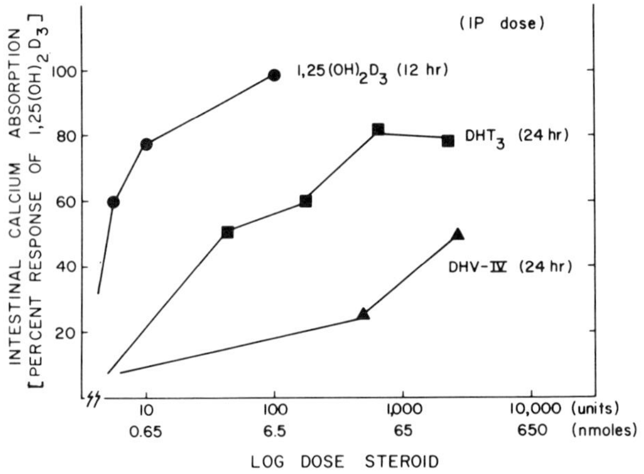

Figure 7-14. Biological response obtained for A-ring analog epimers DHT_3 and DHV_3-IV. Stimulation of intestinal calcium absorption and bone calcium mobilization was determined according to the methods described by Hibberd and Norman (1969). The equatorial/axial ratios of the pseudo 1α-OH for the epimers are given in the text.

There are several reports that the cytosol receptor for steroid hormones exists in solution as an allosteric protein capable of two basic conformations (Samuels and Tomkins, 1970; Marver *et al.*, 1974). It has been suggested that only one form of the receptor protein may be capable of undergoing "activation" prior to entry of the steroid–receptor complex into the nucleus. If this is actually the case for the $1,25(OH)_2D_3$ steroid hormone–receptor system, then, because of the complications introduced by the unique aspects of the dynamic interconversion of the A ring, it is difficult to analyze precisely the consequence of the interaction of these steroid species with the putative allosteric forms of the cytoplasmic receptor. Each of these two conformers may have a different basic intrinsic affinity for the presumed allosteric forms of the cytoplasmic receptor for $1,25(OH)_2D_3$.

Figure 7-18 illustrates two separate model systems that attempt to accommodate and integrate the consequences of the conformationally mobile A ring of $1,25(OH)_2D_3$ as it interacts with its intestinal receptor system. Figure 7-19A gives an example of how the two chair–chair conformers might interact with the two putative allosteric forms of the cytoplasmic receptor. It follows logically from what has been said above that the intracellular sequence of receptor events must contain an irreversible step. Otherwise the "inactive steroid conformer" could be reversibly transformed back to the "active steroid conformer," thus negating any differences due to these two structural orientations. Experimental support for this model requires further comparison of the biological activities of a number of structural stereoisomers that differ in the relative proportions of A-ring conformers as well as a rigorous biochemical characterization of the intestinal cytosol receptor protein.

It is usually presumed that the magnitude or intensity of maximal biological response would not be a function of steroid structure. Under simple conditions the natural steroid and related analogs would produce the same total magnitude response, perhaps with differing concentrations required for production of this maximal response, but in the light of the elegant studies of Samuels and Tomkins (1970) it is apparent that the situation may not be this simple. In experiments comparing the ability of analogs of glucocorticoids to induce the enzyme tyrosine aminotransferase in HTC cells grown in tissue culture, it was apparent that there were at least three different levels of maximal response obtainable, which could be related to the structural class of the analog being tested. These structural classes were referred to as (a) optimal inducers, or those that give an expected normal magnitude of response; (b) suboptimal inducers, or those that generate only a fraction of the maximal response produced by the optimal inducers; and (c) inactive analogs. Samuels and Tomkins (1970) proposed that the molecular basis for the different behavior of these classes of compounds depended on the fact that the cytoplasmic receptor for glucocorticoids in the HTC cells was present as two allosteric species. A further condition was imposed in that only

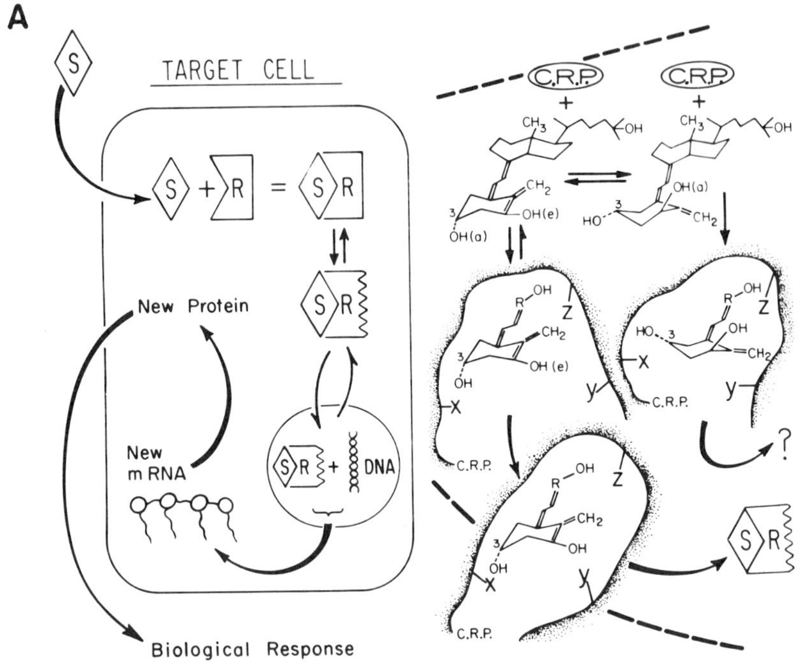

Figure 7-18. Model for the interaction of $1,25(OH)_2D_3$ with its intestinal cytosol–chromatin receptor system. Panel (A) indicates how the two chair–chair conformers might interact with two allosteric forms of the receptor, while (B) emphasizes the key role of the 25-OH functional group in facilitating preliminary capture of the secosteroid; (C) suggests that in the absence of the 25-OH group "capture" of the A ring is much more difficult.

one of the two allosteric species could be "activated" and transported to the nucleus for generation of the biological response. Thus, the magnitude of the maximal response produced by various steroids was dependent on the relative affinity of these two forms of the cytoplasmic receptor for the various analogs. Clearly, such a relationship could also exist between the intestinal cytosol receptor and vitamin D metabolites and their analogs. In view of the rapid equilibration of the two chair–chair conformers of the secosteroids in solution and since the equilibrium for this interconversion is a function of the nature of functional groups on the A ring, it is possible to envision a family of analogs that have differing equatorial/axial population ratios, which in turn might vary in their interaction with the intestinal cytosol receptor. Thus, it may be possible to chemically synthesize analogs of $1,25(OH)_2D_3$ that are optimal inducers, suboptimal inducers, or inactive in the intestinal receptor system. Since the equatorial/axial (e/a) ratio for the 1α-OH of $1,25(OH)_2D_3$ is only 1.0, it is even conceivable that one could synthesize an analog with a greater maximal biological response

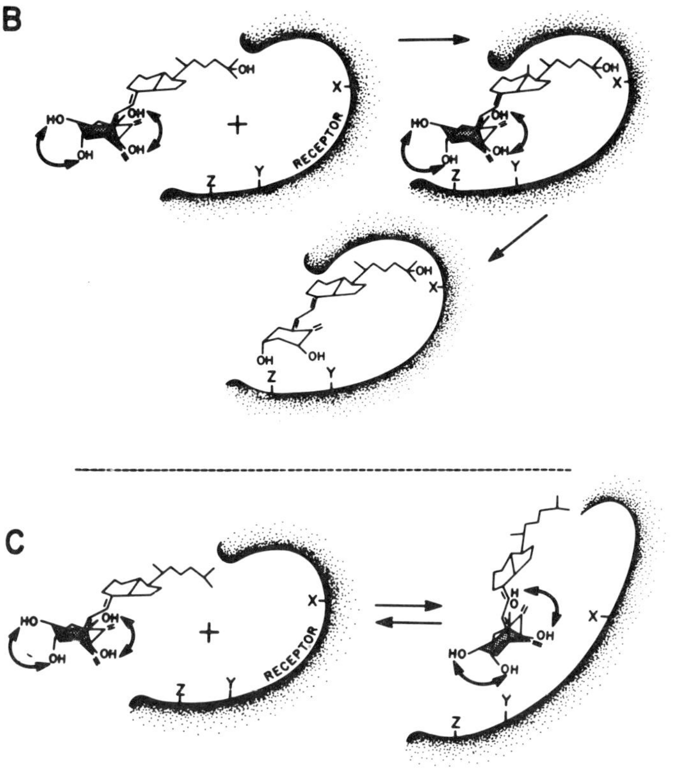

than 1,25(OH)$_2$D$_3$. If this were possible, we would be presented with the unusual circumstance that the naturally occurring form of the steroid hormone is only a suboptimal inducer.

Figure 7-18B shows an alternative model to explain certain aspects of the structural requirements of 1,25(OH)$_2$D$_3$ as they pertain to its unique conformationally mobile A ring. This model emphasizes the key contribution of the 25-hydroxyl on a side chain of precisely the optimal length. One conclusion obtained from data given in Table 7-12 is that 1,25(OH)$_2$D$_3$, as it binds to its cytosolic receptor, forms regions of "interaction" with the receptor protein on both the A ring and the side chain. Thus, both ends of the molecule are involved intimately with the cytosol receptor system. An important point that cannot be resolved at present is whether the A ring continues to be conformationally mobile during association with the receptor protein. By comparing the appropriate data in Table 7-12 it can be predicted that most likely the A ring is ultimately "frozen out" when the final version of the steroid–receptor complex is formed. This can be presumed to be the case, since the competition for 1α(OH)D$_3$ with

1α(OH)-epi-D_3 (in which orientation of the 3-OH group in the A ring is α versus β) is shown to affect the ligand binding. It would seem obvious that the difference in these steroid analogs is as great as that between the two extremes in the equatorial–axial orientation of the 1α-hydroxyl of 1,25$(OH)_2D_3$. Thus, a major problem for the intestinal cytosol receptor system may be to properly "capture" the dynamically active A ring portion of the 1,25$(OH)_2D_3$ molecule. It is in this regard that the important contribution of the 25-OH functional group may be apparent. Figure 7-18B shows that the 25-OH functional group may function as a preliminary recognition site, which forms the first basis of interaction between the 1,25$(OH)_2D_3$ molecule and the receptor system. After this interaction is effectively established, the protein receptor can ultimately capture and "freeze out" the oscillating A-ring portion of the ligand. This result would be consistent with the extreme inactivity of analogs that lack the 25-OH functional group even though they may have optimal functionalities in the A ring, e.g., $1\alpha(OH)D_3$. In the absence of the 25-OH functional group there can be no preliminary "capture process" of the side chain, and accordingly much higher concentrations of the analog are required to permit the random "freezing-out process" of the A ring. Only further experimentation will validate either of the interesting models diagrammed in Fig. 7-18 (see also Norman and Henry, 1978).

D. Effects of Vitamin D and 1,25$(OH)_2D_3$ on RNA Metabolism

The logical extension of the results described above concerning the proposed steroid hormone mechanism of action of 1,25$(OH)_2D_3$, particularly its nuclear and chromatin localization, is that a significant contribution to the time lag in action of 1,25$(OH)_2D_3$ may be the "activation" of information in the genome that is necessary for expression of the biological response. Table 7-13 summarizes the effects of vitamin D as well as its metabolite 1,25$(OH)_2D_3$ on the biosynthesis of intestinal RNA. Both steroids are capable of stimulating the incorporation of nucleotide precursors into messenger RNA fractions of the intestinal mucosa (typical data are shown in Fig. 7-19). To date, no assessment has been made as to whether this represents an increased biosynthesis of mRNA, tRNA, or rRNA. Clearly, the presumption is that it must in part represent increased synthesis of RNA for calcium-binding protein and other proteins possibly related to the biological response.

Emtage *et al.* (1973a,b) and Spencer *et al.* (1976a,b) obtained definitive evidence for an increased level of "messenger" RNA for calcium-binding protein (CaBP) by evaluating the ability of polysomes isolated from rachitic chicks and chicks administered either vitamin D_3 or 1,25$(OH)_2D_3$ to synthesize CaBP in

TABLE 7-13
Effects of Vitamin D and Metabolites on Intestinal RNA Metabolism

RNA system studied	Reference
A. Intestine	
Stimulating effects mediated by vitamin D occurring *in vivo*	Norman (1966b), Zull *et al.* (1966), Stohs *et al.* (1967)
Stimulating effects mediated by $1,25(OH)_2D_3$	
Measured *in vivo*	Tsai and Norman (1973a)
Measured *in vitro*	
Elevation of RNA polymerase II activity	Zerwekh *et al.* (1976)
Chromatin template activity	Zerwekh *et al.* (1974)
"Messenger" RNA for CaBP	Emtage *et al.* (1973a,b)
B. Kidney	
$1,25(OH)_2D_3$-stimulated [^{3}H]uridine incorporation into RNA	Chen and DeLuca (1973b)
Dependence of $25(OH)D_3$ 1-hydroxylase on RNA synthesis	Tanaka *et al.* (1972)

an *in vitro* cell-free system. Chick intestinal polysomes were isolated from a postmitochondrial supernatant by sedimentation through a discontinuous sucrose gradient and then incubated in an incubation medium capable of supporting *de novo* protein synthesis. The presence of CaBP was assessed by measuring the radioactivity present in an immunoprecipitate prepared using antisera monospecific for CaBP. Emtage and co-workers (1974; Spencer *et al.*, 1976a) isolated RNA fractions from intestinal polysomes of vitamin D-treated chicks and measured their ability to direct the *in vitro* synthesis in a rabbit reticulocyte lysate of immunoprecipitable CaBP protein. Collectively, these results strongly support the concept that the action of $1,25(OH)_2D_3$ is analogous to that of other steroid hormones.

Other supportive data totally consistent with this view were obtained by Zerwekh *et al.* (1974, 1976), who measured the ability of $1,25(OH)_2D_3$ to elevate the activity of RNA polymerase II as well as to increase chromatin "template activity." Both of these assays are exceedingly difficult to carry out in a reliable fashion, and the results of these workers strongly attest to the actions of $1,25(OH)_2D_3$ in increasing enzyme activity in the nuclear chromosomal region in a manner consistent with stimulation of "genetic information."

What is not clear at this point is the precise molecular sequence of events concerning the interaction of the $1,25(OH)_2D_3$ steroid–protein receptor complex with the genome. However, our understanding in this regard is not any more deficient than our understanding of the action of other steroid hormones in their respective target tissue nuclear regions on a molecular level.

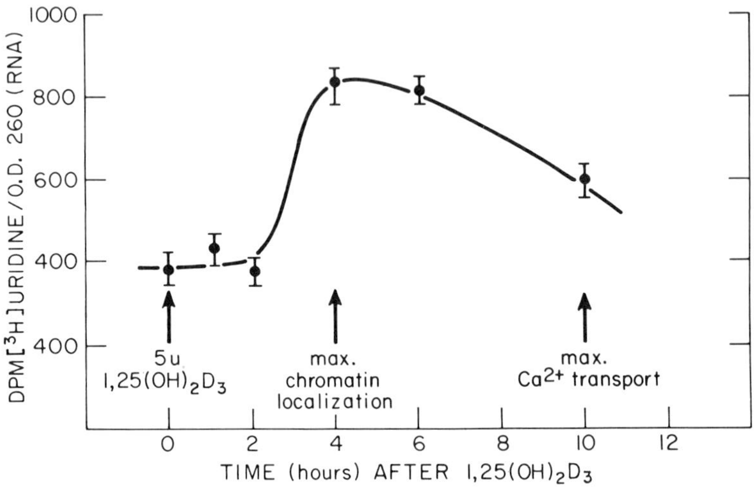

Figure 7-19. Effect of 1,25(OH)$_2$D$_3$ on *in vivo* incorporation of [^{3}H]uridine into intestinal mucosal RNA. Groups of rachitic chicks were given doses of 325 pmoles of 1,25(OH)$_2$D$_3$ intracardially. At various times after administration of the steroid, 5 μCi of [^{3}H]uridine were administered intracardially, and 20 min later the chicks were killed, the total RNA of the intestinal mucosa was isolated, and its radioactivity content was determined. (From Tsai and Norman, 1973.)

E. Effects of Vitamin D and 1,25(OH)$_2$D$_3$ on Protein Synthesis

Figure 7-20 shows the effect of administering small quantities of 1,25(OH)$_2$D$_3$ *in vivo* on the incorporation of [^{3}H]leucine into protein present in the intestinal mucosa. The protein fraction with maximal incorporation was partially purified using the protocol for preparation of CaBP as described by Wasserman and Taylor (1968). It is not yet known whether this apparent increase in synthesis of protein is accounted for exclusively by new CaBP or whether there are in addition other proteins synthesized *de novo*. Wasserman and Taylor (1968) were the first to describe the production of a specific protein in response to the administration of vitamin D; this was identified as a calcium-bonding protein. (See Chapter 10.)

IV. SUMMARY

This chapter summarizes the current evidence supporting the steroid hormone concept as a basis for a description of the action of 1,25(OH)$_2$D$_3$ as the biologically active form of vitamin D. The key element of data supporting this view is the nuclear localization of 1,25(OH)$_2$D$_3$ in the target tissue, particularly the intestinal mucosal epithelial cells. These cells are presumed to be the site of synthesis of intestinal CaBP. In the absence of $1,25(OH)_2D_3$ this protein is not biosynthesized and, as the population of intestinal epithelial cells turns over and is sloughed off, the CaBP present in the intestine decays away. The only positive signal that is known to be capable of initiating the biosynthesis of this protein is the presence of the steroid hormone $1,25(OH)_2D_3$. It is not known with certainty whether CaBP is the only protein or one of a family of proteins that are concerned with the initiation of maintenance of vitamin D-mediated intestinal calcium absorption. From Fig. 10-5, it is apparent that there is a reasonably good correlation of chronology between the onset of stimulation of the appearance of CaBP and the onset of stimulation of intestinal calcium absorption. In this regard, Spencer *et al.* (1976b) presented evidence consistent with the view that there is not a requirement for CaBP in all vitamin D-mediated calcium transport. They reported kinetic evidence that there was a measurable stimulation of intestinal calcium absorption after administration of $1,25(OH)_2D_3$ prior to the definitive onset of the appearance of messenger RNA for CaBP as well as the *de novo* synthesis of CaBP.

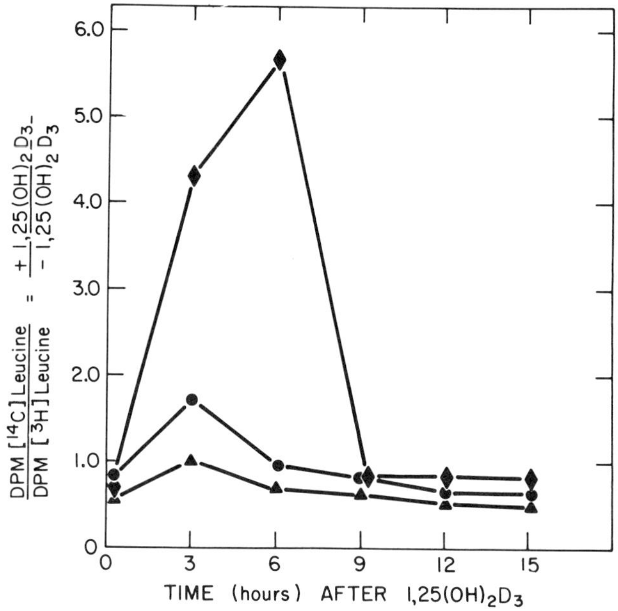

Figure 7-20. Effect of $1,25(OH)_2D_3$ on *in vivo* incorporation of radioactive leucine into proteins of the intestine. Groups of rachitic chicks were given doses of 325 pmoles of $1,25(OH)_2D_3$ intracardially. At various times after administration of the steroid, 15 μCi of ^{3}H- or ^{14}C-labeled leucine were given intracardially to either steroid-treated or nontreated birds. One hour later the birds were killed, and the incorporation of isotope into subcellular fractions of the intestine was assessed. Key: ◆—◆, calcium-binding protein fraction; ●—●, brush borders; ▲—▲, homogenate. (From Norman, 1975.)

Table 7-14 compares the amount of $1,25(OH)_2D_3$ localized in the nucleus of its target tissues with that reported for other steroid hormone systems. In the case of $1,25(OH)_2D_3$ and its target receptor organ, the intestinal mucosa, it can be calculated that there are approximately 2300 molecules of metabolite per intestinal mucosa cell, which is comparable to a metabolite concentration of 1.5 to 4.5×10^{-9} *M* in the entire intestinal mucosa. This concentration of $1,25(OH)_2D_3$ in the intestine is quite comparable to that previously reported for other steroid hormones in their target tissues (Buller and O'Malley, 1976).

Although some attention has been directed toward methods of postranscriptional control as a basis for steroid hormone-induced protein synthesis (Tomkins *et al.*, 1969), it now seems abundantly clear on the basis of data obtained from all steroid hormones that most exert their primary effects at the level of transcription. Administration of aldosterone, glucocorticoid, estrogen, progesterone, dihydrotestosterone, $1,25(OH)_2D_3$, or thyroid hormones under conditions that encourage localization of the hormones *in vivo* in their target tissues results in measurable increases in RNA synthesis. At present, the detailed biochemical steps involved in this stimulation of RNA synthesis are not clearly understood. There are a number of possible mechanisms: (a) New initiation sites for RNA polymerase may be created on the genome as a consequence of the presence of the steroid hormone–receptor complex; (b) the rate of RNA chain elongation may be greatly enhanced as a consequence of the presence of the steroid hormone–receptor complex; or (c) the fundamental enzyme activity of the RNA polymerase may be directly modified by physical interaction with the steroid hormone–receptor complex. It is the goal of all scientists concerned with the mechanism of steroid hormone action to devise definitive experiments that will permit critical evaluation of each of the above-listed possibilities. The ultimate proof of any mechanism by which steroids may modify RNA synthesis will

TABLE 7-14
Amounts of Steroids Accumulated by Target Organs

Steroid hormone	Target organ	Estimated molecules per cell	Reference
$1,25(OH)_2D_3$	Rachitic chick intestine chromatin	2,300	Procsal *et al.* (1975)
Aldosterone	Rat kidney chromatin	600	Swaneck *et al.* (1970)
Estrogens	Rat uterus (immature) nuclei	7,700	Higgins *et al.* (1973)
Progesterone	Chick oviduct nuclei	9,000	Buller *et al.* (1975)
	Chick oviduct chromatin	3,400	Buller and O'Malley (1976)
Glucocorticoids	Rat liver nuclei	10,000	Kalimi *et al.* (1973)
	HTC cell nuclei	15,500	Higgins *et al.* (1973)
Androgens	Rat ventral prostate	2,000	Fang and Liao (1971)
	Rat ventral prostate nuclei	6,000	Mainwaring and Peterken (1971)

require the use of protein receptors that have been purified to homogeneity. This will permit a step-by-step study of the details of how all hormones, including 1,25$(OH)_2D_3$, exert their biological actions.

REFERENCES

Adams, T. H., and Norman, A. W. (1970). *J. Biol. Chem.* **245,** 4421.

Bachelet, M., Ulmann, A., Cloix, J. F., and Funk-Brentano, J. L. (1977). *J. Steroid Biochem.* **8,** 1047.

Blumberg, A., Schönholzer, G., and Aebi, H. (1959). *Helv. Physiol. Pharmacol. Acta* **17,** 16.

Blumberg, A., Aebi, H., Hurni, H., and Schönholzer, G. (1960). *Helv. Physiol. Pharmacol. Acta* **18,** 56.

Bosmann, H. B., and Chen, P. S., Jr. (1966). *J. Nutr.* **90,** 405.

Brumbaugh, P. F., and Haussler, M. R. (1973). *Biochem. Biophys. Res. Commun.* **51,** 74.

Brumbaugh, P. F., and Haussler, M. R. (1974). *J. Biol. Chem.* **249,** 1258.

Brumbaugh, P. F., and Haussler, M. R. (1975a). *J. Biol. Chem.* **250,** 1588.

Brumbaugh, P. F., and Haussler, M. R. (1975b). *Life Sci.* **16,** 353.

Brumbaugh, P. F., Haussler, M. R., and Hughes, M. R. (1975). *Proc. Natl. Acad. Sci. U.S.A.* **72,** 4871.

Buller, R. E., and O'Malley, B. W. (1976). *Biochem. Pharmacol.* **25,** 1.

Buller, R. E., Schrader, W. T., and O'Malley, B. W. (1975). *J. Biol. Chem.* **250,** 809.

Canterbury, J. M., Lerman, S., Claflin, A. J., Henry, H. L., Norman, A. W., and Reiss, E. (1978). *J. Clin. Invest.* **59,** 1375.

Chen, T. C., and DeLuca, H. F. (1973a). *J. Biol. Chem.* **248,** 4890.

Chen, T. C., and DeLuca, H. F. (1973b). *Arch. Biochem. Biophys.* **156,** 321.

Chen, T. C., Weber, J. C., and DeLuca, H. F. (1970). *J. Biol. Chem.* **245,** 3776.

Chertow, B. S., Baylink, D. J., Wergedal, J. E., Su, M. H. H., and Norman, A. W. (1975). *J. Clin. Invest.* **56,** 668.

Corradino, R. A. (1973). *Nature (London)* **243,** 41.

Cousins, R. J., DeLuca, H. F., and Gray, R. W. (1970a). *Biochemistry* **9,** 3649.

Cousins, R. J., DeLuca, H. F., Suda, T., Chen, T., and Tanaka, Y. (1970b). *Biochemistry* **9,** 1453.

DeKloet, R., Wallach, G., and McEwen, B. S. (1975). *Endocrinology* **96,** 598.

DeLuca, H. F. (1969). *Am. J. Clin. Nutr.* **22,** 412.

Eisenstein, R., and Passavoy, M. (1964). *Proc. Soc. Exp. Biol. Med.* **117,** 77.

Eisman, J., and DeLuca, H. F. (1977). *Steroids* **30,** 246.

Emtage, J. S., Lawson, D. E. M., and Kodicek, E. (1973a). *Nature (London)* **246,** 100.

Emtage, J. S., Lawson, D. E. M., and Kodicek, E. (1973b). *Biochem. J.* **140,** 239.

Emtage, J. S., Lawson, D. E. M., and Kodicek, E. (1974). *Biochem. J.* **144,** 339.

Fang, S., and Liao, S. (1971). *J. Biol. Chem.* **246,** 16.

Friedlander, E. J., Henry, H. L., and Norman, A. W. (1977). *J. Biol. Chem.* **252,** 8677.

Frolik, C. A., and DeLuca, H. F. (1975). *Steroids* **26,** 683.

Gray, R. W., and DeLuca, H. F. (1971). *Arch. Biochem. Biophys.* **145,** 276.

Greaves, J. D., and Schmidt, C. L. A. (1933). *J. Biol. Chem.* **102,** 101.

Harrison, H. E., and Harrison, H. C. (1964). *Metab., Clin. Exp.* **13,** 952.

Harrison, H. E., and Harrison, H. C. (1966). *Proc. Soc. Exp. Biol. Med.* **121,** 312.

Haussler, M. R., and Norman, A. W. (1967). *Arch. Biochem. Biophys.* **118,** 145.

Haussler, M. R., and Norman, A. W. (1969). *Proc. Natl. Acad. Sci. U.S.A.* **62,** 155.

Haussler, M. R., Myrtle, J. F., and Norman, A. W. (1968). *J. Biol. Chem.* **243,** 4055.

Haussler, M. R., Thomson, W. W., and Norman, A. W. (1969). *Exp. Cell Res.* **58,** 234.
Haussler, M. R., Boyce, D. W., Littledike, E. T., and Rasmussen, H. (1971). *Proc. Natl. Acad. Sci. U.S.A.* **69,** 177.
Havinga, E., and Botts, J. P. L. (1954). *Recl. Trav. Chim. Pays-Bas Belg.* **73,** 393.
Henry, H., and Norman, A. W. (1975). *Biochem. Biophys. Res. Commun.* **62,** 781.
Henry, H., Midgett, R. J., and Norman, A. W. (1974). *J. Biol. Chem.* **249,** 7584.
Henry, H. L., Taylor, A. N., and Norman, A. W. (1977). *J. Nutr.* **107,** 1918.
Heymann, W. (1936). *J. Pediatr.* **8,** 480.
Heymann, W. (1937a). *J. Biol. Chem.* **118,** 371.
Heymann, W. (1937b). *J. Biol. Chem.* **122,** 249.
Heymann, W. (1937c). *J. Biol. Chem.* **122,** 257.
Hibberd, K. A., and Norman, A. W. (1969). *Biochem. Pharmacol.* **18,** 2347.
Higgins, S. J., Rousseau, G. G., Baxter, J. D., and Tomkins, G. M. (1973). *J. Biol. Chem.* **248,** 5873.
Holick, M. F., Schnoes, H. K., DeLuca, H. F., Suda, T., and Cousins, R. J. (1971). *Biochemistry* **10,** 2799.
Hughes, M. R., and Haussler, M. R. (1978). *J. Biol. Chem.* **253,** 1065.
Imrie, M. H., Neville, P. F., Snellgrove, A. W., and DeLuca, H. F. (1967). *Arch. Biochem. Biophys.* **120,** 525.
Irving, J. T. (1944). *J. Physiol. (London)* **103,** 9.
Johnson, R. L., Okamura, W. H., and Norman, A. W. (1975). *Biochem. Biophys. Res. Commun.* **67,** 797.
Kalimi, M., Beato, M., and Feigelson, P. (1973). *Biochemistry* **12,** 3365.
Knobler, C., Romers, C., Braum, P. B., and Hornstra, J. (1972). *Acta Crystallog., Sect. B* **28,** 2097.
Kodicek, E. (1955). *Biochem. J.* **60,** XXV.
Kodicek, E. (1956). *Bone Struct. Metab., Ciba Found. Symp., 1955* p. 161.
Kodicek, E., and Thompson, G. A. (1965). *Struct. Funct. Connect. Skeletal Tissue, Proc. Adv. Study Inst., 1964* p. 369.
Kodicek, E., Lawson, D. E. M., and Wilson, P. W. (1970). *Nature (London)* **228,** 763.
Kream, B. E., Jose, M. F. L., and DeLuca, H. F. (1977a). *Arch. Biochem. Biophys.* **179,** 462.
Kream, B. E., Yamada, S., Schnoes, H. K., and DeLuca, H. F. (1977b). *J. Biol. Chem.* **252,** 4501.
Kream, B. E., Jose, M., Yamada, S., and DeLuca, H. F. (1977c). *Science* **197,** 1086.
Kunin, A. S., and Krane, S. M. (1965). *Endocrinology* **76,** 343.
Lawson, D. E. M., and Wilson, P. W. (1974). *Biochem. J.* **144,** 573.
Lawson, D. E. M., Wilson, P. W., Barker, D. C., and Kodicek, E. (1969a). *Biochem. J.* **115,** 263.
Lawson, D. E. M., Wilson, P. W., and Kodicek, E. (1969b). *Biochem. J.* **115,** 269.
Lawson, D. E. M., Wilson, P. W., and Kodicek, E. (1969c). *Nature (London)* **222,** 171.
Lawson, D. E. M., Fraser, D. M., Kodicek, E., Morris, H. R., and Williams, D. H. (1971a). *Nature (London)* **230,** 228.
Lawson, D. E. M., Bell, P. A., Pelc, B., Wilson, P. W., and Kodicek, E. (1971b). *Biochem. J.* **121,** 673.
Lumb, G., and Stanbury, S. W. (1974). *Am. J. Med.* **56,** 833.
Lund, J., DeLuca, H. F., and Horsting, M. (1967). *Arch. Biochem. Biophys.* **120,** 513.
McEwen, B. S., DeKloet, R., and Wallach, J. (1976). *Brain Res.* **105,** 129.
McEwen, B. S., Weiss, J., and Schwartz, L. (1970). *Brain Res.* **17,** 471.
Mainwaring, W. I. P., and Peterken, B. M. (1971). *Biochem. J.* **125,** 285.
Marushige, K., and Bonner, J. (1966). *J. Mol. Biol.* **15,** 160.
Marver, D., Stewart, J., Funder, J. W., Feldman, D., and Edelman, I. S. (1974). *Proc. Natl. Acad. Sci. U.S.A.* **71,** 1431.

Mawer, E. B., Backhouse, J., Holman, C. A., Lumb, G. A., and Stanbury, S. W. (1972). *Clin. Sci.* **43,** 413.
Milhaud, G., Moukhtar, M. S., Cherian, A. G., and Perault, A. M. (1964). *C. R. Hebd. Seances Acad. Sci.* **259,** 896.
Mirsky, A., and Pollister, A. W. (1964). *J. Gen. Physiol.* **30,** 117.
Morgan, A. F., and Shimotori, N. (1943). *J. Biol. Chem.* **147,** 189.
Moriuchi, S., Watanabe, T., and Hosoya, N. (1970). *J. Vitaminol.* **16,** 58.
Myrtle, J. F., and Norman, A. W. (1971). *Science* **171,** 78.
Myrtle, J. F., Haussler, M. R., and Norman, A. W. (1970). *J. Biol. Chem.* **245,** 1190.
Nair, P. P., and Bucana, C. (1966). *Biochim. Biophys. Acta* **124,** 254.
Neville, P. F., and DeLuca, H. F. (1966). *Biochemistry* **5,** 2201.
Norman, A. W. (1965). *Science* **149,** 184.
Norman, A. W. (1966a). *Am. J. Physiol.* **211,** 829.
Norman, A. W. (1966b). *Biochem. Biophys. Res. Commun.* **23,** 335.
Norman, A. W. (1967). *Clin. Orthop. Relat. Res.* **52,** 249.
Norman, A. W. (1968). *Biol. Rev. Cambridge Philos. Soc.* **43,** 97.
Norman, A. W. (1974). *Am. J. Med.* **57,** 21.
Norman, A. W. (1975). *Vitam. Horm. (N.Y.)* **32,** 325.
Norman, A. W., and DeLuca, H. F. (1963). *Biochemistry* **2,** 1160.
Norman, A. W., and DeLuca, H. F. (1964). *Arch. Biochem. Biophys.* **107,** 69.
Norman, A. W., and Henry, H. L. (1974). *Recent Prog. Horm. Res.* **30,** 431.
Norman, A. W., and Henry, H. L. (1979). *Trends Biochem. Res.* **4,** 14.
Norman, A. W., Lund, J., and DeLuca, H. F. (1964). *Arch. Biochem. Biophys.* **108,** 12.
Norman, A. W., Myrtle, J. F., Midgett, R. J., Nowicki, H. G., Williams, V., and Popjak, G. (1971). *Science* **173,** 51.
Norman, A. W., Johnson, R. L., Osborn, T. W., Procsal, D. A., Carey, S. C., Hammond, M. L., Mitra, M. N., Pirio, M. R., Rego, A., Wing, R. M., and Okamura, W. N. (1976). *Clin. Endocrinol. N.Y.* **5,** 1215.
Notides, A. (1970). *Endocrinology* **87,** 987.
Okamura, W. H., Norman, A. W. and Wing, R. M. (1974). *Proc. Natl. Acad. Sci. U.S.A.* **71,** 4194.
Okamura, W. H., Hammond, M. L., Rego, A., Norman, A. W., and Wing, R. M. (1977). *J. Organic Chem.* **42,** 2284.
Oldham, S., Arnaud, C., and Jowsey, J. (1973). *Endocrinol., Proc. Int. Symp., 4th, 1973* p. 261.
Ponchon, G., and DeLuca, H. F. (1969). *J. Clin. Invest.* **48,** 1273.
Procsal, D. A., Okamura, W. H., and Norman, A. W. (1975). *J. Biol. Chem.* **250,** 8382.
Procsal, D. A., Okamura, W. H., and Norman, A. W. (1976). *J. Clin. Nutr.* **29,** 1271.
Rasmussen, H., DeLuca, H. F., Arnaud, C., Hawker, C., and von Stedingk, M. (1963). *J. Clin. Invest.* **42,** 1040.
Rasmussen, H., Arnaud, C., and Hawker, C. (1964). *Science* **144,** 1019.
Redel, J., Bazely, N., Tanaka, Y., and DeLuca, H. F. (1978). *FEBS Lettr.* **94,** 228.
Rosenstreich, S. J., Rich, C., and Volwiller, W. (1971). *J. Clin. Invest.* **50,** 679.
Samuels, H. H., and Tomkins, G. M. (1970). *J. Mol. Biol.* **52,** 57.
Schaltegger, H. (1960). *Helv. Chim. Acta* **43,** 1148.
Shain, S. A. (1972). *J. Biol. Chem.* **247,** 4404.
Spencer, R. M., Charman, P., Emtage, J., and Lawson, D. E. M. (1976a). *Eur. J. Biochem.* **71,** 399.
Spencer, R. M., Charman, P., Wilson, E., and Lawson, D. E. M. (1976b). *Nature (London)* **263,** 161.
Spielvogel, A. M., Farley, R. D., and Norman, A. W. (1972). *Exp. Cell Res.* **74,** 359.
Stohs, S. J., Zull, J. E., and DeLuca, H. F. (1967). *Biochemistry* **6,** 3338.

Swaneck, G. E., Chu, L. L. H., and Edelman, I. S. (1970). *J. Biol. Chem.* **245,** 5382.
Tanaka, Y., and DeLuca, H. F. (1971). *Proc. Natl. Acad. Sci. U.S.A.* **68,** 605.
Tanaka, Y., DeLuca, H. F., Omdahl, J., and Holick, M. F. (1971). *Proc. Natl. Acad. Sci. U.S.A.* **68,** 1286.
Tanaka, Y., Chen, T. C., and DeLuca, H. F. (1972). *Arch. Biochem. Biophys.* **152,** 291.
Tanaka, Y., DeLuca, H. F., Ikekawa, N., Morisaki, M., and Koizumi, N. (1975). *Arch. Biochem. Biophys.* **170,** 620.
Tashjian, A. H., Ontjes, D. A., and Goodfriend, T. L. (1964). *Biochem. Biophys. Res. Commun.* **16,** 209.
Tashjian, A. H., Jr. (1965). *Endocrinology* **77,** 375.
Tomkins, G. M., Gelehrter, T. M., Granner, D., Martin, D., Samuels, H. H., and Thompson, E. V. (1969). *Science* **166,** 1474.
Tsai, H. C., and Norman, A. W. (1973a). *Biochem. Biophys. Res. Commun.* **54,** 622.
Tsai, H. C., and Norman, A. W. (1973b). *J. Biol. Chem.* **248,** 5967.
Tsai, H. C., Wong, R. G., and Norman, A. W. (1972). *J. Biol. Chem.* **247,** 5511.
Tsai, H. C., Midgett, R. J., and Norman, A. W. (1973). *Arch. Biochem. Biophys.* **157,** 339.
Vollmer, H. (1939). *Am. J. Dis. Child.* **57,** 343.
Warkany, J., Guest, G. M., and Graybill, F. J. (1945). *J. Lab. Clin. Med.* **27,** 557.
Wasserman, R. H., and Taylor, A. N. (1968). *J. Biol. Chem.* **243,** 3987.
Weber, J. C., Pons, V., and Kodicek, E. (1971). *Biochem. J.* **125,** 147.
Wecksler, W. R. (1978). Ph.D. Dissertation, University of California, Riverside.
Wecksler, W. R., and Norman, A. W. (1978). *J. Miner. Electrolyte Metab.* **1,** 99.
Wecksler, W. R., and Norman, A. W. (1979). "Pediatric Diseases Related to Calcium." North-Holland Publ. Amsterdam.
Wecksler, W. R., Henry, H. L., and Norman, A. W. (1977). *Arch. Biochem. Biophys.* **183,** 168.
Wecksler, W. R., Okamura, W. H., and Norman, A. W. (1978). *J. Steroid Biochem.* **9,** 929.
Wecksler, W. R., Mason, R. S., and Norman, A. W. (1979). *J. Clin. Endocrin. Metab.* **48,** 715.
Wezeman, F. H. (1976). *Science* **194,** 1069.
Wing, R. M., Okamura, W. H., Pirio, M. R., Sine, S. M., and Norman, A. W. (1974). *Science* **186,** 939.
Wing, R. M., Okamura, W. H., Rego, A., Pirio, M. R., and Norman, A. W. (1975). *J. Am. Chem. Soc.* **97,** 4980.
Wise, P., and Payne, A. (1975). *Mol. Cell. Endocrinol.* **3,** 385.
Wong, R. G., Myrtle, J. F., Tsai, H. C., and Norman, A. W. (1972). *J. Biol. Chem.* **247,** 5728.
Zerwekh, J. E., Haussler, M. R., and Lindell, T. J. (1974). *Proc. Natl. Acad. Sci. U.S.A.* **71,** 2337.
Zerwekh, J. E., Lindell, T. J., and Haussler, M. R. (1976). *J. Biol. Chem.* **251,** 2388.
Zile, M., Bunge, E. C., Barsness, L., Yamada, S., Schnoes, H. K., and DeLuca, H. F. (1978). *Arch. Biochem. Biophys.* **186,** 15.
Ziporin, Z. A., Isaac, G. J., Liddle, C. G., and Waring, P. P. (1973). *Calcif. Tissue Res.* **13,** 187.
Zull, J. E., Czarnowska-Misztal, E., and DeLuca, H. F. (1965). *Science* **149,** 182.
Zull, J. E., Czarnowska-Misztal, E., and DeLuca, H. F. (1966). *Proc. Natl. Acad. Sci. U.S.A.* **55,** 177.

CHAPTER 8

Binding Proteins and Receptors for Vitamin D and Its Metabolites

I. VITAMIN D

A. Binding Proteins[1]

In view of our current understanding of the complex metabolic conversion of vitamin D_3 to its hormonally active form(s), particularly 1,25$(OH)_2D_3$, it is not unreasonable to anticipate the existence of plasma binding proteins for the parent vitamin as well as its metabolites. Such proteins would be essential for the orderly translocation of these hydrophobic steroids through the aqueous internal milieu. The physical properties of these secosteroids would also dictate the existence of specific binding proteins for the vitamin D steroids in all their various target tissues, e.g., liver [vitamin D_3 and 25(OH)D_3], kidney

[1]In the study of vitamin D-binding proteins and steroid competition assays, consideration must be given to whether the assay can or cannot distinguish between the side chains of D_2 and D_3. Thus, in this chapter a subscript to vitamin D or its metabolites is included only when the study focused on D_2 versus D_3 differences or the assay could distinguish between D_2 and D_3.

[$25(OH)D_3$, $1,25(OH)_2D_3$, and $24,25(OH)_2D_3$], plasma [vitamin D, $25(OH)D_3$, $1,25(OH)_2D_3$, and $24,25(OH)_2D_3$], intestine [$1,25(OH)_2D$ and possibly $25(OH)D_3$], and bone (as yet unspecified metabolites).

Before the diversity of the metabolism of vitamin D was apparent, investigators were concerned with how vitamin D was transported in the blood. Several reports in recent years have demonstrated that vitamin D is transported systemically bound to specific carrier proteins (see Table 8-1).

Vitamin D is absorbed chiefly via the lymphatic system (Schachter *et al.*, 1964) and is distributed widely in various body tissues but is accumulated in highest concentration in the liver (Norman and DeLuca, 1963). The chief excretory route of vitamin D is through bile (Katz and Cooper, 1974). Two steps can be distinguished in the transport across the intestine: uptake at the mucosal surface, which is relatively rapid, and transfer to the lymphatic system, which is relatively slow. The jejunum and the ileum of the intestine are believed to differ in their absorption of the vitamin primarily in the mucosal uptake step (Schachter *et al.*, 1964). Vitamin D_2 (ergocalciferol) is also known to be absorbed by the lymphatic system but at a slower rate than cholecalciferol. It is interesting that there is no intrinsic necessity for the existence of a specific intestinal absorptive mechanism for either the natural cholecalciferol or the synthetic ergocalciferol. During evolution, animals presumably generated a process for resorbing the required amounts of vitamin D from the site of photochemical production in the epidermis and would not have evolved an intestinal absorptive mechanism. This simply reflects the fact that vitamin D can normally be produced via endogenous mechanisms and is not truly a vitamin. Thus, it might be anticipated that the absorption of vitamin D could follow the pathways normally taken by hydrophobic drugs or other pharmaceutical agents.

As indicated in Table 8-1, vitamin D is associated with certain plasma proteins as well as with the cytosol proteins of the liver (Rojanasathit and Haddad, 1976). After the administration of radioactive vitamin D, as much as 50% of the radioactivity of the blood is associated with the lipoprotein fractions. Incubation of blood obtained from rachitic animals with radioactive vitamin D also results in association with the lipoprotein fractions (DeLuca, 1967). However, as time passes after the intravenous injection, there is a progressive shift of the radioactivity from the lipoprotein fraction to the α_2-globulin fraction (Rikkers and DeLuca, 1967).

Using vitamin D_2, Bukin and Areshkina (1958) first showed that the vitamin was associated with the protein fraction of plasma after the administration of physiological quantities as well as of pharmacological doses that induced hypervitaminosis D. Morgan *et al.* (1958), Thomas *et al.* (1959), and DeCrousaz *et al.* (1965) separated by electrophoresis on starch and agar gel the serum proteins from patients given large doses of vitamin D_2. The protein fractions on the gels were evaluated for antirachitic activity by the rat line test, and it was noted that the activity migrated with α_2-globulins and albumins.

TABLE 8-1
Compilation of Vitamin D Binding to Different Tissues[a]

Tissue[b]	Species	References
Serum	Human	Bukin and Areshkina (1958), Morgan *et al.* (1958), Thomas *et al.* (1959), DeCrousaz *et al.* (1965), Peterson (1971), Haddad and Chyu (1971c), Smith and Goodman (1971), Nilsson *et al.* (1972), Daiger *et al.* (1975), Kida and Goodman (1976)
	Chick	Rikkers and DeLuca (1967), Edelstein *et al.* (1973), Belsey *et al.* (1974c), Edelstein (1974), Daiger (1975)
	Rat	Rikkers and DeLuca (1967), Chalk and Kodicek (1961), Oku *et al.* (1972), Belsey *et al.* (1975), Daiger (1975)
	Dog	Chen and Lane (1965)
	Baboon	Rosenstreich *et al.* (1971)
	Rabbit	Daiger (1975)
	Mouse	Juo and Isenberg (1972), Daiger (1975)
	Cow	Daiger (1975)
	Monkey	Edelstein *et al.* (1973), Daiger (1975), Hay (1975)
Lymph	Rat	Schachter *et al.* (1964)
Liver	Human	Rojanasathit and Haddad (1976)
Kidney	Human	Greenberg *et al.* (1974)
Urine	Human	Peterson (1971)
Cerebrospinal fluid	Human	Peterson (1971)
Intestine	Rat	Hosoya *et al.* (1970)
Mammary tissue	Rat	Edelstein *et al.* (1976)

[a] Binding of vitamin D to the tissue in question was determined by charcoal–dextran assay, electrophoresis, or autoradiography.

[b] Tritium-labeled vitamin D is distributed in a wide variety of other human tissues such as spleen, lung, bone, adipose, marrow, skin, muscle, thyroid, pancreas, adrenal, and intestinal mucosa (Mawer *et al.*, 1972). The vitamin was found in these tissues by organic solvent extraction.

In later studies the fate of vitamin D in terms of its plasma binding was followed by using either ^{14}C- or ^{3}H-labeled molecules. [^{14}C]Vitamin D_2 was added to rat serum, and the protein was subsequently fractionated by starch-block electrophoresis; the radioactivity was found by Chalk and Kodicek (1961) to be associated with the albumin and α_2-globulin fraction. In other studies the serum from dogs given [^{3}H]vitamin D_3 was analyzed by ultracentrifugal flotation techniques. Whereas 80% of the radioactivity in the serum was sedimentable, the remaining 20% floated and was associated with the lipoprotein fractions (Chen and Lane, 1965). In rats the vitamin was associated with the α-globulin fraction *in vivo*, with 80% being bound 15 min after an intravenous dose (Chen and Lane, 1965).

The existence of specific vitamin D-binding proteins in other tissues has been reported by many investigators (see Table 8-1). Rojanasathit and Haddad (1976) observed a specific binding of tritiated vitamin D as well as 25(OH)D_3 to a protein fraction present in the 100,000 *g* supernatant fraction of the liver. Peterson (1971) reported the existence of vitamin D-binding proteins in serum, urine, and the cerebrospinal fluid of normal human beings. These proteins were identified by Outchterlony immunodiffusion analyses with the use of specific antisera against the purified human serum vitamin D-binding protein.

There is little evidence that the concentration of vitamin D–binding proteins in the plasma varies or adapts to reflect the dietary intake of the vitamin. Juo and Isenberg (1972) used disc-gel electrophoresis to study serum proteins from mice that had been injected subcutaneously with excessive doses of vitamin D_2. Although the total protein concentration was not significantly different, there had been some qualitative changes in the pattern of vitamin D-binding proteins in the animals receiving high doses of vitamin D. Jacob and Ray (1968) evaluated the ability of human serum to transport large amounts of vitamin D. They determined that the maximal binding capacity was approximately 6700 IU (436 nmoles) of vitamin D per milligram of serum protein.

Peterson (1971) carried out a rigorous purification of the vitamin D-binding protein present in human plasma by sequential steps of ammonium sulfate precipitation followed by chromatography on columns of Sephadex G-200, DEAE-Sephadex, sulfethyl-Sephadex, and finally Sephadex G-100. This protein was recognized by its high affinity constant (association constant $K_a = 2.8 \times 10^8$ M^{-1}) for vitamin D_3 as determined under completely specified *in vitro* conditions. The molecular weight was approximately 53,000 daltons. The electrophoretic mobility was that of an α_1-globulin. The sedimentation coefficient was reported to be 3.8S, and it was found in the human serum in concentrations of 5 μg/ml. The physical properties of the vitamin D serum binding protein are summarized in Table 8-2. It is now apparent from the more recent work of Bouillon *et al.* (1975, 1976b) and Kida and Goodman (1976) that human serum contains only a single binding protein for both vitamin D_3 and 25(OH)D_3. Thus, the Peterson purification described above for the vitamin D-binding protein also represents the first purification of the 25(OH)D-binding protein.

Nilsson *et al.* (1972) carried out a detailed quantitative evaluation, by fluorescence spectroscopy, of the comparative association constants (K_a) for the binding of vitamin D_3 and vitamin D_2 to their highly purified human vitamin D-binding protein. The K_a values for vitamin D_3 and vitamin D_2 were found to be, respectively, 2.8×10^8 and 1.3×10^8 M^{-1}. This is the first evidence that vitamin D_3 and vitamin D_2 bind to the human vitamin D-binding protein with similar if not identical affinities. The same workers further noted that the binding of 2-p-toluidinylnaphthalene 6-sulfonate (TNS) to human vitamin D serum protein was associated with a strong increase in fluorescence intensity. Concomitantly, a shift occurred in the wavelength of maximal emission, and interestingly, both vitamin D_3 and D_2 were noted to quench the TNS fluorescence. The observed binding satisfied a mechanism of noncompetitive interaction, suggesting

TABLE 8-2
Physical Properties of Serum Binding Protein for Vitamin D

Properties	Unit	Human[a]	Chick[b]
Molecular weight	Daltons	53,000	60,000
Sedimentation constant	S	3.8	3.5
Electrophoretic mobility		1	—
Association constant (K_a)	m^{-1}		
Vitamin D_3		2.8×10^8	—[c]
Vitamin D_2		1.21×10^8	—
Hydrated density	g/ml	1.21	—
Frictional ratio (f/f_0)		1.22	—
Stokes molecular radius	Å	31	—
Subunits		No	—

[a] Peterson (1971) and Nilsson *et al.* (1972).
[b] Edelstein *et al.* (1972, 1973) and Edelstein (1974).
[c] Association constant (K_a) for 25(OH)D_3 was reported to be $4.3 \times 10^8 M^{-1}$ at 4°C.

that TNS and vitamin D did not bind to the same site. These results also suggested to Nilsson *et al.* (1972) that vitamin D binding to its plasma carrier protein is associated with a conformational change in the environment of the receptor site, which produces the corresponding fluorescence changes.

Chick serum contains two vitamin D_3-binding proteins, one of which binds primarily vitamin D_3 and the other both vitamin D_3 and 25(OH)D_3 (Edelstein *et al.*, 1972; 1973; Edelstein, 1974). The proteins have been partially purified by means of Cohn fractionation (Cohn *et al.*, 1950), followed by ammonium sulfate precipitation, gel filtration on Sephadex G-200, ion-exchange chromatography on DEAE-Sephadex, and an additional gel filtration step on Sephadex G-100. Some of the physical properties of the vitamin D_3-binding protein have been determined and are summarized in Table 8-2. The molecular weight was found to be approximately 60,000 daltons. The protein possessed β-globulin mobility on analytical polyacrylamide disc-gel electrophoresis and a sedimentation coefficient of 3.5 S. The association constant for binding vitamin D was not determined. However, thin-layer chromatographic analysis of the lipid extracts of the protein peaks obtained from ion-exchange and DEAE-Sephadex chromatography indicated that 83% of the peak I radioactivity was due to 25(OH)D_3 and 10% due to vitamin D_3. In contrast, the recovered radioactivity of peak II consisted mainly of vitamin D_3 (55%) and a lesser amount of 25(OH)D_3. Peak II was stated by Edelstein and co-workers (1972, 1973) to be the vitamin D_3 serum binding protein for the chick.

An interesting role for the transcalciferin of birds has been proposed by Fraser and Emtage (1976). Egg yolk contains significant quantities of vitamin D_3 (see

Table 13-2) and low levels of 25(OH)D_3. These authors suggest that, in the hen, vitamin D_3 bound to its transcalciferin forms a complex with Ca^{2+} and the yolk phosphoprotein, phosvitin, which is then incorporated into the yolk by the thecal cells of the ovarian follicle.

B. Competitive Binding Assay

To date there has been only one competitive binding protein assay developed that measures circulating concentrations of vitamin D present in plasma. This was first reported by Belsey *et al.* (1971). Their competitive binding assay was developed for the measurement of either vitamin D or 25(OH)D that was obtained from the chromatographic separation of lipid extracts of plasma. The assay utilized a specific vitamin D-binding β-lipoprotein present in rat sera that had a sufficiently high association constant for both vitamin D and 25(OH)D. The β-lipoprotein was partially purified from human plasma. Samples containing the vitamin D from silicic acid columns or standard amounts of vitamin D were incubated with the appropriate amount of β-lipoprotein plus carrier vitamin D-deficient rat serum for a period of 10 days at 4°C; after this period, the bound vitamin D had to be separated from the unbound vitamin D by precipitation of the lipoprotein fraction with heparin and $MnCl_2$. After standing for 15 min in the cold, the mixture was centrifuged for 15 min at 3000 rpm, 4°C, the supernatant decanted, and the radioactivity quantitated. This fraction represented the "free" steroid. Belsey *et al.* (1971) reported that it was possible to detect 1–2 ng/ml of vitamin D and that the assay was capable of accommodating up to 400 ng/ml of either vitamin D or 25(OH)D. The assay, however, has not been widely adopted as a means of measuring plasma levels of vitamin D, undoubtedly because of the extraordinarily long incubation period (10 days) required for establishing equilibrium between the bound and free fractions of vitamin D. Belsey *et al.* (1971) reported that the circulating concentration of vitamin D in normal human beings ranged from 24 to 40 ng/ml.

II. 25(OH)D

A. Binding Proteins

Vitamin D is taken up by the liver and undergoes 25-hydroxylation to give 25(OH)D. In most species, including man, the principal circulating forms of vitamin D are the unchanged parent molecule and 25(OH)D with somewhat lower concentrations of 24,25$(OH)_2$D. The fact that 95% of these molecules in the plasma circulate in association with proteins of a density greater than 1.21

was claimed by Smith and Goodman (1971) as presumptive evidence for the existence of a specific transport protein(s) for these two steroids.

Since it is now known (Bouillon *et al.*, 1975, 1976b; Kida and Goodman, 1976) that both vitamin D and 25(OH)D and possibly also $24{,}25(OH)_2D$ and $1{,}25(OH)_2D$ are transported in the serum by the same binding protein in mammals, the generic name *transcalciferin* has been proposed for this protein, analogous with other serum binding proteins, e.g., transcortin, transferrin, and transcobalamin. In some literature this protein is referred to as DBP for D-binding protein.

Haddad and Chyu (1971a) labeled human plasma binding proteins, *in vivo* and *in vitro,* with tritiated $25(OH)D_3$ and observed that the bulk of the radioactivity was associated with a protein of α-globulin mobility as determined by disc-gel electrophoresis. They suggested that the protein had a molecular weight of 40,000 to 50,000 daltons and a sedimentation coefficient of 3.1 S. These results were consistent with the report of Smith and Goodman (1971) on the human plasma binding protein for $25(OH)D_3$, which had a mobility slightly greater than that of plasma albumin and a molecular weight of 50,000 to 60,000 daltons. More recently Kida and Goodman (1976) carefully evaluated the simultaneous transport of D_3 and $25(OH)D_3$ in human plasma. They concluded that human serum contains only a single binding protein for the normal transport of both vitamin D_3 and $25(OH)D_3$. Also, Edelstein *et al.* (1973) reported that serum obtained from rat, pig, monkey, and man contained a single protein that is responsible for the transport of both vitamin D and 25(OH)D. (See also Hay, 1975 and Hay and Watson, 1975).

Hay and Watson (1976a,b, 1977) carried out a remarkably thorough study of the phylogenic distribution of plasma transport proteins for $25(OH)D_3$ in 22 species of fish, 12 species of amphibians, 5 species of reptiles, 19 species of birds, as well as 72 species from 14 separate orders of mammals. They found that fish with cartilaginous skeletons and amphibians use lipoproteins for the transport of $25(OH)D_3$ and that bony fish and reptiles carry this steroid in the plasma bound to an α-globulin. In 12 species of birds, however, $25(OH)D_3$ is bound to the β-globulin transport proteins, whereas in 4 species of birds it is carried on albumin and in 3 species $25(OH)D_3$ is bound to an α-globulin. Of the 72 species of mammals studied, 65 have an α-globulin transport protein for $25(OH)D_3$, whereas a few species scattered among several orders (including 3 species of *Cebus* monkeys) use albumin as their transport protein for $25(OH)D_3$.

Bouillon *et al.* (1976c) studied in detail the transport of $25(OH)D_3$ in the *Cebus* monkey. In contrast with the α-globulin mobility of the transcalciferin of other primates, the transcalciferin of the *Cebus* monkey has the electrophoretic mobility of albumin. However, careful immunocross-reactivity studies clearly indicated to these workers that the transport of 25(OH)D in the *Cebus* monkey is not by albumin itself, but by a transcalciferin with albumin-like electrophoretic mobility.

The remarkable study of Hay and Watson (1976a,b, 1977) is complementary to the evaluation by Henry and Norman (1975) of the species distribution of the renal $25(OH)D_3$ 1-hydroxylase. They reported the presence of this key enzyme system in 17 classes of animals. Thus, from the combined results of these two studies it is apparent that transport proteins for the intermediate form of vitamin D, $25(OH)D_3$, as well as the enzyme to convert this to the hormonally active form, $1,25(OH)_2D_3$, are widely distributed among the various classes and orders of higher animals. Clearly, vitamin D must play an integral role in normal calcium and phosphorus metabolism in all these widely differing species.

Daiger *et al.* (1975), Cavalli-Sforza *et al.* (1977), and Daiger and Cavalli-Sforza (1977) also carried out a polyacrylamide disc-gel electrophoretic analysis of the plasma proteins that have the capability of binding vitamin D_3 and $25(OH)D_3$ in several species. Their studies demonstrated that most species have plasma ($25(OH)D_3$-binding proteins of the same mobility.

Furthermore, in 25 human sera ^{14}C-labeled vitamin D_3 was bound to a protein with the same electrophoretic mobility as "group-specific component" (Gc) (Daiger *et al.*, 1975). Both radioactive D_3 and $25(OH)D_3$ added to human serum could be precipitated by incubation with an equal amount of anti-GC antiserum. Most significantly, Bouillon *et al.* (1976a) showed that pure human $25(OH)D_3$-binding protein also is immunochemically identical with this human Gc. Therefore, convincing evidence now exists for the identity between the transcalciferin and Gc of serum.

This Gc protein was first isolated by Hirschfeld in 1959. The α-globulin has been extensively studied all over the world (Cleve, 1973), and the three common Gc's are determined by a pair of autosomal alleles (*Gc 1* and *Gc 2*). This Gc system is one of the routinely applied markers in studies of human population, in cases of disputed paternity, and in the diagnosis of twin pairs. Until 1976 (Bouillon *et al.*, 1976c) its function was unknown.

Table 8-3 summarizes the physical properties of the 25(OH)D-binding protein for human beings (Bouillon *et al.*, 1976b; Haddad and Walgate, 1976), rats (Edelstein *et al.*, 1972, 1973), and chicks (Edelstein *et al.*, 1972, 1973; Obsorn, 1976). Only a 500-fold purification was required by Bouillon *et al.* (1976b) to obtain a pure protein as judged by the presence of a single band on both cellulose acetate and acrylamide gel electrophoresis. Clear evidence was obtained indicating that the apo- and holotranscalciferins [i.e., saturated with $25(OH)D_3$] had different chromatographic mobilities. This is suggestive of a conformational change occurring upon binding of the ligand to the transcalciferin. No evidence for subunits was found. The amino acid analysis reported (Bouillon *et al.*, 1976b) is quite similar to that given previously for Gc proteins (Simons and Bearn, 1967).

TABLE 8-3
Physical Properties of Serum Binding Protein for 25(OH)D

Properties	Human[a]	Rat	Chick[b]	Chick[c]
Number of binding proteins	1	1	1	2–3
Molecular weight (approx.)	56,000	?	54,000	60,000
Sedimentation coefficient	4.1 S	6.8 S[d]	3.5 S	4.1 S
Association constant (M^{-1})	1.2×10^{10}	1.8×10^{9}	3.0×10^{8}	6×10^{6}
			0.9×10^{8}	1×10^{8}
Isolectric point	4.89			
Binding capacity (sites/molecule)	0.8			
pH optimum	8–9[c]	8.6[e]	—	8–9

[a]Bouillon *et al.* (1976b); Haddad and Walgate (1976).
[b]Edelstein *et al.* (1972, 1973); Edelstein (1974).
[c]Osborn (1976).
[d]Oku *et al.* (1972).
[e]Belsey *et al.* (1974c).

Sharpe *et al.* (1977) were the first to employ affinity chromatography to purify the chick 25(OH)D transcalciferin. They used a column of Sepharose-aminohexylsuccinyl-25(OH)D_3 to effect a 1000-fold purification.

Haddad and Walgate (1976), Bouillon *et al.* (1976b, 1977) and Imawari *et al.* (1977) developed radial immunodiffusion assays to quantitate plasma levels of human transcalciferin. The mean serum 25(OH)D-binding protein concentration obtained by Haddad and Walgate for 40 normal adults was 525 ± 24 μg/ml, or 6×10^{-6} *M*. It was calculated that only 3% of the available binding sites for 25(OH)D, vitamin D, and 24,25$(OH)_2$D were occupied. Furthermore, there were no fluctuations in the concentration of the binding protein in a wide variety of vitamin D-related disease states. Bouillon *et al.* (1977a) also compared the levels of transcalciferin in maternal and cord serum without finding large differences. This protein is unique among other hormone-binding proteins and vitamin-binding proteins since it combines a high capacity with high affinity for its ligand(s). The direct implication is that the free concentration of 25(OH)D_3 and other metabolites must be extremely low.

The bulk of the physiological responses to vitamin D are currently thought to be mediated through the action of its hormonally active form, 1,25$(OH)_2D_3$. However, 25(OH)D_3, the major circulating metabolite of the vitamin, is found in many tissues of man, rat, and chick. Haddad *et al.* (1973a,b, 1976) incubated tritiated 25(OH)D_3 with 105,000 *g* supernatants of homogenates of rat brain, lung, heart, skeletal muscle, cartilage, liver, intestinal mucosa, kidney, testes, and erythrocytes and obtained evidence for a specific steroid binding with a mobility on a sucrose gradient of 5.85. The widespread specific high-affinity tissue binding of 25(OH)D_3 is summarized in Table 8-4; here the association constants (K_a, M^{-1}) are given for different tissues.

Until the brilliant work of Bouillon and Van Baelen (Van Baelen *et al.*, 1977) the significance of the widespread tissue binding proteins for 25(OH)D_3 was most puzzling. Some felt that this indicated the existence of specific receptors for 25(OH)D in many tissues (Haddad *et al.*, 1973a, 1976) which were suggestive of specific biological actions of this metabolite in these locations. However, Van Baelen *et al.* (1977) presented unequivocal evidence that the 5.8 S cytosol receptor for 25(OH)D_3 is formed from two proteins: a heat-stable 4.1 S 25(OH)D-binding protein, which is identical to the serum 25(OH)D transcalciferin, and a cytosolic heat-labile protein, which sediments around 4 S and does not show any binding properties for 25(OH)D_3 (Fig. 8-1). The 5.8 S complex

TABLE 8-4
Summary of 25(OH)D Binding to Various Tissues

Tissue	Human	Chick (M^{-1})[a]	Rat[b] (M^{-1})[a]
Bone	—	+[c,d]	4.0×10^{9}[e]
Brain	—	—	+[c]
Cartilage	—	—	+[c]
Heart	—	—	+[c]
Intestinal mucosa	—	+[f]	2.0×10^{9}[e]
Kidney	+[c,g]	3.6×10^{8}[d]	1.1×10^{9}[e]
Liver	—	+[f]	+[b,c]
Lung	—	—	+[b,c]
Skeletal muscle	—	+[f]	1.7×10^{9}[e]
Skin	—	—	1.0×10^{9}[e]
Testis	—	—	+[b,c]
Serum	+[c,h]	3.0×10^{8}[f,i] 1.9×10^{8}[d]	1.8×10^{9}[e]
Erythrocytes	—	—	No[e]

[a]Values for the association constants, K_a were taken from Haddad and Birge (1975) and Haddad and Chyu (1971).

[b]See Van Baelen *et al.* (1977) for a detailed evaluation of this subject. Also Oku *et al.* (1972) have made preliminary studies.

[c]The + indicates saturable binding of 25(OH)D_3 demonstrated by competitive binding assay.

[d]Greenberg *et al.* (1974), Osborn (1976).

[e]Edelstein (1974), Hosoya and Oku (1971).

[f]Haddad and Birge (1971, 1974) and Wecksler and Norman (1978).

[g]Greenberg *et al.* (1974).

[h]Bouillon *et al.* (1976b).

[i]Edelstein *et al.* (1973).

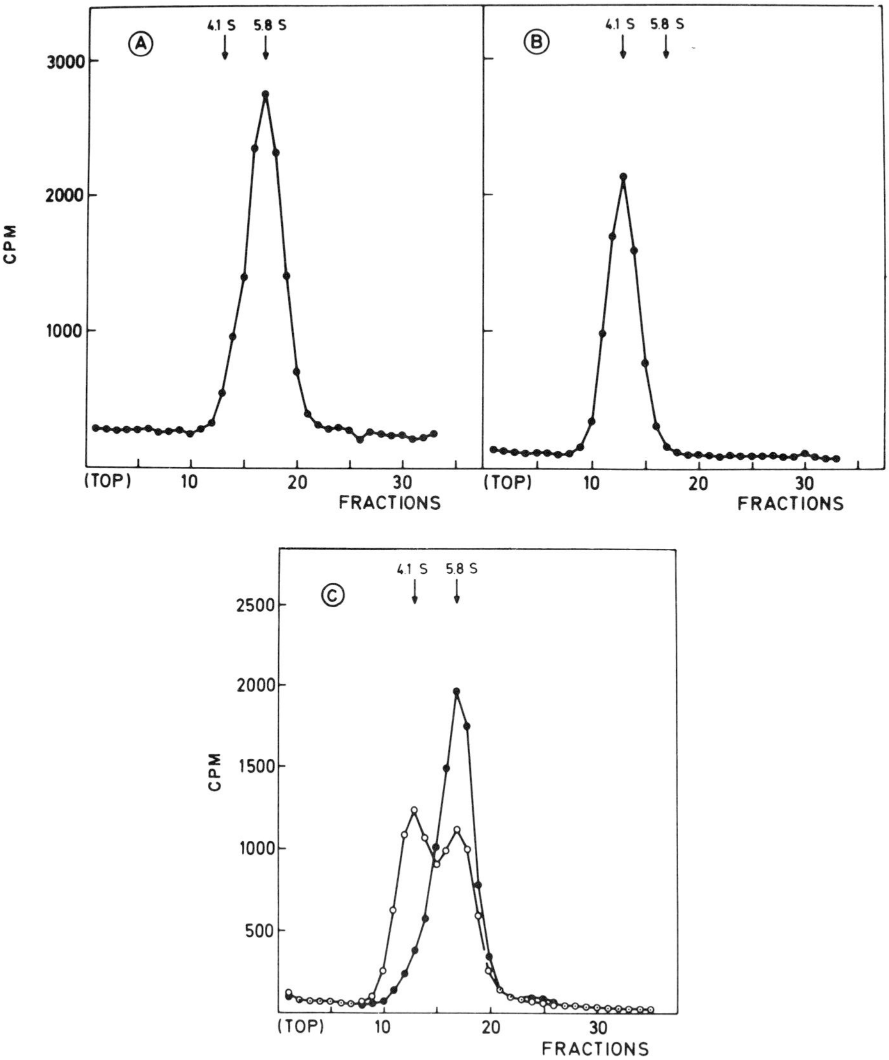

Figure 8-1. Sucrose gradient analysis of tissue and plasma binding proteins for $25(OH)D_3$. (A) Complex formation of rat serum $25(OH)D_3$-binding protein with rat kidney cytosol. Equal volumes of rat kidney cytosol (protein content 6 mg/ml) and 20-fold diluted rat serum previously incubated with tritiated $25(OH)D_3$ were mixed and incubated at 0°C for 30 min. (B) The kidney cytosol employed in the experiment in (A) was first heated at 60°C for 60 min. The 4.1 S peak is identical to that of the plasma transcalciferin for $25(OH)D_3$. (C) Saturation study of rat serum $25(OH)D_3$-binding protein with rat kidney cytosol. Complexes were formed in an ice bath by mixing equal volumes of 20-fold diluted serum previously incubated with 20 pmoles of tritiated $25(OH)D_3$ per milliliter and 20-fold (○—○) or 10-fold (●—●) diluted kidney cytosol. Reproduced by permission of the publisher and author; from Van Baelen *et al.* (1977).

could be formed *in vitro* by incubating cytosol with appropriate amounts of serum. The widespread occurrence of the 4 S cytosolic protein in nucleated tissues raises the possibility that these high-affinity binding proteins for 25(OH)D are largely the result of plasma contamination.

B. Competitive Binding Assays

The existence of natural binding proteins in serum and tissues of mammals and birds along with the availability of high specific activity tritiated 25(OH)D_3 has permitted the development of competitive binding radioassays for 25(OH)D (see Table 8-5). The first usable competitive protein binding assay for 25(OH)D was that reported by Haddad and Chyu (1971a). The source of the specific binding protein was the 100,000 *g* cytosol fraction of rachitic rat kidneys. It is essential for lipid extracts from plasma (samples 1–5 ml) to be chromatographed on columns of either silicic acid or Sephadex LH-20 prior to submission of the 25(OH)D region for assay (Dorantes *et al.*, 1978). This sample or standard 25(OH)D_3 was incubated with the rachitic kidney cytosol protein fraction at 25°C for 60 min and then the "bound" steroid was separated from the "free" by addition of dextran-coated charcoal. This was followed by centrifugation for 20 min at 5°C (see Fig. 8-2A). When 21 pairs of duplicate plasma samples were analyzed on different days, the mean difference of duplicates was 15.4 ± 9.1% (S.D.). The mean plasma 25(OH)D level in 40 volunteers was 27.3 ± 11.8 (S.D.) ng/ml. Since that time, as documented in Table 8-5, a plethora of assays have been developed which employ binding proteins from chick and rat kidney cytosol as well as chick, rat, and human plasma. The recognized insensitivity of chicks to vitamin D_2 can be correlated with the failure of avian sera to bind

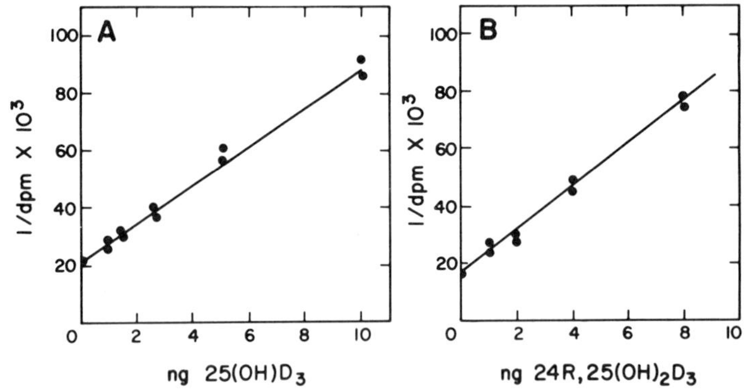

Figure 8-2. Standard curve for steroid competition assay for 25(OH)D_3 (A) and 24,25$(OH)_2D_3$ (B). In each instance the nonradioactive steroid is competing with tritiated 25(OH)D_3 for binding to a standard amount, 10–20 μg, of normal rat serum proteins.

TABLE 8-5
Summary of Results of Competitive Binding Assays for 25(OH)D

Source of binding protein	Normal range of serum 25(OH)D (ng/ml)	Chromatographic technique	Reference
Rat serum	20–40	Silicic acid	Belsey *et al.* (1971)
Rat kidney cytosol	10–50	Silicic acid	Haddad and Chyu (1971a)
Human serum	10–20	Thin-layer plates with silica gel	Bayard *et al.* (1972)
Chick, rat, and human kidney cytosol	—	Silicic acid	Greenberg *et al.* (1974), Caldas *et al.* (1978)
Rat serum	5–30	Sephadex LH-20	Edelstein *et al.* (1974)
	20–100	None	Belsey *et al.* (1974b)
	5–30	Silicic acid	Preece *et al.* (1974a)
	20–40	Sephadex LH-20	Osborn and Norman (1975)
	—	No chromatography	Offermann and Ditmar (1974)
Human serum	5–20	Sephadex LH-20	Bouillon *et al.* (1976a)
Rat serum	20–60	None	Garcia-Pascual *et al.* (1976)
	20–50	HPLC (direct measurement)	Lambert *et al.* (1977), Schaefer and Goldsmith (1978), Koshy and VanDerSlik (1978), Eisman *et al.* (1977)
Bovine globulin	30–50	Sephadex LH-20	Hollis *et al.* (1977)

25(OH)D_2 as avidly as 25(OH)D_3 (Belsey *et al.*, 1974a,b; Preece *et al.*, 1974a,b; Osborn and Norman, 1975). This observation has allowed the development of specific assays for 25(OH)D that can differentiate between the side chains of vitamin D_2 and D_3. Therefore, assays utilizing rat serum or rat kidney cytosol are capable of measuring both D_2 and D_3 hydroxy metabolites, whereas those employing binding proteins obtained from the chick are capable of measuring preferentially 25(OH)D_3 (Osborn, 1976). As can be anticipated, this assay for the determination of the circulating levels of 25(OH)D has had widespread application in a variety of clinical and physiological studies related to vitamin D. A summary of some of these applications is provided in Table 8-6.

III. 1,25(OH)$_2$D

A. Binding Proteins

Extensive studies by Tsai and Norman (Tsai *et al.*, 1972; Tsai and Norman, 1973a,b) and more recently by Haussler and associates (Brumbaugh and Haus-

TABLE 8-6
Applications of Assay for 25(OH)D

Nature of study	Reference
Normal man	Haddad and Chyu (1971c), Hahn *et al.* (1972), Stamp *et al.* (1972), Haddad *et al.* (1973b), Haddad and Hahn (1973), Hillman and Haddad (1974), Lambert *et al.* (1977), Bjorkhem and Holmberg (1976), Stamp *et al.* (1977)
Human perinatal states	Hillman and Haddad (1977), Haddad and Stamp (1974), Davies *et al.* (1978)
Chronic renal failure	Bayard *et al.* (1973), Roginsky *et al.* (1974), Offermann *et al.* (1974), Norman *et al.* (1978)
Seasonal changes	Stamp and Round (1974), McLaughlin *et al.* (1974), Gupta *et al.* (1974), Preece *et al.* (1974b), Neer *et al.* (1977)
Chronic anticonvulsant therapy	Hahn *et al.* (1975), Bouillon *et al.* (1975), Baud *et al.* (1974)
Hyperthyroidism	Mosekilde *et al.* (1977)
Fractures of the proximal femur	Lund *et al.* (1975)
Pregnancy	Dent and Gupta (1975), Turton *et al.* (1977)
Chronic alcoholics	Velentzas *et al.* (1977)
Nutrition (vegetarian versus nonvegetarian diet)	Dent and Gupta (1975)
Urolithiasis (kidney stones)	Velentzas *et al.* (1977)
Liver disease	Long *et al.* (1976), Skinner *et al.* (1977), Seino *et al.* (1978)

sler, 1973, 1974a,b; Brumbaugh *et al.,* 1974a,b) indicate that the intestinal mucosa has two separate components, the cytoplasm and the nuclear chromatin fraction, which selectively and tightly bind $1,25(OH)_2D_3$. This sterol remains bound to the cytosol fraction at 0°C, and a dramatic movement to the nuclear chromatin fraction occurs at room temperature, indicating that the subcellular localization of the sterol is temperature dependent (Brumbaugh *et al.,* 1974a). Tsai and Norman (1973b) also obtained evidence for a tissue specificity for both the chick cytoplasmic receptor and the chromatin binding; neither liver, kidney, or spleen cytosol was able to effectively transfer $1,25(OH)_2D_3$ to intestinal chromatin, nor were liver or kidney nuclei able to accept the steroid from the intestinal cytosol receptor (see also Fig. 7-4). Haddad *et al.* (1973a) identified a soluble macromolecule fraction from the cytosol of the intestinal mucosa of rats capable of specific *in vitro* binding for both $25(OH)D_3$ and $1,25(OH)_2D_3$. Its sedimentation behavior on linear 5–20% sucrose gradients suggested a molecular weight of approximately 100,000 daltons and a sedimentation coefficient of 5 S. The association constant K_a for $25(OH)D_3$ was $2 \times 10^9\ M^{-1}$, and that for

1,25(OH)$_2$D$_3$ was 7.1 × 10^8 M^{-1}. Brumbaugh and Haussler (1974b), working with chick intestinal cytosol, reported that the cytosol–steroid receptor complex sedimented at 3.5 S in the presence of 0.15 M KCl. They also determined the K_a to be 4.5 × 10^8M^{-1}.

In principal any tissue which contains a vitamin D-dependent calcium binding protein (see Table 10-10 for a summary) should contain specific high-affinity binding proteins/receptors for 1,25(OH)$_2$D$_3$. Recently Norman's laboratory has presented evidence for the existence of 1,25(OH)$_2$D$_3$ receptors in human intestine (Wecksler *et al.*, 1979a), chick parathyroid and human parathyroid adenoma (Wecksler *et al.*, 1979b), and chick kidney and pancreas (Christakos and Norman, 1979).

B. Competitive Binding Assays

Two different types of steroid competition assays have been developed for 1,25(OH)$_2$D. The first method employs incubation of tritiated 1,25(OH)$_2$D$_3$ with intestinal cytosol plus the nuclear chromatin fraction (Brumbaugh and Haussler, 1974a,b; Procsal *et al.*, 1975), whereas the second approach, more recently developed by Eisman *et al.* (1976a,b), simply involves incubation of the steroid with chick intestinal cytosol. These assays will be discussed separately.

The procedure of Brumbaugh and Haussler was the first assay to be developed that could provide some insight into the circulating levels of 1,25(OH)$_2$D in the plasma. As originally described by these workers (Brumbaugh and Haussler, 1974b), this assay necessitated a laborious three-stage chromatography of organic solvent extracts of plasma samples (15–25 ml). These chromatographic steps involved successively silicic acid, Sephadex LH-20, and liquid–liquid partition on columns of celite. The 1,25(OH)$_2$D region from the last column then was submitted for assay in a system containing chick intestinal mucosal cytosol plus purified chromatin fraction and standardized amounts of tritiated 1,25(OH)$_2$D$_3$. The putative 1,25(OH)$_2$D in the sample would then displace the tritiated hormone from the cytosol–chromatin receptor preparation. Separation of bound and free steroid was carried out by filtration of the incubation media through glass filters that specifically bind the steroid associated with the chromatin–cytosol receptor. As originally described, this assay had a sensitivity of 80 pg of 1,25(OH)$_2$D$_3$. More recently there have been some improvements, based largely on an increased specific activity of the tritiated steroid employed in the assay, as well as further refinements in technique (Haussler *et al.*, 1976, 1977). Table 8-7 summarizes the clinical applications of this important assay as well as the results of other assays currently available for 1,25(OH)$_2$D.

The assay described by Procsal *et al.* (1975) is essentially identical to that of Brumbaugh and colleagues (1974a,b) except that the separation of the bound steroid from the free is effected by high-speed differential centrifugation. These

TABLE 8-7
Applications of Assays for $1,25(OH)_2D_3$ in Disease States Related to Vitamin D

Nature of study	Average circulatory level of $1,25(OH)_2D_3$ (pg/ml ± S.D.) (*n*)	Reference
Normal adult man	33.9±1.8 (25)	Eisman *et al.* (1976a,b)
	33±6 (58)	Haussler *et al.* (1976)
	35±3 (10)	Lambert *et al.* (1977)
	25.1±2.2 (15)	Stern *et al.* (1977, 1978)
	33 (25)	Schaefer *et al.* (1978)
	34±5 (37)	Caldas *et al.* (1978)
	32±10 (12)	Norman *et al.* (1978)
	44±9 (15)	Bishop *et al.* (1979)
Normal children	64±9 (4)	Haussler *et al.* (1977)
Chronic renal failure	4±4 (50)	Haussler *et al.* (1976), Schaefer *et al.* (1978)
	12±5 (12)	Norman *et al.* (1978)
Anephric man	3±2 (8)	Haussler *et al.* (1977)
Sarcoidosis	36±13 (4)	Haussler *et al.* (1977)
Hypervitaminosis D	36±15 (5)	Hughes *et al.* (1976)
Idiopathic hypercalciuria	50±16 (40)	Kaplan *et al.* (1977)
Familial hypophosphatemic rickets (VDRR)	33±14 (11)	Haussler *et al.* (1977)
Anticonvulsant-induced osteomalacia	47±36 (25)	Jubiz *et al.* (1977)
Postmenopausal osteoporosis	34±12 (32)	Haussler *et al.* (1977)
	28±1.9	Riggs and Gallagher (1977)
Primary hyperparathyroidism	54±21 (26)	Kaplan *et al.* (1977)
Hypoparathyroidism	28±9 (11)	Haussler *et al.* (1977)
Pseudohypoparathyroidism	29±14 (8)	Haussler *et al.* (1977), Diezner *et al.* (1976)
Diabetes (streptozotocin-induced in the rat)		
Control:	67±15 (4)	Schneider *et al.* (1977)
Diabetic:	8±4 (4)	
Tumoral calcinosis	80 (5)	Schaefer *et al.* (1978)
Nephrolithiasis	55±15 (22)	Caldas *et al.* (1978)

workers have employed this assay largely to carry out a detailed structure–function study of the structural requirements for the interaction of $1,25(OH)_2D_3$ and closely related analogues with the chick intestinal receptor system. Figure 7-17 shows the standard curve for $1,25(OH)_2D_3$ and the competition effected by various analogues of this steroid. From studies such as this it has been possible to define in great detail the functional group modifications of vitamin D secosteroids that are tolerated by the chick intestinal receptor system.

More recently Eisman *et al.* (1976a,b) and Kream *et al.* (1976) developed an assay for $1,25(OH)_2D$ that involves incubation of steroid or highly purified plasma samples with chick intestinal cytosol. Then the bound steroid is separated from free steroid by addition of propylene glycol. The propylene glycol precipitates the protein-bound 1,25(OH)$_2$D, leaving the "free" steroid in the supernatant. However, prior to assay, the organic solvent extract of the 5- to 6-ml plasma sample must be subjected to rigorous chromatographic purification. In this instance purification on two columns of Sephadex LH-20 followed by submission of the 1,25(OH)$_2$D region to high-pressure liquid chromatography (HPLC) is required. An assay with comparable sensitivity has recently been developed by Bishop *et al.* (1979). It, too, employs only chick intestinal cytosol as the source of the binding protein, but it separates bound from free steroid by addition of hydroxylapatite. Sample purification is a modification of that described by Eisman *et al.* (1976a). A typical standard curve is given in Fig. 8-3. Both this assay and the Eisman *et al.* (1976a,b) procedure have a sensitivity of 1 pg and require 2–3 ml of serum for triplicate sample assay.

Although the application of radioimmunoassay (RIA) has proved invaluable to the quantitation of other classic steroids, this approach has not yet been successful for vitamin D steroids. There are only two preliminary reports which suggest that it is possible to prepare antisera directed against any vitamin D compound. Both Schaefer *et al.* (1978) and Clemens *et al.* (1978) described the development of an RIA for 1,25(OH)$_2$D$_3$. Unfortunately, the specificity of the antisera each group employed was such that significant cross-reaction occurred with both 25(OH)$_2$D$_3$ and 24,25(OH)$_2$D$_3$ besides the 1,25(OH)$_2$D$_3$. Accordingly, it was necessary to subject plasma samples to organic solvent extraction and HPLC separation prior to assay for 1,25(OH)$_2$D$_3$. It can be anticipated that there will be important developments in the near future with the RIA approach to assessment of the circulating levels of all the vitamin D metabolites.

IV. 24,25(OH)$_2$D Assay

Although the precise physiological role of 24,25(OH)$_2$D remains to be elucidated, the methodology has already been developed to determine the plasma level of this steroid. Taylor *et al.* (1976) were the first to report the development of a steroid competition assay for 24,25(OH)$_2$D. The binding protein may be obtained either from the cytosol of rachitic rat kidneys or from the serum of rachitic rats. The assay is carried out by measuring the ability of standard 24,25(OH)$_2$D$_3$ or sample 24,25(OH)$_2$D to compete with tritiated 25(OH)D$_3$ rather than tritiated 24,25(OH)$_2$D$_3$. This is possible since 24,25(OH)$_2$D$_3$ is virtually equipotent to 25(OH)D$_3$ in the competitive displacement of tritiated 25(OH)D$_3$ (compare Fig. 8-2A and B). The limits of detection are approximately 50 pg of 24,25(OH)$_2$D per assay tube.

The fact that 24,25(OH)$_2$D and 25(OH)D are equally effective competitors for both binding proteins dictates that any sample being submitted for assay must be

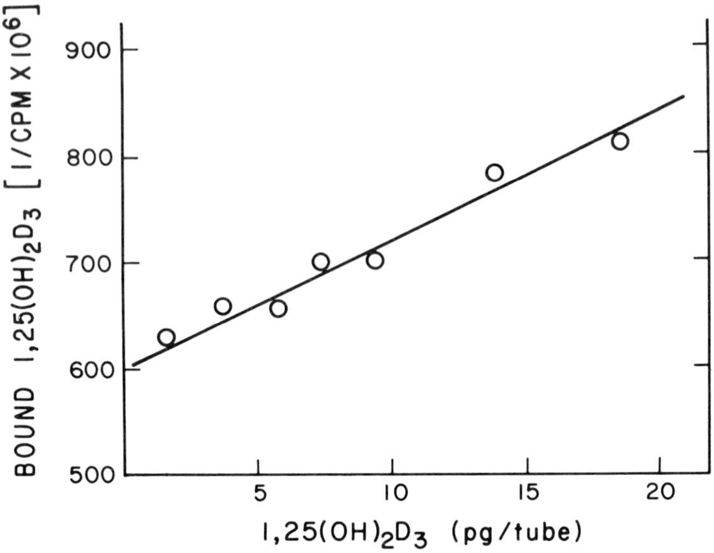

Figure 8-3. Standard curve for steroid competition assay for 1,25(OH)$_2$D. Rachitic chick intestinal cytosol is incubated at room temperature in 100 μl with a standard amount of very high specific activity tritiated 1,25(OH)$_2$D$_3$ (90 Ci/nmole) and either defined amounts of nonradioactive 1,25(OH)$_2$D$_3$ or 25 μl of a serum extract (rigorously purified by ether extraction, 3x backwash with 0.1M Na_2HPO_4, pH 10.5 and HPLC chromatography). After incubation, 0.3 ml of a 50% slurry of hydroxylapatite is added, and a second incubation for 15 min at 0°C is carried out. The pellet is collected by centrifugation in a microfuge and washed three times with Tris–Triton X-100 (1%). The radioactivity in the pellet (representing specifically bound 1,25(OH)$_2$[^{3}H]D$_3$) is extracted with methanol–chloroform (2 : 1) and quantitated by liquid scintillation counting. Values are the mean ± S.D.

first subjected to chromatographic separation of the two metabolites. This can readily be accomplished on a 0.8 × 23 cm Sephadex LH-20 column employing chloroform–hexane (1 : 1) as a solvent. Small spikes of both 25(OH)[^{3}H]D$_3$ and 24,25(OH)$_2$[^{3}H]D$_3$ are added to the plasma sample prior to organic solvent extraction and column chromatography to quantitate the recovery of these steroids in the 25(OH)D and 24,25(OH)$_2$D regions of the chromatogram. Although the 25(OH)D region from the Sephadex column can be assayed directly, the 24,25(OH)$_2$D region ideally must be further purified by HPLC chromatography prior to assay.

Taylor *et al.* (1976; Taylor, 1977) reported that the circulating level of 24,25(OH)$_2$D in normal man is 1.63 ± 0.19 ng/ml (S.E.) ($n = 19$). Haddad *et al.* (1976; Haddad, 1977), utilizing a similar but independently developed methodology, found that the concentration of 24,25(OH)$_2$D$_3$ in normal serum is

TABLE 8-8
Application of Assays for 24,25(OH)$_2$D

Nature of study	Average circulatory level (ng/ml ± S.D.) (*n*)	Reference
Normal adult man	1.6±0.2 (19)	Taylor *et al.* (1976)
	3.7±.02 (42)	Haddad *et al.* (1976, 1977), Haddad (1977)
	2.1±0.5 (20)	Lambert *et al.* (1977)
	1.8±0.2 (36)	Caldas *et al.* (1978)
	5.0±0.7 (4)	Hollis *et al.* (1977)
	5.4±2.0 (12)	Norman *et al.* (1978)
	1.7	O'Riordan *et al.* (1977)
	4.5±0.4 (10)	Bishop *et al.* (1979)
Nephrolithiasis	1.5±0.8 (23)	Caldas *et al.* (1978)
Chronic renal failure	0.8±0.4	Taylor (1977)
	3.5±0.7	Haddad *et al.* (1977)
	0.8±0.5 (12)	Norman *et al.* (1978)
Chronic renal failure (anephric)	0	Taylor (1977)
	3.7±1.2 (7)	Haddad *et al.* (1977)
Hyperparathyroidism	2.3±0.4 (19)	Taylor (1977)

approximately 3.7 ± 0.2 ng/ml (n = 42). These and other results are summarized in Table 8-8.

The possibility exists that the circulating level of 24,25(OH)$_2$D may be affected in certain disease states related to vitamin D. This could be determined since there is an apparent reciprocal relationship between the conversion of 25(OH)D_3 to 1,25(OH)$_2D_3$ or 24,25(OH)$_2D_3$ (see Chapter 6). Some disease states might generate physiological signals that favor 1,25(OH)$_2D_3$ over 24,25(OH)$_2D_3$, whereas other disease states might bring about the reverse. Also, since the assay for 1,25(OH)$_2$D is so tedious, time-consuming, and not generally available, it is conceivable that ultimately information obtained from the 24,25(OH)$_2$D assay might be informative from a clinical viewpoint. For example, Taylor (1977) found significantly higher levels of 24,25(OH)$_2$D in patients with hyperparathyroidism and reduced levels of 24,25(OH)$_2$D in serum from patients with chronic renal failure.

V. BONE CALVARIA ASSAY FOR VITAMIN D METABOLITES

Organ cultures of bone have been used for histological and biochemical studies related to vitamin D for over half a century (Fell, 1928, 1956), but only in recent years have attempts been made to utilize this technique as a quantitative approach to evaluating the synthesis and resorption of both the inorganic and organic phases of bone in culture. Raisz (1965) was the first to develop an *in vitro* system in which the movement of calcium out of and into bone could be examined as a function of hormonal stimuli. This technique was further refined by Reynolds and Dingle (1970), who developed a sensitive *in vitro* method for studying the induction and inhibition of bone resorption. It has been used to evaluate (in a structure–function manner) the interaction of metabolites and analogues of vitamin D with the bone system. Half-calvaria from 6-day-old mice that were pulsed 4 days previously with ^{45}Ca are explanted into separate dishes of liquid medium and maintained *in vitro;* one of the half-calvaria serves as a control, and the other is employed for experimentation of the bone mobilizing effects of the vitamin D-related compound. The time course of steroid action is then followed by removing small samples from the media and evaluating the release of ^{45}Ca into the media. This technique has been employed by a number of investigators to evaluate the bone resorptive effects of vitamin D metabolites and analogues. Raisz *et al.* (1972) were the first to evaluate the effects of $1{,}25(OH)_2D_3$ on bone calcium mobilization; they reported that $1{,}25(OH)_2D_3$ was 100 times as potent on a weight basis as $25(OH)D_3$ (in this system the parent vitamin D has no biological activity). Reynolds, in collaboration with DeLuca and colleagues, further evaluated the role of vitamin D metabolites and analogs in bone calcium mobilization (Reynolds *et al.*, 1973, 1974; Reynolds, 1974). Shown in Figure 8-4 is an

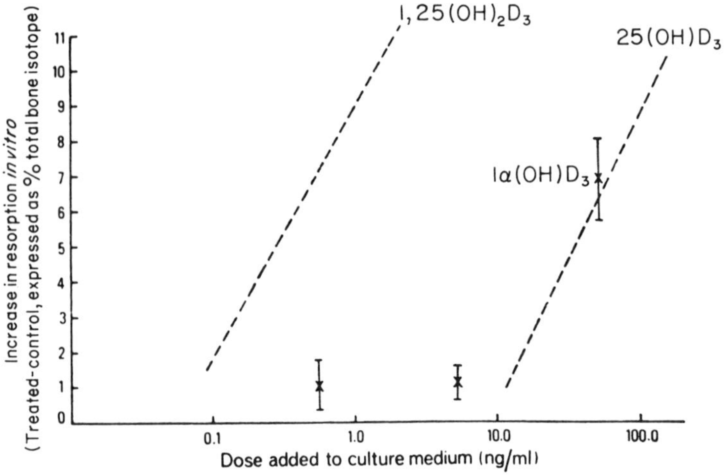

Figure 8-4. Comparison of the response of bone explants to three doses *in vitro* of $1\alpha(OH)D_3$, $25(OH)D_3$, and $1{,}25(OH)_2D_3$. The points are the mean ± S.E., and five pairs of explants were used for each dose level. The response to vitamin D is also indicated. Modified from Fig. 1 of Reynolds *et al.* (1974).

evaluation of the impressive actions of vitamin D metabolites in mediating bone calcium mobilization in this bioassay system. It should be apparent that this assay technique is capable of distinguishing the various structural features of several vitamin D secosteroids.

Stern *et al.* (1975a,b, 1976) have employed this technique to evaluate the relative calcium-mobilizing activities of the two epimers (*R* and *S*) of $24,25(OH)_2D_3$. This technique has also been used by Stern (Stern *et al.*, 1977, 1978) as a means of carrying out a biological evaluation of the circulating levels of $1,25(OH)_2D$ in plasma. It is reassuring that values for plasma $1,25(OH)_2D$ determined by this assay are in good agreement with those obtained from the steroid competition assays (see Table 8-7).

REFERENCES

Baud, L., Paunier, L., Preece, M. A., O'Riordan, J. L. H., Sizonenko, P. C., and Tchicaloff, M. (1974). *Schweiz. Med. Wochenschr.* **104,** 1908.

Bayard, F., Bec, P., and Louvet, J. P. (1972). *Eur. J. Clin. Invest.* **2,** 195.

Bayard, F., Bec, P., Ton That, H., and Louvet, J. P. (1973). *Eur. J. Clin. Invest.* **3,** 447.

Belsey, R. E., DeLuca, H. F., and Potts, J. T. (1971). *J. Clin. Endocrinol. Metab.* **33,** 554.

Belsey, R. E., Clark, M. B., Bernat, M., Glowacki, J., Holick, M. F., DeLuca, H. F., and Potts, J. T. (1974a). *Am. J. Med.* **57,** 50.

Belsey, R. E., DeLuca, H. F., and Potts, J. T. (1974b). *J. Clin. Endocrinol. Metab.* **38,** 1046.

Belsey, R. E., DeLuca, H. F., and Potts, J. T. (1974c). *Nature (London)* **247,** 208.

Bjorkhem, I., and Holmberg, I. (1976). *Clin. Chim. Acta* **68,** 215.

Bishop, J. E., Norman, A. W., Roberts, P. A., Coburn, J. W., and Henry, H. L. (1979). *J. Mineral. Electrolyte Metab.* (in press).

Bouillon, R., Reynaert, J., Claes, J. H., Lissens, W., and DeMoor, P. (1975). *J. Clin. Endocrinol. Metab.* **41,** 1130.

Bouillon, R., Van Kerkhove, P., and DeMoor, P. (1976a). *Clin. Chem.* **22,** 364.

Bouillon, R., Van Baelen, H., Rombauts, W., and DeMoor, P. (1976b). *Eur. J. Biochem.* **66,** 285.

Bouillon, R., Van Baelen, H., and DeMoor, P. (1976c). *Biochem. J.* **159,** 463.

Bouillon, R., Van Baelen, H., and DeMoor, P. (1977). *J. Clin. Endocrinol. Metab.* **45,** 225.

Brumbaugh, P. F., and Haussler, M. R. (1973). *Biochem. Biophys. Res. Commun.* **51,** 1973a.

Brumbaugh, P. F., and Haussler, M. R. (1974a). *J. Biol. Chem.* **249,** 1251.

Brumbaugh, P. F., and Haussler, M. R. (1974b). *J. Biol. Chem.* **249,** 1258.

Brumbaugh, P. F., Haussler, D. H., Bursac, K. M., and Haussler, M. R. (1974a). *Biochemistry* **13,** 4091.

Brumbaugh, P. F., Haussler, D. H., Bressler, R., and Haussler, M. R. (1974b). *Science* **183,** 1089.

Bukin, U. N., and Areshkina, Y. L. (1958). *Proc. Int. Symp. Enzyme Chem., 1957,* p. 475.

Caldas, A. E., Gray, R. W., and Lemann, J., Jr. (1978). *J. Lab. Clin. Med.* **91,** 840.

Cavalli-Sforza, L. L., Daiger, S. P., and Rummel, D. P. (1977). *Am. J. Hum. Genet.* **29,** 581.

Chalk, K. J. J., and Kodicek, E. (1961). *Biochem. J.* **79,** 1.

Chen, P. S., Jr., and Lane, K. (1965). *Arch. Biochem. Biophys.* **112,** 70.

Christakos, S., and Norman, A. W. (1979). *Biochem. Biophys. Res. Commun.* **87,** in press.

Clemens, T. L., Hendy, G. N., Graham, R. F., Baggiolini, E. G., Uskoković, M. R., and O'Riordan, J. L. (1978). *J. Endocrin.* **77,** 49P.

Cleve, H. (1973). *Isr. J. Med. Sci.* **9,** 1133.

Cohn, E. J., Gurd, F. R. N., Surgener, D. M., Barnes, B. D., Brown, R. K., Deronaux, G., Gillespie, J. M., Kahrt, F. W., Lever, W. F., Liu, C. H., Mittelman, D., Monton, R. M., Schmid, K., and Uroma, E. (1950). *J. Am. Chem. Soc.* **72,** 465.

Daiger, S. P. (1975). Ph.D. Dissertation, Stanford University, Stanford, California.

Daiger, S. P., and Cavalli-Sforza, L. L. (1977). *Am. J. Hum. Genet.* **29,** 593.

Daiger, S. P., Schanfield, M. S., and Cavalli-Sforza, L. L. (1975). *Proc. Natl. Acad. Sci. U.S.A.* **72,** 2076.

Davies, D. P., Hughes, C. A., and Moore, J. R. (1978). *Arch. Dis. Child.* **53,** 88.

DeCrousaz, P., Blanc, B., and Antener, I. (1965). *Helv. Odontol. Acta* **9,** 151.

DeLuca, H. F. (1967). *Vitam. Horm. (N.Y.)* **25,** 315.

Dent, C. E., and Gupta, M. M. (1975). *Lancet* **2,** 1057.

Diezner, M. K., Neelson, F. A., Haussler, M., McPherson, N. T., and Lebovitz, H. E. (1976). *J. Clin. Endocrinol. Metab.* **42,** 621.

Dorantes, L. M., Arnaud, S. B., and Arnaud, C. D. (1978). *J. Lab. Clin. Med.* **91,** 791.

Edelstein, S. (1974). *Biochem. Soc. Spec. Publ.* **3,** 43.

Edelstein, S., Lawson, D. E. M., and Kodicek, E. (1972). *Biochim. Biophys. Acta* **270,** 570.

Edelstein, S., Lawson, D. E. M., and Kodicek, E. (1973). *Biochem. J.* **135,** 417.

Edelstein, S., Charman, M., Lawson, D. E. M., and Kodicek, E. (1974). *Clin. Sci. Mol. Med.* **46,** 231.

Edelstein, S., Eizenberg, Z., and Harell, A. (1976). *FEBS Lett.* **62,** 245.

Eisman, J. A., Hamstra, A. J., Kream, B. E., and DeLuca, H. F. (1976a). *Science* **193,** 1021.

Eisman, J. A., Hamstra, A. J., Kream, B. E., and DeLuca, H. F. (1976b). *Arch. Biochem. Biophys.* **176,** 235.

Eisman, J. A., Shepard, R. M., and DeLuca, H. F. (1977). *Anal. Biochem.* **89,** 298.

Fell, H. B. (1928). *Arch. Exp. Zellforsch. Besonders Gewebezuecht.* **7,** 390.

Fell, H. B. (1956). *In* "The Biochemistry and Physiology of Bone" (G. H. Bourne, ed.), 1st ed., p. 401. Academic Press, New York.

Fraser, D. R., and Emtage, J. S. (1976). *Biochem. J.* **160,** 671.

Garcia-Pascual, B., Peytremann, A., Courvoisier, B., and Lawson, D. E. M. (1976). *Clin. Chim. Acta* **68,** 99.

Greenberg, P. B., Hillyard, C. J., Galante, L. S., Colston, K. W., Evans, I. M. A., and MacIntyre, I. (1974). *Clin. Sci. Mol. Med.* **46,** 143.

Gupta, M. M., Round, J. M., and Stamp, T. C. B. (1974). *Lancet* **1,** 586.

Haddad, J. G. (1977). *In* "Vitamin D: Biochemical, Chemical and Clinical Aspects Related to Calcium Metabolism" (A. W. Norman *et al.*, eds.), p. 463. de Gruyter, Berlin.

Haddad, J. G., and Birge, S. J. (1971). *Biochem. Biophys. Res. Commun.* **45,** 829.

Haddad, J. G., and Birge, S. J. (1974). *Endocrinology* **94,** 178.

Haddad, J. G., and Birge, S. J. (1975). *J. Biol. Chem.* **250,** 299.

Haddad, J. G., and Chyu, K. J. (1971a). *J. Clin. Endocrinol. Metab.* **33,** 992.

Haddad, J. G., and Chyu, K. J., (1971b). *Biochim. Biophys. Acta* **248,** 471.

Haddad, J. G., and Chyu, K. J. (1971c). *Clin. Res.* **19,** 49.

Haddad, J. G., and Hahn, T. J. (1973). *Nature (London)* **244,** 515.

Haddad, J. G., and Stamp, T. C. B. (1974). *Am. J. Med.* **57,** 57.

Haddad, J. G., and Walgate, J. (1976). *J. Clin. Invest.* **51,** 1217.

Haddad, J. G., Hahn, T. J., and Birge, S. F. (1973a). *Biochim. Biophys. Acta* **329,** 93.

Haddad, J. G., Chyu, K. J., Hahn, T. H., and Stamp, T. C. B. (1973b). *J. Lab. Clin. Med.* **81,** 22.

Haddad, J. G., Min, C., Walgate, J., and Hahn, T. (1976). *J. Clin. Endocrinol. Metab.* **43,** 712.

Haddad, J. G., Min, C., Mendelsohn, M., Slatopolsky, E., and Hahn, T. J. (1977). *Arch. Biochem. Biophys.* **182,** 390.
Hahn, T. B., Hindin, B. A., Scharp, C. R., and Haddad, J. G. (1972). *N. Engl. J. Med.* **287,** 900.
Hahn, T. J., Hindin, B. A., Scharp, C. R., Boisseau, V. C., and Haddad, J. G. Jr. (1975). *N. Engl. J. Med.* **292,** 550.
Haussler, M. R., Baylink, D. J., Hughes, M. R., Brumbaugh, P. F., Wergedal, J. E., Shen, F. H., Nillsen, R. L., Counts, S. J., Bursac, K. M., and McCain, T. A. (1976). *Clin. Endocrinol. (N.Y.)* **5,** 1515.
Haussler, M. R., Hughes, M. R., Pike, J. W., and McCain, T. A. (1977). *In* "Vitamin D: Biochemical, Chemical and Clinical Aspects Related to Calcium Metabolism" (A. W. Norman *et al.,* eds.), p. 473. de Gruyter, Berlin.
Hay, A. W. M. (1975). *Biochem. J.* **151,** 193.
Hay, A. W. M., and Watson, G. (1975). *Nature (London)* **256,** 150.
Hay, A. W. M., and Watson, G. (1976a). *Comp. Biochem. Physiol. B* **53,** 163.
Hay, A. W. M., and Watson, G. (1976b). *Comp. Biochem. Physiol. B* **53,** 167.
Hay, A. W. M., and Watson, G. (1977). *Comp. Biochem. Physiol. B* **56,** 131.
Henry, H., and Norman, A. W. (1975). *Comp. Biochem. Physiol. B* **50,** 431.
Hillman, L., and Haddad, J. G. (1974). *J. Pediatr.* **84,** 742.
Hillman, L., and Haddad, J. G. (1977). *J. Pediatr.* **125,** 196.
Hirschfeld, J. (1959). *Acta Pathol. Microbiol. Scand.* **47,** 160.
Hollis, B. W., Burton, J. H., and Draper, H. H. (1977) *Steroids* **30,** 285.
Hosoya, N., and Oku, T. (1971). *J. Vitaminol.* **17,** 119.
Hosoya, N., Oku, T., and Moriuchi, S. (1970). *Vitamins* **41,** 325.
Hughes, M. R., Baylink, D. J., Jones, P. G., and Haussler, M. R. (1976). *J. Clin. Invest.* **58,** 61.
Imawari, M., Kida, K., and Goodman, D. S. (1976). *J. Clin. Invest.* **58,** 514.
Jacob, R. L., and Ray, R. D. (1968). *Clin. Orthop. Relat. Res.* **56,** 275.
Jubiz, W., Haussler, M. R., McCain, T. A., and Tolman, K. G. (1977). *J. Clin. Endocrinol. Metab.* **44,** 617.
Juo, P., and Isenberg, G. R. (1972). *C. R. Hebd. Seances Acad. Sci.* **46,** 59.
Kaplan, R. A., Haussler, M. R., Deftos, L. J., Bone, H., and Pak, C. Y. C. (1977). *J. Clin. Invest.* **59,** 756.
Katz, M., and Cooper, B. A. (1974). *J. Clin. Invest.* **54,** 733.
Kida, K., and Goodman, D. S. (1976). *J. Lipid Res.* **17,** 485.
Koshy, K. T., and VanDerSlik, A. L. (1978). *Anal. Biochem.* **85,** 283.
Kream, B., Reynolds, R. D., Knutson, J. C., Eisman, J. A., and DeLuca, H. F. (1976). *Arch. Biochem. Biophys.* **176,** 779.
Lambert, P. W., Syverson, B. F., Arnaud, C. D., and Spelsburg, T. C. (1977). *J. Steroid Biochem.* **8,** 929.
Long, R. G., Skinner, R. K., Meinhard, E., Wills, M. R., and Sherlock, S. (1976). *Gut* **17,** 824.
Lund, B., Sorensen, O. H., and Christensen, A. B. (1975). *Lancet* **2,** 300.
McLaughlin, M. A., Lester Fairney, E., Raggatt, P. R., Brown, D. J., and Wills, M. R. (1974). *Lancet* **1,** 536.
Mawer, E. B., Backhouse, J., Holman, C. A., Lumb, G. A., and Stanbury, S. W. (1972). *Clin. Sci.* **43,** 413.
Morgan, H. G., Thomas, W. C., Haddock, L., and Eager, J. (1958). *Trans. Assoc. Am. Physicians* **71,** 93.
Mosekilde, L., Lund, B., Sorensen, O., Christensen, M. S., and Melsen, F. (1977). *Lancet* **1,** 806.
Neer, R. M., Clark, M. B., Sweeney, M. T., Belsey, R. E., and Potts, J. T. (1977). *In* "Vitamin D: Biochemical, Chemical and Clinical Aspects Related to Calcium Metabolism" (A. W. Norman *et al.,* eds.), p. 595. de Gruyter, Berlin.

Nilsson, S. F., Ostberg, L., and Peterson, P. A. (1972). *Biochem. Biophys. Res. Commun.* **46,** 1380.
Norman, A. W., and DeLuca, H. F. (1963). *Biochemistry* **3,** 1160.
Norman, A. W., Henry, H. L., Bishop, J. E., and Coburn, J. W. (1978). *Clin. Res.* **26,** 432A.
Norman, A. W., Schaefer, K., von Herrath, D., Grigoleit, H.-G., Mawer, E. B., Suda, T., DeLuca, H. F., and Coburn, J. W., eds. (1979). "Vitamin D. Recent Basic Advances and their Clinical Application (Proceedings of the Fourth Workshop on Vitamin D)" Walter de Gruyter Publishing Company, Elmsford, New York.
Offermann, G., and Dittmar, F. (1974). *Horm. Metab. Res.* **6,** 534.
Offermann, G., von Herrath, D., and Schaefer, K. (1974). *Nephron* **13,** 269–277.
Oku, T., Matsura, J., and Hosoya, N. (1972). *Vitamins* **45,** 90.
O'Riordan, J. L. H., and Aurbach, G. D. (1968). *Endocrinology* **82,** 377.
O'Riordan, J. L. H., Graham, R. F., and Dolev, D. (1977). *In* "Vitamin D: Biochemical, Chemical and Clinical Aspects Related to Calcium Metabolism" (A. W. Norman *et al.,* eds.), p. 519, de Gruyter, Berlin.
Osborn, T. W., and Norman, A. W. (1975). *Clin. Res.* **23,** 113A.
Osborn, T. W. (1976). Ph.D. Dissertation, University of California, Riverside.
Peterson, P. A. (1971). *J. Biol. Chem.* **246,** 7748.
Preece, M. A., O'Riordan, J. L. H., Lawson, D. E. M., and Kodicek, E. (1974). *Clin. Chim. Acta* **54,** 245.
Preece, M. A., Tomlinson, S., Ribot, C. A., Pietrek, J., Korn, H. T., Davies, D. M., Ford, J. A., Dunnigan, M. G., and O'Riordan, J. L. H. (1975). *Q. J. Med.* **44,** 575.
Procsal, D. A., Okamura, W. H., and Norman, A. W. (1975). *J. Biol. Chem.* **250,** 8382.
Raisz, L. G. (1965). *J. Clin. Invest.* **44,** 103.
Raisz, L. G., Trummel, C. L., Holick, M. F., and DeLuca, H. F. (1972). *Science* **175,** 768.
Reynolds, J. J. (1974). *Biochem. Soc. Spec. Publ.* **3,** 91.
Reynolds, J. J., and Dingle, J. T. (1970). *Calcif. Tissue Res.* **4,** 329.
Reynolds, J. J., Holick, M. F., and DeLuca, H. F. (1973). *Calcif. Tissue Res.* **12,** 295.
Reynolds, J. J., Holick, M. F., and DeLuca, H. F. (1974). *Calcif. Tissue Res.* **15,** 333.
Riggs, B. L., and Gallagher, J. C.)1977). *In* "Vitamin D: Biochemical, Chemical and Clinical Aspects Related to Calcium Metabolism" (A. W. Norman *et al.,* eds.), p. 639, de Gruyter, Berlin.
Rikkers, H., and DeLuca, H. F. (1967). *J. Physiol. (London)* **213,** 380.
Roginsky, M., Moo, H. F., and Abesamis, C. (1974). *Lancet* **1,** 1235.
Rojanasathit, S., and Haddad, J. G. (1976). *Biochim. Biophys. Acta* **421,** 12.
Rosenstreich, S. J., Volwiler, W., and Rich, C. (1971). *Am. J. Clin. Nutr.* **24,** 897.
Schachter, D., Finkelstein, J. D., and Kowarski, S. (1964). *J. Clin. Invest.* **43,** 787.
Schaefer, P. C., and Goldsmith, R. S. (1978). *J. Lab. Clin. Med.* **91,** 104.
Schaefer, P. C., Lifschitz, M. D., Fadens, S. Z., and Goldsmith, R. S. (1978). *Abstr. 60th Meet. U.S. Endocr. Soc.* pp. 235 and 320.
Schneider, L. F., Schedl, H. P., McCain, T., and Haussler, M. R. (1977). *Science* **196,** 1452.
Seino, Y., Shimotsuji, T., Kai, H., Ikehara, C., and Yabuuchi, H. (1978). *Acta Paediatr. Scand.* **67,** 39.
Shany, S., Yagil, R., and Berlyne, G. M. (1978). *Comp. Biochem. Physiol. B* **59,** 139.
Sharpe, R., Hillyard, C. J., Szelke, M., and MacIntyre, I. (1977). *FEBS Lett.* **75,** 265.
Simons, K., and Bearn, A. G. (1967). *Biochim. Biophys. Acta* **133,** 499.
Skinner, R. K., Long, R. G., Sherlock, S., and Wills, M. R. (1977). *Lancet* **1,** 720.
Smith, J. E., and Goodman, D. S. (1971). *J. Clin. Invest.* **50,** 2159.
Stamp, T. C. B., and Round, J. M. (1974). *Nature (London)* **247,** 563.
Stamp, T. C. B., Round, J., Rowe, D., and Haddad, J. G. (1972). *Br. Med. J.* **4,** 9.

Stamp, T. C. B., Haddad, J. G., and Twigg, C. A. (1977). *Lancet* **1,** 1341.

Stern, P. H., Trummel, C. L., Schnoes, H. K., and DeLuca, H. F. (1975a). *Endocrinology* **97,** 1552.

Stern, P. H., DeLuca, H. F., and Ikekawa, N. (1975b). *Biochem. Biophys. Res. Commun.* **67,** 965.

Stern, P. H., Mavreas, T., Trummel, C. L., Schnoes, H. K., and DeLuca, H. F. (1976). *Mol. Pharmacol.* **12,** 8979.

Stern, P. H., Phillips, T. E., Lucas, S. V., Hamstra, A. J., DeLuca, H. F., and Bell, N. H. (1977). *In* "Vitamin D: Biochemical, Chemical and Clinical Aspects Related to Calcium Metabolism" (A. W. Norman *et al.*, eds.), p. 531. de Gruyter, Berlin.

Stern, P. H., Hamstra, A. J., DeLuca, H. F., and Bell, N. (1978). *J. Clin. Endocrinol. Metab.* **46,** 891.

Taylor, C. M. (1977). *In* "Proceedings of the Third Workshop on Vitamin D: Biochemical, Chemical and Clinical Aspects Related to Calcium Metabolism" (A. W. Norman *et al.*, eds.), p. 546. de Gruyter, Berlin.

Taylor, C. M., Hughes, S. E., and deSilva, P. (1976). *Biochem. Biophys. Res. Commun.* **70,** 1243.

Thomas, W. C., Morgan, H. G., Connor, T. B., Haddock, L., Bills, C. E., and Howard, J. E. (1959). *J. Clin. Invest.* **38,** 1078.

Tsai, H. C., and Norman, A. W. (1973a). *Biochem. Biophys. Res. Commun.* **54,** 622.

Tsai, H. C., and Norman, A. W. (1973b). *J. Biol. Chem.* **248,** 5967.

Tsai, H. C., Wong, R. G., and Norman, A. W. (1972). *J. Biol. Chem.* **247,** 5511.

Turton, C. W. G., Stanley, P., Stamp, T. C. B., and Maxwell, J. O. (1977). *Lancet* **1,** 222.

Velentzas, C., Oreopoulos, D. G., Brandes, L., Wilson, D. R., and Marquez-Julio, A. (1977). *Ann. Intern. Med.* **86,** 198.

Van Baelen, H., Bouillon, R., and DeMoor, P. (1977). *J. Biol. Chem.* **252,** 2515.

Wecksler, W. R., and Norman, A. W. (1978). *J. Mineral Electrolyte Metab.* **1,** 99.

Wecksler, W. R., Mason, R. S., and Norman, A. W. (1979a). *J. Clin. Endocrin. Metab.* **48,** 715.

Wecksler, W. R., Ross, F. P., Mason, R. S., Posen, S., and Norman, A. W. (1979). *Arch. Biochem. Biophys.* (in press).

White, A., Handler, P., and Smith, E. L. (1968). "Principles of Biochemistry," 4th ed., pp. 942 and 948. McGraw-Hill, New York.

CHAPTER

9

Interrelationships between Vitamin D and Other Hormones

I. INTRODUCTORY COMMENTS

A. Physiological Roles of Vitamin D, Parathyroid Hormone, and Calcitonin

Any consideration of the interrelationships between vitamin D and other hormones must take into account the known physiological effects of vitamin D as well as of parathyroid hormone and calcitonin on calcium and phosphorus metabolism. The purpose of this chapter is not so much to describe calcium and phosphorus homeostasis in detail, but to point out the major interactions of parathyroid hormone, calcitonin, and several other hormones with vitamin D. Table 9-1 summarizes the physiological effects of the three principal hormones of calcium and phosphorus metabolism.

The intertwining actions of the three hormones of calcium and phosphorus homeostasis clearly reflect the crucial roles of both calcium and phosphate in the biological processes of higher animals. It is of utmost importance to maintain extracellular calcium ion concentration within narrow limits; accordingly, the higher the phylogenetic order, the greater the complexity of sophisticated endocrinological interrelationships and mechanisms developed to ensure ion homeostasis.

Calcium is essential to a great number of cellular processes (see Table 10-1). One need only recall the important role of calcium in muscle contraction, its key role in the process of blood clotting, its obligatory association with a number of enzyme activities, its possible role as a "second messenger" in many cyclic AMP-mediated responses, and its obvious contribution to the skeleton as well as to the formation of eggshell in birds to gain insight into the *raison de être* of its stringent regulation.

Calcium homeostasis may be disturbed in a wide variety of disease states (see Chapter 13), so a working knowledge of calcium and phosphorus regulation is essential to the treatment of many clinically important diseases. It is not within the province of this chapter to discuss the abnormalities in the endocrine interrelationships between vitamin D and other hormones that relate to the pathophysiology of these disorders. Chapter 13 discusses these disorders in relation to perturbations in vitamin D function.

The three prime target tissues related to calcium and phosphorus homeostasis are the intestine, where these ions enter into the physiological milieu, the bone, where they are stored and made available for minute-by-minute regulation of the serum levels of these ions, and the kidney, where their principal rate of excretion can be affected. The maintenance of calcium and phosphorus homeostasis thus involves the delicate interrelationships of absorption by the intestine, accretion and reabsorption by bone tissue, and urinary excretion by the kidney.

Calcium in plasma exists in three forms: free and ionized, complexed to organic ions such as citrate, and protein bound. The total concentration of calcium in plasma is normally 2.5 m*M*, or 10 mg per 100 ml. Under normal circumstances approximately 46% of the total plasma calcium is bound to protein (primarily to serum albumin), the remaining 54% being ultrafilterable. Thus, there are two basic mechanisms for generating free or ionized calcium in the plasma: that which can be manipulated by endocrine mechanisms and that which can occur by changing the concentrations of plasma protein. It is assumed that

TABLE 9-1
Physiological Effects of Calcitonin, Parathyroid Hormone, and Vitamin D (and Metabolites) Related to Mineral Metabolism

Effect	Calcitonin	Parathyroid hormone	Vitamin D
Intestinal			
Calcium absorption	↓?	↑	↑
Phosphate absorption	?	?	↑
Renal[a]			
Phosphate excretion	↑	↑	↓
Calcium excretion	↑	↓	↓
Hydrogen excretion	→	↓	?
Potassium excretion	Slight ↑	↑	?
Sodium excretion	↑	↑	?
Adenyl cyclase activity	→	↑	?
Skeletal			
Calcium mobilization	↓	↑	↑
Mineralization of bone matrix	—	—	↑
Other			
Plasma levels of calcium	↓	↑	↑
Plasma levels of phosphate	↓	↓	—
Body weight	?	?	Increases

[a]Abstracted from Rasmussen (1974).

the useful and therefore regulated portion of calcium is the ionized species, since there is no evidence that endocrinological changes affect the protein binding of calcium.

The plasma concentrations of the several ionic species of phosphate are not so stringently regulated; rather, they are manipulated in concert with the endocrine perturbation which may have effected changes in calcium concentration. Under normal circumstances phosphate is present in plasma at a level of 1.2 m*M*, or in the range of 2.5 to 4.3 mg per 100 ml (of phosphorus). Approximately 10% of the plasma phosphate is protein bound; the remainder exists as free phosphate, either as HPO_4^{2-} or $H_2PO_4^-$. The relative proportions of these two species, of course, are dependent on plasma pH. There are many biological uses of phosphate extending from its role as an inorganic ion to its multiple involvements as organic phosphate in a plethora of both enzymatic and structural proteins as well as in nucleic acids.

It is apparent from Table 9-1 that vitamin D plays a dominant role in increasing the intestinal absorption of calcium and phosphorus; however, it should be appreciated that this uptake process is regulated according to the needs of the animal and is dictated by certain physiological signals. Once calcium and phosphate are made available in the plasma, a delicate balancing operation occurs between accretion and mobilization in the bone and excretion by the kidney. In the event that the dietary intake or availability of calcium and phosphorus is diminished or increased, it is possible to tip the balance in favor of increased bone mobilization or increased bone accretion to meet the stringent prerequisite of a constant serum calcium level. Thus, serum calcium may become elevated via stimulation of bone calcium mobilization or via parathyroid hormone stimulation of the tubular reabsorption of calcium at the kidney. Concomitantly, PTH also stimulates phosphate excretion so that as serum calcium concentration increases there is usually an associated fall in the plasma phosphate level. In contrast, if serum calcium levels become too elevated the action of calcitonin may come into play. Simply speaking, calcitonin is believed to block many of the actions of PTH at the skeletal level, thereby preventing further elevation of serum calcium levels. Also associated with increased secretion of calcitonin is an increase in calcium excretion by the kidney, which can contribute to a reduction in circulating levels of serum calcium.

It is clear that bone is the central organ in calcium metabolism, acting as both a source of and a reservoir for calcium and phosphorus. Information concerning the role of vitamin D and its metabolites and bone metabolism is discussed in Chapter 12. However, it is apparent that bone remodeling processes may contribute to both short and long time intervals necessary for calcium and phosphorus homeostasis. Both are under intimate endocrine regulation by parathyroid hormone, calcitonin, and possibly vitamin D or its metabolites.

In recent years an important concept has been developed regarding the role of vitamin D in calcium homeostasis. The major theme of this book is that vitamin D is in reality a steroid hormone and that its mode of action is analogous to that of other steroid hormones. It has further become evident that it is informative to analyze the role of vitamin D in calcium and phosphorus homeostasis from an endocrinological perspective. As a consequence, certain conceptual advances have occurred that have made it possible to integrate the actions of vitamin D on calcium and phosphate metabolism with the more classic endocrinological actions of parathyroid hormone and calcitonin on these ions. It has been conclusively shown that vitamin D_3 is first metabolized by the liver to produce $25(OH)D_3$ and that this compound in turn is metabolized by the kidney to produce $24,25(OH)_2D_3$ and $1,25(OH)_2D_3$. There are now increasing examples of the existence of hormone relationships between vitamin D and its metabolites and other more classic endocrine systems.

B. Dynamics and Requirements of Calcium and Phosphate Metabolism

Figure 9-1 is a schematic diagram illustrating calcium and phosphorus metabolism in a normal adult male. Calcium and phosphorus are both absorbed into the body primarily in the duodenum and jejunum (for details, see Chapter

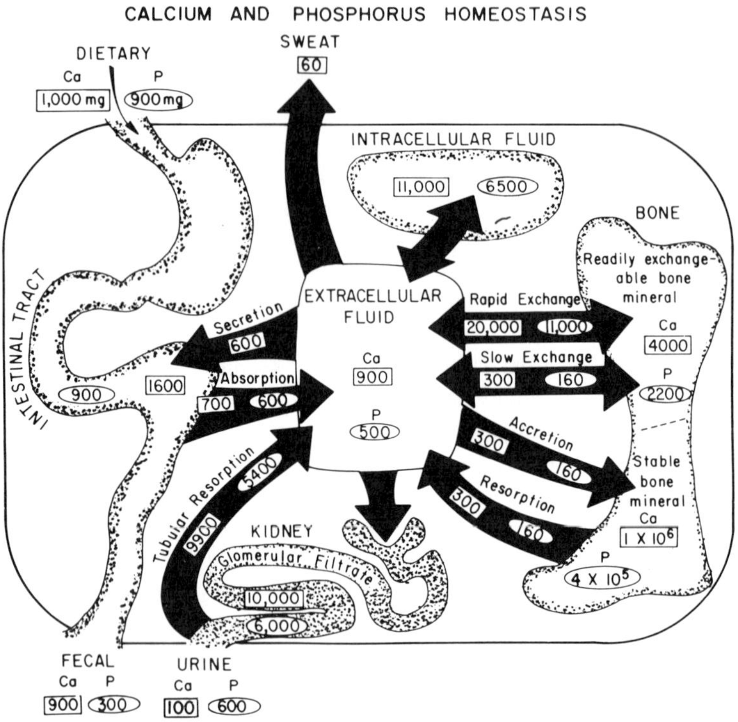

Figure 9-1. A schematic model of calcium and phosphorus metabolism in an adult man having a calcium intake of 1.0 g/day and a phosphorus intake of 0.8 g/day. All numerical values are milligrams per day. All entries relating to phosphate are calculated as phosphorus and are enclosed in ovals. Entries related to calcium are enclosed in boxes.

10). In addition to the calcium ingested in the diet (for normal man, the dietary requirements range from 400 to 1200 mg/day), approximately 600–700 mg is added to the intestinal contents via intestinal secretions. Thus, of the approximate total of 1600 to 1700 mg of calcium present in the lumen of the intestine, shown in the model in Fig. 9-1, approximately 700 mg is reabsorbed, or absorbed into the bloodstream, leaving the remaining 900–1000 mg to be excreted in the feces. After calcium has entered the extracellular pool, it is in constant flux or exchange with the calcium already present in the extra- and intracellular fluids and in certain compartments of the bone and the glomerular filtrate. The entire extracellular pool of calcium turns over between 40 and 50 times per day. On a daily basis the glomerulus filters some 10,000 mg of calcium, but the renal tubular reabsorption of this ion is so efficient that under normal circumstances only between 100 and 150 mg appear in the urine. In the event of hypercalcemia, the urinary excretion of calcium rises in a compensatory fashion. However, it rarely exceeds a value of 400 to 600 mg/day. The renal tubular reabsorption of calcium

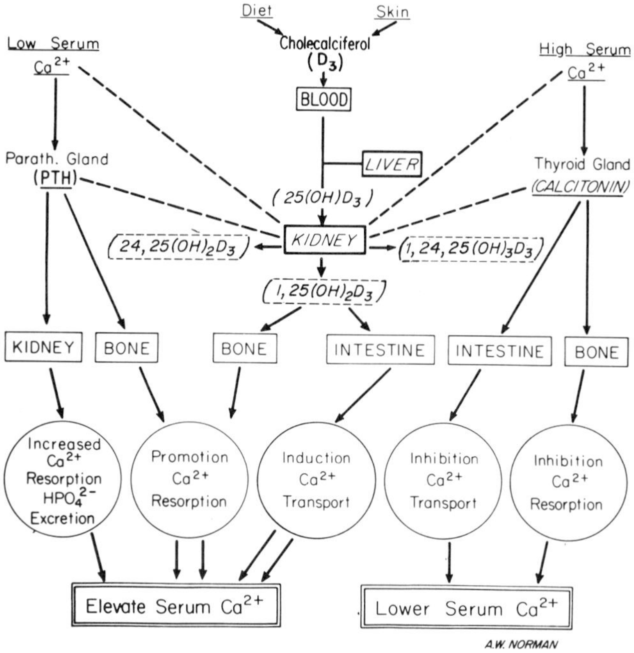

Figure 9-2. Summary of calcium homeostasis.

is stimulated by parathyroid hormone and possibly by vitamin D or one of its metabolites. The increased urinary excretion of calcium is stimulated by phosphate deprivation, acidosis, adrenal steroids, and saline diuresis. Also, it should be noted that an additional 30–100 mg of calcium is lost per day through the skin via sweating.

The term "readily exchangeable bone pool" is not definable explicitly in anatomical terms. It simply represents that fraction of calcium in bone that is in rapid equilibrium with calcium in the plasma, where "rapid" implies the capability of exchange on a minute-by-minute basis. Of the total bone calcium of 1000 to 1200 g in a 70-kg man, approximately 0.4%, or 4000 mg, is present in the readily exchangeable bone pool compartment.

The dynamics of phosphate metabolism are not particularly different from that of calcium. Under normal circumstances, approximately 70% of the phosphate in the diet is absorbed. Absorption of phosphate is interrelated in a complex fashion with the presence of calcium and can be stimulated by a low-calcium diet as well as by vitamin D or its metabolites. The intestinal absorption of phosphate is inhibited by high dietary calcium levels, aluminum hydroxide ingestion,[1] and

[1]Aluminum hydroxide capsules are often given to individuals with chronic renal failure to diminish the level of intestinal phosphate absorption.

beryllium poisoning. Phosphate in the body is also partitioned among three major pools: the kidney ultrafiltrate, the readily exchangeable fraction of bone, and the intracellular compartments in the various soft tissues.

As indicated in Fig. 9-1, the major excretory route for phosphate is via the kidney. The handling of phosphate by the kidney is determined by the rate of glomerular filtration, tubular reabsorption, and possibly tubular secretion. Thus, the glomerulus filters some 6000–10,000 mg of phosphorus per day. A normal man given a diet of 900 mg of phosphorus excretes approximately 600 mg/day in the urine. As indicated above, the major endocrine function of PTH is to regulate the tubular reabsorption of phosphate. Thus, high circulating levels of PTH stimulate the urinary excretion of phosphate by blocking the tubular reabsorption of the inorganic ion present in the glomerular filtrate. The urinary excretion of inorganic phosphate may be decreased by kidney failure, hypoparathyroidism, phosphate deficiency, and Addison's disease. A detailed discussion of the physiological handling of calcium and phosphate is given by Rasmussen (1974). (See also Figure 9-2.)

II. PARATHYROID HORMONE AND CALCITONIN

A. Effects of Parathyroid Hormone on Vitamin D Metabolism

A detailed discussion of the regulation of vitamin D metabolism is presented in Chapter 6. As indicated in Chapter 6 there appear to be at least two mechanisms by which the output of $1,25(OH)_2D_3$ by the kidney can be modulated: (a) a short-time-scale regulatory process in which, on a minute-by-minute basis, changes in the ionic environment of the mitochondria effect a change in the activity of the $25(OH)D_3$ 1-hydroxylase; (b) a regulatory scheme involving hours during which changes occur in the absolute level of active 1-hydroxylase molecules in the mitochondria. It is entirely probable but has not yet been proved that the effects of parathyroid hormone may be manifest on both general regulatory processes. That is, if PTH has the capability of changing the concentration of a critical ionic regulator in renal cortical cells then it could inhibit or stimulate the production of $1,25(OH)_2 D_3$. Furthermore, it is suggested in Chapter 6 that PTH is a trophic stimulator of the biosynthesis of the 25(OH)D 1-hydroxylase, and accordingly there is proposed a major endocrine interaction between the peptide hormone PTH and the biosynthesis of the steroid hormone $1,25(OH)_2D_3$. The view has been advanced that the simplest model of regulation of the production of $1,25(OH)_2D_3$ that accounts for the bulk of published observations in the literature is that in which the rate of synthesis of the $25(OH)D_3$ 1-hydroxylase is dependent on a ratio of PTH to vitamin D status. This is not intended to imply that it is simply the ratio of the circulating levels of these hormones that is the determining factor, but to indicate an empirical relationship based on the collected available results. This is one way of expressing the concept that the action of one regulator cannot be compensated for exclusively by reciprocal changes in the other; each hormone can carry out its regulation only in the presence of some finite amount of the other. As the amount of either PTH or vitamin D becomes very low (parathyroidectomy or vitamin D deficiency, respectively), the rate of biosynthesis of the $25(OH)D_3$ 1-hydroxylase approaches its lower or upper limit, respectively. Furthermore, it is not vitamin D itself that is involved in the regulatory process, but $1,25(OH)_2D_3$ or another metabolite or some unidentified parameter that has yet to be characterized.

Figure 9-3 is a generalized scheme integrating many of the published data concerning potential regulators of the production of $1,25(OH)_2D_3$.

In general two approaches have been employed. The first involves experiments carried out *in vivo* in which the endocrine function of the animal may be perturbed followed by subsequent evaluation *in vitro* of the effects of $1,25(OH)_2D_3$ on renal production. The second approach involves preparation of

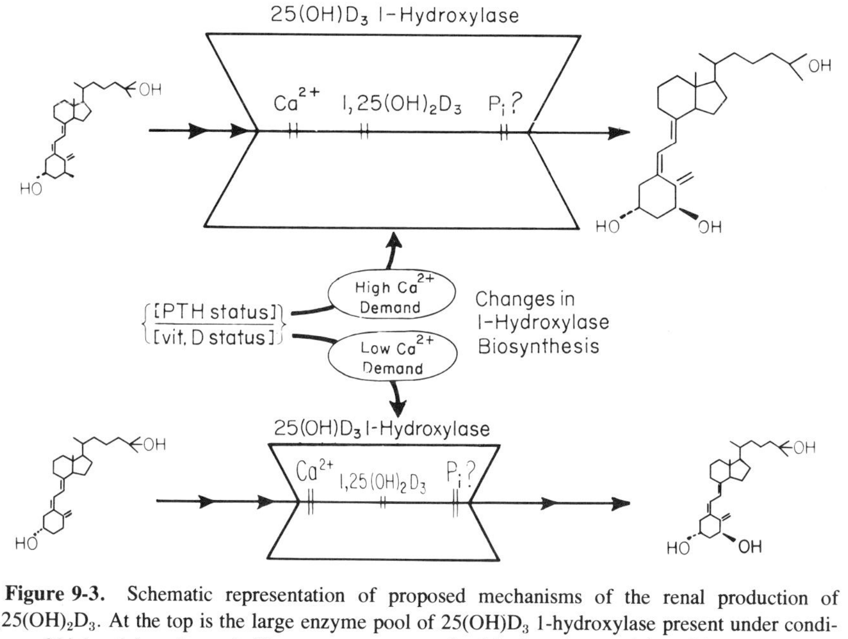

Figure 9-3. Schematic representation of proposed mechanisms of the renal production of $1,25(OH)_2D_3$. At the top is the large enzyme pool of $25(OH)D_3$ 1-hydroxylase present under conditions of high calcium demand. The consequences on the 1-hydroxylase activity of low calcium demand are shown at the bottom. Calcium demand is "coupled" to the 1-hydroxylase specific activity by the [PTH status]/[vitamin D status] ratio of the animal. In both instances there may be direct inhibitory effects of the product $1,25(OH)_2D_3$ and of the calcium and phosphate ions.

renal tubules or homogenates of kidney or mitochondria, which are then subjected to a variety of putative endocrine signals *in vitro* such as the presence of PTH or cAMP.

Fraser and Kodicek (1973) were the first to directly implicate PTH as a potential stimulator of the production of $1,25(OH)_2D_3$ by the kidney. They carried out parathyroidectomy on vitamin D-deficient chicks and then determined the effect of replacement PTH extracts on the levels of the $25(OH)D_3$ 1-hydroxylase. Also, Garabedian *et al.* (1972) reported that thyroparathyroidectomy of rats on a diet low in calcium reduced production of $1,25(OH)_2D_3$ from $25(OH)D_3$ as measured by chromatographic evaluation of the pattern of radioactive metabolites in the plasma. Furthermore, they reported that the administration of the parathyroid extract at a level of 20 units/day prevented these changes. The results of Garabedian *et al.* (1972) and Fraser and Kodicek (1973) were immediately challenged by Galante *et al.* (1972a,b), who found exactly the reverse; that is, the administration of parathyroid extract to intact animals suppressed the conversion of $25(OH)D_3$ to $1,25(OH)_2D_3$. For a period of time a controversy raged as to whether parathyroid hormone inhibited or stimulated the production of $1,25(OH)_2D_3$. It was subsequently shown by DeLuca and co-workers that the results of Galante and co-workers (1972a,b), suggesting an inhibitory effect of PTH, was due to the hypercalcemia-induced stimulation of calcitonin which was mediated by the administration of large exogenous levels of PTH extract.

Perhaps the greatest initial impetus for the suggestion that PTH was a trophic factor for the stimulation of $1,25(OH)_2D_3$ came from the *in vitro* studies of Rasmussen *et al.* (1972). Isolated chick renal tubules to which PTH and cyclic AMP were added *in vitro* were reported to show an approximately two- to threefold stimulation of the 1-hydroxylase. However, a dilemma that has never been resolved is that at virtually the same time that the Rasmussen paper appeared there were reports by Shain (1972a,b), working in Rasmussen's laboratory, that PTH addition to chick tubule preparations *in vitro* had no effect on the level of the 1-hydroxylase.

Henry *et al.* (1974) reported that in the vitamin D-deficient chick, which has high steady-state levels of the $25(OH)D_3$ 1-hydroxylase, surgical removal of the parathyroid gland resulted in the prompt fall, within 6 hr, of the level of 1-hydroxylase measured *in vitro*.

Favus *et al.* (1974) reported the results of an interesting study on the capacity of thyroparathyroidectomized (TPTX) or sham-operated rats to adapt the level of intestinal calcium absorption to differing levels of dietary calcium. They administered radioactive vitamin D to their rats immediately after surgery to evaluate the effects of the ablative technique on vitamin D metabolism. They found that, in spite of the severely reduced plasma levels of $1,25(OH)_2D_3$ (presumably indicative of the effect of the absence of PTH on the output of this steroid), the amount of tritiated $1,25(OH)_2D_3$ localized in the intestine was similar in both sham-operated and TPTX animals. Thus, the interesting circumstance exists that, although PTH may have a major trophic action in the production of $1,25(OH)_2D_3$, its effect is not at absolute one; that is, even in the absence of the parathyroid gland certain basal levels of $1,25(OH)_2D_3$ are still produced. In contrast to these results, Seymour and DeLuca (1974) concluded that the hypoparathyroid rat cannot synthesize appreciable quantities of $1,25(OH)_2D_3$.

As a consequence of the development of the steroid competition assay for measuring circulating levels of $1,25(OH)_2D_3$, Haussler (1975) noted correlations between parathyroid gland activity and the circulating levels of $1,25(OH)_2D_3$. Whereas the plasma levels of $1,25(OH)_2D_3$ in man are normally 25–30 pg/ml, in hypoparathyroidism the values detected were as low as 1–5 pg/ml and in hyperparathyroidism 30–40 pg/ml (see Table 8-7).

Thus, although it is generally accepted by most workers in the field that PTH is a trophic factor for $1,25(OH)_2D_3$ production, a note of caution should be interjected. Since the key observation of the *in vitro* stimulatory effects of PTH on the $25(OH)D_3$ 1-hydroxylase (Rasmussen *et al.*, 1972) could not be readily repeated, it may be that PTH is not really the direct mediator. Through the study of the regulation of the 25(OH)D 1-hydroxylase in isolated cells grown in tissue culture it will be possible to establish the identity of the direct regulators of this important enzyme system.

The proposed interrelationship between vitamin D and PTH is not a new one. The first hints of such a relationship actually came from a consideration of phosphate metabolism rather than calcium metabolism. In particular, investigators were concerned with physiological mechanisms regulating the renal excretion of inorganic phosphate. It was apparent from earlier studies on rickets, both in man and in experimental animals, that there were certain perturbations in phosphate excretion (Howland and Kramer, 1921). However, it was not until Nicolaysen (1937) reported that vitamin D could promote the intestinal absorption of both calcium and phosphate that it became possible to postulate the first tentative types of interrelationships between vitamin D, ion metabolism, and hormones that might also affect these ionic substances. Thus, Harrison and Harrison (1941) reported that the administration of vitamin D to rachitic dogs produced a marked increase in the maximal rate of reabsorption of phosphate by the renal tubules. They further noted that the effects of parathyroid extract on the tubular reabsorption of phosphate were exactly opposite to those observed for vitamin D. This landmark study identified in a preliminary fashion the complex nature of the interrelationship between vitamin D and PTH.

Over the years the Harrisons pursued, in clinical studies as well as in studies on experimental animals, the interrelations of these two calcium-regulating hormones. One of their prime observations pertained to a possible effect of vitamin D on PTH action (Harrison and Harrison, 1964). They stated that "there is an interrelationship between the functions of the parathyroid hormone and vitamin

D so that in the absence of vitamin D there is little or no response of rats to amounts of parathyroid hormone which produce a marked effect in a vitamin D-treated animal. This response involves both the calcium mobilizing and phosphaturic actions of parathyroid hormone.''

At the same time, Toverud (1964) was studying the effect of PTH and parathyroidectomy on the intestinal absorption of calcium and secretion of calcium into the lumen of the intestine in rats. He reported that parathyroidectomy caused a decrease in intestinal absorption and transport of calcium several days after the operation. These results were similar to those reported by Cramer in 1963, who studied the effect of PTH on calcium absorption in intestinal loops in dogs.

Rasmussen *et al.* (1963) studied the effect of parathyroidectomy and PTH administration on the concentration of plasma calcium and phosphorus in vitamin D-deficient and vitamin D-fed animals. These studies were followed by a report from the same laboratory by Arnaud *et al.* (1966). Both papers emphasized that the response of the vitamin D-deficient, parathyroidectomized animal to the infusion of PTH differed from that of the vitamin D-fed control. Qualitatively similar changes occurred in plasma phosphate levels as well as in the urinary excretion of calcium, phosphate, magnesium, sodium, and potassium, but in the vitamin D-deficient animals there was a sustained phosphaturia and secondary hypercalciuria and a hypercalcemia, which did not develop in the vitamin D-treated animal. It was concluded that vitamin D was necessary for the physiological actions of PTH to mobilize calcium and phosphate from bone but that vitamin D was not required for the action of PTH on the renal tubule. These results and conclusions have in part been challenged by the work of Ney *et al.* (1965) and Harrison and Harrison (1964). Evidence supporting the view of Arnaud *et al.* (1966), however, was reported by Hertelendy and Taylor (1960), who found that PTH administration to vitamin D-deficient chickens had no hypercalcemic actions.

B. Effects of Vitamin D Metabolites on Parathyroid Gland

1. Parathyroid Gland Size

Hypertrophy and hyperplasia of the parathyroid glands have been recognized since the report of Nonidez and Goodale (1927). More recent studies have been carried out to investigate the relationship between dietary calcium, vitamin D, and gland size and activity. Mueller *et al.* (1970) reported that there was an inverse relationship between dietary calcium and parathyroid gland size and gland ''activity'' as measured by the uptake of α-aminoisobutyric acid. However, all the chicks in that study were fed vitamin D, so it was not possible to independently assess the effect of the steroid or its metabolites on the gland size.

In a study by Bar *et al.* (1972), it was demonstrated that vitamin D increases serum calcium levels and decreases parathyroid gland weight, regardless of the dietary calcium or phosphorus level. There was, however, no evidence of an inverse relationship between gland weight and serum calcium levels when the data in the presence or absence of vitamin D_3 were considered separately. Also, Au and Raisz (1965) concluded that increased parathyroid gland size and activity were the result only of hypocalcemia per se and that vitamin D had no effect on parathyroid function.

In retrospect, it is only fair to indicate that all of these workers carried out their studies without the knowledge we have today of vitamin D metabolism and the putative role of PTH in stimulating $1,25(OH)_2D_3$ production. In view of the model of regulation of $1,25(OH)_2D_3$ production proposed above (Fig. 9-3), which emphasizes the interaction of vitamin D status and PTH status in the determination of the level of this enzyme, there are many possible points at which the interaction might occur. One possibility is the parathyroid gland itself, wherein the final metabolite $1,25(OH)_2D_3$ might exert a feedback effect, decreasing PTH secretion. This would have at least two consequences: (a) a decrease in the stimulatory actions of PTH on the renal $25(OH)D_3$ 1-hydroxylase and (b) a decrease in the entry of calcium into the blood from the intestine [stimulated by $1,25(OH)_2D_3$] and from bone (stimulated by both the steroid and PTH). Thus, a major advance was made in 1975 by Henry and Norman. Utilizing high specific activity radioactive preparations of $1,25(OH)_2D_3$, they were able to report the uptake of this steroid hormone by the parathyroid gland of vitamin D-deficient chicks (Henry and Norman, 1975). The parathyroid glands were capable of concentrating $1,25(OH)_2D_3$ at least fourfold over the circulating levels in the plasma. Further support for the existence of specific binding of $1,25(OH)_2D_3$ by the parathyroid gland came from the observations of Brumbaugh *et al.* (1975) and Wecksler *et al.* (1977; Wecksler, 1978). These investigators incubated tritiated $1,25(OH)_2D_3$ with homogenates of parathyroid glands from vitamin D-deficient chicks; employing sucrose gradient centrifugation, they obtained evidence of the existence of a 3.1 S receptor in the cytosol for the steroid. Wecksler (1978) extended these studies to include a detailed biochemical and kinetic analysis (association and dissociation of ligand) of the $1,25(OH)_2D_3$ cytosol receptor in the parathyroid gland obtained from both chicks and human adenomas. The discovery of a unique $1,25(OH)_2D_3$-binding component in the parathyroid gland is consistent with a steroid hormone action for this vitamin D metabolite at this site and its possible involvement in the regulation of PTH synthesis and/or secretion.

It should be recalled, however, that $1,25(OH)_2D_3$ is not the only metabolite produced by the kidney; a second metabolite produced in some physiological circumstances is $24,25(OH)_2D_3$, a steroid that is not particularly biologically active in terms of stimulation of intestinal calcium transport or bone calcium mobilization. From the work of Omdahl *et al.* (1972), however, it appears that the production of 24,25$(OH)_2D_3$ is regulated reciprocally with that of 1,25$(OH)_2D_3$, suggesting the physiological importance of this steroid. Henry *et al.* (1977) reported the possible combined actions of 1,25$(OH)_2D_3$ and 24,25$(OH)_2D_3$ in parathyroid gland activities. Their studies involved the feeding either separately or in combination of these two steroids to vitamin D-deficient chicks (for which there is no assay for the circulating levels of PTH) and evaluating the regression of enlarged chick parathyroid glands. After 7 days of vitamin D_3 treatment (100 IU/day; 6.5 nmoles) parathyroid gland weight was significantly lower than that of vitamin D-deficient controls whereas the serum calcium level increased from 6.3 to 8.6 mg per 100 ml. 1,25$(OH)_2D_3$ (1.3 nmoles/day) raised the serum calcium level to 8.6 mg per 100 ml but did not affect the weight of the parathyroid glands; at the same time vitamin D_3 and 1,25$(OH)_2D_3$ separately stimulated the production of intestinal calcium-binding protein. When 1,25$(OH)_2D_3$ and 24,25$(OH)_2D_3$ (3.9 nmoles/day) were fed together for 7 days, there was a significant reduction in gland weight comparable to that observed in the control vitamin D-treated group. These workers concluded that parathyroid gland regression, possibly involving loss of cells, occurs within a few days of treatment with vitamin D metabolites and that this regression does not obligatorily follow an increase in serum calcium. Under circumstances in which 1,25$(OH)_2D_3$ is present in low concentration the presence of 24,25$(OH)_2D_3$ is required to mediate gland reduction. These results suggest that vitamin D metabolites, in particular 1,25$(OH)_2D_3$ and 24,25$(OH)_2D_3$, may play a role in modulating parathyroid gland functions as well as intestinal functions. A summary of these results is given in Fig. 9-4.

It is unfortunate that in the experimental animal systems, the rat and chick, there are no routinely available radioimmunoassays capable of measuring circulating levels of PTH. Thus, there is the dilemma of attempting to equate the rather morphological alterations on parathyroid gland size reported above which are mediated by vitamin D metabolites, with studies on man and other higher animals in which efforts have been made to document the effects of vitamin D status on the actual secretion rate of PTH.

2. *Parathyroid Hormone Secretion*

With the development of our understanding of the role of the endocrine system in processing vitamin D and a demonstration of its intimate interrelationship with PTH and calcium metabolism, the intriguing prospect has arisen that vitamin D or one of its metabolites may modulate the secretion of PTH by the gland. Classic feedback actions of hypercalcemia in diminishing the secretion of PTH have been repeatedly documented (Arnaud *et al.*, 1971). However, only more recently has it been speculated that there may be more than one feedback regulator, i.e., both the calcium ion itself and the products of the kidney, 1,25$(OH)_2D_3$ and

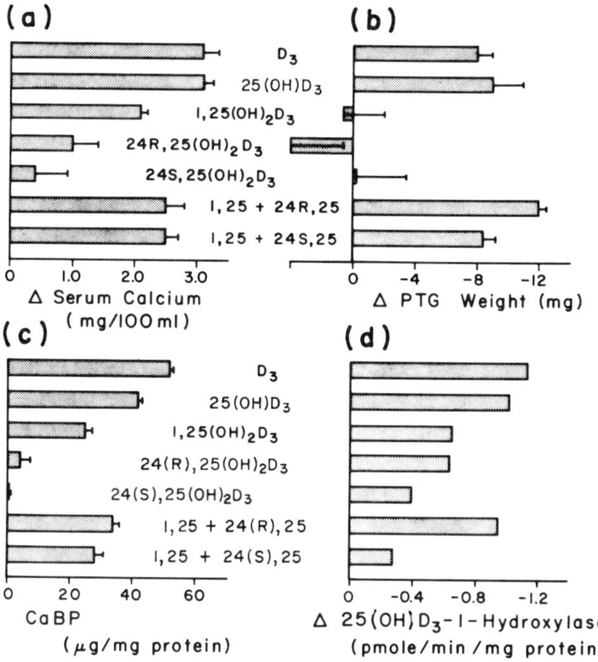

Figure 9-4. Changes in (a) serum calcium, (b) parathyroid gland weight, (c) intestinal calcium-binding protein, and (d) kidney $25(OH)D_3$ 1-hydroxylase brought about by vitamin D metabolites alone and in combination. The daily doses of each steroid were as follows: vitamin D_3, 6.5 nmoles; $25(OH)_2D_3$, 4.9 nmoles; $1,25(OH)_2D_3$, 1.3 nmoles; 24 (*R*)- or 24(*S*),$25(OH)_2D_3$, 3.9 nmoles. Two groups of chicks received combined doses of 1.3 nmoles $1,25(OH)_2D_3$ and 3.9 nmoles 24(*R*)- or 24(*S*),$25(OH)_2D_3$. All values are expressed as the change from the vitamin D-deficient control group and are the mean ± S.E.M. of five chicks per group. From Henry *et al.* (1977).

$24,25(OH)_2D_3$. The most definitive studies to date have been those reported by Chertow *et al.* (1975). Figure 9-5 shows some of their pertinent results. They evaluated the effects of $1,25(OH)_2D_3$ administration in physiological quantities on the circulating levels of immunoreactive PTH measured in normal rats and noted that within 4 hr after administration of the steroid there was a 40% reduction in the circulating level of PTH that was measured by the antiserum employed.

Figure 9-6 presents the results of Canterbury and co-workers (1978), who studied the effects of either $1,25(OH)_2D_3$ or $24,25(OH)_2D_3$ infusion into the artery leading to the parathyroid gland of normal dogs. They followed the level of PTH in the vein draining the vascular bed of the parathyroid gland. The results show an intriguing relationship: Administration of $1,25(OH)_2D_3$ and $24,25(OH)_2D_3$ results in each case in a perturbation of the circulating level of iPTH. These effects, however, appear to be obtained by distinctly different

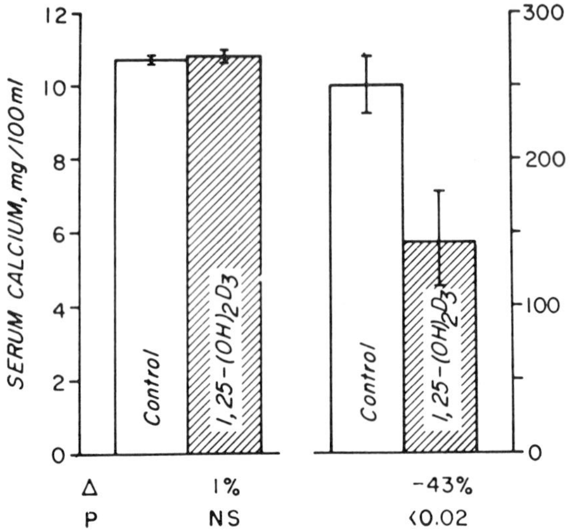

Figure 9-5. Effect of $1,25(OH)_2D_3$ treatment on serum Ca^{2+} and PTH in normal rats. Taken from Chertow *et al.* (1975).

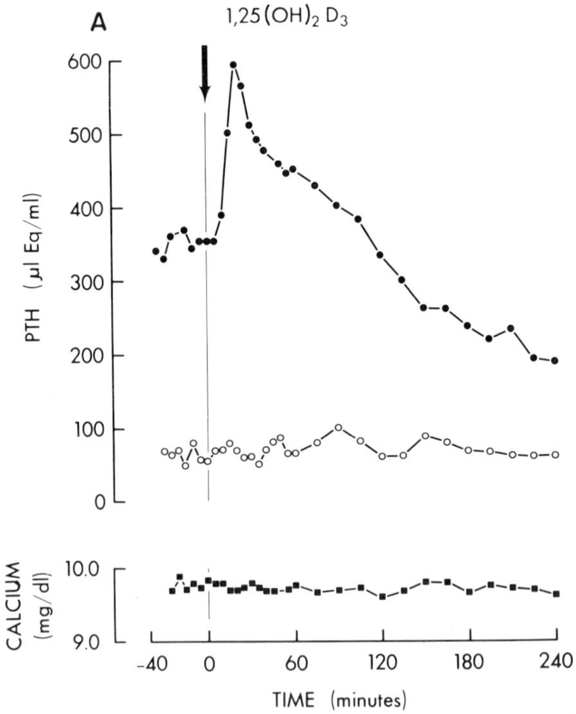

Figure 9-6. Effects of administration of $1,25(OH)_2D_3$ (A) and $24,25(OH)_2D_3$ (B) on secretion of PTH in the normal dog. Taken from Canterbury *et al.* (1978).

mechanisms for each steroid. Administration of 1,25$(OH)_2D_3$ acutely stimulates the release of preexisting PTH in the gland, followed by apparent inhibition of the biosynthesis of the additional hormone. Conversely, the administration of 24,25$(OH)_2D_3$ results in an acute decrease in the secretion of iPTH, followed by an intermediate time period of increased secretion of iPTH and then by a chronic achievement of reduced PTH levels. Similar results were reported by Care *et al.* (1975) and Oldham *et al.* (1976). More recently, using a tissue culture system of cells obtained from either porcine parathyroid glands or human parathyroid adenoma tissue, Altenahr *et al.* (1977) found that addition of 1,25$(OH)_2D_3$ to the system *in vitro* resulted in a 63% inhibition of immunoreactive PTH.

3. *Feedback Mechanisms*

With the demonstration of the potential stimulatory effects of PTH on the production of 1,25$(OH)_2D_3$ and the associated feedback regulation of 1,25$(OH)_2D_3$ and 24,25$(OH)_2D_3$ in parathyroid hormone secretion the possibility of a classic endocrine regulatory mechanism exists, particularly when considered in concert with the well-documented feedback actions of elevated serum calcium levels on the parathyroid gland. As shown in Fig. 9-7 the analogy between this

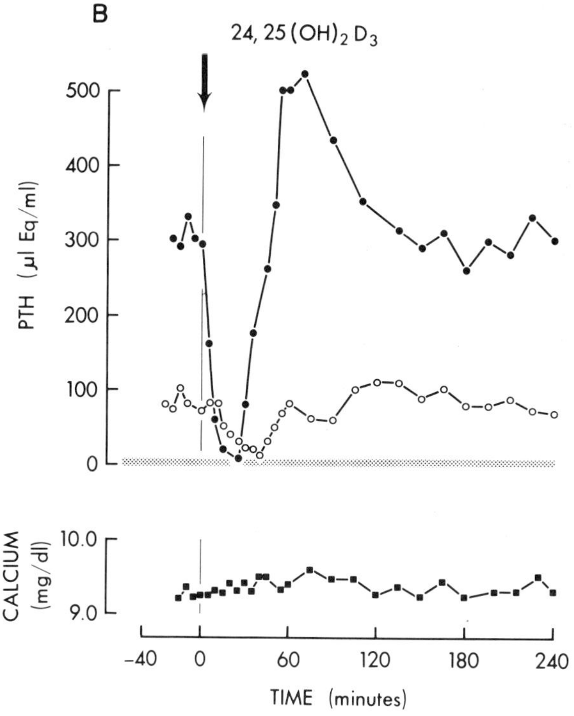

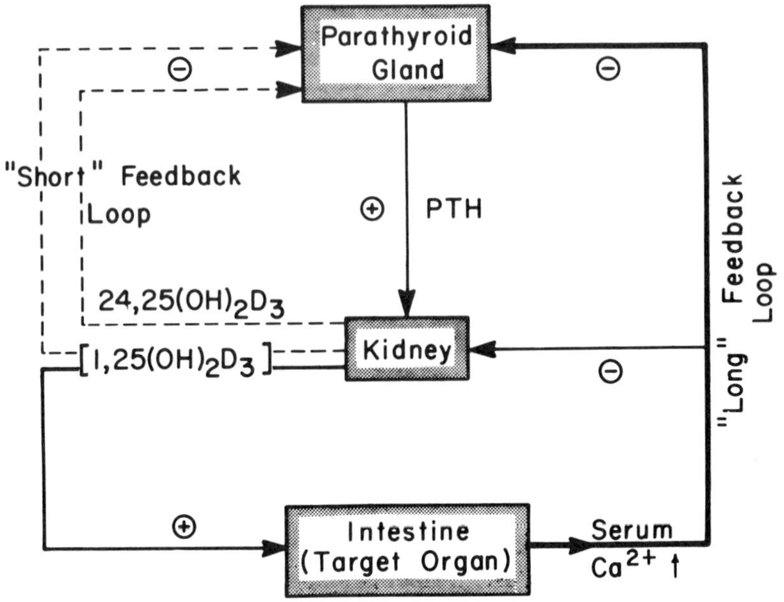

Figure 9-7. Postulated feedback loops for the parathyroid–kidney calcium endocrine system. This is modeled on similar systems related to the neurohypophysis.

calcium endocrine system and the neurohypophysis relay systems is striking. There are "short-loop" and "long-loop" feedback relationships in both systems. It is well known that feedback and feedforward controls in biochemical and endocrine systems represent mechanisms for the transfer of information. Chemical messengers indicate to one part of the cell or organism the state of or activity in another part of the cell or organism. In order to ensure the proper flow of information throughout the biological system specific chemical messengers or transmitters must exist. In endocrine systems, this implies the existence of specific hormonal receptors on or within the relevant cells of the endocrine glands so that they can respond to incoming information.

The primary attribute of an endocrinological system is that it exists and operates as a "closed-loop system" rather than as an "open-loop system." The distinction between the two systems, although simple, has profound implications for the mechanisms that are operative therein and the consequences of the operation. With a closed-loop system, the output influences the behavior of the system, which becomes, in terms of its responses, a "feedback input." That is, stimulus (input) leads to a response, but response (output) must ultimately influence the original stimulus. In this regard the most important aspect of the closed-loop operation is one of the "feedback control" and particularly "negative feedback control."

It has become increasingly apparent in recent years that one of the hallmarks in the regulation of integrated peptide hormone and steroid hormone endocrine systems are feedback loops. Thus, peptide hormones are known in several systems to have a trophic action on the production of steroid hormones, e.g., ACTH on adrenal cortical hormones and leutinizing hormone on estrogen or testosterone production. These steroid hormones then initiate specific biological functions, which produce defined biological responses. These responses in some way feed back and diminish both the secretion of the steroid hormone and that of the trophic peptide hormone. In addition to this long loop of "feedback" there is a short loop of feedback wherein the steroid hormone itself feeds back directly on the endocrine gland of its trophic stimulator, i.e., the endocrine gland that secretes the peptide hormone. Thus, as shown in Fig. 9-7, one can identify the "long-loop" and "short-loop" feedback steps in both the calcium arena and the pituitary axis. It should be apparent that this is an area of investigation that is far from complete. At present, there are only the barest outlines in biochemical and molecular terms of the stimulatory actions of PTH on the renal production of $1,25(OH)_2D_3$ as well as the putative feedback action of renal vitamin D metabolites on the actions of the parathyroid gland.

C. Calcitonin

The present understanding of the relationship between vitamin D, its metabolism, and its interrelationship with calcitonin is even less well defined than that for PTH. Tashjian (1965) was one of the first to study the interrelationships between PTH, calcitonin, and calcium homeostasis. He reported that 1 hr after subcutaneous administration of calcitonin to rats, the plasma calcium concentration reached its lowest level; the same acute hypocalcemic effect was observed in rats that had been given actinomycin D or that were parathyroidectomized. He further noted that the plasma calcium concentration returned to normal in the control rats within 1–3 hr, whereas in actinomycin D-treated or parathyroidectomized rats the plasma calcium concentration did not return to normal at all. His data demonstrated that in an actinomycin D-treated rat, parathyroid glands cannot maintain a normal plasma calcium concentration and that the short duration of the hypocalcemic effect of calcitonin is due in large part to the actions of the parathyroid gland. In retrospect, it can be appreciated that the failure of the actinomycin D-treated animals, which also received calcitonin, to respond normally was due to a blockage of the responses generated by the vitamin D metabolite $1,25(OH)_2D_3$. Exactly at this time the effects of actinomycin D in blocking the response to vitamin D were reported by Norman (1965) and Zull *et al.* (1965).

Shortly thereafter, Morii and DeLuca (1967) studied the relationship between vitamin D deficiency, calcitonin, and PTH. They reported that calcitonin was capable of lowering serum calcium levels in vitamin D-deficient animals, whereas PTH was incapable of acting in a hypercalcemic fashion. These results tend to support the view that calcitonin can act in the absence of vitamin D. These studies were followed by a report by Melançon and DeLuca (1969) that calcitonin produced hypocalcemic response in rats with hypercalcemia due to hypervitaminosis D. Thus, calcitonin was capable of mediating hypocalcemic effects in the presence of excess vitamin D as well as in its absence. Still later, Olson *et al.* (1972) reported putative effects of calcitonin in inhibiting vitamin D-induced intestinal calcium absorption. The latter results, however, were not supported by the work of Cramer (1973), who studied the effects of calcitonin administration in thyroparathyroidectomized but PTH-supplemented (i.e., calcitonin-deficient) rats and noted that subsequent administration of purified salmon calcitonin either in physiological or pharmacological doses failed to alter the absorption of calcium by the intestine. They noted further that restoration of PTH enhanced the calcium absorption above that of the parathyroid-deficient animals. In retrospect, this could be interpreted simply in terms of PTH stimulating the production of $1,25(OH)_2D_3$, which would further elevate the baseline level of intestinal calcium absorption.

An interesting relationship between calcitonin and intestinal calcium absorption concerns the apparent stimulation of calcitonin secretion by any process that can stimulate intestinal calcium absorption, e.g., the ingestion of a meal. Thus, in a classic endocrine study, Munson and Gray (1970) administered calcium by gavage to rats and found a rapid increase in blood calcium levels in thyroidectomized rats with transplanted parathyroids, but not in sham-operated rats. The results suggest that there is a simultaneous secretion of calcitonin with the slight incremental increase in serum calcium levels occurring following absorption of significant quantities of calcium. Other studies have suggested a possible interrelationship between the secretion of gastrin and the subsequent secretion of calcitonin (Cooper *et al.*, 1972).

More recent developments pertaining to the relationship between vitamin D and calcitonin concern the possible effects of the peptide hormone in regulating vitamin D metabolism. Galante *et al.* (1972b) reported that in rats the administration of exogenous calcitonin dramatically enhanced the conversion of $25(OH)D_3$ to $1,25(OH)_2D_3$, as determined by evaluation of the pattern of radioactive metabolites in the plasma. However, this result was immediately challenged by a number of laboratories (Rasmussen *et al.*, 1972; Garabedian *et al.*, 1972). Shortly thereafter, MacIntyre's laboratory reported (Larkins *et al.*, 1974) the results of studies carried out with isolated renal tubules prepared from vitamin D-deficient and vitamin D-replete chicks. They found that synthetic salmon calcitonin enhanced the production of $1,25(OH)_2D_3$, whereas human calcitonin was without effect. These effects of calcitonin on vitamin D metabolism, however, are still not generally accepted by most research workers in the field.

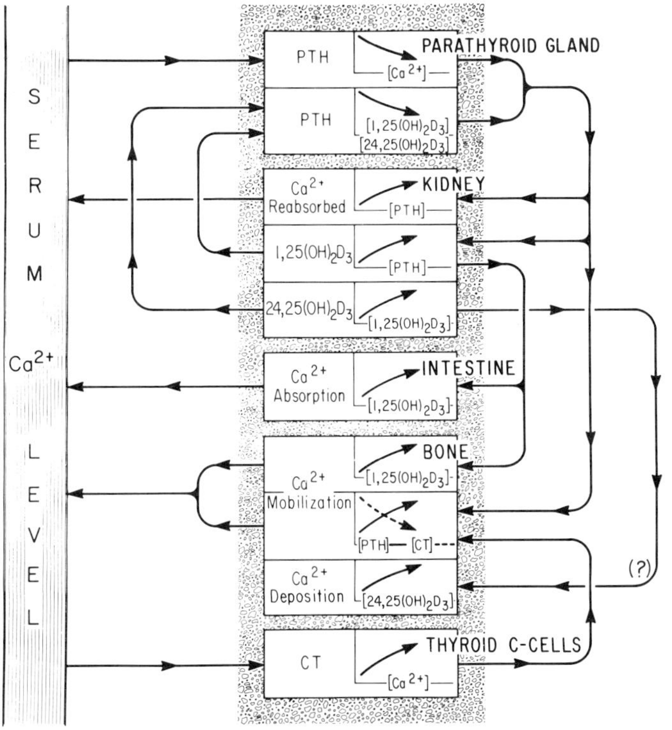

Figure 9-8. Current understanding of calcium homeostasis.

D. Integrated View of Calcium Homeostasis

Figure 9-8 gives an integrated view of calcium homeostasis that attempts to interrelate the known actions of calcitonin, PTH, and $1,25(OH)_2D_3$ on calcium metabolism. It is not yet possible to include in equivalent detail the actions of these hormones on phosphorus homeostasis. The reader is referred to reviews that address this complex subject in more detail (Rasmussen, 1971, 1974; Copp, 1970; Raisz and Bingham, 1972).

III. ADRENAL CORTICAL STEROIDS

A. Background

The relation of adrenal steroids to calcium and bone metabolism has been well documented. Osteoporosis is often a prominent sign of Cushing's disease, which is, in essence, an overproduction of adrenal glucocorticoids. The bone disease osteoporosis also occurs frequently after prolonged adrenal corticoid therapy, which is often associated with rheumatoid arthritis. It is known that administration of cortisol or other adrenal steroids may cause a decrease in intestinal absorption of calcium and also in the renal tubular reabsorption of calcium. In addition, cortisol and related steroids are known to have effects on bone resorption and bone accretion. The mode of action of cortisol in any of these target tissues (intestine, kidney, and bone) remains to be elucidated; however, there is some evidence that cortisol or steroid treatment has antivitamin D-like activity.

B. Hydrocortisone–Parathyroid Hormone Interaction

It has been known since the 1940's that in instances of overdosage or administration of pharmacological doses of vitamin D a predominant cause of hypercalcemia is excessive mobilization of calcium from bone. It was first noted by Anderson *et al.* (1954) that this hypercalcemia could be corrected by cortisone administration. Also, hypercalcemia and hypercalciuria had been reported in 10–40% of the patients with sarcoidosis, nephrolithiasis, and nephrocalcinosis. The defect has been suggested to be excessive intestinal absorption of calcium, and this may also be corrected by cortisone or treatment with other glucocorticoids (Henneman *et al.*, 1956; Bell *et al.*, 1964).

Some support has come from animal studies for antagonism of PTH action by glucocorticoids. In particular, it was shown by Stoerk *et al.* (1963), Canas *et al.* (1967), and Magargal *et al.* (1969) that administration of adrenal corticoids to rats tends to lower plasma calcium concentration; however, detectable hypocalcemia was manifest only in the parathyroidectomized animals. This suggested that in the intact animals a compensatory increase in PTH prevented hypocalcemia. More recent studies by Williams *et al.* (1974) demonstrated that, in intact rats, PTH caused not only an increase in plasma calcium concentration but also an adrenocortical hyperplasia and an increase in circulating levels of corticosterone. The same workers reported that cortisone acetate caused parathyroid gland hyperplasia and an increase in serum immunoreactive PTH without associated changes in circulating calcium levels. Williams *et al.* (1974) interpreted these results as showing that PTH-induced hypercalcemia leads to increased adrenocortical function, which partially inhibits the hypercalcemia, and that the hypocalcemic action of cortisol leads to increased parathyroid function, which prevents significant hypocalcemia. Consistent with this hypothesis of PTH–adrenocortical hormone interaction is the frequent association of Cushing's syndrome with hyperparathyroidism (Schmidt *et al.*, 1961).

In the more recent study of Fucik *et al.* (1975) the effects of glucocorticoids on PTH secretion in man were evaluated. These data indicate that in man, as shown previously in the rat, an increase in cortisol, with its associated hypocalcemic effect, causes stimulation of the parathyroid glands with a measurable increase in PTH secretion. These observations are also consistent with the view that the bone loss that often occurs with excessive glucocorticoid treatment may be partially caused by an induced elevation of PTH secretion.

Thus, an important new dimension in the study of calcium homeostasis may exist if there are direct actions of the glucocorticoids on PTH function as well as possible effects of PTH on adrenocortical activity. In view of the recent evidence of vitamin D metabolites affecting the regulation of PTH actions, it is clear that this topic will receive much further attention in the future.

C. Hydrocortisone Inhibition of Intestinal Calcium Absorption

As indicated above, glucocorticoid administration dramatically lowers the serum calcium level in clinical situations associated with vitamin D overdosage or hypersensitivity to vitamin D. It has been proposed that serum calcium reduction occurs via a concomitant reduction in the intestinal absorption of calcium. Williams *et al.* (1961) measured intestinal calcium absorption in the rat by the everted gut sac technique to determine whether the presence or prior administration of cortisone would inhibit vitamin D-mediated calcium absorption. They observed that the prior subcutaneous administration of 2.5 mg of cortisone acetate completely abolished the response of increased stimulation of intestinal calcium absorption that occurred after the administration of pharmacological doses of 20,000 IU of vitamin D. Harrison and Harrison (1960) also reported antagonistic effects of glucocorticoids on the stimulation of intestinal calcium transport in the rat. It might be anticipated that, if glucocorticoids inhibit vitamin D-mediated intestinal calcium transport, then bilateral adrenalectomy should modestly increase active calcium transport in rats (Kimberg *et al.*, 1961).

Several hypotheses have been advanced to explain the apparent ''antagonistic'' actions that glucocorticoids have on intestinal calcium absorption (Kimberg, 1969). These hypotheses include the following. (a) Cortisone administration could interfere with the metabolism of vitamin D by preventing the formation of necessary active metabolites or by facilitating its metabolic degradation; (b) the administration of glucocorticoids could lead to metabolic alterations in tissues normally responsive to vitamin D quite independently of direct interaction with the vitamin; (c) cortisone could be a competitive inhibitor of vitamin D or its metabolites.

D. Effects of Glucocorticoids on Vitamin D Metabolism

Efforts have been made to evaluate the effects of cortisone treatment on vitamin D metabolism. Avioli *et al.* (1968) studied vitamin D_3 metabolism in normal adults before and during periods of prednisone administration and came to the conclusion that the observed antagonism of glucocorticoids in man is related to the increased metabolic turnover of vitamin D that occurs as a consequence of the steroid treatment. In their studies prednisone induced a decrease in the plasma half-time of vitamin D and a decrease in the accumulation in the plasma of 25(OH)D. However, these results, obtained in man, have not been supported by studies in experimental animal models. Particularly, the elegant work of Kimberg *et al.* (1971; Favus *et al.,* 1973a,b) has clearly shown that in the rat glucocorticoid administration does not alter vitamin D metabolism. The first report of Kimberg *et al.* (1971) indicates that cortisone administration affects the cellular mechanisms mediating calcium transport in a manner opposite to that of vitamin D, but is independent of any direct interaction with the parent vitamin or its metabolites. Measurement of the levels of vitamin D-dependent calcium-binding protein and the subcellular distribution of vitamin D metabolites in the intestinal mucosa failed to indicate any effects of hydrocortisone. Furthermore, the same authors reported that glucocorticoid administration also inhibited the transport of iron and D-galactose, neither of which is known to be dependent on vitamin D. This suggests that cortisone treatment may be responsible for more than a simple antagonism of just the effects of vitamin D. The fact that there are normal or increased levels of calcium-binding protein in the intestinal mucosa of animals treated with cortisone clearly indicates that there is no impairment in intestinal events related specifically to vitamin D.

However, more recent studies by Carré *et al.* (1974) and Miravet *et al.* (1975) indicate that, contrary to the previous reports, adrenal corticoids may indeed alter the intestinal accumulation and possible metabolism of $1,25(OH)_2D_3$. These workers reported that the prior administration of prednisolone to rats altered the subsequent metabolism of radioactive $1,25(OH)_2D_3$ in the intestine so that there were increased quantities of a polar, biologically inactive metabolite in the intestine. Their data suggested that the polar metabolite was derived directly from $1,25(OH)_2D_3$ and not from $25(OH)D_3$. This would be consistent with the view that the more polar metabolite occurred as a consequence of the further metabolism of $1,25(OH)_2D_3$ in the intestinal mucosa of the treated rats. Clearly, additional studies pertaining to glucocorticoid effects on vitamin D and, perhaps more importantly, $1,25(OH)_2D_3$ metabolism are warranted.

The recent report by Spanos *et al.* (1977) is puzzling. They found that administration of glucocorticoids (2 mg) to vitamin D-replete chicks inhibited the production of $24,25(OH)_2D_3$ and stimulated the production of $1,25(OH)_2D_3$. Surprisingly, a similar stimulation of $1,25(OH)_2D_3$ production was noted when glucocorticoids were added *in vitro* to kidney tubule preparations.

There are also a limited number of reports on the effect of hydrocortisone on vitamin D-related events in bone. Kunin and Meyer (1969) and Meyer and Kunin (1969) reported that cortisone treatment of rats interferes with the intermediary metabolism of epiphyseal cartilage in rats, specifically by decreasing their glycolytic enzyme activity. Also, Reynolds (1966) evaluated the effect of hydrocortisone on the growth of chick bone rudiments in a chemically defined growth medium. Hydrocortisone was observed to cause a progressive inhibition of growth of the chick bone rudiments when present in quantities of 1 to 10 mg per milliliter of growth medium. Hydrocortisone also progressively inhibited the synthesis of polysaccharide in the bone matrix. Thus, the possibility exists that glucocorticoids may directly interfere with certain aspects of bone organic matrix metabolism.

IV. OTHER HORMONES

A. Estrogens

The effect of estrogens on bone metabolism has been of interest for at least 30 years, largely because of the therapeutic use of this sex steroid in the treatment of osteoporosis. It is well known that with the onset of the menopause the secretion of estradiol is limited and that many postmenopausal women develop osteoporosis.

The reports of Kenny *et al.* (1976) as well as Tanaka *et al.* (1976) and Castillo *et al.* (1977) that estrogen and testosterone administration to Japanese quail and chicks, respectively, interferes with $25(OH)D_3$ conversion to $1,25(OH)_2D_3$ are consistent with the foregoing observations. There is the possibility that sex steroids may indeed be intimately involved in the regulation of vitamin D metabolism and action.

B. Thyroxine

The thyroid hormones thyroxine and triiodothyronine are known to influence mineral metabolism and bone calcium turnover. Thus, certain abnormalities of bone metabolism are noted in the disease states of hypothyroidism and hyperthyroidism (Michie *et al.*, 1971). It has been shown that patients who suffer from hyperthyroidism also have an associated hypercalcemia. It is not clear whether the hypercalcemia is related to an associated hyperparathyroidism that occurs from nearest-neighbor perturbation or whether some long-range physiological signals are generated to produce the hypercalcemia in another manner. Velentzas *et al.* (1977) and Mosekilde *et al.* (1977) reported that patients with thyrotoxicosis have significantly lowered levels of plasma $25(OH)D_3$.

C. Growth Hormone—Somatomedin

One of the major target organs for the action of growth hormone in the developing animal is the skeleton. In the absence of growth hormone skeletal development is markedly slowed and, in the extreme, dwarfism may result. It has been shown that most of the effects of growth hormone are in fact mediated by somatomedin. Thus, a critical need may develop for one of these hormones during the period of developent, during which time there is a marked increase in calcium demand by the animal. However, it is known that in the adult animal human growth hormone is not necessary for normal mineral homeostasis.

It is to be anticipated that new relationships between growth and endocrine signals related to generation of growth may intervene in some aspect of calcium and phosphorus homeostasis. Whether such effects will be manifest via alterations in vitamin D metabolism is not yet apparent.

D. Insulin/Diabetes

It was shown by Levin *et al.* (1976) that individuals with either juvenile-onset or adult-onset diabetes have a reduced bone mass as compared with age-matched controls. A similar observation was made by Ringe *et al.* (1976). Abnormalities of skeletal mass can also be produced by inducing diabetes in experimental animals (Ramurthy *et al.*, 1973). As yet the pathogenesis of the reduced bone mass in diabetic man is not clearly known.

A series of experiments on diabetic rats implicated a defect in vitamin D metabolism in the production of calcium malabsorption in these animals. It was shown that in this experimental model there was intestinal malabsorption of calcium (Schneider and Schedl, 1972) and a decreased quantity of a specific intestinal calcium-binding protein which is similar to the protein induced by the administration of vitamin D (Schneider *et al.*, 1974). The transport defect could be corrected by the administration of $1,25(OH)_2D_3$ but not by the administration of $25(OH)D_3$ or vitamin D_3 itself, suggesting that there was a defect in production of $1,25(OH)_2D_3$ (Schneider *et al.*, 1975a). The defect could also be corrected by administration of *Solanum malacoxylon* (Schneider *et al.*, 1975b). More recently Schneider *et al.* (1977) reported that the serum level of $1,25(OH)_2D_3$ is significantly lowered in rats with streptozoticin-induced diabetes. No studies of vitamin D metabolism or calcium absorption have been done as yet in human diabetics, but it can be anticipated that this will be a fertile field of investigation in the future.

E. Prolactin

An exciting new development concerns the possible involvement of the vitamin D–endocrine system with changes in hormonal concentrations that occur during pregnancy and lactation. Spanos *et al.* (1976a) reported that a single acute dose or chronic administration of ovine prolactin to the chick was effective increasing the activity of the renal $25(OH)D_3$ 1-hydroxylase as measured *in vitro*. Further support for this action was obtained by measuring changes in the plasma levels of $1,25(OH)_2D_3$ that occurred after prolactin administration. As reported by Spanos *et al.* (1976b), there was a significant elevation in plasma $1,25(OH)_2D_3$ levels. Care must be taken in the interpretation of these results since an action of ovine prolactin in chicks may not necessarily reflect an action of the hormone in mammals.

The report by Osborn and Norman (1977) of the presence of a $25(OH)D_3$-like substance in human, bovine, and equine milk is also suggestive of possible vitamin D-endocrine system interactions during pregnancy and lactation. Edelstein *et al.* (1976), in a preliminary report, noted the existence of a binding protein for vitamin D_3 in the mammary glands of lactating rats. Also, Weisman *et al.* (1976) reported the existence of a possible maternal–perinatal relationship in vitamin D metabolism in rats. Similarly, Dent and Gupton (1975) reported no change, whereas Turton *et al.* (1977) reported a decrease in the circulating level of 25(OH)D during pregnancy.

REFERENCES

Altenahr, E., Dietel, M., and Montz, R. (1977). *Acta Endocrinol. (Copenhagen)* **86,** 533.

Anderson, J., Harper, C., Dent, C. E., and Philpot, G. R. (1954). *Lancet* **2,** 720.

Arnaud, C., Rasmussen, H., and Anast, C. (1966). *J. Clin. Invest.* **45,** 1955.

Arnaud, C., Tsao, H. S., and Sizemore, G. W. (1971). *J. Clin. Invest.* **50,** 21.

Au, W. Y., and Raisz, L. G. (1965). *Am. J. Physiol.* **209,** 637.

Avioli, L. V., Birge, S. J., and Lee, S. W. (1968). *J. Clin. Endocrinol. Metab.* **28,** 1341.

Bar, A., Hurwitz, S., and Cohen, I. (1972). *Comp. Biochem. Biophys. A* **43,** 519.

Bell, N. H., Gill, J. R., Jr., and Bartter, F. C. (1964). *Am. J. Med.* **36,** 500.

Blonner, T., Hopkins, T. R., Thomas, W. C., Carey, R. A., and Howard, J. E. (1956). *J. Clin. Endocrinol. Metab.* **16,** 945.

Brumbaugh, P. F., Haussler, M. R., and Hughes, M. R. (1975). *Proc. Natl. Acad. Sci. U.S.A.* **72,** 4871.

Canas, F. M., Bergström, W. H., and Churgin, S. J. (1967). *Metab., Clin. Exp.* **16,** 670.

Canterbury, J., Lerman, S., Claflin, A. J., Henry, H. L., Norman, A. W., and Reiss, E. (1978). *J. Clin. Invest.* **61,** 1375.

Care, A. D., Bates, R. F. L., Swaminathan, R., Scanes, C. G., Peacock, M., Taylor, C. M., DeLuca, H. F., Tomlinson, S., and O'Riordan, J. (1975). *In* "Calcium Regulating Hormones" (R. Talmage, M. Owen, and J. Parsons, eds.), Int. Congr. Ser. No. 346, p. 100. Exerpta Med., Found. Amsterdam.

Carré, M., Ayigbede, O., Miravet, L., and Rasmussen, H. (1974). *Proc. Natl. Acad. Sci. U.S.A.* **71,** 2996.

Castillo, L., Tanaka, Y., DeLuca, H. F., and Sunde, M. L. (1977). *Arch. Biochem. Biophys.* **179,** 211.

Chertow, B. S., Baylink, D. J., Wergedal, J. F., Su, H. H., and Norman, A. W. (1975). *J. Clin. Invest.* **56,** 668.

Cooper, C. W., Schwesinger, W. H., Mahgoub, A. M., Antjes, D. A., Gray, T. K., and Munson, P. L. (1972). *In* "Calcium, Parathyroid Hormone and the Calcitonins" (R. V. Talmage and

P. L. Munson, eds.), Int. Congr. Ser. No. 243, p. 128. Exerpta Med., Found. Amsterdam.
Copp, D. H. (1970). *Annu. Rev. Physiol.* **32,** 161.
Cramer, C. F. (1963). *In* "The Transfer of Calcium and Strontium across Biological Membranes" (R. H. Wasserman, ed.), p. 75. Academic Press, New York.
Cramer, C. F. (1973). *Calcif. Tissue Res.* **13,** 169.
Dent, C. E., and Gupta, M. M. (1975). *Lancet* **2,** 1057.
Edelstein, S., Eizenberg, Z., and Harrell, A. (1976). *FEBS Lett.* **62,** 245.
Evans, I. M. A., Colston, K. W., Galante, L., and MacIntyre, I. (1975). *Clin. Sci. Mol. Med.* **48,** 227.
Favus, M. J., Kimberg, D. V., Millar, G., and Gershon, E. (1973a). *J. Clin. Invest.* **52,** 1328.
Favus, M. J., Walling, M. W., and Kimberg, D. V. (1973b). *J. Clin. Invest.* **52,** 1680.
Favus, M. J., Walling, M. W., and Kimberg, D. V. (1974). *J. Clin. Invest.* **53,** 1139.
Fraser, D. R., and Kodicek, E. (1973). *Nature (London), New Biol.* **241,** 163.
Fucik, R. F., Kukreja, S. C., Hargis, G. K., Bower, E. N., Henderson, W. J., and Williams, G. A. (1975). *J. Clin. Endocrinol. Metab.* **40,** 152.
Galante, L., MacAuley, S., Colston, K., and MacIntyre, I. (1972a). *Lancet* **1,** 985.
Galante, L., Colston, K. W., MacAuley, S. J., and MacIntyre, I. (1972b). *Nature (London)* **238,** 271.
Galante, L. S., Colston, K. W., Evans, I. M. A., Byfield, P. G. H., Matthews, E. W., and MacIntyre, I. (1973). *Nature (London)* **244,** 438.
Garabedian, M., Holick, M. F., DeLuca, H. F., and Boyle, I. T. (1972). *Proc. Natl. Acad. Sci. U.S.A.* **69,** 1673.
Harrison, H. E. (1966). *Yale J. Biol. Med.* 393.
Harrison, H. E., and Harrison, H. C. (1941). *J. Clin. Invest.* **20,** 47.
Harrison, H. E., and Harrison, H. C. (1960). *Am. J. Physiol.* **199,** 265.
Harrison, H. E., and Harrison, H. C. (1964). *Metab., Clin. Exp.* **13,** 952.
Haussler, M. R. (1975). *In* "Proceedings of the Second Workshop on Vitamin D and Problems Related to Uremic Bone Disease" (A. W. Norman *et al.,* eds.), p. 25. de Gruyter, Berlin.
Henneman, P. H., Dempsey, E. F., Carroll, E. L., and Albright, F. (1956). *J. Clin. Invest.* **35,** 1229.
Henry, H. L., Midgett, R. J., and Norman, A. W. (1974). *J. Biol. Chem.* **249,** 7584.
Henry, H. L., Taylor, A. N., and Norman, A. W. (1977). *J. Nutr.* **107,** 1918.
Henry, H. L., and Norman, A. W. (1975). *Biochem. Biophys. Res. Commun.* **62,** 781.
Hertelendy, F., and Taylor, T. G. (1960). *Biochim. Biophys. Acta* **44,** 200.
Horiuchi, N., Suda, T., Sasaki, S., Ezawa, I., Sano, Y., and Ogata, E. (1974). *FEBS Lett.* **43,** 353.
Howland, J., and Kramer, B. (1921). *Am. J. Dis. Child.* **22,** 105.
Kenny, A. D., Baksi, S. N., and Pang, P. K. (1976). *Am. J. Physiol.* **230,** 1609.
Kimberg, D. V. (1969). *N. Engl. J. Med.* **280,** 1396.
Kimberg, D. V., Schacter, D., and Schenke, H. (1961). *Am. J. Physiol.* **200,** 1256.
Kimberg, D. V., Baerg, R. D., Gershon, E., and Graudusius, R. T. (1971). *J. Clin. Invest.* **50,** 1309.
Kunin, A. S., and Meyer, W. L. (1969). *Arch. Biochem. Biophys.* **129,** 421.
Larkins, R. G., MacAuley, S. J., Rapoport, A., Martin, T. J., Tulloch, B. R., Byfield, P. G. H., Matthews, E. W., and MacIntyre, I. (1974). *Clin. Sci. Mol. Med.* **46,** 569.
Levin, M. E., Boisseau, V. C., and Avioli, L. V. (1976). *N. Engl. J. Med.* **294,** 241.
Lukert, B. P., Stanbury, S. M., and Mawer, E. B. (1973). *Endocrinology* **93,** 718.
Magargal, L. E., Magargal, H., and Reidenberg, M. M. (1969). *J. Pharmacol. Exp. Ther.* **169,** 138.
Melançon, M. J., Jr., and DeLuca, H. F. (1969). *Endocrinology* **85,** 704.
Meyer, W. L., and Kunin, A. S. (1969). *Arch. Biochem. Biophys.* **129,** 431.
Michie, W., Stowers, J. M. (1971). *Lancet* **1,** 508.

Miravet, L., Carré, M., Ayigbede, O., and Rasmussen, H. (1975). *In* "Proceedings of the Second Workshop on Vitamin D and Problems Related to Uremic Bone Disease" (A. W. Norman *et al.*, eds.), p. 59. de Gruyter, Berlin.
Morii, H., and DeLuca, H. F. (1967). *Am. J. Physiol.* **213,** 358.
Mosekilde, L., Lund, B., Sorensen, O., Christensen, M. S., and Melsen, F. (1977). *Lancet* **1,** 806.
Mueller, G. L., Third, W., Anast, C. S., and Breitenback, R. P. (1970). *Am. J. Physiol.* **218,** 1718.
Munson, P. L., and Gray, T. K. (1970). *Fed. Proc., Fed. Am. Soc. Exp. Biol.* **29,** 1206.
Ney, R. L., Au, W. Y. W., Kelly, G., Radde, I., and Bartter, F. C. (1965). *J. Clin. Invest.* **44,** 2003.
Ney, R. L., Kelly, G., and Bartter, F. C. (1968). *Endocrinology* **82,** 760.
Nicolaysen, R. (1937). *Biochem. J.* **31,** 122.
Nonidez, J. F., and Goodale, H. D. (1927). *Am. J. Anat.* **38,** 319.
Norman, A. W. (1965). *Science* **142,** 184.
Oldham, S., Smith, J., Hartenbower, D., Henry, H. L., Norman, A. W., and Coburn, J. W. (1976). *Fed. Proc., Fed. Am. Soc. Exp. Biol.* **35,** 302.
Olson, E. B., Jr., DeLuca, H. F., and Potts, J. T., Jr. (1972). *Endocrinology* **90,** 151.
Omdahl, J. L., Gray, R. W., Boyle, I. T., Knutson, J., and DeLuca, H. F. (1972). *Nature (London), New Biol.* **237,** 63.
Osborn, T. W., and Norman, A. W. (1977). *In* "Proceedings of the Third Workshop on Vitamin D: Biochemical, Chemical and Clinical Aspects Related to Calcium Metabolism" (A. W. Norman *et al.*, eds.), p. 523. de Gruyter, Berlin.
Raisz, L. G., and Bingham, P. J. (1972). *Annu. Rev. Pharmacol.* **12,** 337.
Raker, J. W., Henneman, P. H., and Grafi, W. S. (1962). *J. Clin. Endocrinol. Metab.* **22,** 273.
Ramurthy, N. S., Zebrowski, E. J., Baker, C., and Golub, L. M. (1973). *Res. Commun. Chem. Pathol. Pharmacol.* **5,** 614.
Rasmussen, H. (1971). *Am. J. Med.* **50,** 567.
Rasmussen, H. (1974). *In* "Textbook of Endocrinology" (R. H. Williams, ed.), 5th ed., Chapter 13, p. 660. Saunders, Philadelphia, Pennsylvania.
Rasmussen, H., DeLuca, H. F., Arnaud, C., Hawker, C., and von Stedingk, M. (1963). *J. Clin. Invest.* **42,** 1940.
Rasmussen, H., Wong, M., Bikle, D., and Goodman, E. B. P. (1972). *J. Clin. Invest.* **51,** 2502.
Reynolds, J. J. (1966). *Exp. Cell Res.* **41,** 174.
Ringe, J. D., Kuhlencordt, F., and Kruse, H. P. (1976). *Am. J. Roentgenol.* **126,** 1300.
Schmidt, J. R., Labhart, A., and Rossier, P. H. (1961). *Am. J. Med.* **31,** 343.
Schneider, H., Schedl, H. P., McCain, T., and Haussler, M. R. (1977). *Science* **196,** 1452.
Schneider, L. E., and Schedl, H. P. (1972). *Am. J. Physiol.* **223,** 1319.
Schneider, L. E., Wilson, H. D., and Schedl, H. P. (1974). *Am. J. Physiol.* **227,** 832.
Schneider, L. E., Omdahl, J., and Schedl, H. P. (1975a). *Physiologist* **18,** 381.
Schneider, L. E., Wasserman, R. H., and Schedl, H. P. (1975b). *Endocrinology* **97,** 649.
Seymour, J. L., and DeLuca, H. F. (1974). *Endocrinology* **94,** 1009.
Shain, S. A. (1972a). *J. Biol. Chem.* **247,** 4393.
Shain, S. A. (1972b). *J. Biol. Chem.* **247,** 4404.
Spanos, E., Colston, K. W., Evans, I. M. A., Galante, L. S., MacAuley, S. J., and MacIntyre, I. (1976a). *Mol. Cell. Endocrinol.* **5,** 163.
Spanos, E., Pike, J. W., Haussler, M. R., Colston, K. W., Evans, I. M. A., Goldener, A. M., McCain, T., and MacIntyre, I. (1976b). *Life Sci.* **19,** 1751.
Spanos, E., Colston, K. W., and MacIntyre, I. (1977). *FEBS Lett.* **75,** 73.
Stoerk, H. C., Peterson, A. C., and Jelinek, V. C. (1963). *Proc. Soc. Exp. Biol. Med.* **114,** 690.
Tanaka, Y., and DeLuca, H. F. (1973). *Arch. Biochem. Biophys.* **154,** 566.
Tanaka, Y., and DeLuca, H. F. (1974). *Science* **183,** 1198.

Tanaka, Y., Castillo, L. and DeLuca, H. F. (1976). *Proc. Natl. Acad. Sci. U.S.A.* **73,** 2701.
Tashjian, A. H., Jr. (1965). *Proc. Soc. Exp. Biol. Med.* **77,** 375.
Toverud, S. U. (1964). *Acta Physiol. Scand.* **62,** 3.
Turton, C. W. G., Stanley, P., Stamp, T. C. B., and Maxwell, J. D. (1977). *Lancet* **1,** 222.
Velentzas, C., Oropoulos, D. G., From, G., Porret, B. V., and Rapoport, A. (1977). *Lancet* **1,** 370.
Wecksler, W. R. (1978). Ph.D. Dissertation, University of California, Riverside.
Wecksler, W. R., Henry, H. L., and Norman, A. W. (1977). *Arch. Biochem. Biophys.* **183,** 168.
Weisman, Y., Sapir, R., Harell, A., and Edelstein, S. (1976). *Biochim. Biophys. Acta* **428,** 385.
Williams, G. A., Bowser, E. N., Henderson, W. J., and Uzgiries, V. (1961). *Proc. Soc. Exp. Biol. Med.* **106,** 664.
Williams, G. A., Peterson, W. C., Bowser, E. N., Henderson, W. J., Hargis, G. K., and Martinez, N. J. (1974). *Endocrinology* **95,** 707.
Zull, J. E., Czarnowska-Misztal, E., and DeLuca, H. F. (1965). *Science* **149,** 182.

CHAPTER 10

Intestinal Effects of Vitamin D

I. BACKGROUND CONSIDERATIONS

A. Introduction

Calcium and phosphorus are the most abundant of the inorganic elements in the body (Widdowson and Dickerson, 1964). Accordingly, it is quite appropriate that these substances have been a topic of major concern for biologists, biochemists, physiologists, and endocrinologists over the past three-quarters of a century. As can be seen in Table 10-1, these two elements play key roles in a wide spectrum of biological processes. Obviously a problem of major significance to the living organism is one of ensuring an adequate supply of calcium and phosphorus to meet these bodily needs. It is essential to life that calcium and phosphorus be supplied on a continuing daily basis.

The primary means of acquisition of phosphorus and calcium is via dietary intake. The focus of this chapter is a review of the current understanding of the

TABLE 10-1
Biological Calcium and Phosphorus

Calcium	Phosphorus
Utilization	
Body content: 70-kg man has 1200 g Ca^{2+}	Body content: 70-kg man has 770 g P
Structural: Bone has 95% of body Ca	Structural: Bone has 90% of body P_i
Plasma [Ca^{2+}] is 2.5 mM, 10 mg%	Plasma [P_i] is 2.3 mM
Muscle contraction	Intermediary metabolism (phosphorylated intermediates)
Nerve pulse transmission	Genetic information (DNA and RNA)
Blood clotting	Phospholipids
Membrane structure	Enzyme/protein components (phosphohistidine, phosphoserine)
Enzyme cofactors (amylase, trypsinogen, lipases, ATPases)	Membrane structure
Eggshell (birds)	
Daily requirements (70-kg man)	
Dietary intake: 700[a]	Dietary intake: 1200[b]
Fecal excretion[c]: 300–600[a]	Fecal excretion[c]: 350–370[b]
Urinary excretion[c]: 100–400[a]	Urinary excretion[c]: 200–600[b]

[a]Taken from Bronner (1964). Values in milligrams per day.
[b]Taken from Bartter (1964). Values in milligrams per day.
[c]Based on the indicated level of dietary intake.

mechanisms involved in the intestinal absorption of calcium and phosphorus and the important role played by vitamin D and its metabolites in this process. However, it would be naive to simply focus on the intestine without the realization that the problem of calcium and phosphorus absorption is interrelated with the larger problems of phosphorus and calcium homeostasis. Since these two elements are so important to the organism and since the problem of dietary excess in some ways may present as many potential problems as a dietary paucity, the organism has evolved a ''total body solution'' to these most important problems. This is in fact the system of calcium and phosphorus homeostasis. This process involves the integrated actions of the site of uptake, the intestine, with those of the site of major deposition of these ions, the bone, and of the major site of excretion of these minerals, the kidney. The coordinated operation of these three organs provides the minute-to-minute basis for calcium and phosphorus homeostasis.

The subject of calcium and phosphorus homeostasis has been discussed in a multitude of reviews over the years. For example, see the following for other viewpoints and emphasis: Borle (1972), Bronner (1964, 1973), Comar and Bronner (1969), Corradino and Wasserman (1971), Eanes and Posner (1970), Martonosi *et al.* (1971), Neuman and Neuman (1958), Nichols and Wasserman (1971), Nicolaysen and Eg-Larsen (1953), Nicolaysen *et al.* (1953), Norman 1968),

Rahaminoff (1970), Rasmussen and DeLuca (1963), Wasserman (1963, 1972, 1974), Wasserman and Corradino (1971), Wasserman and Kallfelz (1970), and Wasserman and Taylor (1969, 1972).

It has been traditional to consider calcium and phosphorus separately; however, it is obvious that in terms of many of their physiological interactions these ions are regulated in a coordinated manner. In man, the concentration of calcium in the blood is remarkably constant; major endocrinological efforts are exerted by the organism to maintain this constancy at a level of 2.3 to 2.5 m*M*. The acceptable phosphorus range in plasma is somewhat wider, i.e., 0.8–2.2 m*M*. This is not surprising since phosphorus is in equilibrium not only with bone phosphate but with the phosphorus that is associated with the many organic phosphorus-containing compounds involved in intermediary metabolism.

To determine the dietary requirements of calcium and phosphorus is complicated since the requirement for one ion is dependent on the amounts of the other ion present in the diet. In many instances the requirements have been proved to vary markedly from species to species. The calcium intake of most human beings varies between 200 and 1500 mg calcium per day (Bronner, 1964). As discussed in Section III,A, the fraction of this dietary calcium that is absorbed is under stringent regulation via physiological mechanisms that are dictated by "the calcium demand" of the organism. Dietary phosphate intake in man ranges from 600 to 2000 mg/day (Irving, 1964; Bartter, 1964). At present no specific evidence is available, suggesting that adaptation is a component of the intestinal absorption process for phosphorus. One complication related to determining the availability of dietary calcium and phosphorus is their propensity for precipitation. When calcium and phosphorus are both present in relatively large quantities in the diet, their coprecipitation in the lumen of the intestine may interfere with efficient and quantitative absorption.

B. Intestinal Morphology and Cytology

Any studies designed to elucidate the biochemical parameters of intestinal calcium and phosphorus absorption must take into account the unique morphology of the intestinal columnar epithelial cells. These cells are highly differentiated for their special role in various absorptive processes. The lumen of the small intestine is composed of a multitude of fingerlike projections, which are termed villi. Typically these villi range from 0.5 to 1.5 nm in length. They are composed principally of two types of cells: the columnar epithelial cell and the goblet or mucus-secreting cell. The latter is believed to be involved with the secretion of mucopolysaccharide components into the lumen of the intestine.

The cells on the villus are rapidly renewed. The mucosal cells originate in a progenitor population in the crypt of Lieberkuhn, and the cells migrate toward the villi tips, where they are extruded into the lumen. Only after epithelial cells enter the villus do they differentiate into fully functional absorptive cells. This differentiation process is characterized by a change in the RNA/protein ratio and a change in the activity of various enzymes as a function of the position of the epithelial cell on the villus. The undifferentiated cells in the crypt possess a high content of RNA (Webster and Harrison, 1969), mainly in the form of free ribosomes. Their microvilli are sparse and blunted and contain several enzymes with low activity, e.g., esterases, disaccharidases, and alkaline phosphatase (Palade, 1958; Dahlquist and Nordstrom, 1966; Nordstrom *et al.*, 1968). The enzymatic activities of esterase, leucine aminopeptidase, invertase, and alkaline phosphatase increase in a regular pattern with migration of epithelial cells toward the villus (Padykula, 1962; Lipkin and Bell, 1968). Intestinal epithelial cell turnover times of 30 to 48 hr have been reported in mice, rats, and human beings. The rate of epithelial cell renewal increases when there is an increased demand for new cells, as in recovery from radiation injury, response to parasite infestation, or adaptation to partial intestinal resection (Crane *et al.*, 1965).

Figure 10-1 is a diagrammatic representation of the intestinal villus. Figure 10-2 shows the remarkable trophic effect of vitamin D on the length of the intestinal villi. Spielvogel *et al.* (1972) and Birge and Alpers (1973) reported that in the chick and rat, respectively, chronic administration of physiological levels of vitamin D increases the length of the villus by 20–30%. In the chick the turnover time of cells on the villus was found to be 90–92 hr in both vitamin

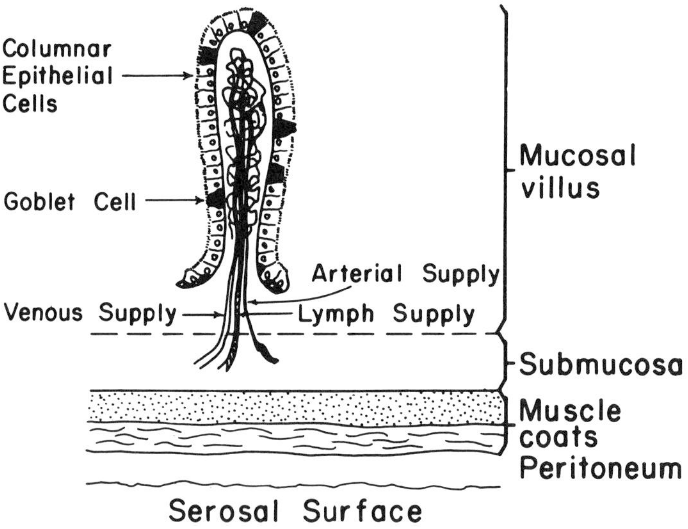

Figure 10-1. Schematic diagram of a small intestinal villus in longitudinal section.

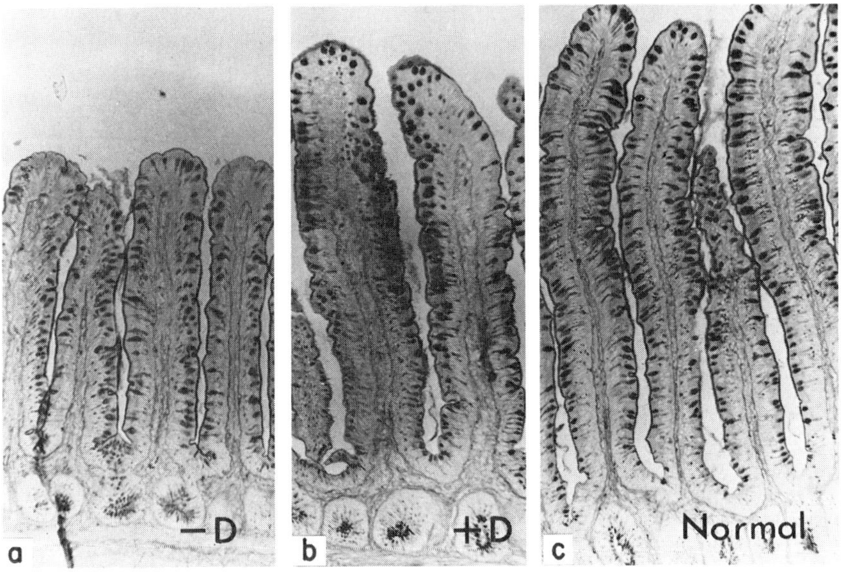

Figure 10-2. Morphology of chick intestinal mucosa as revealed by the light microscope. Longitudinal sections of the ileum of 4-week-old chicks that were (a) vitamin D-deficient, (b) treated with 500 IU (32.5 nmoles) vitamin D_3 every 48 hr starting 120 hr before they were killed (+D), (c) fed 50 IU (3.25 nmoles) vitamin D_3 every 48 hr starting at hatch (normal). (A, B, C) × 180. (From Spielvogel *et al.*, 1972.)

D-deficient and vitamin D_3-replete birds. Since the +D villus was 30% longer, this has the interesting consequence that the cells on the +D villus must migrate from the crypts of Lieberkuhn to the villus tip significantly more rapidly than the cells on the −D villus.

The rate of cell renewal is regulated by the cell proliferation in the crypt and cell loss at the extrusion zone. The molecular basis of this regulation is as yet poorly understood, but it is interesting to consider the possible intervention of vitamin D or its active metabolite, $1,25(OH)_2D_3$, in this process.

Figure 10-3 is an electron micrograph of the intestinal columnar epithelial cells. The apical surface of these cells, which is exposed to the lumen, is referred to as the brush border or microvillar membrane. These microvilli are approximately 1 μm long and 0.1 μm wide. As a consequence the surface area of the mucosa is increased 600-fold, as compared to the total area of a simple cylinder (Wilson, 1962). A variety of carbohydrate hydrolyases and an alkaline phosphatase of the intestinal mucosal cell are specifically associated with this brush border region (Miller and Crane, 1962; Norman *et al.*, 1970). This is believed to be the region of localization of permeases that are postulated as being involved in the absorption of materials into the cell.

Beneath the columnar epithelial cell lie the lymphatic and blood vascular systems, which project into each villus and thus provide an efficient mechanism for the translocation of a substrate once it exits from the epithelial cells.

The outermost surface of the columnar epithelial cell, i.e., the microvilli or brush border region, is covered with a filamentous mucopolysaccharide coat termed the glycocalyx or "fuzzy coat" (Ito, 1965). The function of the glycocalyx is not specifically known. Some workers have reported that the glycocalyx is impregnated with knobs or spherical particles 40–60 Å in diameter (Forstner, 1971), which can be stained by dyes that are specific for polysaccharides (Forstner, 1969). It has been suggested by Forstner (1971) that these surface knobs and filaments are identical with glycoproteins exhibiting disaccharidase, naphthalamidase, and alkaline phosphatase enzymatic activity.

The intestinal brush border region can be seen in the electron micrograph of Fig. 10-3. In Fig. 10-3A the substructure, or "core," of the microvilli, as well as the overlying glycocalyx, is clearly evident. In Fig. 10-3B (a cross-sectional plane of the brush border) the complex membrane architecture is apparent. At present little is known concerning the possible relationship between the membrane ultrastructure and its role in intestinal transport processes.

Jande (1976) carried out the first freeze-fracture evaluation of the duodenal absorptive cell membranes. He found that vitamin D_3 (500 IU for 24 hr) given to rachitic chicks resulted in an increase in the number of randomly scattered particles on the interior faces of the plasma membrane.

C. Intestinal Calcium and Phosphorus Absorption—The Problem

It is possible to identify in a flow chart the various steps that one may anticipate should or could be associated with the multistep and multicompartmental problem of intestinal calcium and phosphorus absorption (Fig. 10-4). The problem reduces to the simple transfer of the ion in question from the lumen of the intestine across the intervening membranes to the plasma. Kinetically one can follow this as disappearance of ion from the lumen or appearance of ion in the plasma. However, consideration of the various intervening membranes and compartments that one can postulate should be involved suggests that a simple, straightforward kinetic analysis may not expose the sophistication and details of the overall process.

There are basically three steps involved in the transport process: uptake across the extracellular membrane of the intestinal cell, transport across the cell, and efflux out of the cell across another cell membrane. One must be concerned with the state of the ion as it is transported, keeping in mind that calcium may be chelated by an endogenous substance such as citrate and that phosphate is capable of forming covalent bonds with organic molecules. Also, the charge on the

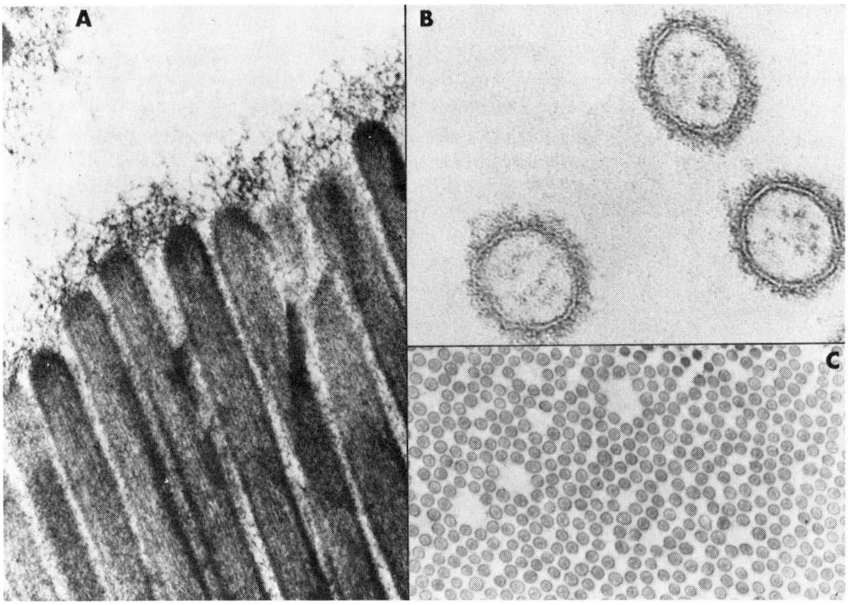

Figure 10-3. Electron microscopic evaluation of chick intestinal brush border region. (A) "Core" region of the brush border; the adhering glycocalyx on the tips of the microvilli is also apparent. (B, C) Cross section of microvilli. A, B × 40,000; C × 8000. (From Wong, 1972.)

phosphate ion may be of importance since Borle (1972) has shown that renal membranes are severalfold more permeable to HPO_4^{2-} than to $H_2PO_4^-$. The first step concerns the possible interaction of these substances with the negatively charged glycocalyx mucopolysaccharide, which has exposed sulfate groups. Then at some point interaction with the microvillar membrane should occur. In this respect a pertinent question is whether passive diffusion, carrier-mediated transport, or active transport across this membrane is the means of ion translocation. Related to this is the fact that the electric potential of the inside of the cell is negative with respect to the exterior and thus, for calcium, is an attractive force, whereas for phosphate it is a repulsive force. Similar considerations, with the charges reversed, would apply to the exit step at the basal side of the cell.

Inside the cell a multitude of interactions may occur. A pertinent question involves the role of mitochondrial and microsomal membranes in the transcellular migration of phosphate and calcium. The movement of the substances through the membrane at the basal side of the cell and the possible intervention of a sodium/potassium-activated ATPase have been studied by a number of investigators. Having exited from the cell, the ions in question then must move through interstitial space until they finally encounter the endothelial cells of the

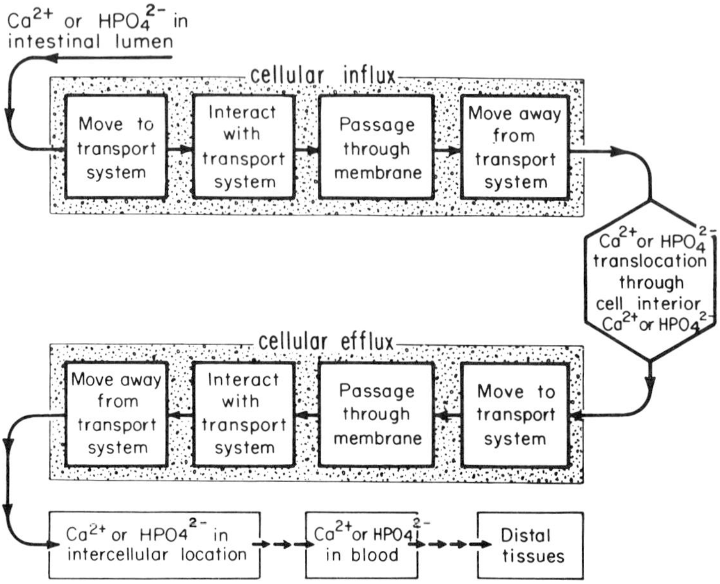

Figure 10-4. Flow chart analysis of the process of transfer of calcium and phosphorus from the lumen of the intestine across the intestinal cell to the blood.

blood capillaries. In terms of the three potential regulators or mediators of intestinal absorption of these substances, e.g., vitamin D and its metabolites, parathyroid hormone, and calcitonin, it is apparent that there are numerous possible sites on which they exert putative, specific actions enabling the translocation of calcium and phosphorus into the body.

It has also been suggested by Diamond and Wright (1969) that a significant fraction of materials absorbed by the intestine may be transported via diffusional pathways between cells rather than through cells.

Administration of vitamin D to rachitic animals mediates a 2.5- to 3.5-fold increase in intestinal calcium transport (Adams and Norman, 1970), with the increase occurring only after a time lag of 24 to 48 hr (Norman, 1966). The present concept of the mechanism of action of vitamin D involves at least two major time-dependent processes which partially account for this time lag: (a) the time required for the two-step metabolism of vitamin D to $1,25(OH)_2D_3$; (b) the time required for interaction of $1,25(OH)_2D_3$ with its intestinal cytoplasmic and nuclear receptor (Norman and Henry, 1974), resulting in subsequent *de novo* synthesis or induction of proteins including calcium-binding protein (Wasserman *et al.*, 1968), alkaline phosphatase (Norman *et al.*, 1970), and an ATPase activated by calcium (Melançon and DeLuca, 1970; Holdsworth, 1970). The activity of all these proteins has been shown to increase in intestinal mucosal cells after administration of vitamin D or 1,25$(OH)_2D_3$. The important point, however, is that the appearance and loss of these proteins could be dependent on the rate of turnover of the mucosal cells themselves.

The following questions can be asked concerning the effect of calciferol on intestinal calcium transport. (a) Does vitamin D affect the physiology of the intestine? (b) Is such a change a prerequisite for the increase of intestinal calcium transport? (c) Is the turnover time of the intestinal epithelial cells a determinant factor in the gradual increase or the decrease in calcium transport after a single dose of calciferol?

Another pertinent fact is that the increase in intestinal calcium transport and the rise in brush border enzyme activities are maximal 35–40 hr after a single dose of vitamin D or in only 12–20 hr when 1,25$(OH)_2D_3$ is given to chicks (Fig. 10-5). At this time the villus size and rate of migration in the vitamin D- or metabolite-treated birds would not be significantly different from that of the vitamin D-deficient birds. It is of some interest that the stimulation of intestinal

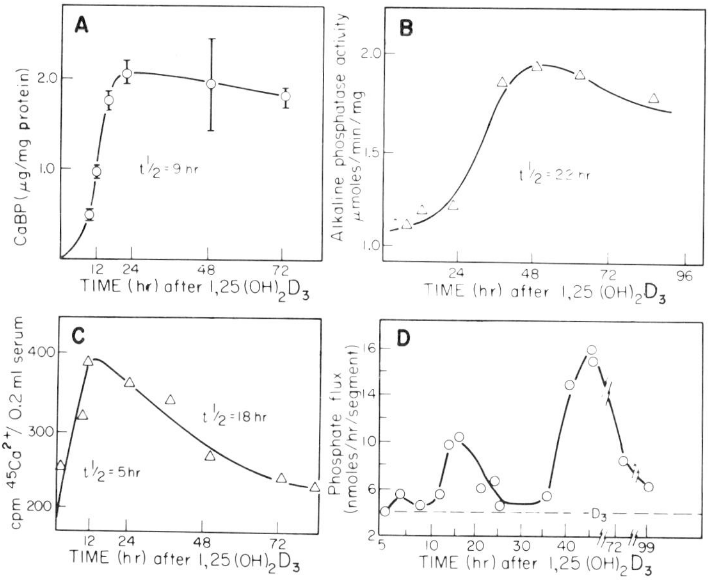

Figure 10-5. Time course of several intestinal responses after treatment with 1,25$(OH)_2D_3$. In (A), (B), and (C), chicks were treated orally with 325 pmoles (5 U) of 1,25$(OH)_2D_3$ dissolved in 1,2-propanediol. (A) Appearance of calcium-binding protein; CaBP was determined by radial immunoassay in the laboratory of Professor R. H. Wasserman, Cornell University. (B) Increase in alkaline phosphatase activity of the intestinal brush border (Norman *et al.*, 1970). (C) Increase in intestinal Ca^{2+} transport measured *in vivo* (Myrtle and Norman, 1971). (D) Increase in stimulation of intestinal absorption of phosphate after administration of 1,25$(OH)_2D_3$ (R. Mitsuyasu and A. W. Norman, unpublished observations).

calcium transport by 1,25$(OH)_2D_3$ in the rat is markedly slower than in the chick [compare 24–36 hr for maximal response in the rat (M. W. Walling, unpublished results) versus 10–14 hr for the chick] (Figure 10-5). Brickman and co-workers observed that oral administration of 65 pmoles of 1,25$(OH)_2D_3$ to man stimulates the intestinal absorption of calcium within 6–8 hr. Thus, the result obtained in the chick indicates that the primary action of vitamin D—increased calcium transport—is not integrally dependent on a change at the cellular level of the increase in cell size, number, or migration rate. Clearly, vitamin D and its metabolites have effects on the villus size and migration rate; however, these are not absolute prerequisites for stimulation of intestinal calcium transport.

D. Methods of Study

Over the years many techniques have been devised for quantitating various facets of the intestinal absorption of phosphorus and calcium. An excellent review of this subject has appeared (Berger, 1960). These methods are summarized in Table 10-2.

Basically two approaches have been used: those in the intact animal and those in which a portion of the intestinal cells have been removed for study under more defined conditions *in vitro*. Prior to the 1940's almost all techniques depended on the use of stable isotopes and conventional nutritional balance measurements by which the input and output of calcium and phosphorus by the animal were quantitated.

At present two radioactive isotopes of calcium are available. Calcium-45, a β emitter (0.252 meV max) has a half-life of 152 days; ^{47}Ca is a γ emitter (1.31 meV, 0.81 meV, and 0.49 meV) and a β emitter (1.98 meV and 0.67 meV) with a half-life of 4.53 days. Two radioactive isotopes of phosphorus are also available. Phosphorus-32 is primarily used as a strong β emitter (1.7 meV) with a half-life of 14.3 days; ^{33}P is a weak β emitter (0.248 meV) with a half-life of 24.5 days (Lederer *et al.*, 1967).

In experimental animals the primary *in vivo* technique has been the procedure of Coates and Holdsworth (1961) as modified by Hibberd and Norman (1969). In this technique radioactive calcium or phosphorus is placed in an isolated loop in a selected region of the small intestine of an anesthetized animal; at various times the appearance of the isotope in the plasma is monitored. Care must be exercised to obtain the plasma sample in a relatively short period of time after the isotope is placed in the intestine, since there is rapid exchange of both plasma calcium and phosphate with the readily exchangeable pools of these substances in the bone. Thus, if the appearance of the isoptope in the plasma is to be a measure of "intestinal absorption," these measurements must be taken before significant exchange and dilution of the isotope has occurred with nonradioactive ions in the bone. Alternatively, it is possible, as Wasserman and Taylor (1973b) have done,

TABLE 10-2
Methods for Measuring Calcium and Phosphorus Absorption by the Intestine

Method	Reference
In vivo	
A. Experimental animals	
1. Perfusion, *in situ*	Olsen and DeLuca (1969)
2. Isolated loops, *in situ*	Coates and Holdsworth (1961), Scott (1965), Hibberd and Norman (1969)
B. Man	
1. Fecal recovery of radiocalcium	Blair *et al.* (1954), Rich and Ivanovich (1964)
2. Metabolic balance studies	Liu and Chu (1943), Stanbury and Lumb (1962)
3. Plasma appearance after oral radiocalcium	Heany and Whedon (1958)
4. Double-isotope method (one given orally and the other i.v.)	
a. Two separate doses of ^{47}Ca with external counting	Curtis *et al.* (1967), Litwak (1969)
b. ^{47}Ca and ^{45}Ca measured in plasma and/or urine	DeGrazia and Rich (1964), Szymender *et al.* (1972)
In Vitro	
A. Transcellular transport	
1. Everted intestinal sacs	Wilson and Wiseman (1954), Schacter and Rosen (1959)
2. Short-circuit conditions	Ussing (1949), Walling and Rothman (1969), Adams and Norman (1970), Walling (1977)
3. Glass perfusion apparatus	Adams and Norman (1970)
a. Unidirectional tissue uptake	Martin and DeLuca (1969b)

either to measure disappearance of isotope from the intestinal loop or to measure the isotopic accumulation by the intestinal tissue over a 30- to 40-min period.

Conventional techniques for *in vitro* studies on the intestinal absorption of calcium and phosphorus use either an everted intestinal sac as pioneered by Wilson and Wiseman (1954) or the short-circuit conditions as originally defined by Ussing (1949). The sac technique necessitates everting the segment of the small intestine, which presumably facilitates the oxygenization of mucosal cells when they are incubated in a bath with solution available to both sides. Such sac preparations have been shown to maintain a number of physiological functions for at least 1 hr or longer. However, the technique does have certain drawbacks. Usually only one sample per sac is obtained, and the serosal volume is quite small, about 0.5 ml, so that significant errors due to adsorption and absorption may occur. Furthermore, the value obtained is not a rate but an equilibrium ratio of ion concentration in the inside to ion concentration on the outside. Another problem associated with the small volume in the serosal compartment is that it may gain up to 0.2–0.3 ml of water in the course of the incubation period. This large volume change makes it difficult to ascertain whether one is studying the effect of water movement on phosphorus transport or on calcium transport.

A significant improvement in technique is the apparatus originally described by Helbock *et al.* (1966), which is a modification of an earlier apparatus described by Ussing (1949). Walling and Rothman (1969) and Adams and Norman (1970) previously commented on the numerous advantages of this technique. which include the fact that the experiments can be run under short-circuit conditions and thus remove the extraneous effect of other electropotentials and that multiple samples can be taken as a function of time so that a rate of transport is quantitatively determined. Walling (1977) made elegant use of this technique to simultaneously study the transport *in vitro* of ^{45}Ca and $^{32}P_i$.

An additional *in vitro* technique is that described by Martin and DeLuca (1969b). They can measure the rate of uptake of ions into the cell across the brush border membrane. The "uptake apparatus" consists of two Lucite sheets, one of which has a small orifice of approximately 0.5 cm diameter. An ileal segment of the tissue is placed serosal side down on the solid Lucite sheet, and the second sheet with the orifice is placed over the tissue with the hole centered over the tissue. The slides are held together with rubber bands and the edges pressed firmly together with a silicone gasket forming a seal around the edges. The slide is then emersed in a beaker for incubation with isotope. After incubation the slides are transferred to a second beaker containing wash buffer, which is kept ice cold. The slides are then blotted dry, and the exposed tissue is cut out with a ¼-in. cork borer. Thus, one can measure the isotope in the excised piece of tissue which is present only by virtue of uptake across the exposed cellular membrane.

II. EARLY WORK ON THE INTESTINAL ABSORPTION OF CALCIUM AND PHOSPHORUS

Before the availability of radioactive calcium and phosphorus in the 1940's, it was difficult to establish that one of the primary actions of vitamin D was to promote or facilitate the intestinal absorption of calcium. One of the first papers to report studies concerned with defining the mechanism of intestinal absorption of calcium and phosphorus was that of Bergheim (1926). Bergheim pointed out that both phosphorus and calcium were secreted by the intestine and then subject to reabsorption in a different intestinal location. Other investigators in this period utilized primarily balance studies in which the intake and the fecal and urine levels of calcium and phosphorus were monitored. These studies were carried out on children (Findley *et al.*, 1920), the rat (McClendon, 1922; Brown *et al.*, 1932), the chick (Bethke *et al.*, 1929), and the dog (Jones, 1927). It was generally agreed that there was an increased loss of phosphorus and calcium in vitamin D deficiency, which resulted primarily from an increased output of these elements into the feces.

It was not until the pioneering and thorough studies of Nicolaysen that the first direct causal relationship between vitamin D and calcium absorption was established. In a notable series of experiments he demonstrated the following. (a) When a Thiery Vella fistula was made of the entire colon in the rat, there was no alteration in the amount of calcium or phosphorus excreted into the feces by vitamin D-deficient or normal rats (Innes and Nicolaysen, 1937). (b) Intravenous injection of calcium was not followed by increased fecal calcium but by a concomitant increase in renal excretion of calcium in the urine. These results were independent of the vitamin D status of the rats (Innes and Nicolaysen, 1937). (c) Under conditions of dietary phosphorus deprivation, vitamin D markedly stimulated intestinal calcium absorption whereas, when dietary calcium was withheld, vitamin D had no enhancing or inhibiting effect on phosphorus absorption (Nicolaysen, 1937a,b). This result was obtained irrespective of whether dietary phosphorus was inorganic or organic phosphate. (d) In a pioneering experiment utilizing isolated, ligated jejunal loops of rachitic and normal rats *in vivo,* Nicolaysen (1937a) found that the rate of absorption of calcium was markedly increased in normal rats as compared to vitamin D-deficient rats. Under similar conditions the absorption of calcium from the abdominal cavity was identical in normal and vitamin D-deficient rats. This study clearly demonstrated for the first time the stimulatory effect of vitamin D on intestinal calcium absorption.

Thus, when radioactive calcium and phosphorus became available in the early 1940's, the groundwork was laid for more sophisticated studies. Greenberg (1945) concluded from one of the early tracer experiments utilizing both orally and intraperitoneally administered $^{45}Ca^{2+}$ that the intestinal excretion of calcium was not affected by the vitamin D status of the animal. Other studies by Migicovsky and Emslie (1947, 1949) in the chick, and by Carlsson (1951) and Lindquist (1952) in the rat utilizing radioactive calcium, substantiated the earlier conclusion of Nicolaysen that vitamin D had a significant effect on intestinal calcium absorption in the rat.

Very little work was done from 1920 to 1950 that was specifically concerned with defining the mechanism of phosphate absorption. One of the first studies was conducted by Nicolaysen (1937a,b), utilizing ligated intestinal loops *in vivo.* He found that inorganic phosphate and sodium glycerol phosphate were absorbed equally well in normal and vitamin D-deficient rats. Later studies of Dols *et al.* (1938) in the rachitic chick, Cohn and Greenberg (1939) and Manley and

Morgareidy (1939) in the rat, and Shimotori and Morgan (1943) in the dog with orally administered radioactive inorganic phosphorus reported no effect of vitamin D on phosphorus absorption.

III. MODERN ERA

A. Adaptation of Intestinal Ca^{2+} Absorption

The modern era of experimental investigations into phosphorus and calcium absorption can be appreciated only in the recent context of the metabolism and proposed steroid hormone mechanism of action of cholecalciferol. The development of this model is based on the concept that, in terms of its structure and mode of action, vitamin D is similar to other steroid hormones. It is now possible to correlate changes in the metabolism of the fat-soluble vitamin D to the active steroid hormone, $1,25(OH)_2D_3$, which are dictated by the calcium demands of the organism, with changes in the efficiency of intestinal calcium transport (Norman, 1975).

Figure 10-5 summarizes several intestinal responses that result from treating vitamin D-deficient chicks with small quantities of the active form of vitamin D, $1,25(OH)_2D_3$. As can be seen in Fig. 10-5C,D, $1,25(OH)_2D_3$ is capable of stimulating the intestinal absorption of both calcium (maximal stimulation at 12 hr) and phosphorus (maximum stimulation at 40 hr). However, since there is a dramatic difference in the time required for onset of action, these two processes are probably dissociated from one another. Figure 10-5A shows a time course of stimulation of intestinal calcium-binding protein and Fig. 10-5B the time course of stimulation of intestinal brush border alkaline phosphatase. Thus, there seems to be a complex pattern of time-dependent responses to $1,25(OH)_2D_3$ in the intestinal mucosa. It should be noted that similar response patterns can be obtained with the parent vitamin D, although the times involved are longer due to the required metabolism.

Another aspect of the complexity of interaction of $1,25(OH)_2D_3$ and the parent vitamin with the intestine and the subsequent stimulation of calcium transport is illustrated in Fig. 10-6, where three different examples of the adaptation of the intestinal transport system are shown. Figure 10-6A (Coburn *et al.*, 1973) indicates how the absorption of calcium varies in man, depending on its dietary availability. When lower amounts are available, there is a higher fractional absorption of calcium. Figure 10-6B indicates that a similar situation exists in the chick. When there is a high dietary level of calcium (1.8%) there is, in a vitamin D-replete bird, a relatively low level of intestinal calcium absorption; when the dietary calcium content is low ($<0.05\%$), there is an approximate threefold increase in the rate of calcium transport when vitamin D is administered. Thus,

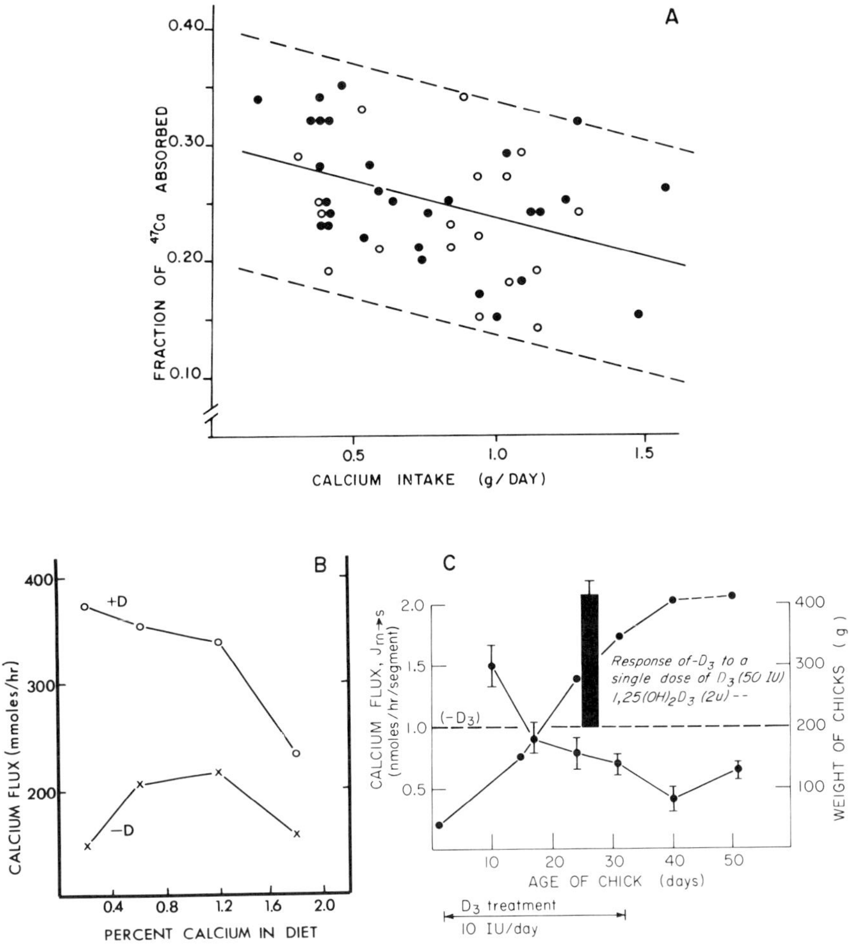

Figure 10-6. (A) The relationship between the fraction of ^{47}Ca absorbed and the previous habitual dietary intake of calcium in normal human beings. Each point represents a separate individual (●, males; ○, females; the dashed lines encompass the 95% confidence limits for individual values). Reproduced by the permission of the authors (Coburn *et al.*, 1973). (B) Adaptation of calcium trasnport in chicks. Chicks were raised for 20 days on a standard rachitogenic diet, 0.6% Ca^{2+} (Norman and Wong, 1972). (Reprinted from Kidney International.) Then they were changed to diets containing 0, 0.6, 1.2, or 1.8% calcium with 0.4% phosphate. Half the birds received 15 IU of vitamin D_3 (+D) daily; the other half received only 1,2-propanediol. After 5 days the rate of calcium flux was measured in ileal segments *in vitro,* as described by Adams and Norman (1970). (C) Changes in the activity of intestinal calcium transport with age and vitamin D status. Groups of chicks were placed on a diet of 0.6% calcium, 0.4% phosphate and received 10 IU (0.65 nmole) of vitamin D_3 per day, from day 1 to day 32. The rate of intestinal calcium transport was measured *in vitro* in an apparatus similar to that of Ussing as described by Adams and Norman (1970). Other groups of chicks received no vitamin D_3 for 21 days, at which time they exhibited the classic symptoms of rickets. At this point they received either 50 IU (3.25 nmoles) of vitamin D_3 or 2 units (0.13 nmole) of $1{,}25(OH)_2D_3$ and their intestinal transport was measured either 24 or 8 hr later, respectively.

the bird is able to adapt its rate of intestinal calcium transport to reflect inversely the amount of calcium in the diet. It is also apparent that the "adaptation process" is dependent on the presence of vitamin D. In the absence of cholecalciferol (Fig. 10-6B) there is no marked change in the rate of transport of calcium as the dietary content of calcium is varied. Figure 10-6C shows the adaptation of intestinal calcium transport with an increase in the rate of growth of chicks. For the first 30 days after hatching, during which time the birds are actively growing and presumably have a high demand for calcium, there is a surprising fall in the rate of calcium transport when there is a ready dietary source of vitamin D. Thus, the presence of the dietary vitamin D ensures that the intestinal calcium transport system may respond in an adaptive fashion to meet the demands of the calcium absorption system. Figure 10-6C also documents the response of a vitamin D-deficient, rachitic young chick given a single dose of cholecalciferol or the vitamin D metabolite 1,25$(OH)_2D_3$. There are as yet no reports concerning attempts to assess a possible adaptation of the intestinal absorption of phosphorus.

B. Contrasting Views on the Mechanism of Calcium and Phosphorus Transport

The physiological studies demonstrating the enhancing effect of vitamin D on intestinal absorption of calcium and possibly on phosphorus have laid the groundwork for a rigorous biochemical examination of the detailed mechanism by which these two substances are moved across the small intestine. The problem is basically one of determining whether the transport of calcium and/or phosphorus is an active transport, i.e., transport against an electrochemical gradient (Ussing, 1949), or passive transport, and what the detailed role of vitamin D and/or its metabolites may be in these processes. Does the vitamin or its metabolite (a) act as a direct effector(s) and bind to some crucial membrane to change the conformation of protein components so that the membrane has an increased permeability, thus in essence facilitating a passive transfer, or (b) induce the synthesis of the appropriate enzyme systems involved in an active transport system or (c) induce the synthesis of a modified, more permeable membrane (to calcium and/or phosphate)? Although the vitamin or its metabolite might not directly be involved in calcium transport, it is still an intriguing question as to how these cations and anions actually cross the cell membrane and interior of the cell. If vitamin D induces the production of a transport system, either active or passive, it is pertinent also to know whether the parameters of the induced system are identical or different from those of the noninduced system (vitamin D-deficient animal). Does vitamin D induce additional quantities of the same preexisting system, alter components of an existing system, or initiate the production of a second calcium or phosphate transport system? There have been a multitude of papers and interpretations of data that bear on the subject. The conclusions concerning vitamin D-mediated calcium transport reached by major laboratories are summarized in Table 10-3.

Schacter's group began a series of investigations on intestinal calcium transport in 1959. These studies were a departure from the original intact-animal experiments mentioned earlier that had been performed by Nicolaysen, Greenberg, and others since Schacter used the everted sac technique to study calcium transport *in vitro*. He found that calcium was transported against a concentration gradient (Schacter and Rosen, 1959). According to the criterion of Rosenberg and Wilbrandt (1957) this is indicative of active transport. Schacter's group later became interested in evaluating the role of vitamin D in the system when they found that vitamin D deprivation decreased intestinal calcium transport. Using the everted sac method, they observed that the concentration ratio (serosal/mucosal) was 2.9 for the vitamin D-treated animals and only 1.1 for the vitamin D-deficient animals. Cyanide, azide, dinitrophenol, iodoacetamide, and malonate were effective inhibitors of calcium transport *in vitro;* suggesting that metabolic energy was required for both uptake and release (Schacter and Rosen, 1959).

In other studies by Schacter and co-workers, efforts were made to define subcomponents of the overall transport process by studying separately uptake and release of calcium from intestinal slices. The mechanism was described as having a facilitated diffusion step at the mucosal surface and an active pump located at the basal membrane of the columnar epithelial cells (Kimberg *et al.*, 1961).

Wasserman and colleagues determined flux rates *in vivo* in the normal rat by the method of Curran and Solomon (1957) and provided evidence that the flux rate was greater than unity at all levels of calcium concentration. This indicated to these workers that calcium was actively transported in the intact animal (Wasserman *et al.*, 1961). Wasserman's laboratory also studied calcium flux *in vitro* in intestines from rachitic rats and chicks. They found that vitamin D administration increased the plasma-to-ileum calcium flux in the chick ileum 2.7-fold and that in the rat duodenum 1.9-fold. As expected, the lumen-to-plasma flux was also increased, but it was increased only 1.3-fold in both the chick and the rat. These data suggested that the major effect of vitamin D was not on a unidirectional transport system, but that it operated only to increase diffusional permeability. It was proposed that this could be caused by a change in membrane structure or by the synthesis of proteins specific for calcium (Wasserman *et al.*, 1966). (Calcium-binding protein is discussed in Section III,F.)

Harrison and Harrison (1960) found that the effect of vitamin D on calcium transfer *in vitro* in rat intestine is not blocked by inhibitors of oxidative metabolism. This observation led to the conclusion that vitamin D increases the rate of diffusion of calcium across the intestine. Harrison and Harrison (1965) also found that calcium is actively transported in rat duodenum as judged by the

TABLE 10-3
Summary of Studies on Vitamin D-Mediated Calcium Transport

Effect of vitamin D on calcium transport	Comment	Investigator	Reference
Active transport stimulated	There is a Ca^{2+}-stimulated ATPase in the intestinal brush borders that responds to vitamin D treatment	DeLuca	Martin and DeLuca (1969a,b), Martin *et al.* (1969)
Altered permeability	The action of vitamin D may be a permeability change, which potentiates an active calcium pump by the increased availability of calcium	Harrison and Harrison	Harrison and Harrison (1960, 1965)
Active transport stimulated	Vitamin D inhibits a metabolically operated pump that returns calcium from the mucosal cell to the lumen	Holdsworth	Sallis and Holdsworth (1962), Holdsworth (1965)
Increased permeability of brush border membrane for Ca^{2+} but not P_i	Transport of Ca^{2+} from lumen to serosa is energy dependent and active in both +D and −D states; chief effect of vitamin D is to improve uptake of Ca^{2+} but not P_i across brush border membrane	Norman	Adams and Norman (1970), Adams *et al.* (1970), Wong *et al.* (1970), Wong and Norman (1975)
Vitamin D effect is at a site adjacent to microvillar membrane	Uptake of Ca^{2+} by cell consists of two steps; the first is very rapid and unaffected by vitamin D_3, and the second is slower and affected by vitamin D_3	O'Donnel and Smith	O'Donnel and Smith (1973a,b)

Not active (effect of vitamin D not investigated)	Calcium transport in mature rats was found to be nonactive according to the method of Ussing; P_i transport was active and could cause calcium to be actively transported	Saltman	Helbock *et al.* (1966)
Active transport stimulated	Two-step mechanism involving an uptake and release of Ca^{2+} with a vitamin D effect on both processes	Schachter	Schachter and Rosen (1959), Schachter *et al.* (1960), Kimberg *et al.* (1961)
Vitamin D acts at both brush border and basal membrane sites	Studies of Ca^{2+} transport in the small intestine perfused *in vivo;* transport against concentration gradient seen in all segments	Schedl	Krawitt and Schedl (1968), Urban and Schedl (1969a,b, 1970), Youngoszai *et al.* (1972a,b, 1973)
Active transport process adapts to calcium needs of the animal	Calcium transport, according to the method of Ussing, gave flux ratios of 2.2 for +D and 1.4 for −D in rats; the "active" component is internal to the adaptive uptake process	Walling and Rothman	Walling and Rothman (1969, 1970, 1973), Walling (1977)
Increased diffusional permeability across brush border	Isolated CaBP implicated in Ca^{2+} transport. CaBP is localized in the brush border region; amount of CaBP adapts to reflect Ca needs of the animal	Wasserman	Wasserman *et al.* (1961, 1966, 1968), Wasserman and Taylor (1968, 1969, 1973a,b), Wasserman and Corradino (1971)

criterion of Rosenberg and Wilbrandt (1957). In later studies in which calcium transfer was measured in tissue that had its mucosa removed (i.e., only the underlying serosa was present) there was no difference due to vitamin D administration. This indicated that the difference due to vitamin D treatment lay in the mucosal tissue rather than serosal tissue. In related studies by the Harrisons, active transport of calcium was observed when the everted intestinal loops were incubated in a buffer with a sodium concentration of 26 m*M* but not in the presence of 145 m*M* sodium. Similar results were reported by DeLuca's laboratory (Martin and DeLuca, 1969a; Martin *et al.*, 1969). Vitamin D stimulated intestinal calcium transport even when the experiment was performed *in vitro* with *N*-ethylmaleimide present in the incubation solution (Hurwitz *et al.*, 1967). All of these results supported the original contention of Harrison and Harrison that the vitamin D effect is not on a unidirectional pump for calcium, but rather that the membrane permeability of calcium is altered by vitamin D treatment.

Sallis and Holdsworth (1962) studied calcium transport *in vitro* in vitamin D-treated and vitamin D-deficient chicks. Using everted sacs they found that metabolic inhibitors were able to inhibit calcium transport. Transport was not inhibited by the cardiac glycoside ouabain in the mucosal solution, but *N*-ethylmaleimide was an effective inhibitor of calcium transport, as were low incubation temperatures.

In everted sacs incubated at 38°C, vitamin D_3 increased the amount of calcium transferred to the serosal fluid and the amount of calcium in the mucosal compartment. On the basis of this and other results, these workers concluded that calcium is pumped out of the epithelial cells by a process that is dependent on the metabolic energy. A model was formulated in which vitamin D was proposed to inhibit an active pump which returns calcium from the mucosal cell to the lumen, thus bringing about a unidirectional transport of calcium (Holdsworth, 1965).

Walling and Rothman (1969, 1970, 1973) have carried out the most detailed kinetic studies to date of the transport of calcium *in vitro*. They employed the Ussing chamber under short-circuit conditions, in which they were able to monitor both M→S[1] and S→M fluxes and obtained evidence for an energy-dependent, phosphate-independent, saturable transport process for calcium. The K_m for M→S Ca^{2+} transport was calculated to be 1.25 m*M*. They also demonstrated that the M→S but not S→M flux of Ca^{2+} could be increased by feeding a low-calcium diet and that the affinity, or K_m, decreased to 0.6 m*M* under these conditions. This finding is reminiscent of studies on substrate-induced transport pathways in bacterial systems. In the view of Walling and Rothman, the primary effect of vitamin D administration is to increase via inductive processes the uptake of calcium across the brush border membrane of the intestinal cell. Similar conclusions have been reached by O'Donnel and Smith (1973a,b).

[1]M→S denotes flux or rate of transfer from the mucosal (M) to the serosal (S) surface of the cell; S→M, flux in the reverse direction.

Urban and Schedl (1969a,b; 1970) and Schedl and co-workers (Krawitt and Schedl, 1968; Youngoszai and Schedl, 1972a,b; Youngoszai *et al.*, 1973) reported extensive studies on the role of vitamin D in intestinal Ca^{2+} transport. In their view, vitamin D has a unidirectionally oriented action on transmural calcium transport; it increases lumen-to-plasma but not plasma-to-lumen fluxes 1.6-fold. The obvious conclusion here is that the net effect of vitamin D can not be explained simply by increases in the bidirectional passive permeability of the uptake calcium across the brush border membrane. In contrast, these workers found that vitamin D treatment resulted in a 9-fold increase in *both* mucosa-to-plasma and plasma-to-mucosa fluxes at the basal membrane of the columnar epithelial cell. This is consistent with a bidirectionally operative membrane permeability change at this cellular site.

There are a variety of conflicting reports concerning the effect of vitamin D on phosphorus absorption. Carlsson (1954) noted a possible positive effect of vitamin D on phosphate absorption in studies carried out in rats. Under circumstances in which the animals were fed a calcium-deficient diet, he felt that the increase in phosphate absorption was due to a "general improvement of the condition of the animal" and not due to a direct effect of vitamin D. In the more modern era, Harrison and Harrison (1961) reported that the absorption of phosphorus was activated by the presence of calcium and that phosphate absorption was less efficient in vitamin D-deficient animals than in vitamin D-treated controls. Sallis and Holdsworth (1962), using rachitic chick intestinal loops perfused *in vivo,* reported that the steroid had no effect on the intestinal absorption of radioactive phosphate.

Kowarsky and Schacter (1969) reported the effects of vitamin D on the transport of inorganic phosphate into and across the intestinal mucosa. Vitamin D given to intact rats was found to increase phosphate transport *in vitro* selectively in the direction of mucosa to serosa. They further claimed that the sterol acted directly in the intestine without prior activation; however, this proposition seems untenable in light of much more recent information on the metabolism of vitamin D. Kowarsky and Schacter also stated that phosphate transport was restricted to "selective channels" in the mucosa; this conclusion was based on a complex interpretation of the relative specific activities of differing phosphate pools present in this tissue. Hence, these workers reported that the effect of vitamin D on calcium transport was maximal in the duodenum and independent of the presence of phosphate and, since phosphate transport was found to be maximal in the jejunum and independent of the presence of calcium, they concluded that vitamin D influences separately these two intestinal transport mechanisms.

More recently, Wasserman and Taylor (1973b) and Taylor (1974a) studied the effects of vitamin D on the intestinal absorption of radioactive phosphate in the chick. They observed that phosphate was rapidly translocated across all segments of the small intestine and that vitamin D administration stimulated the process in each segment. The absorption of phosphate was claimed to be inhibited by the presence of arsenate, ethane diphosphonate (EHDP), and L-phenylalanine (an inhibitor of alkaline phosphatase). These investigators stated that they could not detect the existence of a phosphate-binding protein comparable to the calcium-binding protein. The stimulation of phosphate uptake by vitamin D in mucosal tissue was maximal at 16 hr, whereas stimulation of the complete transfer of phosphate from lumen to blood became maximal only at 48 hr.

Hurwitz and Bar (1972) also believe that vitamin D stimulates phosphate absorption independent of calcium absorption. Their conclusion is based on results similar to those reported above by Kowarski and Schacter; i.e., the vitamin D-enhanced calcium absorption in the chick occurred mainly in the duodenum and that of phosphate mainly in the jejunum.

Chen *et al.* (1974) found that vitamin D and the metabolites $25(OH)D_3$ and $1,25(OH)_2D_3$, but not $24,25(OH)_2D_3$, stimulated phosphate transport independently of calcium transport in the rat. In the jejunum phosphate transport was completely independent of the presence of calcium in the medium. Furthermore, these workers concluded that, since $25(OH)D_3$ did not stimulate phosphate transport in an anephric animal, the active form of vitamin D that stimulated phosphate transport was the renal metabolite $1,25(OH)_2D_3$.

Walling (1977) has clearly carried out the most definitive study of the differential effects of vitamin D_3, $1,25(OH)_2D_3$, and $24,23(OH)_2D_3$ on both calcium and phosphate absorption in the rat intestine. These studies were carried out *in vitro* in an Ussing chamber in the absence of an electrochemical gradient. $1,25(OH)_2D_3$ increased the active absorption of calcium in all segments of the small intestine, with duodenum > jejunum > ileum. $1,25(OH)_2D_3$ also increased net P_i absorption, but the transport was greatest in the jejunum followed by the duodenum and then the ileum. $24(R),25(OH)_2D_3$ had similar effects on the transport of both calcium and P_i but was less potent. Walling's results seem most compatible with a differential distribution of vitamin D-responsive calcium, and P_i-absorptive cells with a predominance of cells with calcium-absorptive sites occurring in duodenum, more P_i-absorbing cells in jejunum, and a nearly equal ratio of each type in the ileum.

Birge and Miller (1977) examined the response of chick intestine to vitamin D and its metabolites in organ culture preparations of chick ileum explants. From their studies they postulate the novel view that the primary action of vitamin D and its metabolites in the intestine is to enhance the ability of the mucosal cell to accumulate phosphate. The elevated cellular levels of phosphate then permit further expression of the cell responses to vitamin D-related sterols, i.e., induction of CaBP.

Figure 10-5D presents the results obtained in the laboratory of the author indicating that $1,25(OH)_2D_3$ does have the capability of stimulating intestinal phosphate transport. What is puzzling is the kinetics of the stimulation of phosphate transport after administration of the steroid. The basis for the slow response of phosphate transport to this metabolite as compared to the relatively more rapid stimulation of calcium transport is not known.

Finally, it should be noted that Tanzer and Navia (1973) reported that treatment of rats with calcitonin can inhibit the intestinal absorption of phosphate.

C. Factors That Affect Intestinal Absorption of Calcium and Phosphorus

Over the years an incredible array of substances have been found to have an effect on the intestinal absorption of calcium and phosphorus. These range from compounds as simple as lactose and ethanol to antibiotics as complex and diverse in action as actinomycin D and Filipin. Table 10-4 is a compilation of many of these effectors and the appropriate literature citations. In a review by Wasserman and Taylor (1969) is a detailed description of the effect of lactose and related carbohydrates, amino acids, and detergents, including bile acids and cetrimide. The reader is referred to this review for a detailed discussion of the mode of

TABLE 10-4
Factors Affecting Intestinal Absorption of Calcium or Phosphorus

Factor	Reference
Amino acids	Wasserman *et al.* (1956)
Antibiotics	
Gene-active	
Actinomycin D	Norman (1965, 1966), Zull *et al.* (1965), Eisenstein and Passavoy (1964)
α-Amanitin	Corradino (1973)
Membrane-active	
Filipin	Adams *et al.* (1970), Wong *et al.* (1970), Wong and Norman (1975)
Ethane diphosphonate	Krawitt *et al.* (1974), Bonjour *et al.* (1972, 1973)
Ethanol	Krawitt *et al.* (1973)
Glucocorticoids	Krawitt (1972)
Lactose and other carbohydrates	Wasserman and Comar (1959)
Metabolic poisons	
2,4-Dinitrophenol, cyanide, iodoacetamide	Schacter and Rosen (1959), Adams and Norman (1970)
Peptide hormones	
Parathyroid hormone	Rasmussen (1959), Shah and Draper (1966)
Calcitonin	Olsen *et al.* (1972), Tanzer and Navia (1973)
Solanum (glaucophyllum) malacoxalon	Humphreys (1973), Ferraro *et al.* (1977)
Vitamin D	Walling (1977), Taylor (1974b), Wasserman and Taylor (1973b)

action of these substances. Our attention in this chapter is devoted to the remaining entries in Table 10-4.

It is already apparent from discussion in Chapter 1 that the gene-active antibiotics (inhibitors of messenger RNA synthesis) actinomycin D (Norman, 1965) and α-amanitin (Corradino, 1973) and the protein synthesis inhibitors cycloheximide and puromycin (inhibitors of messenger RNA translation) inhibit intestinal calcium transport by virtue of blocking the $1,25(OH)_2D_3$-induced expression of gene information that is essential for the biological response.

There have been numerous reports in the literature of the ability of diphosphonates to inhibit vitamin D-stimulated intestinal calcium transport (Bonjour *et al.*, 1972, 1973). The administration of 10 mg of EHDP to rats was shown by Bonjour *et al.* (1972) to inhibit bone mobilization and hypercalcemia and to dramatically decrease the intestinal absorption of calcium. The present basis of understanding of the mode of action of EHDP is that it inhibits the conversion of vitamin D to its active form, $1,25(OH)_2D_3$. Thus, the administration of $1,25(OH)_2D_3$, but not vitamin D, to vitamin D-deficient animals treated with EHDP results in a marked stimulation of intestinal calcium transport. These results suggest that the basis of action of this drug is not at the intestinal level, but is principally at the renal level (Krawitt *et al.*, 1973), where the metabolic transformation of $25(OH)D_3$ to $1,25(OH)_2D_3$ occurs. [See Chapter 6 for a discussion of the effects of EHDP, both *in vivo* and *in vitro,* on the metabolism of vitamin D and/or $25(OH)D_3$.]

Krawitt *et al.* (1973) reported that chronic administration of ethanol effects an inhibition of the intestinal absorption of calcium by the duodenum. However, at present, the mechanism underlying this inhibition of calcium transport and the possible clinical implications of the known occurrence of calcium malabsorption by chronic alcoholic patients are not known.

It is also well established that an excess of glucocorticoids can reduce the intestinal absorption of calcium (Harrison and Harrison, 1960; Kimberg *et al.*, 1961), and it has been postulated by several investigators that the glucocorticoids are "antagonistic" to the action of vitamin D. It has been shown by Kimberg *et al.* (1961), Krawitt (1972), and Lukert *et al.* (1973) that glucocorticoids reduce the active transport of calcium by the duodenum of rats, suppress brush border alkaline phosphatase activity, and abolish the appearance of calcium-binding protein. Originally there was some discussion as to whether this antagonistic effect was a result of interference with the metabolism of vitamin D to its active form, $1,25(OH)_2D_3$, or whether it was the result of an independent "end organ action" on the intestine. The studies by Favus *et al.* (1973) and Lukert *et al.* (1973) indicate that the suppression of calcium transport is mediated independently of any direct intervention in the metabolism of vitamin D.

Another complicated area of endeavor in the field of intestinal calcium and phosphorus absorption is the elucidation of the effects of the peptide hormones calcitonin and parathyroid hormone on these processes. The polypeptide hormone calcitonin is generally believed to act in preventing hypercalcemia, but the mechanisms by which the hormone achieves this are not completely understood. However, one likely action is inhibition by calcitonin of bone resorption. Olson *et al.* (1972) also reported inhibition by calcitonin of vitamin D-induced calcium absorption. An acute infusion of pharmacological doses of purified porcine calcitonin into rats produced an immediate drop in calcium absorption in animals given vitamin D but had no effect on calcium absorption in vitamin D-deficient animals. Also, Tanzer and Navia (1973) found that administration of calcitonin can inhibit the intestinal absorption of phosphate.

The possible role of parathyroid hormone in the overall process of intestinal calcium absorption is perhaps somewhat clearer. Several reports have appeared in the literature that support the view that the regulation of intestinal calcium absorption and the adaptation to dietary calcium in deprivation is mediated in part by parathyroid hormone. Until recently the site of action of the hormone on the transport process was unknown. However, it now appears that parathyroid hormone is a trophic factor capable of stimulating the output by the kidney of $1,25(OH)_2D_3$ (Henry *et al.*, 1974). Under periods of high calcium demand—dictated possibly by a low level of dietary calcium—serum calcium would most likely fall. This would result in an increased secretion of parathyroid hormone and concomitant increased renal production of $1,25(OH)_2D_3$. The increased availability of $1,25(OH)_2D_3$ to the intestine would potentially result in an increased biosynthesis of calcium-binding protein and other transport components and hence an increased intestinal absorption of calcium. In the event that $1,25(OH)_2D_3$ also is a direct stimulator of intestinal phosphate absorption, parathyroid hormone would be capable of eliciting changes in intestinal phosphate absorption also. However, this point has not yet been tested directly.

D. Effects of Plant Extracts

The effects of ingestion of the leaves of the plant *Solanum glaucophyllum (malacoxalon)* represent an interesting new area in the study of vitamin D-mediated calcium transport. It has been conclusively shown that an aqueous extract from this plant is capable of producing a rapid hypercalcemia and hyperphosphatemia as a result principally of the rapid stimulation of intestinal calcium and phosphate absorption. The molecular basis of its action is believed to be related to the fact that the aqueous extract of the *Solanum* plant contains an analog of $1,25(OH)_2D_3$ (Wasserman, 1974b; Uribe *et al.*, 1974; Procsal *et al.*, 1976).

The presence of a calcemic agent in the South American plant *S. glaucophyllum* was first reported by Worker and Carrillo (1969). This was followed shortly by reports from Mautalen and Rossi (1970), Camberos *et al.* (1970), and Mautalen (1972). In South American cattle the disease produced by ingestion of *S. glaucophyllum* is referred to as "Enteque seco." The primary symptoms of Enteque seco are an elevated Ca × P ion-product, soft-tissue calcification, and calcinosis. It is now apparent that there are several species of plants that have in their leaves a substance(s) with vitamin D-like activity. These include *Cestrum diurnum,* which is found in Florida (Forsyth *et al.*, 1972), and *Trisetum flavescens,* present in pastures of the Black Forest region of West Germany (Dirksen *et al.*, 1975).

Figure 10-7B documents the time course of the stimulation of intestinal calcium transport in chicks after being fed aqueous extracts of *S. glaucophyllum* (Procsal *et al.*, 1976). When these results are compared with those for 1,25(OH)$_2$D$_3$ (Fig. 10-7A), it is clear that both substances are capable of generating an extremely rapid onset of stimulation of intestinal calcium transport in the vitamin D-deficient animal. This is one of the hallmarks of the actions of

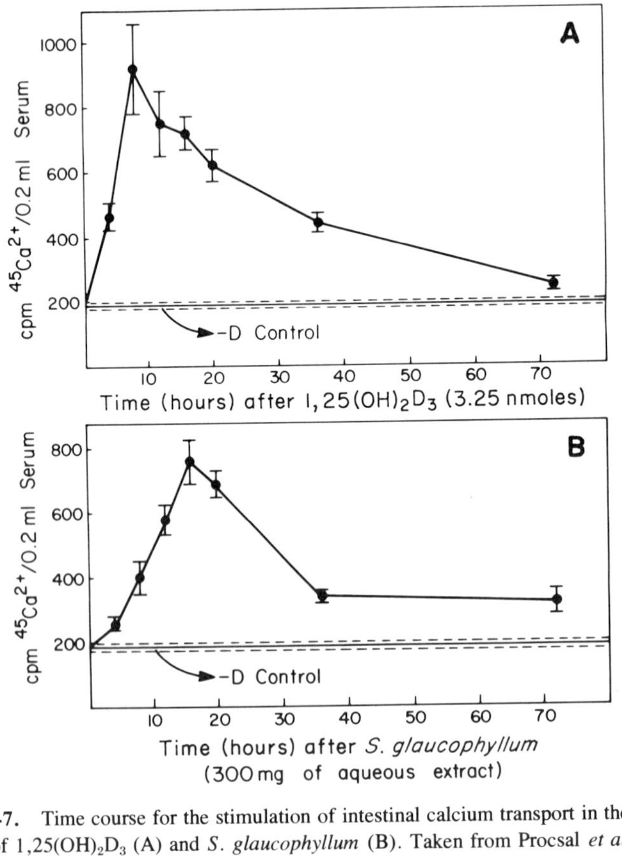

Figure 10-7. Time course for the stimulation of intestinal calcium transport in the chick after a single dose of 1,25(OH)$_2$D$_3$ (A) and *S. glaucophyllum* (B). Taken from Procsal *et al.* (1976).

$1,25(OH)_2D_3$. As might be predicted, extracts of *S. glaucophyllum* are fully active in anephric rats (Walling *et al.*, 1975a,b). This strongly suggests that no further metabolism by the kidney is required prior to the onset of biological response.

The similarity of action for extracts of *S. glaucophyllum* with $1,25(OH)_2D_3$ has also been strikingly demonstrated by the following observations: (a) Actinomycin D blocks the generation of a *S. glaucophyllum*-induced biological response for calcium absorption (Ferraro *et al.*, 1977); (b) extracts of *S. glaucophyllum* are capable of inducing the *de novo* synthesis of calcium-binding protein in isolated organ cultures of embryonic chick duodenum (Corradino and Wasserman, 1974); (c) extracts of the plant bypass the dietary strontium block (see Chapter 6) of calcium absorption (Wasserman, 1974b); and (d) administration of plant extracts initiates bone calcium resorption in mouse calvaria grown *in vitro* in tissue culture (Walling *et al.*, 1975a,b).

These results are supported by the data given in Fig. 10-7, which are the results of experiments (Procsal *et al.*, 1976) in which the ability of aqueous extracts of *S. glaucophyllum* to fill the intestinal receptor for $1,25(OH)_2D_3$ were determined. Aqueous extracts of *S. glaucophyllum* or physiological amounts of $1,25(OH)_2D_3$ (50 units or 3.25 nmoles) were given orally at various times prior to assessment of the extent of filling of the intestinal chromatin receptors for $1,25(OH)_2D_3$ by the receptor assay for the steroid described in Chapter 8 and by Procsal *et al.* (1976). A similar report was made by Napoli *et al.* (1977). Clearly, the properties of both substances in this assay are quite similar.

In 1976 the collaborative efforts of Wasserman and Haussler (Peterlik *et al.*, 1976; Wasserman *et al.*, 1976; Haussler *et al.*, 1976) resulted in the chemical identification of the aglycone portion of the *S. glaucophyllum* extract as definitely having the chemical structure of $1,25(OH)_2D_3$. This is a noteworthy achievement in that it represents the first clear-cut demonstration of vitamin D activity in the plant world.

E. Use of the Polyene Antibiotic Filipin as a Tool to Study Calcium Transport

Since the intestinal transport mechanism for phosphorus and calcium is so incredibly complicated, it is incumbent on the researcher to find means that will help explain the functioning of the various components or substeps of the process. In this respect, the author's laboratory initiated a systematic study of the effects of a variety of antibiotics on intestinal calcium and phosphorus absorption. We found that the polyene antibiotic Filipin is a specific tool with which to study calcium transport in the vitamin D-deficient chick. The results of Filipin treatment *in vitro* are remarkably similar to the effect induced by administration of cholecalciferol or $1,25(OH)_2D_3$ *in vivo* (Adams *et al.*, 1970).

The structure of Filipin is given in Fig. 10-8. There are some 40 polyene antibiotics described in the literature (Norman *et al.*, 1975). Of these, amphotericin B, pimaricin, Filipin, etruscomycin, and nystatin have been most extensively studied (Van Zupthen *et al.*, 1971; Norman *et al.*, 1972a,b; Spielvogel and Norman, 1975). The structure of a polyene is characterized by the presence of a large lactone ring, which has a number of conjugated double bonds on one side and multiple hydroxyl groups on the opposite side of the molecule. The biological effects of polyene antibiotics, including Filipin, have been shown conclusively by Kinsky *et al.* (1967), Demel *et al.* (1972), and Norman *et al.* (1972a,b, 1975) to result as a consequence of their ability to increase the permeability of target membranes to selected small molecules. The molecular basis of this action of Filipin is believed to be mediated by a selective interaction of the polyene antibiotic with membrane-bound sterols, specifically cholesterol. A stoichiometric interaction results between one molecule of the membrane-bound cholesterol and one molecule of Filipin to produce a molecular complex (Katzenstein *et al.*, 1974). This is a noncovalent interaction and is primarily hydrophobic in nature. As a consequence of the polyene antibiotic-membrane-bound sterol interaction, a selective change results in the permeability properties of the membrane. The molecular basis for these changes has been described in detail (Spielvogel and Norman, 1975).

Figure 10-9 shows some of the original data we obtained that suggested the utility of using Filipin *in vitro* as a tool for studying calcium transport *in vitro*. As shown in Fig. 10-9A, Filipin at concentrations of 10 μg/ml (ca. 1.7×10^{-5} *M*) stimulates the calcium flux J_{MS} of ileal tissue from vitamin D-deficient chicks by 150–200% but has little or no effect on J_{MS} of ileal tissue obtained from calciferol-treated birds. As shown in Fig. 10-9B, the Filipin treatment *in vitro* of ileal tissue obtained from calciferol-deficient chicks is surprisingly specific for calcium as compared to water, thiourea, serine, phosphate, sulfate, or rubidium. It should be emphasized that the data presented in Fig. 10-9B reflect transport of

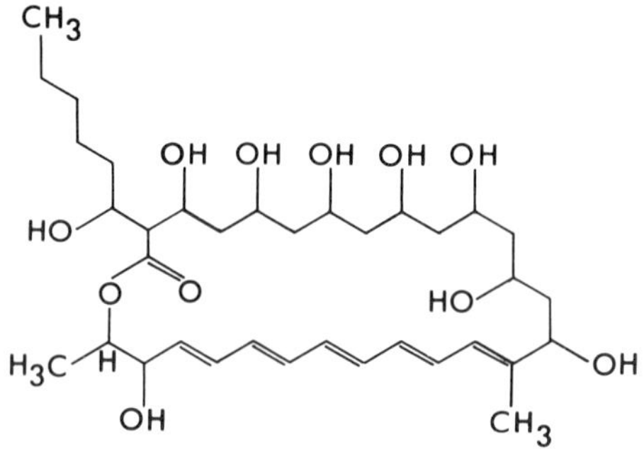

Figure 10-8. Structure of the polyene antibiotic Filipin.

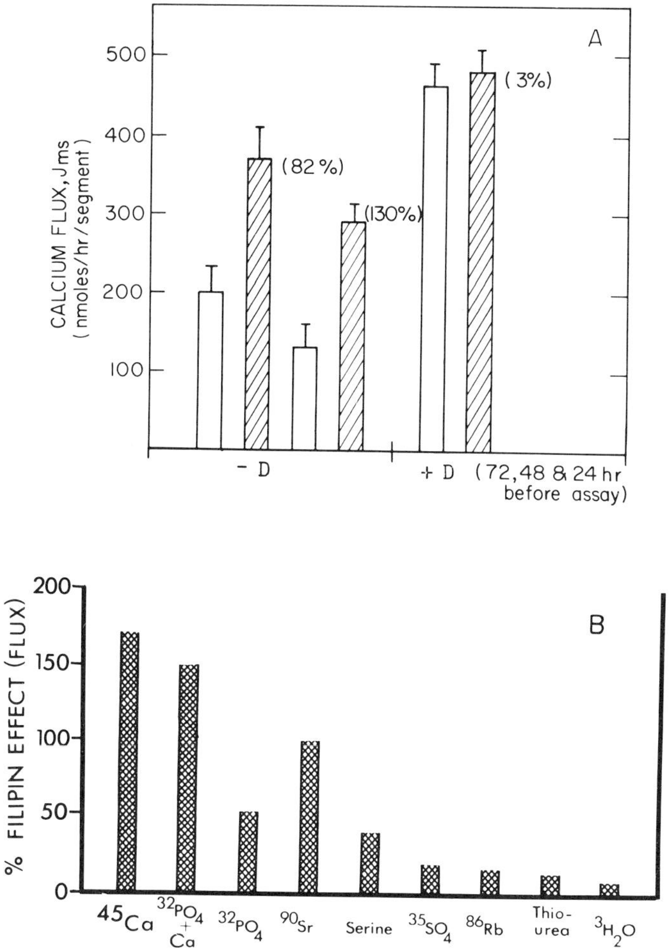

Figure 10-9. Effects of Filipin on transport properties of the chick ileum. (A) Effect of Filipin treatment *in vitro* on the intestinal transport of calcium. Segments of intestinal mucosa tissue were obtained either from vitamin D-deficient (−D) chicks or from chicks which had received 500 IU of vitamin D 72, 48, and 24 hr before death (+D). The intestinal segments were mounted in the transport chambers (see Adams and Norman, 1970) and Filipin, 10 μg/ml (ca. 10^{-5} *M*) placed in the solution bathing only the mucosal surface of the tissue. Thirty minutes later the intestinal transport of calcium was measured, and calculated as calcium flux, J_{MS} nmoles per hr per segment. (B) The effect of Filipin *in vitro* on the ileal flux of various ions and substances in the calciferol-deficient chick intestine. Experiments were performed *in vitro* in the Ussing transport apparatus for all experiments except the strontium and rubidium flux experiments, which were performed in a glass transport apparatus (see Adams and Norman, 1970). The initial concentration of all ions and compounds tested was 0.10 m*M* except Rb^+ (0.2 m*M*) and water. The initial flux determination was made for each isotope for a 20-min period following the initial preincubation period. Filipin was added to the mucosal compartment to give a final concentration of 10 μg/ml. After a 20-min lag, the flux determination was made in the presence of Filipin. The Filipin effect was then measured as the percent increase of the flux rate due to Filipin over the initial flux rate in the absence of Filipin.

the substance in question completely across the mucosal cells, i.e., its disappearance from the mucosal side and its appearance on the serosal side. Filipin was the most effective of all the polyene antibiotics tested. No effect has ever been noted when Filipin has been placed in a solution bathing the serosal surface of the tissue; that is, the effects of Filipin occur only on the brush border or microvillar side of the intestinal columnar epithelial cell.

The results of Filipin incubation *in vitro* with ileal tissue from vitamin D-deficient birds were found to mimic many effects of vitamin D administration on calcium transport (Table 10-5). Filipin, when placed in a solution bathing only the brush border side of the intestinal cell, (a) induces an active translocation of calcium against an electrochemical gradient; (b) confers the property of cold sensitivity on the increased J_{MS} flux; (c) confers sensitivity to the sulfhydryl reagent *N*-ethylmaleimide on the increased J_{MS} flux; and (d) interacts with the membrane-bound carrier on the brush border side of the cell to effect an increased uptake of calcium into the cell (Adams and Norman, 1970; Adams *et al.*, 1970; Wong *et al.*, 1970). Furthermore, Filipin was clearly shown not to be an ionophoretic compound for calcium, so that the enhanced calcium transport could not be ascribed to a direct interaction or chelation of calcium by Filipin. It is also interesting to note the marked specificity of Filipin for calcium in contrast to its lack of effect on phosphate transport.

Although our original studies (Adams *et al.*, 1970; Wong *et al.*, 1970) appeared (on the basis of M→S fluxes) to suggest that Filipin acted preferentially on the brush border membrane of intestines from vitamin D-deficient chicks as compared to vitamin D-treated chicks, the subsequent report by Wong and Nor-

TABLE 10-5
Comparison of Intestinal Calcium Transport When Vitamin D Was Given *in Vivo* or the Polyene Antibiotic Filipin Was Applied *in Vitro*[a]

Property	−D	−D + Filipin (*in vitro*)[b]	+D
Active transport of calcium	No	Yes	Yes
Flux rate, J_{MS}/J_{SM}	0.96	1.8	2.2
Specificity for Ca^{2+} transport	—	Yes	Yes
Sensitivity to low temperature	—	Yes	Yes
N-Ethylmaleimide sensitivity	—	+	+
CaBP present	No	No	Yes
Alkaline phosphatase activity	Low	Unchang.	Incr.
Effect sensitive to actinomycin D	No	No	Yes
Evidence that vitamin D or Filipin mediates an increased cellular uptake of Ca^{2+}	—	Yes	Yes
Calcium transport system is adaptive to dietary Ca^{2+} levels	No	No	Yes

[a] Taken from Adams and Norman (1970), Adams *et al.* (1970), and Wong *et al.* (1970).
[b] Filipin was added *in vitro* to the solution bathing ileal tissue from calciferol-deficient (−D) chicks.

man (1975) showed this not to be the case. When we determined the effect of Filipin treatment *in vitro* on the rate of uptake of calcium into the mucosal cell, we observed that there was a marked enhancement (65–85%) of the uptake of calcium into the cell irrespective of the vitamin D status of the animals from which the tissue preparations were obtained. However, this was not a generalized membrane permeability effect since Filipin effected little or no change in the permeability properties of the brush border membrane with regard to other ions or substances such as thiourea, urea, glycerol, sulfate, phosphate, or rubidium. Thus, these results emphasize strongly that the molecular basis of the action of Filipin in these two tissue preparations is identical. That is, Filipin is capable of effecting the same changes in permeability properties in ileal tissue from vitamin D-deficient and vitamin D-replete animals, and these changes are specific for calcium.

In parallel studies, Spielvogel and Norman (1975) found that, when Filipin was applied to liposomes composed of phospholipids plus cholesterol, there was a generalized increase in permeability for both anions (including phosphate) and cations (including calcium). That is, in model membranes devoid of protein, there was no specific Filipin-mediated enhancement of calcium transport to the exclusion of phosphate transport. This strongly suggests that the protein component of the brush border membrane plays an important role in the determination of the selective calcium and phosphate permeability properties. Filipin is capable of selectively improving the permeability to calcium, as can vitamin D or its metabolites; however, these metabolites have to act *in vivo*.

Figure 10-10 is a schematic diagram showing the possible molecular basis of the action of Filipin in the brush border region of intestinal mucosal cells. The evidence summarized here and reported in detail elsewhere (Spielvogel, 1973; Wong *et al.*, 1970; Spielvogel and Norman, 1975) suggests that Filipin is apparently able to effect a structural reorganization of the brush border membrane of ileal tissue obtained from vitamin D-deficient chicks so that an increased uptake of calcium into the mucosal cell occurs. The consequences of the direct, Filipin-mediated reorganization of the brush border membrane are remarkably similar to the indirect, actinomycin D-sensitive effect brought about by dietary vitamin D or $1,25(OH)_2D_3$. A plausible hypothesis, then, for a portion of the mechanism of action of $1,25(OH)_2D_3$ is that its administration to a vitamin D-deficient animal mediates, by the induction of *de novo* synthesis of proteins, a structural reorganization of the brush border or microvillar membrane. These "new" proteins could function in either a catalytic or structural role in the brush border membrane, resulting in a more efficient translocation of calcium and also possibly phosphate. It is also conceivable that the vitamin D metabolites have independent selective effects on the absorption of phosphate. The finding that Filipin *in vitro* can enhance the uptake of calcium in the ileum of vitamin D-treated chicks but cannot change the overall rate of transport from the mucosal

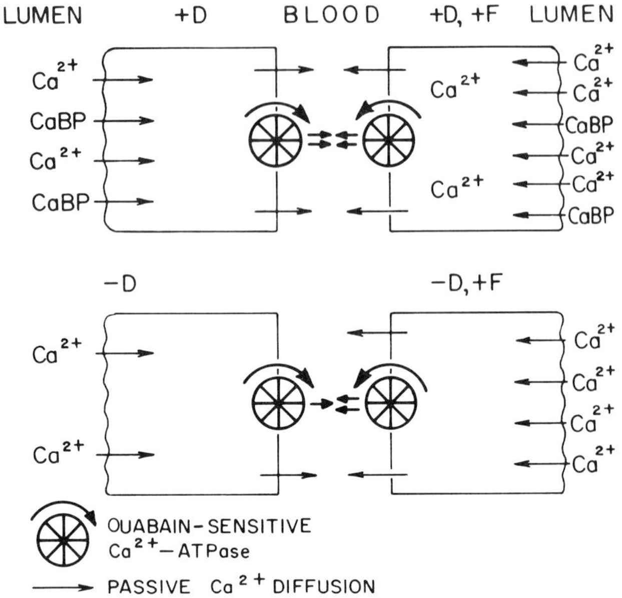

Figure 10-10. Schematic model for the action of Filipin on intestinal calcium absorption (D, calciferol; F, Filipin).

to the serosal side indicates that the rate-limiting step for the transport process is *not* at the brush border membrane. The rate-limiting factor of the overall calcium transport could therefore be intracellular [mitochondria are known to accumulate calcium rapidly (Rossi and Lehninger, 1963; Norman 1967)] or at the basal membrane of the epithelial cells. Wong (1972) proposed that a ouabain-sensitive Na^+, K^+-activated ATPase located at the serosal side of the epithelial cell is involved in the extrusion of calcium from the epithelial cells. This proposal has also been supported by the work of Birge and Alpers (1973), Martin and DeLuca (1969a,b), and Youngoszai *et al.* (1973).

Filipin, upon interaction with a sterol in the brush border membrane, can cause a structural rearrangement of the membrane components. Consequently, some negative binding sites at the mucosal side of the intestinal epithelial cell are perhaps uncovered. The increase in negative binding sites on the brush border membrane of vitamin D-treated ($+D_3$) and vitamin D-deficient ($-D_3$) chicks enhances the concentration of calcium near this membrane. This is shown on the right-hand side of Fig. 10-10. More calcium enters the epithelial cells as a consequence of the Filipin treatment. The calcium-binding protein present in the brush border region of vitamin D-treated chicks (discussed in the next section) may serve a purpose similar to that of Filipin in that it could increase the calcium concentration in the brush border membrane and in the intestinal epithelial cells. The ouabain-sensitive calcium pump located at the serosal side of intestinal epithelial cells actively transports the calcium into the bloodstream. It is assumed that this process is rate limiting in the intestine of vitamin D- or $1,25(OH)_2D_3$-treated chicks. Therefore, identical amounts of calcium are translocated from the mucosal to the serosal side in ileal segments obtained from vitamin D-treated birds (+D) and intestines of calciferol-treated or calciferol-depleted chicks after incubation *in vitro* with Filipin (+D, +F and −D, +F). However, less calcium is transported by the intestinal epithelial cells obtained from vitamin D-deficient chicks (−D).

F. Calcium-Binding Protein

One of the most outstanding and important contributions in the vitamin D field has been the discovery of intestinal calcium-binding protein (CaBP). Wasserman and Taylor (1966) first reported the existence of this vitamin D-dependent protein in 1966. Since that time Wasserman, Taylor, Corradino, and associates have published an impressive series of papers and reviews describing various aspects of this subject (Wasserman, 1973; Wasserman and Taylor, 1973a; Wasserman *et al.*, 1973).

It has been conclusively shown that the presence of CaBP in the intestinal mucosa is totally dependent on the prior administration of vitamin D_3 or one of its biologically active metabolites, e.g., $25(OH)D_3$, $1,25(OH)_2D_3$, or $24,25(OH)_2D_3$. No CaBP is present in the intestine of a vitamin D-deficient chick or rat. Figure 10-5A shows the time course of appearance of CaBP in chick intestinal mucosa after the administration of 325 pmoles of $1,25(OH)_2D_3$. When this result is compared with the time course of stimulation of intestinal calcium transport (as given in Fig. 10-5C), it is possible to understand the cause and effect relationship be tween CaBP and calcium transport that has been proposed by Wasserman and co-workers (Wasserman and Corradino, 1973; Wasserman and Taylor, 1968; Ebel *et al.*, 1969). The *de novo* synthesis of CaBP in response to vitamin D was established by the fact that its appearance was virtually blocked by prior administration of actinomycin D (Corradino and Wasserman, 1968). Experiments by MacGregor *et al.* (1970), who studied the inhibitory effect of actinomycin D on the incorporation of tritiated amino acids into CaBP, confirmed this result. Other aspects of the molecular basis of $1,25(OH)_2D_3$ in promoting the synthesis of CaBP are discussed in Chapter 1.

The properties of chick, bovine, and porcine intestinal CaBP are summarized in Table 10-6. The protein is readily released into solution by homogenization with a Potter–Elvehjem homogenizer and can be purified in high yield to homogeneity in three to four steps (Wasserman *et al.*, 1968; Taylor and Wasserman, 1967; Fullmer *et al.*, 1973; Hitchman *et al.*, 1973). Isolation and

TABLE 10-6
Properties of Representative Vitamin D-Dependent Calcium-Binding Proteins

Property	Chick[a]	Bovine[b]	Porcine[c]
Molecular weight	28,000	11,000	9000
Amino acid residues/mole	242	85	74
Acidic residues (Glu + Asp)	78	24	24
Basic residues (Lys + Arg + His)	32	12	12
Half-cystine	3	0	0
Tryptophan	2	2	0
Number of Ca atoms bound per mole	4	2	?
Affinity constant, K_a, for Ca^{2+}	$2 \times 10^6\ M^{-1}$	?	?
Alkaline earth selectivity	Ca > Sr > Ba > Mg	?	?

[a] Data from Wasserman and Taylor (1968) and Ingersoll and Wasserman (1971).
[b] Data from Fullmer and Wasserman (1973), Huang *et al.* (1975), and Fullmer *et al.* (1975).
[c] Data from Dorrington *et al.* (1974).

purification are facilitated by the fact that CaBP represents about 1% of the soluble protein present in chick intestinal mucosa. The protein has an impressively high affinity ($K_a = 2 \times 10^6\ M^{-1}$) for calcium. It is enriched in acidic amino acid residues. To date all mammalian CaBP's have been found (Table 10-7) to have molecular weights of 9000 to 13,000 daltons, whereas avian CaBP's are approximately 28,000 daltons; no evidence has been obtained to date indicating that the avian CaBP has subunits.

The relative ease of isolation of intestinal CaBP has facilitated a study of the amino acid composition and sequence as well as other physical parameters of the protein. Table 10-8 gives the amino acid composition of the chick, bovine, and porcine CaBP's. It is apparent that there is a high degree of divergence between the mammalian and avian CaBP's. The mammalian intestinal CaBP's lack half-cystine, histidine, methionine, and tryptophan, whereas the avian intestinal CaBP is reported to have all these residues.

A major advance was made in 1975 by the combined efforts of Cohn's and Wasserman's laboratories; together they established the primary amino acid sequence of bovine intestinal CaBP (Huang *et al.*, 1975). This is given in Fig. 10-11. It consists of a single amino acid chain with its NH_2-terminal lysine blocked by an *N*-acetyl group. A comparison of the sequence of intestinal CaBP with the "test" sequence of muscle Ca^{2+}-binding proteins (Tufty and Kretsinger, 1975) suggested to Huang *et al.* (1975) that the bovine CaBP may contain one or two regions of homology (denoted as E–F hands[2]), which account for its calcium-

[2]The E–F hand nomenclature refers to a region of a protein chain consisting of an α helix followed by a loop and then by another α helix. It has been proposed that calcium is bound to the loop region of the E–F structure (Tufty and Kretsinger, 1975).

binding property. Also, a preliminary report has appeared (Moffat *et al.*, 1975) which cites the unit cell dimensions of bovine intestinal CaBP that was crystallized from ammonium sulfate at alkaline pH.

Both Ingersoll and Wasserman (1971) and Dorrington *et al.* (1974) reported the results of circular dichroism studies on chick and porcine CaBP, respectively. Dorrington *et al.* (1974) found spectral evidence that was consistent with a conformational change occurring in the protein as calcium was bound.

A particularly useful system for studying the molecular biology of CaBP has been the organ culture of intestinal segments obtained from 20-day chick embryos (Corradino and Wasserman, 1971).

The embryonic chick intestine is devoid of CaBP; it appears only on the second or third day after hatching. It is possible, however, to put embryonic chick intestine in organ culture and add vitamin D_3 or a metabolite or related analog and induce the synthesis of CaBP. This induction of CaBP in organ culture has been shown to be blocked by the presence of actinomycin D or α-amanitin (Corradino, 1973, 1974). As little as 0.5 nM (5×10^{-10} M)

TABLE 10-7
Species Distribution of Intestinal Calcium-Binding Protein

Species	Molecular weight	Reference
Cow	11,000	Fullmer and Wasserman (1973)
Chick	25,000, 28,000	Wasserman *et al.* (1968)
Dog	—	Taylor *et al.* (1968)
Frog, toad	—	Wasserman and Corradino (1973)
Golden hamster	—	Schachter (1970), Kallfelz and Wasserman (1972)
Guinea pig	—	Chapman *et al.* (1972)
	10,000–12,000	Fullmer and Wasserman (1973)
Horse	10,000–12,000	Fullmer and Wasserman (1973)
Human	12,000–13,000	Hitchman *et al.* (1973)
	21,000	Alpers *et al.* (1972)
	21,500	Piazolo *et al.* (1971)
	—	Menczel *et al.* (1971)
Japanese quail, duck	—	Wasserman and Corradino (1973)
Monkey	—	Wasserman and Taylor (1971)
Pig	—	Forsyth *et al.* (1972)
	12,000–13,000	Hitchman *et al.* (1973)
	9000	Dorrington *et al.* (1974)
	—	Kallfelz *et al.* (1967)
Rat	27,000 and 12,500	Moriuchi *et al.* (1975)
	13,000	Schachter (1970)
	24,000	Oozumi *et al.* (1970)
	8000–9000, 13,000	Drescher and DeLuca (1971)
	12,000–13,000	Hitchman *et al.* (1973)
Turtle	—	Wasserman and Corradino (1973)

TABLE 10-8
Amino Acid Composition of Vitamin D-Dependent Intestinal Calcium-Binding Proteins

Amino acid	Calcium-binding protein (nearest integer residues)		
	Chick[a]	Porcine[b]	Bovine[c]
Alanine	17	5	3
Arginine	5	1	0
Aspartic	34	7	7 (3 amide)
Half-cystine	3	0	0
Glutamic	44	17	18 (8 amide)
Glycine	13	4	6
Histidine	3	0	0
Isoleucine	11	3	2
Leucine	31	10	12
Lysine	24	11–12	13
Methionine	8	0	0
Phenylalanine	13	5	5
Proline	3	0	5
Serine	9	6–7	8
Threonine	9	1	2
Tryptophan	2	0	0
Tyrosine	8	1	1
Valine	5	3	3
	242	85	85
Amide	17	—	11

[a]Taken from Bredderman and Wasserman (1974).
[b]Taken from Dorrington *et al.* (1974).
[c]Taken from Huang *et al.* (1975).

$1,25(OH)_2D_3$ was capable of initiating the synthesis of CaBP, whereas a 10,000 times higher concentration of the parent vitamin D_3 was required for an equivalent effect. The relative effectiveness of steroids was found to be $1,25(OH)_2D_3 > 1\alpha(OH)D_3 > 25(OH)D_3 > 24,25(OH)_2D_3$. This dramatically emphasizes the biological potency of $1,25(OH)_2D_3$ and that it is the primary mediator or vitamin D activator in the intestine.

An exceedingly important point of concern has been to identify the cellular localization of CaBP. Holdsworth (1970) advanced the view that since intestinal CaBP is found in the high-speed supernatant after cell breakage via homogenization, this is the cellular site of action of CaBP. However, this is hardly conclusive proof, since if CaBP were only loosely attached, perhaps via ionic protein interactions to a cellular membrane, it is entirely possible that the CaBP would be released into the cytosol upon homogenization. In contrast, Taylor and Wasserman (1970) found, using immunofluorescent antibody techniques, that although CaBP was highly concentrated inside goblet cells it was outside the columnar epithelial cells immediately adjacent to the brush border region. It is likely that the localization of CaBP in the goblet cell represents the site of its biosynthesis, whereas its external location may be the site of its functional involvement in calcium transport. A. N. Taylor (personal communication) recently confirmed these findings by utilizing the lactoperoxidase technique for electron microscopic evaluation.

There can be little doubt that the presence of CaBP is in some way associated with intestinal calcium absorption. Table 10-9 summarizes the varied means of correlating the upward or downward changes in the level of CaBP with a concomitant and parallel change in the activity of intestinal calcium absorption. In fact, as discussed in detail in Chapters 6 and 7, it is likely that the intensity of intestinal calcium absorption and the amount of CaBP is directly proportional to the rate of production and/or circulating plasma level of $1,25(OH)_2D_3$. Bronner and Freund (1975) proposed that quantification of intestinal CaBP may be employed as an index of vitamin D status.

It has not been possible to date to provide a detailed description at the molecular level of the role of CaBP in intestinal calcium absorption. In this respect there are a number of obvious problems. (a) Calcium-binding protein has an extremely high affinity for calcium, $K_a = 2 \times 10^6\ M^{-1}$. It is not known how Ca^{2+} can be rapidly and efficiently removed or released from CaBP. Does CaBP function dynamically or statically as an ion exchanger? (b) Calcium transport and the effect of vitamin D and/or $1,25(OH)_2D_3$ therein are not so simple as to be explained merely by invoking the presence of only CaBP. (c) There may be and probably should be other vitamin D-dependent components; some evidence for their existence is already available. As shown in Fig. 10-5A, C, 48 hr after the administration of $1,25(OH)_2D_3$ to a rachitic chick, CaBP levels are virtually

```
                                        10
N-Ac-Lys-Gln-Ser-Pro-Leu-Glu-Lys-Tyr-Ala-Ala-Glu-Lys-
Ser- Ile- Gln-Lys-Glu- Ile- Glu-Lys- Gly-Phe-Phe-Lys-Gln-
                    30
Leu-Leu- Val-Ser- Val- Gln-Lys-Ala- Gly-Asp-Lys-Glu-Ser-
   40                                         50
Leu-Gln- Pro-Leu-Phe- Thr-Leu-Leu- Lys-Ser- Gly-Pro- Glu-
                                   60
Glu-Asn-Leu-Lys-Glu- Ser- Gln-Asn-Gly-Pro- Asp-Leu-Lys-
                    70
Ser- Gly- Pro- Gln-Asn- Asp-Leu-Glu- Glu-Lys-Gly-Thr- Asp-
         80
Phe-Val- Lue-Phe-Ser- Leu-Lys-Gln-
```

Figure 10-11. Primary amino acid sequence of bovine intestinal calcium-binding protein. From Huang *et al.* (1975).

TABLE 10-9
Possible Relationships between Calcium Absorption and Intestinal Calcium-Binding Protein

Observation	Reference
Coincident appearance of CaBP and increased Ca absorption in the rachitic chick after administration of	
Vitamin D_3	Ebel *et al.* (1969), Emtage *et al.* (1974a,b)
$25(OH)D_3$	Wasserman *et al.* (1973)
$1,25(OH)_2D_3$	See Fig. 10-5
Correlation between level of CaBP and biological activity of vitamin D-related steroids	Wasserman and Taylor (1968), Omdahl and Thornton (1972), Corradino (1973)
Correlation between level of CaBP and rate of Ca absorption in duodenum, jejunum, and ileum	Taylor and Wasserman (1967), Schacter (1970)
Adaptive correlation between CaBP and change in Ca absorption in animals fed diets of	Wasserman and Taylor (1969), Bronner (1964), Schacter (1970), Hurwitz and Bar (1972)
Low calcium (↑)	Omdahl and Thornton (1972), Hurwitz *et al.* (1973), Arnold *et al.* (1975a,b)
Low phosphorus (↑)	Hurwitz and Bar (1972)
High strontium (↓)	Corradino and Wasserman (1970), Corradino *et al.* (1971a,b)
In egg-laying chickens (↑)	Wasserman and Taylor (1968), Hurwitz *et al.* (1973)
Correlation between affinity of CaBP for alkaline earths (Ca > Sr > Ba > Mg) and the relative intestinal absorption of these ions	Taylor and Wasserman (1967), Schacter (1970)
Measurement of messenger RNA levels for CaBP and production of CaBP	Emtage *et al.* (1974a,b), Spencer *et al.* (1976a,b)

maximal, whereas the rate of Ca^{2+} absorption has increased (maximal at 12–14 hr) and decreased again to a low level. This may be indicative of the rapid turnover of other vitamin D-dependent factors necessary for optimal rates of Ca^{2+} absorption. Kowarski and Schacter (1975) reported the presence of a particulate vitamin D-dependent calcium-binding substance in rat intestine that had a molecular weight of 0.5 to 1.0×10^6. It is likely that important advances will be made in this area in the near future.

It is only fair to indicate, however, that not all workers support the view that intestinal calcium absorption obligatorily involves CaBP. Lawson and co-workers (Spencer *et al.*, 1976a,b, 1978) studied the chronology of onset of stimulated intestinal calcium absorption and the appearance of *de novo* CaBP in vitamin D-deficient chicks given $1,25(OH)_2D_3$. They found that, although calcium absorption was definitely stimulated in 1–2 hr, messenger RNA for CaBP was not produced until after 4 hr, and CaBP could not be detected until after 5–6 hr. Clearly, further work is necessary to confirm and place in perspective these provocative results.

An interesting observation is that CaBP is not confined to the intestine. Table 10-10 reports the tissue distribution of vitamin D-dependent CaBP's reported in the literature. Table 10-11 reports quantitative tissue distribution obtained in the chick by the use of a radioimmunoassay employing antisera prepared in the rabbit against homogeneous chick intestinal CaBP (Christakos and Norman, 1978, 1979). It appears that besides the intestine, the kidney, pancreas, bone, and cerebral cortex all have significant levels of a vitamin D-dependent protein that cross-reacts with antisera to chick intestinal CaBP. As a consequence of these observations it may be appropriate to propose a wider role for CaBP in calcium metabolism than mere intestinal calcium absorption. It will be exciting to observe the unfolding of efforts to determine the involvement of the vitamin and its metabolites in calcium metabolism in these tissues.

G. Alkaline Phosphatase, ATPase, and Phytase

In addition to the effects of vitamin D_3 and $1,25(OH)_2D_3$ on the induction of CaBP, these steroids are known to increase the levels of several other proteins in the intestinal mucosa. These include alkaline phosphatase, calcium-stimulated ATPase, and phytase enzyme activities.

A relationship between vitamin D and alkaline phosphatase activity in the intestine was first noted by Motzok (1950). More recently Haussler *et al.* (1970), Holdsworth (1970), and Norman *et al.* (1970) documented a three- to fourfold

TABLE 10-10
Tissue Distribution of Vitamin D-Dependent Calcium-Binding Protein

Evidence for presence of CaBP	Reference
Intestine	See Tables 10-7 and 10-9
Kidney	Lippiello and Wasserman (1975), Christakos and Norman (1979)
Avian shell gland	Corradino *et al.* (1968), Lippiello and Wasserman (1975)
Brain (cerebellum)	Taylor (1974a, 1977)
Blood	Arnold *et al.* (1975b), Christakos and Norman (1979)
Pancreas	Morrisey (1975), Christakos and Norman (1979)
Mammary tissue	A. N. Taylor (personal communication)
Parathyroid glands	Oldham *et al.* (1974) (vitamin D-dependent), Arnold *et al.* (1975a,b) (not vitamin D-dependent), Christakos and Norman (1977) (vitamin D-dependent)
Bone	Christakos and Norman (1978)

TABLE 10-11

Tissue Distribution of Immunocross-reactivity to Intestinal CaBP in the Chick[a]

Tissue	−D (ng CaBP/mg protein)	n	+D (ng CaBP/mg protein)	n	p value (+D vs. −D)
Jejunum	79±18	6	32,000±5,900	6	<0.001
Duodenum	36±14	6	25,000±4,400	6	<0.001
Ileum	31±5	6	10,000±1,400	6	<0.001
Kidney	490±13	4	3,100±370	5	<0.001
Pancreas	21±7	4	1,500±200	6	<0.001
Bone (tibia)	4±1	6	110±22	6	<0.001
Adrenal	18±1.3	3[b]	46±3	4[b]	<0.001
Lungs	0.75±0.7	5	21±8	6	<0.05
Esophagus	5.5±1	5	11±3	5	<0.05
Liver	1.2±0.3	5	3±0.6	5	<0.1
Skeletal muscle	2.0±0.2	4	4.3±1.5	5	<0.2
Myocardium	1.1±0.15	6	1.7±0.5	4	<0.2
Thyroid	17.6±5	3[c]	11.3±2	3[c]	<0.2
Hypothalamus	275±34	4	340±14	3	<0.2
Parathyroid glands	25±4	4[d]	31.3±3	3[c]	<0.4
Testis	16±3	3[b]	15.4±4	5	<0.5
Cerebral cortex	248±18	4	261±22	2	<0.5
Serum	0	6	49±8 ng/ml (1.1 ng/mg protein)	6	<0.001

[a]The table is arranged in order of decreasing differences for immunocross-reactivities of tissues obtained from either vitamin D-deficient (−D) or vitamin D_3-replete (+D) chicks. Tissues termed −D were obtained from 1-month-old rachitic chicks; tissues termed +D were obtained from 1-month-old chicks that were raised on a rachitogenic diet and had received 1.3 nmoles of vitamin D_3 for the last 2 weeks. Except where indicated, n is the number of animals. Taken from Christakos and Norman (1979).

[b]Each n represents pooled tissue from two animals.

[c]Each n represents pooled tissue from three animals.

[d]Each n represents pooled tissue from eight animals.

rise in the measurable level of intestinal alkaline phosphatase after administration of vitamin D_3 to rachitic chicks. In each instance the bulk of the activity was specifically associated with the brush border fraction. Krawitt *et al.* (1973) found in rats that the level of duodenal alkaline phosphatase increased when the rats were fed diets containing low levels of calcium. Similar results were obtained by Fournier *et al.* (1977). Collectively these results were suggestive of some role of alkaline phosphatase in the complex calcium transport process, particularly entry into the cell. However, as shown in Fig. 10-5B, the time course of an alkaline phosphatase increase after administration of $1,25(OH)_2D_3$ is not consistent with this proposal. Calcium transport was stimulated maximally at 12–14 hr, whereas the increase in alkaline phosphatase was not maximal until 45–55 hr. In fact, since $1,25(OH)_2D_3$-stimulated phosphate absorption was also maximal at 48 hr, the intriguing possibility exists that the vitamin D-related elevation in alkaline phosphatase level is associated with phosphate rather than calcium transport.

Brush borders obtained from chick or rat intestinal mucosa were reported by Martin *et al.* (1969b) and Melançon and DeLuca (1970) to contain a vitamin D-related increase in Ca^{2+}-stimulated ATPase. On the basis of time course studies and inhibitor studies (ouabain, mersalyl acid, and oligomycin), they proposed a role for this enzyme in calcium transport across the brush border membrane.

Haussler *et al.* (1970) and Holdsworth (1970) suggested a molecular identity between Ca-ATPase and alkaline phosphatase. Both enzymes were inhibited by zinc, beryllium, and the amino acid L-phenylalanine. Russell *et al.* (1972) noted a very similar rate of temperature inactivation for these two enzyme activities. Bonjour *et al.* (1972) found that treatment of rats with dietary ethane-1-hydroxyl-1,1-diphosphonate resulted in parallel reductions in intestinal Ca-ATPase, alkaline phosphatase, and CaBP. If these enzyme activities are in fact associated with the same protein, it is possible that the enzyme is complex in nature, i.e., multifunctional or membrane bound. The subject of intestinal brush border alkaline phosphatase is particularly complicated in its own right; Moog (1964) reported the presence of five isoenzymes of brush border alkaline phosphatase.

The chief argument against the coidentity of brush border Ca-ATPase and alkaline phosphatase is the failure of Krawitt *et al.* (1973) to note coordinate adaptive changes in Ca-ATPase with calcium absorption under conditions of restricted dietary calcium.

There are also reports that vitamin D status affects the level of intestinal phytase (Steenbock and Herting, 1955; Davies *et al.*, 1970). Phytase is an enzyme that is assayed by measuring the hydrolysis of myoinositol hexaphosphate. It was proposed by Davies and Motzok (1972) that phytase activity is associated with the same protein as alkaline phosphatase.

It is apparent that since Ca-ATPase, phytase, and alkaline phosphatase are all associated with the highly organized membranous brush border or microvilli (see Fig. 10-3), the elucidation of their relationship to one another and their putative role in calcium transport must await a determination of the membrane structure–function relationships of these important subcellular organelles.

H. Concluding Remarks

Figure 10-12 is an integrated scheme describing the overall process of calcium and phosphate absorption and transport in the intestine and the role of vitamin D metabolites in these processes. The active transport system for calcium is dependent on the intracellular availability of calcium. As the intracellular calcium concentration increases (either by Filipin action *in vitro* or CaBP and other unknown compounds), it is possible to observe increased effluxes of calcium at the basal membrane side. It is known that the intracellular concentration of calcium is very low (10^{-6} to 10^{-7} *M*) and that most of the intracellular calcium is contained in the mitochondria (Borle, 1972). The increase in calcium in the intestinal epithelial cells is reflected by a more efficient supply of calcium to the Na^+, K^+-activated ATPase, which actively transports calcium into the underlying blood vessels. If this serosal pump operated unidirectionally, the ratio of flux of calcium from mucosa to serosa to the flux from serosa to mucosa would

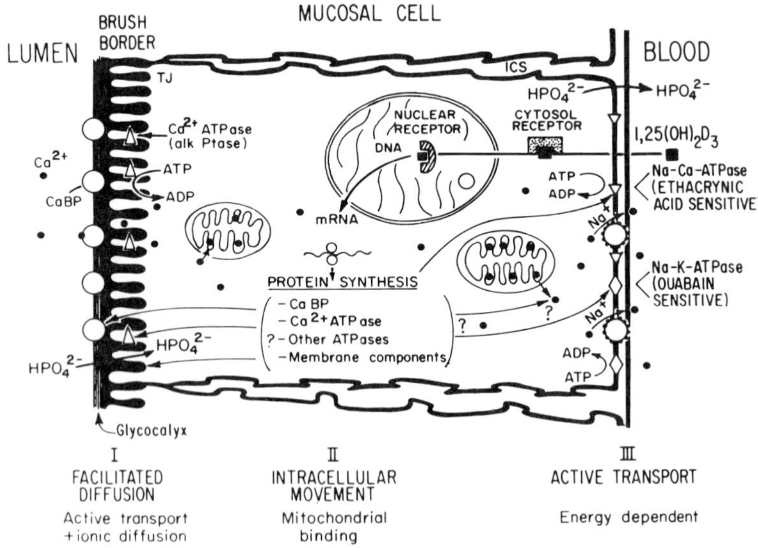

Figure 10-12. Integrated scheme for vitamin D-mediated intestinal calcium and phosphorus absorption.

exceed 1.00 if the tissue were treated with Filipin. It is also conceivable, however, that the K_m of this calcium pump limits the maximal amount of calcium that can be extruded during a given time interval. This would explain the finding that the Filipin-mediated increase in calcium in the ileum of vitamin D-treated chicks was not reflected in an overall increase in calcium translocation. Since this active pump on the serosal side requires metabolic energy, this suggests that any interference with the translocation of substrates for cellular metabolism will inhibit both the vitamin D- and Filipin-mediated active calcium transport in the intestine.

It is clear that a detailed understanding of the intestinal absorption of calcium and phosphorus at the molecular level is a challenging problem to which there is not yet a completely definitive solution. It is apparent that the role of vitamin D and its active metabolite, $1,25(OH)_2D_3$, is firmly established in terms of its ability to stimulate or mediate an increased intestinal absorption of calcium. Furthermore, there are a number of studies that strongly indicate that this steroid hormone also exerts an independent effect on intestinal absorption of phosphate. Many of the "black box" complications of the multistep process for transfer of these substances from the lumen of the intestine to the blood have at least been identified. In some instances, notably the isolation of CaBP, a detailed study at the molecular level of a putative component of the transport system has in fact been accomplished. A project for the future, however, is to provide an equally detailed description of both the function and the composition of other components associated with or intimately involved with the intestinal absorption of phosphorus and calcium.

REFERENCES

Adams, T. H., and Norman, A. W. (1970). *J. Biol. Chem.* **245,** 4421.

Adams, T. H., Wong, R. G., and Norman, A. W. (1970). *J. Biol. Chem.* **245,** 4432.

Alpers, D. H., Lee, S. W., and Avioli, L. V. (1972). *Gastroenterology* **62,** 559.

Arnold, B. M., Kuttner, M., Swaminathan, R., Cane, A. D., Hitchman, A. J. W., Harrison, J. E., and Murray, T. M. (1975a). *Can. J. Physiol. Pharmacol.* **53,** 1129.

Arnold, B. M., Kuttner, M., Willis, D. M., Hitchman, A. J. W., Harrison, J. E., and Murray, T. M. (1975b). *Can. J. Physiol. Pharmacol.* **53,** 1135.

Bartter, F. C. (1964). *Miner. Metab.* **2,** Part A, 315.

Berger, E. Y. (1960). *Miner. Metab.* **1,** Part A, 249.

Bergheim, O. (1926). *Biochem. J.* **70,** 51.

Bethke, R. M., Kennard, D. C., Kik, C. H., and Zinzalian, G. (1929). *Poult. Sci.* **8,** 257.

Birge, S. J., and Alpers, D. H. (1973). *Gastroenterology* **64,** 977.

Birge, S. J., and Miller, R. (1977). *J. Clin. Invest.* **60,** 980.

Blair, M., Spencer, H., Swernov, J., and Laszlo, D. (1954). *Science* **120,** 1029.

Bonjour, J.-P., Russell, R. G. G., Morgan, D. B., and Fleisch, H. A. (1972). *Am. J. Physiol.* **224,** 1011.

Bonjour, J.-P., DeLuca, H. F., Fleisch, H., Trechsel, U., Matejowec, L. A., and Omdahl, J. L. (1973). *Eur. J. Clin. Invest.* **3,** 44.
Borle, A. (1972). *In* "Calcium, Parathyroid Hormone and the Calcitonins" (R. V. Talmage and P. L. Munson, eds.), Int. Congr. Ser. No. 243, p. 484. Excerpta Med. Found., Amsterdam.
Bredderman, P. J., and Wasserman, R. H. (1974). *Biochemistry* **13,** 1687.
Bronner, F. (1964). *Miner. Metab.* **2,** Part A, 341.
Bronner, F. (1973). *In* "Engineering Principles in Physiology" (J. H. V. Brown and D. S. Gann, eds.), Vol. 1, p. 227. Academic Press, New York.
Bronner, F., and Freund, T. (1975). *Am. J. Physiol.* **229,** 689.
Brown, H. B., Shohl, A. T., Chapman, E. E., Rose, C. S., and Saurwein, E. M. (1932). *J. Biol. Chem.* **98,** 207.
Camberos, H. R., Davis, G. K., Djafar, M. J., and Simpson, C. F. (1970). *Am. J. Vet. Res.* **31,** 685.
Carlsson, A. (1951). *Acta Pharmacol. Toxicol.* **7,** Suppl. 1, 1.
Carlsson, A. (1954). *Acta Physiol. Scand.* **31,** 301.
Chapman, M., Pond, W., Taylor, A. N., Krook, L., and Rivers, J. (1972). *J. Anim. Sci.* **35,** 283.
Chen, T. C., Castillo, L., Korycka-Dahl, M., and DeLuca, H. F. (1974). *J. Nutr.* **98,** 1056.
Christakos, S., and Norman, A. W. (1977). *Abstr., Parathyroid Conf. 6th, 1977* Int. Congr. Ser. No. 421.
Christakos, S., and Norman, A. W. (1978). *Science* **202,** 70.
Christakos, S., and Norman, A. W. (1979). *Endocrinology* **104,** 1495.
Coates, M. E., and Holdsworth, E. S. (1961). *Br. J. Nutr.* **15,** 131.
Coburn, J. W., Koppel, M. H., Brickman, A. S., and Massry, S. G. (1973). *Kidney Int.* **3,** 264.
Cohn, W. E., and Greenberg, D. M. (1939). *J. Biol. Chem.* **130,** 625.
Comar, C. L., and Bronner, F., eds. (1969). "Mineral Metabolism: An Advanced Treatise," Vol. 3. Academic Press, New York.
Cooper, C. W., Schwesinger, W. H., Mahgoub, A. M., Ontjes, D. A., Gray, T. K., and Munson, D. L. (1972). *In* "Calcium, Parathyroid Hormone and the Calcitonins" (R. V. Talmage and P. L. Munson, eds.), Int. Congr. Ser. No. 243, p. 128. Excerpta Med. Found., Amsterdam.
Corradino, R. A. (1973). *Nature (London)* **243,** 41.
Corradino, R. A. (1974). *Endocrinology* **94,** 1607.
Corradino, R. A., and Wasserman, R. H. (1968). *Arch. Biochem. Biophys.* **126,** 957.
Corradino, R. A., and Wasserman, R. H. (1970). *Proc. Exp. Biol. Med.* **133,** 960.
Corradino, R. A., and Wasserman, R. H. (1971). *Science* **172,** 731.
Corradino, R. A., and Wasserman, R. H. (1974). *Nature (London)* **252,** 716.
Corradino, R. A., Wasserman, R. H., Publos, M. H., and Chang, S. I. (1968). *Arch. Biochem. Biophys.* **125,** 378.
Crane, R. K., Forstner, G., and Eichholz, A. (1965). *Biochim. Biophys. Acta* **109,** 467.
Curran, P. F., and Solomon, A. K. (1957). *J. Gen. Physiol.* **41,** 143.
Curtis, F. K., Fellows, H., and Rich, C. (1967). *J. Lab. Clin. Med.* **69,** 1036.
Dahlquist, A., and Nordstrom, C. (1966). *Biochim. Biophys. Acta* **113,** 624.
Davies, M. I., and Motzok, I. (1972). *Comp. Biochem. Physiol. B* **42,** 345.
Davies, M. I., Ritcey, G. M., and Motzok, I. (1970). *Poult. Sci.* **49,** 1230.
DeGrazia, J. A., and Rich, C. (1964). *Metab., Clin. Exp.* **13,** 650.
Deller, D. J., Worthley, B. W., and Martin, H. (1965). *Australas. Ann. Med.* **14,** 223.
Demel, R. A., Bruckdorfer, K. R., and van Deenen, L. L. M. (1972). *Biochim. Biophys. Acta* **255,** 311.
Diamond, J. A., and Wright, E. M. (1969). *Annu. Rev. Physiol.* **31,** 581.
Dirksen, G., Plank, P., Hanichan, T., and Simon, W. (1975). *In* "Proceedings of the Second

Symposium on Vitamin D and Problems Related to Uremic Bone Disease'' (A. W. Norman *et al.*, eds.), p. 698. de Gruyter, Berlin.
Dols, M. J. L., Jansen, B. C. P., Sizoo, G. J., and DeVries, J. (1938). *Nature (London)* **139,** 1068.
Dorrington, K. J., Hui, A., Hoffman, T., Hitchman, A. J., and Harrison, J. E. (1974). *J. Biol. Chem.* **249,** 199.
Drescher, D., and DeLuca, H. F. (1971). *Biochemistry* **10,** 2302.
Eanes, E. D., and Posner, A. S. (1970). *In* ''Biological Calcification: Cellular and Molecular Aspects'' (H. Schraer, ed.), p. 1. Appleton, New York.
Ebel, J. G., Taylor, A. N., and Wasserman, R. H. (1969). *Am. J. Clin. Nutr.* **22,** 431.
Eisenstein, R., and Passavoy, M. (1964). *Proc. Soc. Exp. Biol. Med.* **117,** 77.
Emtage, J. S., Lawson, D. E. M., and Kodicek, E. (1974a). *Biochem. J.* **140,** 239.
Emtage, J. S., Lawson, D. E. M., and Kodicek, E. (1974b). *Biochem. J.* **144,** 399.
Favus, M. J., Walling, M. W., and Kimberg, D. V. (1973). *J. Clin. Invest.* **52,** 1680.
Ferraro, C., Ladizesky, M., Cabrejas, M., and Mautalen, C. A. (1977). *Medicina (Buenos Aires)* **37,** 385.
Findley, L., Paton, D. N., and Sharpe, J. S. (1920). *Q. J. Med.* **14,** 352.
Forstner, G. G. (1969). *Am. J. Med. Sci.* **258,** 172.
Forstner, G. G. (1971). *Biochem. J.* **121,** 781.
Forsyth, D. M., Pond, W. G., Wasserman, R. H., and Krook, L. (1972). *J. Nutr.* **102,** 1623.
Fournier, P., Fontaine, N., and Fournier, A. (1977). *Ann. Nutr. Aliment.* **31,** 277.
Fullmer, C. S., and Wasserman, R. H. (1973). *Biochim. Biophys. Acta* **317,** 172.
Fullmer, C. S., Wasserman, R. H., Hamilton, J. W., Huang, W. Y., and Cohn, D. V. (1975). *Biochim. Biophys. Acta* **412,** 256.
Greenberg, D. M. (1945). *J. Biol. Chem.* **157,** 99.
Harrison, H. E., and Harrison, H. C. (1960). *Am. J. Physiol.* **199,** 265.
Harrison, H. E., and Harrison, H. C. (1961). *Am. J. Physiol.* **201,** 1007.
Harrison, H. E., and Harrison, H. C. (1965). *Am. J. Physiol.* **208,** 370.
Haussler, M. R., Nagode, L. A., and Rasmussen, H. (1970). *Nature (London)* **228,** 1199.
Haussler, M. R., Wasserman, R. H., McCain, T. A., Peterlik, M., Bursac, K., and Hughes, M. R. (1976). *Life Sci.* **18,** 1049.
Heaney, R. P., and Whedon, G. D. (1958). *J. Clin. Endocrinol. Metab.* **18,** 1246.
Helbock, H. J., Forte, J. G., and Saltman, P. (1966). Biochim. Biophys. Acta **126,** 81.
Henry, H. L., Midgett, R. J., and Norman, A. W. (1974). *J. Biol. Chem.* **249,** 7584.
Hibberd, K. A., and Norman, A. W. (1969) *Biochem. Pharmacol.* **18,** 2347.
Hitchman, A. J. W., Kerr, M. K., and Harrison, J. E. (1973). *Arch. Biochem. Biophys.* **155,** 221.
Holdsworth, E. S. (1965). *Biochem. J.* **96,** 475.
Holdsworth, E. S. (1970). *J. Membr. Biol.* **3,** 43.
Huang, W., Cohn, D. V., Hamilton, J. W., Fulmer, C., and Wasserman, R. H. (1975). *J. Biol. Chem.* **250,** 7647.
Humphreys, D. J. (1973). *Nature (London), New Biol.* **246,** 156.
Hurwitz, S., and Bar, A. (1972). *Am. J. Physiol.* **222,** 761.
Hurwitz, S., Bar, A., and Cohen, I. (1973). *Am. J. Physiol.* **225,** 150.
Hurwitz, S., Harrison, H. C., and Harrison, H. E. (1967). *J. Nutr.* **91,** 319.
Ingersoll, R. J., and Wasserman, R. H. (1971). *J. Biol. Chem.* **246,** 2808.
Innes, J. R. M., and Nicolaysen, R. (1937). *Biochem. J.* **31,** 101.
Irving, J. T. (1964). *Miner. Metab.* **2,** Part A, 249.
Ito, S. (1965). *J. Cell Biol.* **27,** 475.
Jande, S. S. (1976). *Cytobios* **17,** 171.
Jones, M. R. (1927). *Am. J. Physiol.* **79,** 694.

Kallfelz, F. A., and Wasserman, R. H. (1972). *Proc. Soc. Exp. Biol. Med.* **139,** 77.
Kallfelz, F. A., Taylor, A. N., and Wasserman, R. H. (1967). *Proc. Soc. Exp. Biol. Med.* **125,** 54.
Katzenstein, I. P., Spielvogel, A. M., and Norman, A. W. (1974). *J. Antibiot.* **27,** 943.
Kimberg, D. V., Schachter, D., and Schenker, H. (1961). *Am. J. Physiol.* **200,** 1256.
Kinsky, S. C., Demel, R. A., and van Deenen, L. L. M. (1967). *Biochim. Biophys. Acta* **135,** 835.
Kowarski, S., and Schachter, D. (1969). *J. Biol. Chem.* **244,** 211.
Kowarski, S., and Schachter, D. (1975). *Am. J. Physiol.* **229,** 1198.
Krawitt, E. L. (1972). *Biochim. Biophys. Acta* **274,** 179.
Krawitt, E. L., and Schedl, H. P. (1968). *Am. J. Physiol.* **214,** 232.
Krawitt, E. L., Stubbert, P. A., and Ennis, P. H. (1973). *Am. J. Physiol.* **224,** 548.
Krawitt, E. L., Sampson, H. W., Kunin, A. S., and Matthews, J. L. (1974). *Calcif. Tissue Res.* **15,** 21.
Lederer, C. M., Hollander, J. M., and Perlman, I. (1967). "Table of Isotopes," 6th ed., Wiley, New York.
Lindquist, B. (1952). *Acta Paediatr. (Stockholm)* **41,** Suppl. 86, 1–80.
Lipkin, M., and Bell, T. (1968). *In* "Cell Proliferation" (C. F. Code, ed.), p. 2861. Washington, D.C.
Lippiello, L., and Wasserman, R. H. (1975). *J. Histochem. Cytochem.* **23,** 110.
Litwak, L. (1969). *Am. J. Clin. Nutr.* **22,** 771.
Liu, S. H., and Chu, H. I. (1943). *Medicine (Baltimore)* **22,** 103.
Lukert, B. P., Stanbury, S. W., and Mawer, E. B. (1973). *Endocrinology* **93,** 718.
McClendon, J. F. (1922). *Am. J. Physiol.* **61,** 373.
MacGregor, R. R., Hamilton, J. W., and Cohn, D. V. (1970). *Biochim. Biophys. Acta* **222,** 482.
Manley, M. L., and Morgareidy, K. (1939). *J. Nutr.* **18,** 411.
Martin, D. L., and DeLuca, H. F. (1969a). *Am. J. Physiol.* **216,** 1351.
Martin, D. L., and DeLuca, H. F. (1969b). *Arch. Biochem. Biophys.* **134,** 139.
Martin, D. L., Melançon, M. J., and DeLuca, H. F. (1969). *Biochem. Biophys. Res. Commun.* **35,** 819.
Martonosi, A., Pucell, A. G., and Halpin, R. A. (1971). *In* "Cellular Mechanisms for Calcium Transfer and Homeostasis" (G. Nichols, Jr. and R. H. Wasserman, eds.), p. 175. Academic Press, New York.
Mautalen, C. A. (1972). *Endocrinology* **90,** 563.
Mautalen, C. A., and Rossi, F. M. (1970). *Medicina (Buenos Aires)* **30,** 433.
Melançon, M. J., Jr., and DeLuca, H. F. (1970). *Biochemistry* **9,** 1658.
Menczel, J., Eilon, G., Steiner, A., Karaman, C., Mor, E., and Ron, A. (1971). *Isr. J. Med. Sci.* **7,** 396.
Migicovsky, B. B., and Emslie, A. R. G. (1947). *Arch. Biochem. Biophys.* **13,** 185.
Migicovsky, B. B., and Emslie, A. R. G. (1949). *Arch. Biochem. Biophys.* **20,** 325.
Miller, D., and Crane, R. K. (1961). *Anal. Biochem.* **2,** 284.
Moffat, K., Fullmer, C. S., and Wasserman, R. H. (1975). *J. Mol. Biol.* **97,** 661.
Moog, F. (1964). *Science* **144,** 414.
Moriuchi, S., Yamanovchi, T., and Hosoya, N. (1975). *J. Nutr. Sci. Vitaminol.* **21,** 251.
Morrissey, R. L. (1975) *Fed. Proc., Fed. Am. Soc. Exp. Biol.* **34,** 8881.
Motzok, I. (1950). *Biochem. J.* **47,** 193.
Myrtle, J. F., and Norman, A. W. (1971). *Science* **171,** 79.
Napoli, J. L., Reeve, L. R., Eisman, J. A., Schnoes, H. K., and DeLuca, H. P. (1977). *J. Biol. Chem.* **252,** 2580.
Neuman, W. F., and Neuman, M. W. (1958). "Chemical Dynamics of Bone Mineral." Univ. of Chicago Press, Chicago, Illinois.

Nichols, G., Jr., and Wasserman, R. H., eds. (1971). "Cellular Mechanisms for Calcium Transfer and Homeostasis." Academic Press, New York.
Nicolaysen, R. (1937a). *Biochem. J.* **31,** 107.
Nicolaysen, R. (1937b). *Biochem. J.* **31,** 122.
Nicolaysen, R., and Eeg-Larsen, N. (1953). *Vitam. Horm. (N.Y.)* **11,** 29.
Nicolaysen, R., Eeg-Larsen, N., and Malm, O. J. (1953). *Physiol. Rev.* **33,** 424.
Nordstrom, C., Dahlquist, A., and Josefsson, L. (1968). *J. Histochem. Cytochem.* **15,** 713.
Norman, A. W. (1965). *Science* **149,** 184.
Norman, A. W. (1966). *Am. J. Physiol.* **211,** 829.
Norman, A. W. (1967). *Clin. Orthop. Relat. Res.* **52,** 249.
Norman, A. W. (1968). *Biol. Rev. Cambridge Philos. Soc.* **43,** 97.
Norman, A. W. (1975). *Vitam. Horm. (N.Y.)* **32,** 325.
Norman, A. W., and Wong, R. G. (1972). *J. Nutrit.* **102,** 1709.
Norman, A. W., and Henry, H. L. (1974). *Recent Prog. Horm. Res.* **30,** 431.
Norman, A. W., Haussler, M. R., Adams, T. H., Myrtle, J. F., Roberts, P., and Hibberd, K. A. (1969). *Am. J. Clin. Nutr.* **22,** 396.
Norman, A. W., Mircheff, A. K., Adams, T. H., and Spielvogel, A. M. (1970). *Biochim. Biophys. Acta* **215,** 348.
Norman, A. W., Demel, R. A., DeKruyff, B., and van Deenen, L. L. M. (1972a). *J. Biol. Chem.* **247,** 1918.
Norman, A. W., Demel, R. A., DeKruyff, B., Geurts van Kessel, W. S. M., and van Deenen, L. L. M. (1972b). *Biochim. Biophys. Acta* **290,** 1.
Norman, A. W., Spielvogel, A. M., and Wong, R. G. (1975). *Adv. Lipid Res.* **14,** 127.
O'Donnel, J. M., and Smith, M. W. (1973a). *J. Physiol. (London)* **229,** 733.
O'Donnel, J. M., and Smith, M. W. (1973b). *Biochem. J.* **134,** 667.
Oldham, S. B., Fischer, J. A., Shen, L. H., and Arnaud, C. D. (1974). *Biochemistry* **13,** 4790.
Olsen, E. B., and DeLuca, H. F. (1969). *Science* **165,** 405.
Olsen, E. B., DeLuca, H. F., and Potts, J. T., Jr. (1972). *Endocrinology* **90,** 151.
Omdahl, J. L., and Thornton, P. (1972) *Biochem. Pharmacol.* **21,** 231.
Oozumi, K., Moriuchi, S., and Hosoya, N. (1970). *J. Vitaminol.* **16,** 228.
Padykula, H. A. (1962). *Fed. Proc., Fed. Am. Soc. Exp. Biol.* **21,** 873.
Palade, G. E. (1958). *In* "Frontiers in Cytology" (S. L. Palay, ed.), p. 283. Yale, Univ. Press, New Haven, Connecticut.
Peterlik, M., Bursac, K., Haussler, M. R., Hughes, M. R., and Wasserman, R. H. (1976). *Biochem. Biophys. Res. Commun.* **70,** 797.
Piazolo, P., Schleyer, M., and Franz, H. E. (1971). *Hoppe-Seyler's Z. Physiol. Chem.* **352,** 1480.
Procsal, D. A., Hendrickson, T., and Norman, A. W. (1976). *Endocrinology* **99,** 437.
Rahaminoff, R. (1970). *In* "Calcium and Cellular Function" (A. W. Cuthbert, ed.), p. 131. St. Martin's, New York.
Rasmussen, H. (1959). *Endocrinology* **65,** 317.
Rasmussen, H., and DeLuca, H. F. (1963). *Ergeb. Physiol., Biol. Chem. Exp. Pharmakol.* **53,** 108.
Reiss, E., and Canterbury, J. M. (1974). *Recent Prog. Horm. Res.* **30,** 391.
Rich, C., and Ivanovich, P. (1964). *Northwest Med.* **63,** 792.
Rosenberg, T., and Wilbrandt, W. (1957). *J. Gen. Physiol.* **41,** 289.
Rossi, C. S., and Lehninger, A. L. (1963). *Biochem. Z.* **338,** 698.
Russell, R. G. G., Monod, A., Bonjour, J.-P., and Fleisch, H. (1972). *Nature (London), New Biol.* **240,** 126.
Sallis, J. D., and Holdsworth, E. S. (1962). *Am. J. Physiol.* **203,** 497.
Schachter, D. (1970). *In* "The Fat-Soluble Vitamins" (H. F. DeLuca and J. W. Suttie, eds.), p. 55. Univ. of Wisconsin Press, Madison.

Schachter, D., and Rosen, S. M. (1959). *Am. J. Physiol.* **196,** 357.
Schachter, D., Dowdle, E. B., and Schenker, H. (1960). *Am. J. Physiol.* **198,** 263.
Scott, D. (1965). *Q. J. Exp. Physiol. Cogn. Med. Sci.* **50,** 312.
Segré, V., and Potts, J. T. (1975). *In* "Calcium Metabolism, Bone and Metabolic Bone Disease" (F. Kuhlencordt and H. P. Kruse, eds.), p. 285. Springer-Verlag, Berlin and New York.
Shah, B. G., and Draper, H. H. (1966). *Am. J. Physiol.* **211,** 763.
Shimotori, N., and Morgan, A. F. (1943). *J. Biol. Chem.* **147,** 201.
Spencer, R. M., Charman, P., Emtage, J. S., and Lawson, D. E. M. (1976a). *Eur. J. Biochem.* **71,** 399.
Spencer, R. M., Charman, P., wilson, E., and Lawson, D. E. M. (1976b). *Nature (London)* **263,** 161.
Spencer, R. M., Charman, P., Wilson, E., and Lawson, D. E. M. (1978). *Biochem. J.* **170,** 93.
Spielvogel, A. M. (1973). Ph.D. Dissertation, University of California, Riverside.
Spielvogel, A. M., and Norman, A. W. (1975). *Arch. Biochem. Biophys.* **167,** 335.
Spielvogel, A. M., Farley, R. D., and Norman, A. W. (1972). *Exp. Cell Res.* **74,** 359.
Stanbury, S. W., and Lumb, G. A. (1962). *Medicine (Baltimore)* **41,** 1.
Steenbock, H., and Herting, D. C. (1955). *J. Nutr.* **57,** 449.
Szymender, J., Heaney, R. P., and Saville, P. (1972). *J. Lab. Clin. Med.* **79,** 570.
Tanzer, F. S., and Navia, J. M. (1973). *Nature (London), New Biol.* **242,** 221.
Taylor, A. N. (1974a). *J. Nutr.* **104,** 489.
Taylor, A. N. (1974b). *Arch. Biochem. Biophys.* **161,** 100.
Taylor, A. N. (1977). *J. Nutr.* **107,** 480.
Taylor, A. N., and Wasserman, R. H. (1967). *Arch. Biochem. Biophys.* **119,** 536.
Taylor, A. N., and Wasserman, R. H. (1970). *J. Histochem. Cytochem.* **18,** 107.
Taylor, A. N., Wasserman, R. H., and Jowsey, J. (1968). *Fed. Proc., Fed. Am. Soc. Exp. Biol.* **27,** 675.
Tsai, H. C., Wong, R. G., and Norman, A. W. (1972). *J. Biol. Chem.* **247,** 5511.
Tsai, H. C., Midgett, R. J., and Norman, A. W. (1973). *Arch. Biochem. Biophys.* **157,** 339.
Tufty, R. M., and Kretsinger, R. H. (1975). *Science* **187,** 167.
Urban, E., and Schedl, H. P. (1969a). *Proc. Soc. Exp. Biol. Med.* **132,** 1110.
Urban, E., and Schedl, H. P. (1969b). *Am. J. Physiol.* **217,** 126.
Urban, E., and Schedl, H. P. (1970). *Am. J. Physiol.* **219,** 944.
Uribe, A., Holick, M. F., Jorgensen, N. A., and DeLuca, H. F. (1974). *Biochem. Biophys. Res. Commun.* **58,** 257.
Ussing, H. H. (1949). *Acta Physiol. Scand.* **19,** 43.
Van Zupthen, H., Demel, R. A., Norman, A. W., and van Deenen, L. L. M. (1971). *Biochim. Biophys. Acta* **241,** 310.
Walling, M. W. (1977). *Am. J. Physiol.* **232,** E488.
Walling, M. W., and Rothman, S. S. (1969). *Am. J. Physiol.* **217,** 1144.
Walling, M. W., and Rothman, S. S. (1970). *J. Biol. Chem.* **245,** 5007.
Walling, M. W., and Rothman, S. S. (1973). *Am. J. Physiol.* **225,** 618.
Walling, M. W., and Kimberg, D. A. (1975a). *Endocrinology* **97,** 1567.
Walling, M. W., Kimberg, D. V., Lloyd, W., Wells, H., Procsal, D. A., and Norman, A. W. (1975b). *In* "Proceedings of the Second Symposium on Vitamin D and Problems Related to Uremic Bone Disease" (A. W. Norman *et al.*, eds.), p. 717. de Gruyter, Berlin.
Walling, M. W., Kimberg, D. V., Wasserman, R. H., and Feinberg, M. (1976). *Endocrinology* **98,** 1130.
Wasserman, R. H., ed. (1963). "The Transfer of Calcium and Strontium across Biological Membranes." Academic Press, New York.
Wasserman, R. H. (1972). *In* "Metabolic Transport" (L. E. Hokin, ed.), p. 351. Academic Press, New York.

Wasserman, R. H. (1973). *Hard Tissue Growth, Repair Remineralization, Ciba Found. Symp., 1972* p. 373.
Wasserman, R. H. (1976). *Handb. Physiol., Sect. 7: Endocrinol.* **5,** 137.
Wasserman, R. H. (1974). *Science* **183,** 1092.
Wasserman, R. H., and Comar, C. L. (1959). *Proc. Soc. Exp. Biol. Med.* **101,** 314.
Wasserman, R. H., and Corradino, R. A. (1971). *Annu. Rev. Biochem.* **40,** 501.
Wasserman, R. H., and Corradino, R. A. (1973). *Vitam. Horm. (N.Y.)* **31,** 43.
Wasserman, R. H., and Kallfelz, F. A. (1970). *In* "Biological Calcification: Cellular and Molecular Aspects" (H. Schraer, ed.), pp. 313. Appleton, New York.
Wasserman, R. H., and Taylor, A. N. (1966). *Science* **152,** 791.
Wasserman, R. H., and Taylor, A. N. (1968). *J. Biol. Chem.* **243,** 3987.
Wasserman, R. H., and Taylor, A. N. (1969). *Miner. Metab.* **3,** 321.
Wasserman, R. H., and Taylor, A. N. (1971). *Proc. Soc. Exp. Biol. Med.* **136,** 25.
Wasserman, R. H., and Taylor, A. N. (1972). *Annu. Rev. Biochem.* **41,** 179.
Wasserman, R. H., and Taylor, A. N. (1973a). *Triangle* **12,** 13.
Wasserman, R. H., and Taylor, A. N. (1973b). *J. Nutr.* **103,** 586.
Wasserman, R. H., Comar, C. L., and Nold, M. M. (1956). *J. Nutr.* **59,** 371.
Wasserman, R. H., Kallfelz, F. A., and Comar, C. L. (1961). *Science* **133,** 883.
Wasserman, R. H., Taylor, A. N., and Kallfelz, F. A. (1966). *Am. J. Physiol.* **211,** 419.
Wasserman, R. H., Corradino, R. A., and Taylor, A. N. (1968). *J. Biol. Chem.* **243,** 3978.
Wasserman, R. H., Taylor, A. N., and Fullmer, C. S. (1974). *In* "Metabolism and Function of Vitamin D" (D. Fraser, ed.), pp. 55–74. The Biochemical Society of London, London.
Wasserman, R. H., Corradino, R. A., Krook, L., Hughes, M. R., and Haussler, M. R. (1976). *J. Nutr.* **106,** 457.
Webster, H. L., and Harrison, D. D. (1969). *Exp. Cell Res.* **56,** 245.
Widdowson, E. M., and Dickerson, J. W. T. (1964). *Miner. Metab.* **2,** Part A, 1.
Wilson, T. H. (1962). "Intestinal Absorption." Saunders, Philadelphia, Pennsylvania.
Wilson, T. H., and Wiseman, G. (1954). *J. Physiol. (London)* **123,** 116.
Wong, R. G. (1972). Ph.D. Dissertation, University of California, Riverside.
Wong, R. G., and Norman, A. W. (1975). *J. Biol. Chem.* **250,** 2411.
Wong, R. G., Adams, T. H., Roberts, P. A., and Norman, A. W. (1970). *Biochim. Biophys. Acta* **219,** 61.
Worker, N. A., and Carrillo, B. J. (1969). *Nature (London)* **215,** 72.
Youngoszai, M. K., and Schedl, H. P. (1972a). *Gastroenterology* **62,** 565.
Youngoszai, M. K., and Schedl, H. P. (1972b). *Proc. Soc. Exp. Biol. Med.* **140,** 496.
Youngoszai, M. K., Urban, E., and Schedl, H. P. (1973). *Am. J. Physiol.* **225,** 287.
Zull, J. E., Czarnowska-Misztal, E., and DeLuca, H. F. (1965). *Science* **149,** 182.

CHAPTER 11

Vitamin D Actions in the Kidney (Excluding Vitamin D Metabolism)

I. THE KIDNEY AND MINERAL HOMEOSTASIS

A. Introductory Comments

The aim of this chapter is to review the role of vitamin D and its metabolites in the physiological and other functions of the kidney. The focus is on relating the sophisticated anatomical and physiological aspects of the kidney to calcium and phosphorus homeostasis in light of studies on vitamin D. The aspects governing the regulation of metabolism of 25(OH)D to $1,25(OH)_2D$ and/or $24,25(OH)_2D$ in the renal cortex are not discussed here because they are covered in Chapter 6. It may appear arbitrary to separate the renal metabolism of vitamin D from the physiological actions of the kidney vis-à-vis mineral metabolism, but it has been done to simplify the discussion.

As yet there have been no hypotheses elaborated that explain the presence of 25(OH)D 1-hydroxylase and 25(OH)D 24-hydroxylase in the kidney. The assumption is that their presence reflects the prominent role of the kidney in calcium and phosphorus homeostasis. As stated by Peters (1935), "the kidneys appear to serve as the ultimate guardians of the constitution of the internal environment." It would appear to be eminently logical to place the enzymatic machinery concerned with the production of the biologically active and relevant forms of vitamin D, e.g., $1,25(OH)_2D_3$ and $24,25(OH)_2D_3$, in the same organ, in fact in the same substructures, the kidney tubules, since these are concerned with the minute-by-minute regulation of the ionic composition of the plasma.

The kidney carries out its homeostatic actions by secretion, tubular reabsorption, and glomerular filtration, all processes that regulate the concentration of metabolic end products, the osmotic pressure, the ionic composition, and the volume of the internal environment.

B. Role of the Kidney and Vitamin D in Calcium and Phosphorus Homeostasis

The principal sites of regulation of calcium and phosphorus homeostasis are the intestine, the skeleton, and the kidney (see Fig. 9-1).

The concentration of calcium in the blood, particularly its ionized form, is stringently regulated through complex interactions among (a) the movement of calcium in and out of bone, (b) its absorption by the intestine, and (c) the renal tubular reabsorption of calcium lost into the renal tubule by glomerular filtration. The kidneys of a typical adult male transfer per day some 11,000 mg (275 nmoles) of calcium from the plasma into the glomerular filtrate. However, only 0.5–1.0% of this large amount of filtered calcium is lost in the urine; this is a reflection of the remarkably effective tubular reabsorption mechanism(s) for calcium. Man normally loses 100–200 mg of calcium daily in the urine. It is known that several nonhormonal as well as hormonal factors may alter the renal handling of calcium and its excretory rate.

The concentration of phosphorus in the blood (principally HPO_4^{2-} and $H_2PO_4^-$) is not as stringently regulated as that of calcium. In the case of phosphate, 40–60% of that available in the diet is absorbed by the intestine and, as indicated in Chapter 10, there appears to be only a modest regulation of the intestinal absorptive processes for phosphate. The inorganic phosphate in the blood also is very efficiently filtered at the glomerulus so that in a typical day approximately 6000–10,000 mg of phosphate are transferred from the blood to the glomerular filtrate. Of this amount the renal tubule reabsorbs 80–90%. Man normally loses 700–1500 mg of phosphate daily in the urine. Thus, in comparison to calcium, a significantly larger amount of phosphate is excreted on a daily basis. As will become evident later, both parathyroid hormone and vitamin D play important roles in modulating the amount of phosphate that is actually excreted in the urine. Under circumstances of dietary phosphate restriction, the kidney becomes very efficient in its tubular reabsorption of phosphate from the glomerular filtrate, thus conserving this important anion for the body. In contrast, in situations of a dietary excess of phosphate, the plasma phosphorus concentration may become elevated, resulting ultimately in a significant increase in the amount of phosphorus excreted in the urine.

Figure 11-1 is a schematic diagram of a typical kidney nephron. Indicated in this figure are the sites of reabsorption of the various ions, including calcium and phosphate. Also shown are the putative sites of action of parathyroid hormone and vitamin D and/or its metabolites.

From a consideration of the fluid dynamics of the kidney, it is possible to imagine an increase in urinary excretion of calcium, which may arise either from a decreased tubular reabsorption or from an increased filtered load of calcium or both. An increase in filtered load of calcium that is produced by an elevation in the rate of glomerular filtration normally has only a small effect on calcium excretion (Massry and Kleeman, 1972). However, an increase in the filtered load produced by hypercalcemia may result in a more marked reduction in the tubular reabsorption of calcium (Coburn *et al.,* 1970).

Table 11-1 lists the factors related to the renal handling of calcium and phosphate. Under circumstances in which there is an increase in the intestinal absorption of calcium, an increase in urinary calcium normally results via the production of a mild hypercalcemic condition, which in turn increases the filtered load of calcium. Parathyroid hormone (PTH) is one of the hormonal factors that is capable of altering the tubular reabsorption of calcium. Thus, PTH reduces urinary calcium by increasing the efficiency of reabsorption of the kidney tubule, which results in an increase in the serum calcium level. There is, however, a potential counterbalancing effect because, as the serum calcium increases when PTH increases tubular reabsorption, the resulting hypercalcemia itself may, with time, increasingly inhibit the tubular reabsorption process and thus generate a degree of hypercalciuria.

It is well documented that there is a close association between the renal tubular reabsorption of calcium and that of sodium, and it can readily be shown that circumstances that alter the tubular reabsorption of sodium have a similar effect on calcium handling. These include renal vasodilatation, several diuretics, e.g., ethacrynic acid or furesomide, and saline infusion. An enhanced urinary excretion of calcium will arise from an increase in filtered load as well as from a decreased tubular reabsorption.

It is generally held that the fluxes of calcium from the skeleton and the intestine are the primary determinants of the circulating serum calcium levels (Massry and Coburn, 1973), although some have postulated a more important role for the kidney as a regulator of serum calcium concentration (Nordin and Peacock, 1969; Nordin, 1972).

Several factors are capable of influencing the efficiency of the tubular reabsorption of phosphorus. There is a close interrelationship between the renal handling of sodium and that of phosphate; thus, expansion of extracellular vol-

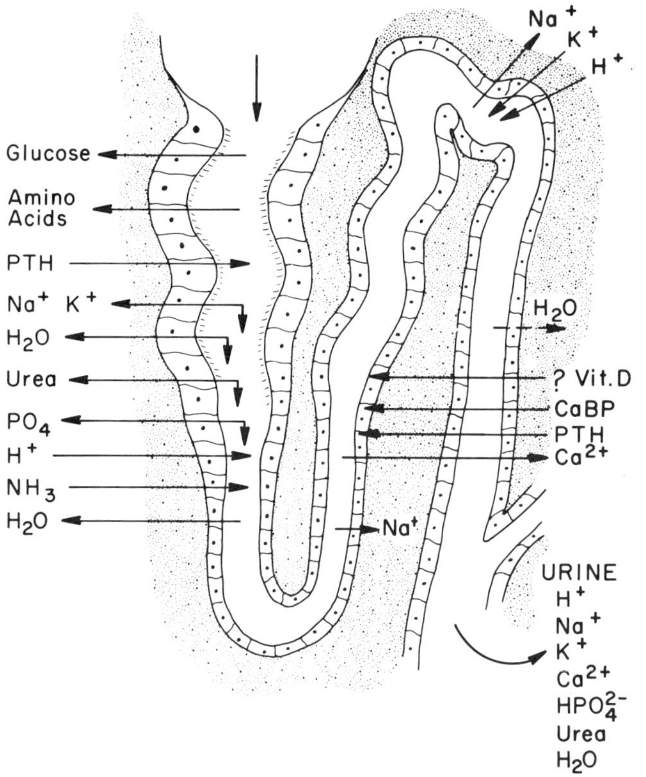

Figure 11-1. Schematic diagram of the kidney nephron. The sites of reabsorption of calcium and phosphate and other ionic substances are indicated as are possible sites of intervention of PTH and vitamin D or its metabolites. The afferent arteriole enters the glomerulus and subsequently is divided into many capillaries, which serve as a filter. The glomerular filtrate may be modified subsequently by both secretory and resorptive events occurring in the proximal tubule. Ultimately the filtrate enters the loop of Henle. Here it slowly becomes further concentrated by diffusion of water into the hypertonic interstitium. In the ascending limb of the loop of Henle, sodium is actively transported from the filtrate (thereby diluting it) to the interstitium, where it is concentrated. The osmolality of the interstitial fluid therefore can increase from approximately 300 to 1100 mOsm/kg H_2O as the papilla is approached. Then, as the distal tubule passes back past the glomerulus, the closely packed cells of the macula densa nestle against the afferent arterioles that are a part of the juxtaglomerular apparatus. Next, in the distal tubule, sodium may be reabsorbed in exchange for hydrogen or potassium ions, and eventually water is reabsorbed from the distal tubule and collecting duct under the influence of vasopressin. See Golden and Maher (1971) for a detailed discussion.

ume by the infusion of saline may cause a marked increase in the amount of urinary phosphate excreted (Puschett *et al.*, 1972a). Another major effector is PTH, which acts on the renal tubules to decrease the amount of tubular reabsorption of phosphate. Thus, the action of PTH is to promote the urinary excretion of phosphorus; i.e., it has a phosphaturic action. Also, changes in blood calcium concentration can affect the processing of phosphate by the kidney. Lavender and

TABLE 11-1
Factors Related to the Renal Handling of Calcium and Phosphate[a]

Factor	Effect on fractional renal tubular reabsorption	Effect on urinary excretion	Reference
Calcium			
Saline infusion (extracellular volume expansion)	↓	↑	Walser (1973), Massry *et al.* (1967)
Renal vasodilatation	↓	↑	Earley and Friedler (1966)
Diuretics, mercurial	↓	↑	Duarte (1968)
(furesomide or ethacrynic acid)	↓	↑	Eknoyan *et al.* (1970)
Increased glomerular filtration rate	↓	↑	Massry and Kleeman (1972)
Parathyroid hormone	↑	↓	Kleeman *et al.* (1961), Bethune *et al.* (1968)
Phosphate depletion	↓	↑	Lotz *et al.* (1968), Coburn and Massry (1970)
Acidosis	↓	↑	Lemann *et al.* (1967)
Carbohydrate ingestion	↓	↑	Hodgkinson and Heaton (1965)
Increase in serum Ca by infusion	↓	↑	Coburn *et al.* (1970), Massry *et al.* (1968)
Calcitonin	↓	↑	Singer *et al.* (1969), Aldred *et al.* (1970)
Vitamin D	↑	↓	Puschett *et al.* (1972b), Ney *et al.* (1968), Sutton (1978)
Phosphorus			
Saline infusion (extracellular volume expansion)	↓	↑	Puschett *et al.* (1972a, 1974)
Parathyroid hormone	↓	↑	
Short-term increase in serum calcium	↑	↓	Lavender and Pullman (1963)
Long-term increase in serum calcium	↓	↑	Eisenberg (1965)
Vitamin D	↑	↓	Puschett *et al.* (1972b), Harrison and Harrison (1942), Bonjour *et al.* (1978)

[a]An extensive discussion of these factors is given by Massry and Coburn (1973).

Pullman (1963) clearly showed that the short-term infusion of calcium into one renal artery was capable of inducing a decrease in excretion of urinary phosphorus by the other or ipsilateral kidney.

Thus, it can be seen by evaluation of Table 11-1 as well as Fig. 11-1 that the kidney makes a critical contribution to the maintenance of normal calcium and phosphorus homeostasis.

II. EFFECTS OF VITAMIN D AND METABOLITES ON RENAL TUBULAR FUNCTION

A. Calcium-Binding Protein

Taylor and Wasserman (1972) first reported the presence of a vitamin D-dependent calcium-binding protein (CaBP) in the kidney of chicks. This was detected not only by the Chelex resin method for a competitive calcium-binding assay, but also by a radial immunodiffusion assay employing highly specific antiserum to chick intestinal CaBP. The possible existence of a renal CaBP activity had been alluded to in an earlier paper of Taylor and Wasserman (1967). There had been previous suggestions of the presence of a ''calcium-binding component'' in dog kidney cortex in a report by Sands and Kessler (1971). However, their studies did not address the possible relation of vitamin D or its metabolites to the presence of this ''activity.''

In subsequent studies carried out by Wasserman *et al.* (1974) a number of tissues and organs from calves and cows were tested immunologically against rabbit antisera prepared against bovine intestinal CaBP. The presence or absence of CaBP was established initially by double-diffusion analysis. The CaBP of bovine kidney was exclusively located in the renal cortex, and it appeared to be present in a concentration approximately one-sixth of that of the duodenum. In other studies (Wasserman *et al.*, 1974), the tubular location of the calf renal CaBP was determined via utilization of fluorescent-labeled antibody sections and comparable, conventionally stained histological sections. These studies indicated that the CaBP was localized largely in the distal tubules with little or no CaBP detectable in the proximal tubules. At the subcellular level the distribution of the fluorescence, which was indicative of the CaBP, suggested its presence at cell boundaries, as has been determined in chick intestinal cells.

The studies of Taylor and Wasserman (1972) conclusively demonstrated the dependence of this renal CaBP on the presence of vitamin D in the chick system. As chicks were fed a vitamin D-deficient diet and as they became progressively more rachitic, there was a concomitant fall in both serum calcium concentration (over an interval of 4 to 5 weeks) and the concentration of renal CaBP. However, as is the case for the intestinal CaBP, no conclusive studies have yet been presented showing a functional involvement of the renal CaBP in the renal metabolism of calcium.

B. Calcium

The effect of vitamin D and its metabolites on the renal tubular reabsorption of calcium varies depending on whether pharmacological doses or physiological doses of the vitamin have been given. Litvak *et al.* (1958), Hanna (1961), and Edwards and Hodgkinson (1965) observed that after the administration of pharmacological doses of vitamin D there was invariably an increase in the urinary excretion of calcium. However, it should be remembered that, in the presence of pharmacological doses of vitamin D, the intestinal absorption of calcium is usually increased, and simultaneously there is an increased resorption of bone calcium with a concomitant elevation of serum calcium concentration. As a result, there is an increased filtered load of calcium available in the renal tubules, and it is not so surprising, therefore, that there is an increased urinary excretion of calcium.

However, it was suggested by Litvak *et al.* (1958) that vitamin D actually might directly inhibit calcium reabsorption or transport by the nephron. This suggestion was based largely on observations that patients with hypoparathyroidism treated with massive doses of vitamin D responded with a marked hypercalciuria and only marginal increases in serum calcium. Bernstein *et al.* (1963) in additional studies on subjects with hypoparathyroidism, whose serum calcium had been increased by either vitamin D treatment or calcium infusion, noted no difference in the fraction of filtered calcium excreted at equivalent levels of serum calcium. Therefore, they concluded that the high rate of calcium excretion in vitamin D-treated patients was not a direct action of vitamin D but was instead induced by an increase in the filtered load of calcium.

Ney *et al.* (1968) in studies carried out in vitamin D-deficient, acutely thyroparathyroidectomized (TPTX) dogs found that large doses of vitamin D were invariably associated within the first two 24-hr periods with a fall in urinary calcium. However, there was, within 6 days, a somewhat higher urinary excretion of calcium; this was probably associated with the higher levels of serum calcium that might be present at that time.

With the elucidation of the metabolic pathway for the transformation of vitamin D into its biologically active forms, and with the dramatic demonstration of the key "endocrine role" of the kidney in the production of $1,25(OH)_2D_3$ and $24,25(OH)_2D_3$, it became possible to evaluate more critically the effects of the specific vitamin D metabolites on kidney function.

Puschett and co-workers (1972a,b, 1974) as well as Sutton (1978) studied the effects of the administration of either $25(OH)D_3$ or $1,25(OH)_2D_3$ on the tubular reabsorption of calcium. These studies were carried out in dogs that had undergone thyroparathyroidectomy and volume expansion with saline; it should be recalled from Table 11-1 that both of these treatments would tend to inhibit calcium reabsorption, i.e., facilitate urinary calcium excretion. These workers found that these vitamin D steroids reduced urinary calcium excretion under the conditions studied. In later studies, Puschett *et al.* (1974) found that the administration of calcitonin, cAMP, or even PTH, as well as the infusion of calcium, all of which raise serum calcium levels to normal, blocked the stimulatory effect of $25(OH)D_3$ on the tubular reabsorption of calcium. In related studies, Costanzo *et al.* (1974) administered 48 hr prior to analysis 100 IU (6.5 nmoles) of vitamin D to vitamin D-deficient TPTX rats and noted that, in instances of comparable levels of sodium clearance, the fractions of filtered calcium excreted were significantly lower in vitamin D-treated than in untreated animals. The bulk of current evidence relating to the effects of $25(OH)D_3$ or the parent vitamin D on the renal handling of calcium suggests that these steroids enhance the tubular reabsorption of calcium.

There have been several reports on the effects of $1,25(OH)_2D_3$ on renal calcium metabolism. Steele *et al.* (1976) as well as Puschett *et al.* (1975) found that, in vitamin D-deficient TPTX rats stabilized on a diet containing either 0.1 or 0.02% phosphorus, a dose of 0.65 to 1.3 nmoles of $1,25(OH)_2D_3$ resulted in a significant lowering of the fraction of filtered calcium that was excreted. Thus, there is a similarity in the reported renal actions of $1,25(OH)_2D_3$ and its precursor $25(OH)D_3$. At present there are no reports concerning the renal effects of $24,25(OH)_2D_3$.

The effects of vitamin D or its metabolites on renal calcium excretion in man are not yet clearly understood. Hall *et al.* (1969), who administered large doses of vitamin D_3 (10,000 IU), and Brickman *et al.* (1974), who gave 1.0–2.5 μg of $1,25(OH)_2D_3$, reported an increase in urinary calcium. In the latter studies this effect was observed within 7–8 hr after a single dose of $1,25(OH)_2D_3$ (Coburn *et al.*, 1975). A possible explanation for these observations, which would account for their apparent disparate actions from those in experimental animals, is as follows. In the event that the vitamin D or $1,25(OH)_2D_3$ mediated an increased tubular reabsorption of calcium, a slight elevation of serum calcium would result, which would present a higher filtered load of calcium to the kidney tubule; the response, then, would most likely be a decrease in the fractional tubular reabsorption of calcium and modest hypercalciuria.

C. Phosphate

In a landmark paper Harrison and Harrison (1942) reported that vitamin D given at a dose of 20,000 IU/day (1300 nmoles) for 3 days mediated a rise in the

T_m[1] for phosphate in vitamin D-deficient dogs (with intact parathyroid glands) with a concomitant fall in urinary excretion of phosphate. In an earlier study Liu *et al.* (1940) noted that after treatment of rachitic children with vitamin D there was a fall in the urinary phosphorus excretion. A similar observation was made 13 years later by Klein and Gow (1953). A possible criticism of these earlier studies is that the observed reduction in phosphate excretion after vitamin D administration might have been mediated by the actions of vitamin D in increasing serum calcium, which generated a concomitant inhibition of PTH secretion.

Thus, it was not surprising that Ney *et al.* (1968) found that the intravenous administration of vitamin D_3 (500 IU; 32.5 nmoles) over a 2-hr period to rachitic dogs that had been previously given an intramuscular dose of 100,000 IU (6.5 μmoles) of vitamin D_3 daily stimulated the urinary excretion of phosphate, i.e., decreased the tubular reabsorption of phosphate. Similarly, Crawford *et al.* (1955) noted the stimulation of urinary phosphate excretion in parathyroidectomized rats that had received 500,000 IU/day (32.5 μmoles/day) of either vitamin D_3 or D_2. The observations of Crawford *et al.* (1955) as well as Ney *et al.* (1968) might be explained by a gradual "escape" from the avid phosphate reabsorption that immediately follows parathyroidectomy. In support of this hypothesis is the study of Eisenberg (1965), who reported that in parathyroidectomized human beings a slow increase in serum calcium from low to normal levels produced a concomitant phosphaturia.

In more recent studies Gekle *et al.* (1971), who evaluated proximal tubular phosphate reabsorption by a sophisticated micropuncture technique, noted a significant increase in phosphate reabsorption following the infusion of vitamin D (20–1800 IU; 1.3–117 nmoles) in parathyroidectomized and intact rats. Furthermore, Costanzo *et al.* (1974) evaluated the renal clearance of both calcium and phosphorus in vitamin D-deficient thyroparathyroidectomized and intact rats and those that had been administered 100 IU (6.5 nmoles) of vitamin D_3 48 hr prior to study. They found that the vitamin D-deficient rats excreted significant quantities of phosphate at low filtered loads, whereas the vitamin D-replete TPTX rats, who had a higher filtered load, excreted no phosphate in the urine.

The modern era was introduced with the studies of Puschett *et al.* (1972a), who evaluated the effect of $25(OH)D_3$ on the renal handling of phosphate in vitamin D-replete TPTX dogs. Extracellular volume expansion was induced with saline infusion so that the tubular phosphate reabsorption would be decreased and phosphaturia would be enhanced. Vitamin D (10,000 IU; 650 nmoles) and $25(OH)D_3$ (100 IU; 6.5 nmoles) when infused over a 15-min period produced

[1] T_m is an abbreviation for transport maximum, a quantitative parameter of renal excretory function. It is (depending on sign) the maximal ability of the kidneys to either resorb or secrete a given material.

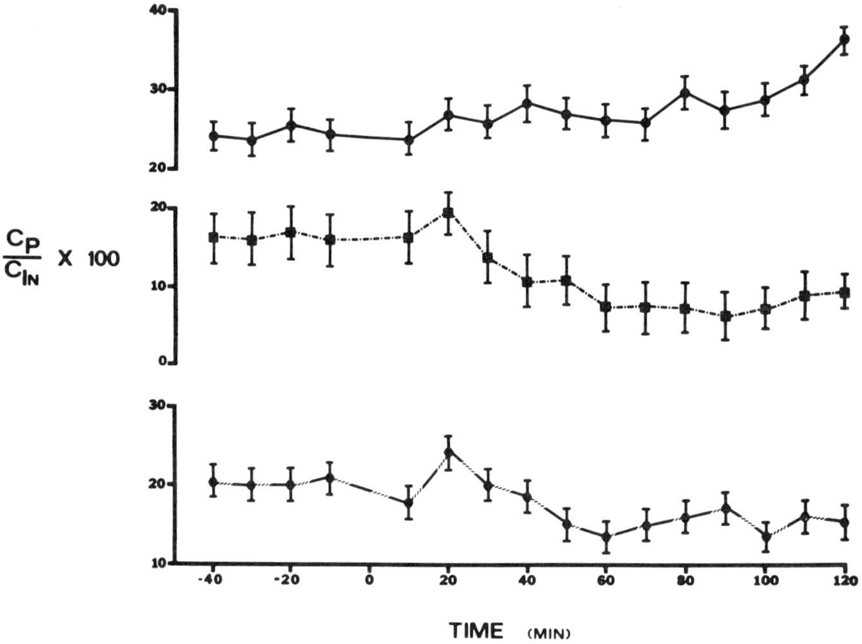

Figure 11-2. Time course of the effects of sustained saline expansion (controls, top), 25–120 units (1.6–8.0 nmoles) of $25(OH)D_3$ (middle), and 10,000 IU (650 nmoles) of vitamin D_3 (bottom) on the percentage of filtered phosphate excreted. Both steroids were given at time zero; each point represents the mean of all animals studied in each group at the times indicated. Reproduced by permission of the publisher and author from Puschett *et al.* (1972a).

within 1 hr a significant fall in phosphate excretion (Fig. 11-2). Puschett *et al.* further noted that in the presence of PTH (also via iv infusion), which produces a phosphaturic effect, there was no effect of $25(OH)D_3$ on the renal tubular absorption of phosphate.

In later studies, Puschett *et al.* (1974) evaluated the effects of cAMP and calcitonin on the ability of $25(OH)D_3$ to modulate the renal handling of phosphate. They reported that cAMP itself produced a phosphaturia and tended to abolish the hypophosphaturic effects of $25(OH)D_3$. They also noted that calcitonin, which by itself is without effect on calcium and phosphate excretion in dogs, abolished the observable effects of $25(OH)D_3$ on phosphate reabsorption.

Similar studies evaluating the effects of $25(OH)D_3$ on renal phosphate metabolism in the rat were carried out by Popovitzer *et al.* (1974). The infusion of 2.4 nmoles/kg per hour of $25(OH)D_3$ caused a decrease in urinary phosphate excretion in animals with intact parathyroid glands but had no effect on the urinary phosphate excretion in those that had undergone parathyroidectomy 2 days before the study. When PTH was infused into vitamin D-deficient TPTX rats, the subsequent treatment with $25(OH)D_3$ resulted in an inhibition of the phosphaturic action of PTH.

The results of Puschett *et al.* (1972a, 1974) regarding the effects of $25(OH)D_3$ on the renal handling of phosphate conflict somewhat with those of Popovitzer *et al.* (1974). Puschett *et al.* found an independent action of $25(OH)D_3$ in improving renal tubular reabsorption of phosphate in TPTX dogs, which was abolished in the presence of PTH. Popovitzer *et al.* (1974) found that in the absence of PTH (i.e., TPTX rats) $25(OH)D_3$ administration had no effect on phosphate clearance. Popovitzer and Robinette (1975) also found that the administration of $25(OH)D_3$ to TPTX rats was effective not only in blocking the phosphaturic action of PTH but also in blocking the usual increase in urinary excretion of cAMP stimulated by PTH. Clearly, further studies should be carried out to resolve this conflict.

Several laboratories have reported the results of studies in which effects of $1,25(OH)_2D_3$ on renal phosphate clearance have been evaluated. Puschett *et al.* (1972a) reported that when 5–20 units (0.32–1.3 nmoles) of $1,25(OH)_2D_3$ were given to TPTX vitamin D-replete dogs, the steroid mediated a reduction in phosphate clearance within 20–30 min. Popovitzer *et al.* (1974) also found that iv administration of $1,25(OH)_2D_3$ in intact rats decreased renal phosphate clearance, whereas it was without effect in TPTX rats. Also, A. S. Brickman, J. W. Coburn, and A. W. Norman (unpublished observations) observed that administration of 2.7 μg of $1,25(OH)_2D_3$ to vitamin D-deficient dogs resulted in a decrease in the urinary phosphate excretion, which occurred prior to changes in the plasma concentrations of phosphorus or calcium. Steele *et al.* (1976) gave 650–1300 pmoles of $1,25(OH)_2D_3$ to TPTX vitamin D-deficient rats and noted no effect of the steroid on the rate of or total urinary phosphate excretion. However, it should be recalled that the rat is particularly efficient in the renal tubular reabsorption of phosphate. For example, in the studies of Steele *et al.* (1976) the phosphate-depleted TPTX rats reabsorbed more than 99% of their filtered phosphate. It would have been experimentally difficult to detect a further improvement due to the effect of $1,25(OH)_2D_3$.

Thus far, the role, if any, of $1,25(OH)_2D_3$ in the day-to-day handling of phosphate by the kidney has not been convincingly established. There is evidence to suggest that the action of $1,25(OH)_2D_3$ is analogous to that which is more firmly established for $25(OH)D_3$, i.e., improving the renal tubular reabsorption of phosphate. However, the precise relationship between the effects of $1,25(OH)_2D_3$, PTH, and cAMP, whether they are permissive or independent, has not yet been determined. The detailed responsibility of $1,25(OH)_2D_3$, and perhaps of $25(OH)D_3$, in maintaining homeostasis of phosphate at the kidney level remains to be clearly established.

D. Other Ions (Na^+, HCO_3^-, K^+)

As described previously, the renal tubular handling of calcium, and to some extent phosphate, is closely interrelated with the renal tubular handling of sodium. However, there is little direct evidence suggesting that vitamin D or any of its metabolites play a role in sodium homeostasis. This problem is complicated in that there are other hormones that intervene in sodium homeostasis, and thus any acute actions of vitamin D metabolites might be quickly obliterated by the equal but opposite effects of the other hormonal systems. In the studies of Costanzo *et al.* (1974) equivalent fractions of filtered sodium were excreted in vitamin D-deficient rats and in animals treated with 1000 IU (65 nmoles) of vitamin D 2 days previously. Also, Puschett *et al.* (1972a,b) found no difference in the renal excretion of sodium in either the absence or presence of vitamin D (10,000 IU; 650 nmoles), $25(OH)D_3$ (100 units; 6.5 nmoles), or $1,25(OH)_2D_3$ (25 units; 1.6 nmoles).

There is even less information available connecting possible actions of vitamin D and its metabolites with the renal handling of potassium. The only relevant data are those of Puschett *et al.* (1974), who noted that $25(OH)D_3$ administration to volume-expanded TPTX dogs decreased the urinary excretion of potassium. However, the situation may be quite complicated in that this effect was blocked by treatment with either cAMP or calcitonin.

The only studies suggesting a relationship between vitamin D and the renal handling of bicarbonate are those of Siegfried *et al.* (1975). They concluded from studies carried out in intact and parathyroidectomized dogs that an inhibition of bicarbonate reabsorption by $25(OH)D_3$ required the presence of PTH.

E. Amino Acids

It has long been known that there is an aminoaciduria in patients with chronic vitamin D deficiency. Jonxis and Huisman (1953) noted that treatment with vitamin D can ultimately lead to a slow decrease in the elevated rates of amino acid excretion. Fraser *et al.* (1967) suggested that this phenomenon was related to secondary hyperparathyroidism. The implication of this would be that in a vitamin D-deficient rat, which is of necessity hyperparathyroid, the excess levels of the peptide hormone stimulate an increased urinary excretion of amino acids. Consistent with this are the observations of Grose and Scriver (1968), who noted that aminoaciduria in vitamin D-deficient rats was dependent on the presence of the parathyroid glands. Also, Short *et al.* (1974) found that administration of PTH to normal males mediated an increased renal excretion of a variety of amino acids. To date there are no reports evaluating the possible effects of any vitamin D metabolites on the renal handling of amino acids.

III. OTHER VITAMIN D–KIDNEY INTERACTIONS

A. Mitochondrial Ion Transport

A number of interactions between the kidney and vitamin D were known before 1966, which was the beginning of the era of studies that uncovered the metabolic pathway of vitamin D. One particularly interesting phase of study focused on the relationship between the *in vitro* uptake and release of calcium by kidney mitochondria and the effects thereon of vitamin D (not its metabolites). DeLuca and co-workers (1960, 1962) reported that there was a relationship between vitamin D status and the ability of kidney mitochondria to metabolize citrate, and as shown in Fig. 11-3 there was in fact a readily demonstrable effect of vitamin D status on the morphology of isolated kidney mitochondria. The mitochondria isolated from the kidneys of vitamin D-deficient rats showed gross morphological alterations, including damaged and swollen cristae. Dietary administration of vitamin D_3 *in vivo* at physiological levels, i.e., 10–30 IU/day (0.65–1.95 nmoles), for a week prevented these morphological changes. It is important to appreciate that the altered morphological appearance was observed only in mitochondria that had been isolated from broken cells. When intact kidney tissue from vitamin D-deficient rats was fixed and evaluated with the electron microscope, no alteration of mitochondrial morphology was apparent. The effect of vitamin D on the morphology of isolated mitochondria was unique to the kidney; the morphology of liver, heart, and intestinal mitochondria was unaffected by vitamin D.

The physiological significance of these observations concerning the effect of vitamin D on the morphology of kidney mitochondria is not yet known. However, it is intriguing that it is the vitamin D-deficient renal mitochondria that when assayed *in vitro* have such remarkably high levels of $25(OH)D_3$ 1-hydroxylase activity. Possibly there is some correlation between kidney mitochondrial morphology and the measurable levels of $25(OH)D_3$ 1-hydroxylase therein.

The study of vitamin D effects on mitochondrial ion metabolism had its origins in the earlier work relating vitamin D to the metabolism of citrate and particularly its oxidation by mitochondria. Mitchell (1961) and Robertson (1960) each suggested that oxidative phosphorylation and ion transport were intimately related phenomena. Since that time the process of mitochondrial ion transport has received much attention by two quite distinct groups of researchers, those interested primarily in active transport of ions and those interested in the mechanism of action of oxidative phosphorylation. The latter have employed mitochondrial ion uptake as a tool, along with inhibitors (antimycin A, rotenone), uncouplers (2,4-dinitrophenol), fractionation studies, and isolation of putative high-energy intermediates, to study the elusive details of mitochondrial

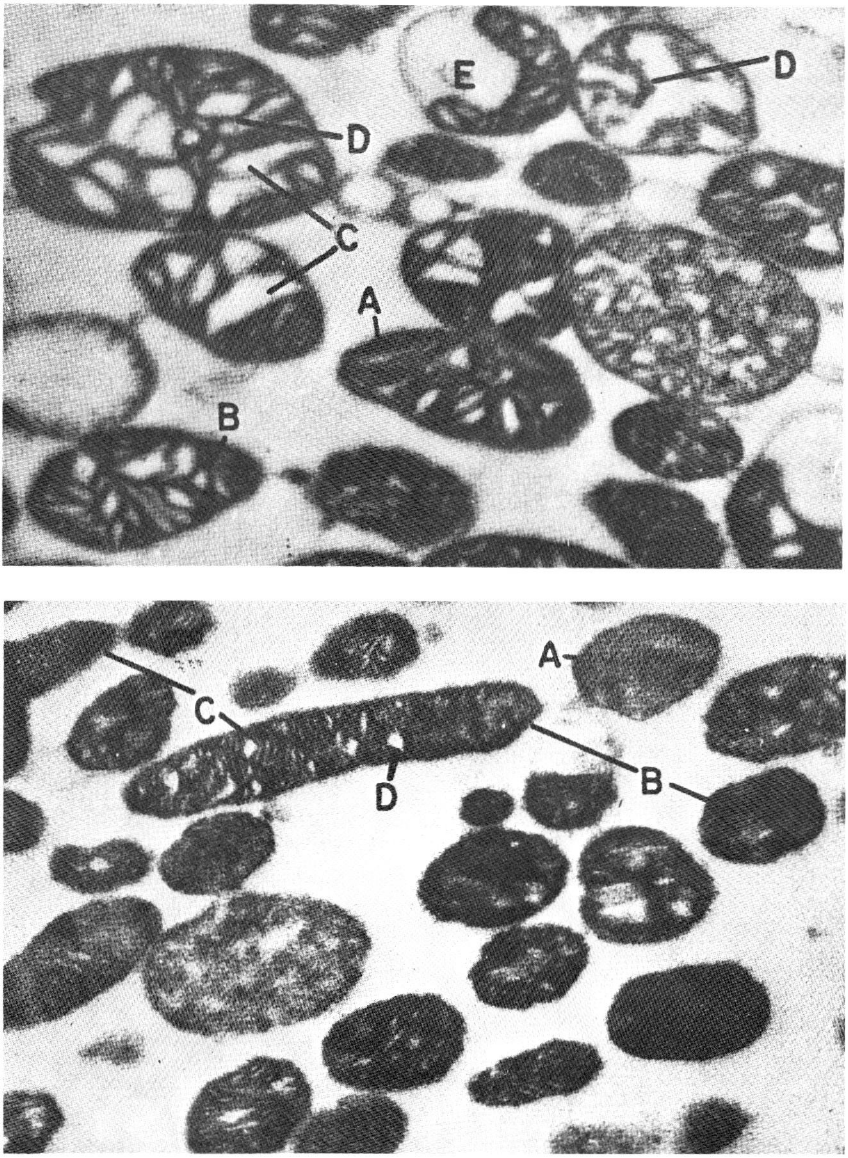

Figure 11-3. Electron micrographic appearance of kidney mitochondria isolated from a vitamin D-deficient rat (top) or a vitamin D-supplemented rat (bottom). In both instances the mitochondria were isolated in 0.44 *M* sucrose and magnification is ×34,000. Top: The outer double membranes are clearly discernible (A), as are the cristae (B). Note the large intercristal spaces (C), the swollen appearance of most mitochondria and the disrupted cristal arrangements (D), and the separation of the cristae from the outer membrane (E). Bottom: The outer double membrane (A) envelops a tightly packed and highly organized cristal system (B). Note the rods (C) and the small intercristal spaces (D), which are poorly visible in most cases. Reproduced by permission of the publisher and authors from DeLuca *et al.* (1960).

oxidative phosphorylation. Mitochondria have been shown capable of an efficient energy-dependent accumulation of calcium (DeLuca and Engström, 1961; Vasington and Murphy, 1962), strontium (Carafoli *et al.*, 1965), barium, manganese, and magnesium (Brierley *et al.*, 1963), potassium and phosphate (Sallis, 1963), acetate (Rasmussen *et al.*, 1964), and arsenate ions. The uptake of these ions is followed in some instances by an energy-dependent ejection of hydrogen ions. It is not within the scope of this chapter to review the details of oxidative phosphorylation and the complex effects of inhibitors and uncouplers on mitochondrial ion uptake and release properties. The reader is referred to a review by Lehninger (1964) for a detailed consideration of these topics.

In 1962 an exciting discovery in the vitamin D field was made by DeLuca and co-workers, who observed that addition of vitamin D *in vitro* to kidney mitochondrial preparations from vitamin D-deficient rats stimulated a prompt release of previously bound calcium (DeLuca and Engström, 1961; DeLuca *et al.*, 1962) (Fig. 11-4). This observation was studied in great detail by Engström and DeLuca (1964) and by Rasmussen and DeLuca (1963). Another provocative observation, made virtually simultaneously, was that PTH added *in vitro* to kidney mitochondria obtained from vitamin D-deficient, parathyroidectomized animals also mediated release of bound calcium.

The effect of vitamin D on the release of mitochondrically bound calcium was specific in a number of respects. (a) The effect of the vitamin D administration was apparent regardless of the calcium and phosphorus content of the diet; (b) it was observable over a wide range of calcium concentrations in the mitochondrial incubation medium; (c) the vitamin D "release effect" was limited primarily to calcium, and the release of strontium and barium from the mitochondria was only slightly stimulated by the presence of the steroid; (d) the "release effect" was not elicited with other vitamin D-related steroids, such as ergosterol, 7-dehydrocholesterol, and, perhaps most importantly, dihydrotachysterol. It should be noted

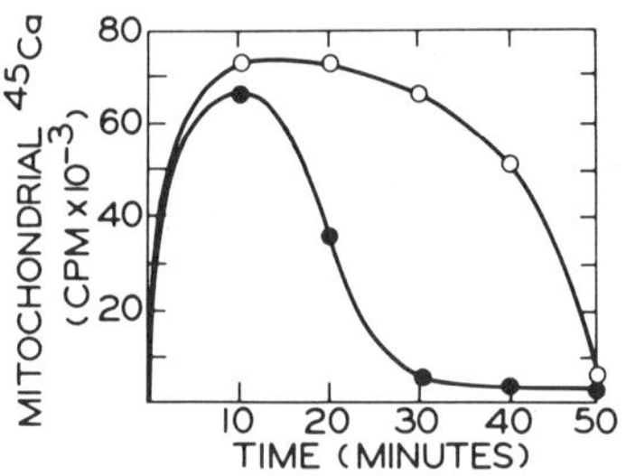

Figure 11-4. Stimulation of calcium release from isolated kidney mitochondria by the addition *in vitro* of vitamin D_3. At time zero 2000 IU (130 nmoles) of vitamin D_3 were added to the incubation medium. The mitochondria were isolated from kidneys obtained from vitamin D-deficient, parathyroidectomized rats (○, no added vitamin D; ●, added vitamin D_3). Reproduced by permission of the publisher and authors from DeLuca *et al.* (1962).

that at this time virtually no analogues of vitamin D were known, and certainly none of the metabolites had yet been recognized or characterized.

Kimberg and Goldstein (1967) brought this era to a close with the observation that liver mitochondria from vitamin D-replete rats accumulated and lost calcium at a more rapid rate than did mitochondria from vitamin D-depleted animals. These studies were followed by the report of Chudapongse and Lowchareonkul (1975), who evaluated the effects *in vitro* of vitamin D on oxidative phosphorylation and ATPase activity in rat liver mitochondria. They observed that both vitamin D_2 and D_3 were capable of depressing ATP synthesis. The effect was specific for the vitamin; it was not obtainable with dihydrotachysterol; vitamin D was not capable of inhibiting dinitrophenol-stimulated ATPase activity.

To date none of the above observations have been repeated using any vitamin D metabolites or analogs, so it is not possible to ascertain the true physiological significance of the parent vitamin D "release phenomenon" in kidney mitochondrial ion metabolism. In evaluating the striking mitochondrial interactions of vitamin D one must remember several pertinent facts. Rather high levels of vitamin D_2 (2000 IU; 130 nmoles) were used *in vitro*. The physiological requirement of vitamin D (see Chapter 4) is only 50–75 IU/week (3.25 nmoles). Normally when vitamin D is administered *in vivo* to a deficient animal, there is a lag of 20 to 40 hr before an increase in serum calcium level or an increase in intestinal absorption of calcium is noted (see Chapter 1). The mitochondrial "release effects" described above were instantaneous. However, the fact does remain that the phenomenon could be readily reproduced, and it is intriguing to speculate on the possible significance of the effects of the parent vitamin D in altering the ionic environment of the kidney mitochondria in which the renal $25(OH)D_3$ 1-hydroxylase and 24-hydroxylase are located. It is still conceivable that the results of studies carried out during this period in the development of our understanding of vitamin D will prove to be important in the elucidation of vitamin D effects in the kidney.

B. Vitamin D and Citric Acid Metabolism

It has been known since the early 1940's that there is an intimate connection between vitamin D, bone biochemistry, and citric acid metabolism. The relationship between vitamin D and citric acid metabolism in bone was first observed by Dickens (1941), who found that the citric acid content of bones from vitamin D-deficient animals was about 50% that of normal bones (see Chapter 12). This relationship was subsequently confirmed by Nicolaysen and Nordbo (1943), Wassjo and Eeg-Larsen (1951a,b), Steenbock and Bellin (1953), and Carlsson and Hollunger (1954) (see Table 11-2). In other work it was shown that dietary vitamin D increases the citrate content of many tissues (Steenbock and Bellin, 1953; Freeman and Chang, 1950) and induces an increased urinary excretion of

TABLE 11-2
Effect of Vitamin D Status on the Citric Acid Content of Rat Tissues[a]

Tissue	Citric acid content		
	−D (μg/g)	+D (μg/g)	Increase due to vitamin D (%)
Blood	13	21	61.5[b]
Heart	43	53	23.2
Kidney	18	38	111[b]
Small intestine	61	76	24.6
Liver	13	12	—
Bone	3.4	5.2	54[b]

[a] Abstracted from a paper of Steenbock and Bellin (1953).
[b] $P < 0.01$.

citrate (Bellin and Steenbock, 1952; Harrison and Harrison, 1951) (see Table 12-5).

It was shown in the laboratory of Steenbock and DeLuca that the addition of vitamin D to the diet of rats lowered the oxidation rates by kidney homogenates and mitochondria of citrate and isocitrate, but not that of other tricarboxylic acid cycle intermediates (DeLuca *et al.*, 1957a,b). This effect was also attained by the addition of vitamin D to systems *in vitro* (DeLuca and Steenbock, 1957). The latter observation was particularly notable in that it was the first reported *in vitro* effect of vitamin D and, as such, at the time it was reported, was believed to provide significant insight into the possible mode of action of vitamin D. As described above, electron microscopy of isolated rat kidney mitochondria revealed that dietary vitamin D had a marked protective effect on the structural integrity of these organelles (DeLuca *et al.*, 1960). It was then postulated that the diminished oxidation of citrate observed previously could be explained in terms of a physical inhibition of citrate penetration into the mitochondria.

However, a contrasting view was put forth by Patwardhan and co-workers (Ramalingaswami *et al.*, 1954; Dikshit *et al.*, 1956; Joshi *et al.*, 1957; Meyer *et al.*, 1959), who suggested that vitamin D increased the synthesis of citrate from acetate in bone. Joshi *et al.* (1957) concluded that the administration of vitamin D induced an increase in the enzyme citrogenase of the cartilage. It was not possible, however, to decide between these alternative explanations for increased tissue accumulation of citric acid as a function of vitamin D until the studies of Norman and DeLuca (1964) and Kunin and Krane (1965). Their results, described in more detail in Chapter 12, supported the hypothesis that vitamin D decreased the rate of conversion of citrate to subsequent intermediates in the tricarboxylic acid cycle.

Other observations suggested that the action of vitamin D on extracellular citrate could be prevented by treatment with pantothenic acid (Guroff *et al.*, 1963) as well as by pyridoxine deficiency or by cortisol administration (Harrison *et al.*, 1958). None of these treatments interfered with the action of vitamin D in elevating serum calcium. Since cortisol had been shown to inhibit the actions of vitamin D on intestinal calcium absorption, the observation that it did not inhibit the elevation of tissue levels of citric acid suggested that the relationship between vitamin D and citrate was not a primary one, but perhaps might occur as a consequence of the action of vitamin D or its metabolites on membrane permeability.

IV. TOXIC EFFECTS OF VITAMIN D ON THE KIDNEY

It is well known that the administration of pharmacological doses of vitamin D for an extended period of time inevitably leads to hypercalcemia and certain concomitant alterations in renal function that are undoubtedly due to the hypercalcemia produced. Epstein (1968) and Massry *et al.* (1973) reviewed in detail the effects of hypercalcemia on renal function. Certain physiological effects are detectable very rapidly after the onset of acute hypercalcemia. Wiedmann *et al.* (1972) reported increased peripheral vascular resistance, i.e., an elevated blood pressure, which is produced rapidly in response to hypercalcemia. A high blood calcium level may also alter the transport of certain ions by the kidney tubules; thus, an increase in the level of calcium in the glomerular filtrate may inhibit tubular reabsorption of sodium (Dibona, 1971) and calcium (Gutman and Gottschalk, 1966). Suki *et al.* (1969) noted that hypercalcemia reduces the reabsorption of sodium in the loop of Henle, and Massry *et al.* (1968) reported similar effects in the proximal tubule. Coburn *et al.* (1970) also observed a decreased tubular reabsorption of magnesium in concert with elevated serum calcium levels.

Another consequence of hypercalcemia is an impaired ability of the kidney to concentrate the urine, leading to polyuria. Epstein *et al.* (1958) and Manitus *et al.* (1960) produced this effect in the dog by the administration of large doses of vitamin D. The extent of the renal concentrating defect appeared to be related to the degree of nephrocalcinosis and the duration of the hypercalcemia rather than to the extent of hypercalcemia. Bennett (1970) advanced the alternative view that the impaired concentrating ability associated with chronic hypercalcemia could be accounted for by a reduced rate of glomerular filtration.

It has also been noted that there are certain similarities in the consequences of prolonged administration of pharmacological doses of vitamin D and those of the hypercalcemia produced by infusion of large doses of parathyroid extract. Both treatments result in degeneration and necrosis of the tubular epithelium of the ascending limb of the loop of Henle and also of the collecting duct and its associated distal convoluted tubule.

Prolonged treatment with pharmacological doses of vitamin D can result in soft-tissue calcification. This is initially observed as intratubular and intracellular calcific casts, which eventually obstruct the lumen and lead to an intrarenal hydronephrosis. As the hypercalcemia continues, deposits of calcium ultimately appear in the renal interstitium. This may result in an infection of the urinary tract as well as in the development of hypertension. These symptoms lead to the identification of the pathological lesions of chronic pyelonephritis and nephrosclerosis. As reported by Ziegler and Delling (1975) the continued ingestion of pharmacological amounts of vitamin D (e.g., 15 mg two times monthly for a period of 10 months) may prove to be fatal. Serum calcium concentrations as high as 19 mg per 100 ml have been reported after such extraordinary levels of vitamin D intake (Ziegler and Delling, 1975).

Another consequence of vitamin D intoxication is an excessive loss of urinary potassium and an associated hypokalemia (Verner *et al.*, 1958; Ferris *et al.*, 1961, 1962). Ferris *et al.* (1961, 1962) reported that in rats that had received 5 mg of vitamin D_2 per day for 4 days there was an inability to conserve potassium when they were subsequently stressed with a low potassium diet. These investigators postulated that the renal potassium wasting and related renal tubular acidosis might be an acquired defect as a result of the chronic hypercalcemia resulting from the rat's state of vitamin D intoxication.

It is clear from the foregoing comments that vitamin D in high doses is quite a toxic substance. Although the relative toxicities of $25(OH)D_3$, $1,25(OH)_2D_3$, and the other metabolites must still be documented, it is to be anticipated, in view of the "protection" that accrues to the animal because of the stringent regulation of vitamin D metabolism at the level of the kidney, that $1,25(OH)_2D_3$ particularly may be quite a hypercalcemic and toxic substance.

REFERENCES

Aldred, J. P., Kleszynski, R. R., and Bastian, J. W. (1970). *Proc. Soc. Exp. Biol. Med.* **134,** 1175.

Bellin, S. A., and Steenbock, H. (1952). *J. Biol. Chem.* **194,** 311.

Bennett, C. M. (1970). *J. Clin. Invest.* **49,** 1447.

Bernstein, D., Kleeman, C. R., and Maxwell, M. H. (1963). *Proc. Soc. Exp. Biol. Med.* **112,** 353.

Bethune, J. E., Turpin, R. A., and Inoue, H. (1968). *J. Clin. Endocrinol. Metab.* **28,** 673.

Bonjour, J.-P., Gloor, H. J., and Fleisch, H. (1978). *Proc. Int. Congr. Nephrol., 7th, 1978* p. 455.

Brickman, A. S., Coburn, J. W., Massry, S. G., and Norman, A. W. (1974). *Ann. Intern. Med.* **80,** 161.

Brierley, G. P., Murer, E., Bachmann, E., and Green, D. E. (1963). *J. Biol. Chem.* **238,** 3482.

Carafoli, E., Weiland, S., and Lehninger, A. L. (1965). *Biochim. Biophys. Acta* **97,** 88.

Carlsson, A., and Hollunger, B. (1954). *Acta Physiol. Scand.* **31,** 317.

Chudapongse, P., and Lowchareonkul, S. (1975). *Biochem. Pharmacol.* **24,** 2127.

Coburn, J. W., and Massry, S. G. (1970). *J. Clin. Invest.* **49,** 1619.
Coburn, J. W., Massry, S. G., and Kleeman, C. R. (1970). *Nephron* **7,** 131.
Coburn, J. W., Brickman, A. S., Llach, F., Kurokawa, K., Canterbury, J., Reiss, E., and Norman, A. W. (1975). *Clin. Res.* **23,** 134A.
Costanzo, L. S., Sheehe, P. R., and Weiner, I. M. (1974). *Am. J. Physiol.* **226,** 1490.
Crawford, J. D., Gribetz, D., and Talbot, N. B. (1955). *Am. J. Physiol.* **180,** 156.
DeLuca, H. F., and Engström, G. (1961). *Proc. Natl. Acad. Sci. U.S.A.* **47,** 1744.
DeLuca, H. F., and Steenbock, H. (1957). *Science* **126,** 258.
DeLuca, H. F., Gran, F. C., and Steenbock, H. (1975a) *J. Biol. Chem.* **224,** 201.
DeLuca, H. F., Gran, F. C., Steenbock, H., and Reiser, S. (1957b). *J. Biol. Chem.* **228,** 469.
DeLuca, H. F., Reiser, S., Steenbock, H., and Kaesberg, P. (1960). *Biochim. Biophys. Acta* **49,** 526.
DeLuca, H. F., Engström, G. W., and Rasmussen, H. (1962). *Proc. Natl. Acad. Sci. U.S.A.* **48,** 1604.
Dibona, G. F. (1971). *Am. J. Physiol.* **221,** 53.
Dickens, F. (1941). *Biochem. J.* **35,** 1011.
Dikshit, P. H., Joshi, J. G., and Patwardhan, V. N. (1956). *Indian J. Med. Res.* **44,** 719.
Duarte, C. G. (1968). *Metab., Clin. Exp.* **17,** 867.
Earley, L. F., and Friedler, R. M. (1966). *J. Clin. Invest.* **45,** 542.
Edwards, N. A., and Hodgkinson, A. (1965). *Clin. Sci.* **29,** 143.
Eisenberg, E. (1965). *J. Clin. Invest.* **44,** 942.
Eknoyan, G., Suki, W. N., and Martinez-Maldonado, M. (1970). *J. Lab. Clin. Med.* **76,** 257.
Engstrom, G. W., and DeLuca, H. F. (1964). *Annu. Rev. Biochem.* **33,** 729.
Epstein, F. H. (1968). *Am. J. Med.* **45,** 700.
Epstein, F. H., Rivera, M. J., and Carone, F. A. (1958). *J. Clin. Invest.* **37,** 1702.
Ferris, T. F., Kasgarian, M., Levitin, H., Brandt, I., and Epstein, F. H. (1961). *N. Engl. J. Med.* **265,** 924.
Ferris, T. F., Levitin, H., Phillips, E. T., and Epstein, F. H. (1962). *J. Clin. Invest.* **41,** 1222.
Fraser, D., Kooh, S. W., and Scriver, C. R. (1967). *Pediatr. Res.* **1,** 425.
Freeman, S., and Chang, T. S. (1950). *Am. J. Physiol.* **160,** 341.
Frick, A. (1969). *Pfluegers Arch.* **313,** 106.
Gekle, D., Stroder, J., and Rostock, D. (1971). *Pediatr. Res.* **5,** 40.
Golden, A., and Maher, J. F. (1971). "The Kidney: Structure and Function in Disease." Williams & Wilkins, Baltimore, Maryland.
Gradowska, L., Caglar, S., Rutherford, E., Harter, H., and Slatopolsky, E. (1973). *Kidney Int.* **3,** 230.
Grose, J. H., and Scriver, C. R. (1968). *Am. J. Physiol.* **214,** 370.
Guroff, G., DeLuca, H. F., and Steenbock, H. (1963). *Am. J. Physiol.* **204,** 833.
Gutman, Y., and Gottschalk, C. Y. (1966). *Isr. J. Med. Sci.* **2,** 243.
Hall, B. D., MacMillan, D. R., and Bronner, F. (1969). *Am. J. Clin. Nutr.* **22,** 448.
Hanna, S. (1961). *Metab., Clin. Exp.* **10,** 735.
Harrison, H. C., Harrison, H. E., and Park, E. A. (1958). *Am. J. Physiol.* **192,** 432.
Harrison, H. E., and Harrison, H. C. (1942). *Am. J. Physiol.* **137,** 171.
Harrison, H. E., and Harrison, H. C. (1951). *Yale J. Biol. Med.* **24,** 273.
Hodgkinson, A., and Heaton, F. W. (1965). *Clin. Chim. Acta* **11,** 354.
Jonxis, J. H. P., and Huisman, T. H. J. (1953). *Lancet* **2,** 428.
Joshi, J. G., Dikshit, P. K., and Patwardhan, V. N. (1957). *Indian J. Med. Res.* **45,** 439.
Kimberg, D. V., and Goldstein, S. A. (1967). *Endocrinology* **80,** 89.
Kleeman, C. R., Bernstein, D., Rockney, R., Dowling, J. T., and Maxwell, M. H. (1961). *Yale J. Biol. Med.* **34,** 1.

Klein, R., and Gow, R. C. (1953). *J. Clin. Endocrinol. Metab.* **13,** 271.
Kunin, A. S., and Krane, S. M. (1965). *Biochim. Biophys. Acta* **111,** 32.
Lavender, A. R., and Pullman, T. N. (1963). *Am. J. Physiol.* **205,** 1025.
Lehninger, A. L. (1964). "The Mitochondrian: Molecular Basis of Structure and Function." Benjamin, New York.
Lemann, J., Jr., Litzon, J. R., and Lennon, E. J. (1967). *J. Clin. Invest.* **46,** 1318.
Litvak, J., Moldawer, M. P., Forbes, A. P., and Henneman, P. H. (1958). *J. Clin. Endocrinol. Metab.* **18,** 246.
Liu, S. H., Chu, H. I., Su, C. C., Yu, T. F., and Cheng, T. Y. (1940). *J. Clin. Invest.* **19,** 349.
Lotz, M., Zisman, E., and Bartter, F. C. (1968). *N. Engl. J. Med.* **278,** 400.
Manitus, A., Levitin, H., Beck, D., and Epstein, F. H. (1960). *J. Clin. Invest.* **36,** 331.
Massry, S. G., and Coburn, J. W. (1973). *Nephron* **10,** 66.
Massry, S. G., and Kleeman, C. R. (1972). *J. Lab. Clin. Med.* **80,** 654.
Massry, S. G., Coburn, J. W., Chapman, L. W., and Kleeman, C. R. (1967). *Am. J. Physiol.* **213,** 1218.
Massry, S. G., Coburn, J. W., Chapman, L. W., and Kleeman, C. R. (1968). *Am. J. Physiol.* **214,** 1403.
Massry, S. G., Friedler, R. M., and Coburn, J. W. (1973). *Arch. Intern. Med.* **131,** 828.
Meyer, J., Bolen, R. J., and Antin, J. (1959). *Arch. Biochem. Biophys.* **81,** 340.
Mitchell, P. (1961). *Nature (London)* **191,** 144.
Ney, R. L., Kelly, G., and Bartter, F. C. (1968). *Endocrinology* **82,** 760.
Nicolaysen, R., and Nordbo, R. (1943). *Acta Physiol. Scand.* **5,** 212.
Nordin, B. E. C. (1972). *In* "Calcium, Parathyroid Hormone and the Calcitonins" (R. V. Talmage and P. L. Munson, eds.), Int. Congr. Ser. No. 243, p. 263. Exerpta Med., Found. Amsterdam.
Nordin, B. E. C., and Peacock, M. (1969). *Lancet* **2,** 1280.
Norman, A. W. (1967). *Clin. Orthop. Relat. Res.* **52,** 249.
Norman, A. W., and DeLuca, H. F. (1964). *Biochem. J.* **91,** 124.
Peters, J. P. (1935). "Body Water." Baillière, London.
Popovitzer, M. M., and Robinette, J. B. (1975). *Am. J. Physiol.* **229,** 907.
Popovitzer, M. M., Robinette, J. B., DeLuca, H. F., and Holick, M. F. (1974). *J. Clin. Invest.* **53,** 913.
Puschett, J. B., Moranz, J., and Kurnick, W. S. (1972a). *J. Clin. Invest.* **51,** 373.
Puschett, J. B., Fernandez, P. C., Boyle, I. T., Gray, R. W., Omdahl, J. L., and DeLuca, H. F. (1972b). *Proc. Soc. Exp. Biol. Med.* **141,** 379.
Puschett, J. B., Beck, W. S., Jr., Jelonek, A., and Fernandez, P. C. (1974). *J. Clin. Invest.* **53,** 756.
Puschett, J. B., Beck, W. S., and Jeloneck, A. (1975). *Science* **190,** 473.
Ramalingaswami, V., Sriramachari, S., Dikshit, P. K., Tulpule, P. G., and Patwardhan, V. N. (1954). *Indian J. Med. Sci.* **8,** 509.
Rasmussen, H., and DeLuca, H. F. (1963). *Ergeb. Physiol., Biol. Chem. Exp. Pharmakol.* **53,** 108.
Rasmussen, H., Sallis, J., Fang, M., DeLuca, H. F., and Young, R. (1964). *Endocrinology* **74,** 388.
Robertson, R. N. (1960). *Biol. Rev. Cambridge Philos. Soc.* **35,** 231.
Sallis, J. D. (1963). *J. Biol. Chem.* **238,** 4098.
Sands, H., and Kessler, R. H. (1971). *Proc. Soc. Exp. Biol. Med.* **137,** 1267.
Short, E. M., Elsas, L. J., and Rosenberg, L. T. (1974). *Metab., Clin. Exp.* **23,** 715.
Siegfried, J. D., Kumar, R., Kurtzman, N. A., and Pillay, V. K. G. (1975). *Clin. Res.* **50,** 2159.
Singer, F. R., Woodhouse, N. J. Y., Parkinson, D. R., and Joplin, G. F. (1969). *Clin. Sci.* **37,** 181.
Steele, T. H., Engle, J. E., Tanaka, Y., Lorenc, R. S., Dudgeon, K. L., and DeLuca, H. F. (1975). *Am. J. Physiol.* **229,** 489.
Steenbock, H., and Bellin, S. A. (1953). *J. Biol. Chem.* **205,** 985.
Suki, W. N., Eknoyan, G., Rector, F. C., and Seldin, D. W. (1969). *Nephron* **6,** 50.

Sutton, R. A. (1978). *Proc. Int. Congr. Nephrol. 7th, 1978* p. 463.
Taylor, A. N., and Wasserman, R. H. (1967). *Arch. Biochem. Biophys.* **119,** 536.
Taylor, A. N., and Wasserman, R. H. (1972). *Am. J. Physiol.* **223,** 110.
Vasington, F. D., and Murphy, J. V. (1962). *J. Biol. Chem.* **237,** 2670.
Verner, J. V., Engel, F. L., and McPherson, H. T. (1958). *Ann. Intern. Med.* **48,** 765.
Waasjo, E., and Eeg-Larsen, N. (1951a). *Acta Physiol. Scand.* **25,** Suppl. 84.
Waasjo, E., and Eeg-Larsen, N. (1951b). *Acta Physiol. Scand.* **25,** Suppl. 89.
Walser, M. (1973). *Handb. Physiol., Sect. 7: Endocrinol.* **2,** 555.
Wasserman, R. H., Corradino, R. A., Fullmer, C. S., and Taylor, A. N. (1974). *Vitam. Horm. (N.Y.)* **32,** 299.
Wiedmann, P., Massry, S. G., Coburn, J. W., Atelson, J. A., Maxwell, M. H., and Kleeman, C. R. (1972). *Ann. Intern. Med.* **76,** 741.
Ziegler, R., and Delling, G. (1975). *In* "Proceedings of the Second Symposium on Vitamin D and Problems Related to Uremic Bone Disease" (A. W. Norman *et al.*, eds.), p. 689. de Gruyter, Berlin.

CHAPTER 12

Vitamin D Actions on Bone

I. BACKGROUND CONSIDERATIONS

A. Introduction

Any discussion of the actions of vitamin D on bone tissue is very complex. This is due in part to the fact that despite our current understanding of the proposed steroid hormone mode of action of $1,25(OH)_2D_3$ in intestinal tissue and our unraveling of the pathway for the regulated production of $1,25(OH)_2D_3$ by the kidney, there are as yet no definitive answers to questions regarding the effects of vitamin D or its metabolites on bone tissue. A second reason has to do with the inherent complexity of the morphology of bone tissue. Although it might be argued that the cellular anatomy of bone is no more complex than that of other body organs, such as the kidney or brain, it is certainly obvious that the intrinsic physical properties of bone have not lent themselves to ready manipulation by the physiologist and biochemist who may wish to probe in detail aspects of various subcomponents.

The possible relationship between vitamin D and bone has been apparent for centuries. For example, see Fig. 1-1, which is taken from the book "De Rachitide" by Frances Glisson, FRCP (1597–1677). This book provided the first comprehensive and medically accurate description of rickets. The drawing portrays a rachitic patient in a physician's examining room; on the wall is a bowed femur and a scoliotic vertebral column.

In fact, the unusual prominence that vitamin D enjoys in a clinical setting is a result of the effects of a deficiency of the steroid on bone metabolism. Vitamin D may be produced photochemically by ultraviolet light from the precursor 7-dehydrocholesterol present in the skin. However, in the absence of sunlight, a dietary requirement for vitamin D develops, and it is in this sense that the steroid vitamin D gains prominence as a vital nutritional substance. As long as people lived or worked primarily outdoors and had access to minimal levels of ultraviolet light, their needs for vitamin D could be largely met by the generation of this steroid in the skin. However, in the 1800's, with the industrial revolution and the expansion of urban life (when exposure to ultraviolet light was greatly reduced), the deficiency aspects of vitamin D in relation to the bone became strikingly apparent. Rickets and osteomalacia were found in virtually epidemic proportions in factory workers in many cities in England (Hess, 1929).

Studies on bone, particularly studies of rickets, have also made an important contribution to our current understanding of the steroid hormone mechanism of action of vitamin D. Rickets was used as a characteristic and quantifiable end point of vitamin D deficiency by Mellanby (1921, 1923) in his brilliant pioneering studies in the 1920's (Fig. 12-1). This work demonstrated that, in the absence of sunlight, vitamin D was truly a trace essential dietary constituent, e.g., a vitamin. The development of the experimental dietary conditions for producing rickets provided investigators the world over with the opportunity to put their studies of the "fat-soluble vitamin" and its relationship to calcium metabolism and the bone disease rickets on a firm experimental basis. These diets are still in use today (see Appendix B), and the appearance of rickets in both the chick and rat is now routinely taken as evidence of the presence of an overt vitamin D deficiency.

It is also informative to consider the origins of the term "rickets." Some hold that it is a Greek derivative, whereas others support the view that it is derived from old English. Professor F. Glisson (1650) in his comprehensive treatise discussed the problem in some detail. He favored the term *rachitis-idis,* which is the Greek word for spine. One can envision the precise Greek term ῥάχις evolving only slightly to the present-day usage of "rickets."

Whistler (1645), however, believed that the term may have sprung from the Dorset County dialect, *to rucket,* which meant to breathe with difficulty. Another old English term that some have considered (Hess, 1929) is *wrick* or the

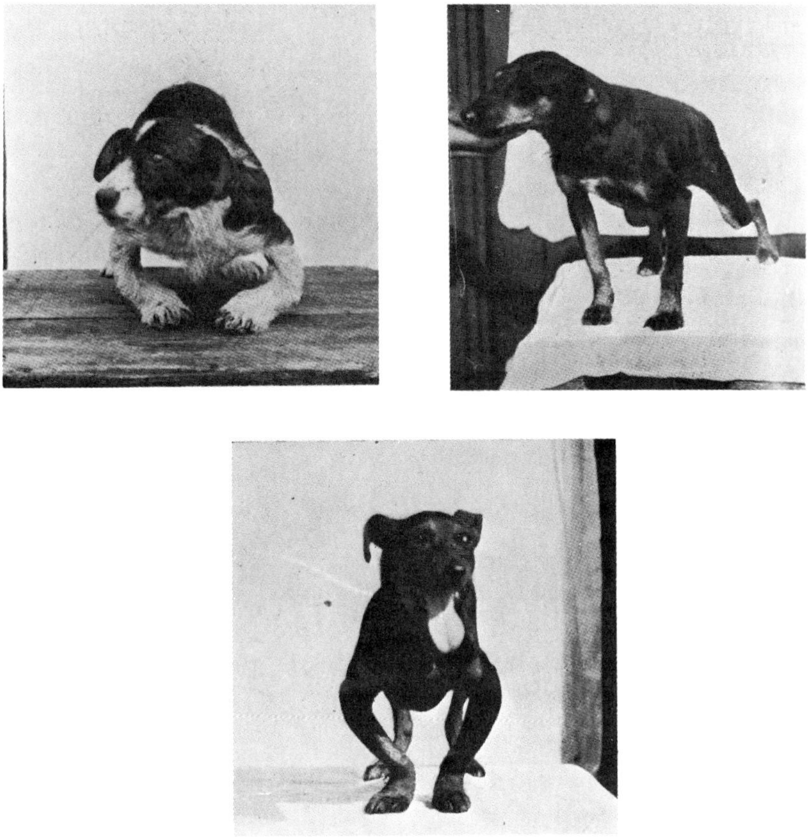

Figure 12-1. Photograph of rachitic dogs raised by Sir Edward Mellanby in his classic studies that led to the first experimental production of rickets. Reproduced by permission from Mellanby (1921).

middle English *wrikken,* both of which mean "to twist" as in "to wrick your ankle." Another alternative is the middle English word *rieg,* which indicates a protuberance. Ultimately the disease even became known as *die englische Krankenheit,* or "English sickness." Today the disorder rickets is referred to in German as *rachitis,* in Italian as *rachitide,* in Russian as *rachit,* in French as *rachitisme,* and in Spanish as *raquitis.* A delightful discussion of this subject, entitled "Rickets, Ruckets, Rekets or Rackets," was provided by Hunter (1972).

The effect on the skeleton of a vitamin D deficiency is a defect in calcification, which affects both the cartilage and bone matrix. In infants this is characterized by the development of the disease state rickets and in adults by the development of osteomalacia. Figure 13-10 shows an example of a child with a severe vitamin

D deficiency. Figure 12-2 shows what has often been referred to as the "rachitic rosary," which is simply a series of enlarged costochondrial joints in the rib cage. Both rickets and osteomalacia can be prevented by an adequate dietary intake of vitamin D or by regular access to sunlight.

B. Calcium and Phosphorus Homeostasis—Role of the Bone

Any discussion of the integrated control of calcium and phosphorus homeostasis must include a detailed consideration of the contributions of bone to this process. The average adult human being contains approximately 1200 g of calcium and 500–600 g of phosphorus (present as inorganic phosphate). Nearly 99% of both of these ions reside in the hydroxyapatite crystals of bone, with the remainder being present in extracellular fluids and other cellular compartments. Thus, bone tissue provides an enormous reservoir of both calcium and phosphorus, and in view of the dynamic movement of these ions into and out of bone

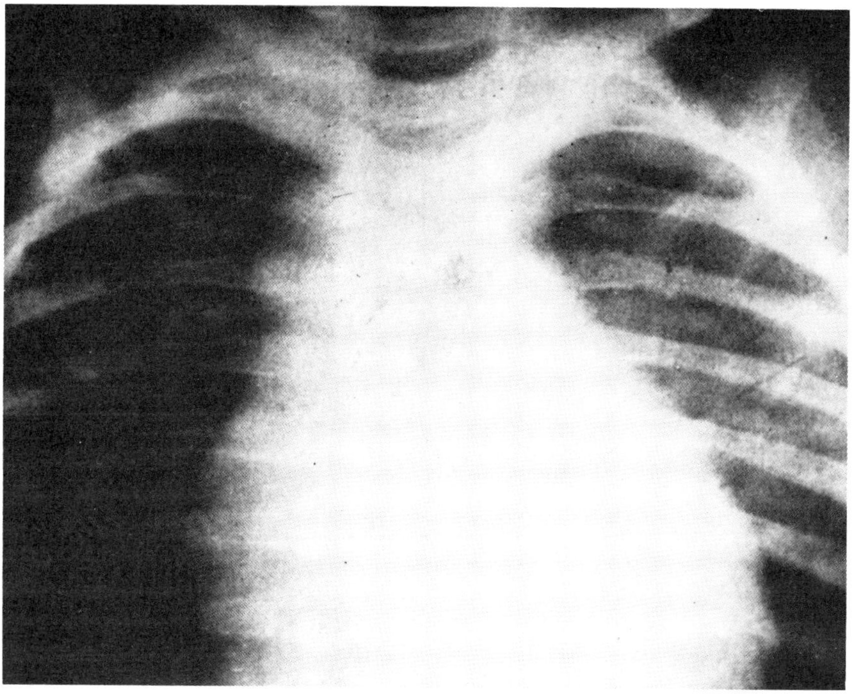

Figure 12-2. X-ray appearance of rib cage and classic rachitic "rosary." The beaded appearance results from enlarged costochondrial regions of the bone.

it is apparent why this organ can play such a prominent role in calcium and phosphorus homeostasis.

Central to considerations of calcium and phosphorus homeostasis is the fact that the endoskeleton of higher organisms serves two important functions: (a) a metabolic role concerned with the maintenance of a dynamic steady state not only of calcium and phosphorus but of many other ionic constituents for the body's extracellular fluids; (b) a mechanical or supportive function integral to locomotion and protection of the organism. A characteristic feature of bone that enables it to fulfill both these functions is that the skeleton normally undergoes a process of continual remodeling throughout life. This remodeling process is governed by changes in the mechanical stresses on the skeleton as well as by effects of metabolic regulators. Bone tissue is responsive to the following hormones: parathyroid hormone, calcitonin, $1,25(OH)_2D_3$, $24,25(OD)_2D_3$, growth hormone, gonadal hormones, thyroxine, and glucocorticoids.

The purpose of this chapter is to review our current understanding of the interactions of vitamin D with bone tissue; it is not the intention to review the integrated actions of vitamin D and its metabolites, parathyroid hormone, calcitonin, or other possible hormones in the bone tissue. This is the subject of numerous papers, and the reader is referred to any of the following reviews and books for in-depth coverage: Rasmussen and Bordier (1974), Vaughan (1970), MacLean and Urist (1961), Collins (1966), Neuman and Neuman (1958), Frost (1964), Bourne (1956, 1971, 1972), and Avioli and Krane (1977).

C. Bone Tissue—Morphology and Physiology

Bone is a complex tissue made up of cells as well as extracellular material; it is composed of both organic and mineral components. The cells are of a wide variety of morphological and functional types, but all have a common origin in the mesenchymal tissue. On a dry weight basis, bone consists of approximately 65–70% inorganic crystals of the salt hydroxyapatite and 30–35% organic matrix, known as osteoid. Thirty-nine percent of osteoid is collagen. It is impossible to proceed with any discussion of the action of vitamin D steroids in bone without at least a minimal understanding of the physiology and morphological organization of these bone components.

The formation of functional bone tissue can be divided roughly into two phases: (a) that concerned with production and secretion of the extracellular collagen bone matrix and (b) the deposition of mineral calcium hydroxyapatite crystals in the matrix. It should be emphasized that bone is a dynamic tissue and that both of these processes occur continuously.

Neither the collagen matrix, the extracellular mineral crystals, or the several different cell types associated with bone determines the behavior of the tissue as a whole. It is the unique combination of the organic and inorganic phases as well as the particular biochemical properties of its cells that confer on bone both its unusual mechanical properties and its ability to serve as a dynamic reservoir for the calcium and phosphorus ions needed for mineral homeostasis in the intact organism. Table 12-1 is an outline of the elements of bone structure and metabolism.

Bone matrix is biosynthesized, secreted, organized, mineralized, and finally destroyed via resorption, all in accordance with the physiological and hormonal signals operative at a particular time. The production of organic matrix by osteoblast cells first involves the intracellular synthesis by the ribosomal system of protocollagen molecules by a conventional protein biosynthetic mechanism. The protocollagen is then polymerized to yield a three-stranded triple helix, each strand of which has a separate, unique amino acid sequence. Next, approximately half of the proline residues and a small number of lysine residues of the protocollagen helix are enzymatically hydroxylated, and these new hydroxyamino acid residues are then glycosylated to yield the macromolecule known as procollagen. The procollagen is secreted into the extracellular space around the osteoblast cells, where it undergoes further conversion to yield tropocollagen via cleavage of an N-terminal fragment of 20,000 daltons from each of the three individual peptide chains of the macromolecule. After proteolysis, the tropocollagen molecule is some 15 Å in diameter. It immediately undergoes polymerization to yield microfibrils, which are several centimeters in length and consist of five tropocollagen molecules across the diameter. These microfibril pentamers further polymerize to yield the final form of collagen fibers, which range in diameter from 150 to 1300 Å. The polymerization process, although spontaneous, is highly ordered and involves principally hydrophobic interactions between adjacent peptide chains. The final phase of formation of "mature collagen molecules" is the generation of covalent chemical bonds either by an aldol condensation or by a Schiff base conjugation. An excellent review of collagen biosynthesis is that of Grant and Prokop (1972a,b,c).

In the normal process of bone formation, there is usually a delay of 5 to 10 days between the synthesis of the extracellular organic matrix and its ultimate mineralization. It is believed that the normal coupling time between matrix formation and subsequent mineralization may depend on the presence of vitamin D and/or its metabolites. After final secretion of protocollagen by the osteoblast and the ultimate formation of mature collagen, these cells are incorporated into the bone matrix as osteocytes, where they differentiate to become cells capable of secreting matrix calcification granules. These granules then may facilitate the extracellular accumlation of calcium and phosphate, which ultimately results in the appearance of amorphous calcium phosphate. This in turn is crystallized into the formal hydroxyapatite structure of bone within the matrix of mature collagen

TABLE 12-1
Outline of Bone Structure and Metabolism[a]

	Comment
I. Structure of bone	
A. Macroscopic level	
1. Spongiosa or cancellous bone	Occurs in metaphyseal region of long bone and is composed of spicules known as trabeculae; is the most metabolically active region
2. Cortical bone	Occurs in cortex and diaphysis of long bone
B. Microscopic level	
1. Collagen fiber distribution	
a. Woven bone	Composed of loosely and randomly arranged collagen bundles; predominant in young bones
b. Lamellar bone	Composed of highly order bundles of collagen fibers arranged in layers interspersed between osteocytes; is characteristic of adult bone
2. Three-dimensional collagen fiber network	Principally characteristic of adult bone
a. Trabecular	Synonymous with cancellous bone
b. Haversian	Occurs as a consequence of remodeling of cortical bone
C. Types of bone cells	
1. Osteoprogenitor	Synonymous with mesenchymal cells
2. Osteoblasts	Cells that synthesize and secrete bone matrix
3. Osteoclasts	Cells that resorb bone; are multinucleate
4. Osteocytes	Precise function not known
II. Inorganic phase	On a dry weight basis bone is 65–70% inorganic material
A. Components	
1. Crystalline calcium hydroxyapatite	Constitutes 55–60% of bone mineral; molecular formula $[(Ca^{2+})_{10-y}(H_3O)^{+}_{2x} \cdot (PO_4^{3})_6(OH^-)_2]$
2. Amorphous calcium phosphate	Constitutes 40–45% of bone mineral; may be formed before crystalline Ca hydroxyapatite, which is then produced with time
B. Ionic composition	Other ions include K^+, Na^+, Mg^{2+}, Sr^{2+}, Cl^-, CO_3^-, F^-, and citrate^{3-} and many trace constituents
III. Organic phase of bone	On a dry weight basis bone is 30–35% organic material, often referred to as bone matrix or osteoid

(*continued*)

TABLE 12-1 (*Continued*)

	Comment
A. Collagen	
1. Biosynthetic steps	
a. Intracellular phase	
(1) Protocollagen biosynthesis	Occurs on ribosome; composed of 20% proline and 33% glycine
(2) Protocollagen hydroxylation	Specific hydroxylation of 50% of proline residues and 5–10% of lysine residues
(3) Glycosylation of protocollagen to yield procollagen	Procollagen molecular weight 360,000; is secreted into extracellular space
b. Extracellular phase	
(1) Conversion of procollagen to tropocollagen	An N-terminal fragment of procollagen of 20,000 daltons is removed; tropocollagen molecule is 3000 × 15 Å
(2) Tropocollagen polymerization into microfibrils	44 Å diameter × several cm length
(3) Polmerization of microfibrils into collagen fibrils	150–1300 Å diameter × several cm length
(4) Cross-linking of strands of collagen fibers	Formation of Schiff bases, followed by aldol condensation
B. Ground substance	5% bone matrix is ground substance
1. Mucopolysaccharide	
2. Mucoproteins	

[a] A more detailed discussion of these topics can be found in Rasmussen and Bordier (1974).

fibers. It has not yet been possible to provide a detailed molecular description of calcification.

Bone tissue is dynamic both in terms of the metabolic activity of the various cell populations present and in terms of the kinetics of mineral flux into and out of various bone compartments. During the process of skeletal remodeling, bone mineral must also turn over. As can be inferred from Table 12-1, mineral deposition eventually follows the elaboration of a suitable organic matrix. This process, whether it takes places at the epiphyseal region or at sites of primary bone formation, is under direct cellular control. It is dependent principally on the presence of sufficient levels of calcium and phosphorus in the extracellular fluids as well as on the presence of appropriate amounts and kinds of vitamin D and its metabolites. The hallmark of a vitamin D deficiency is a failure of mineralization of bone matrix; as a consequence, in rickets or osteomalacia there is an increased accumulation of uncalcified matrix or osteoid.

D. The Problem

In view of the multiplicity of steps summarized in Table 12-1 that are associated with bone morphology, physiology, and metabolism, it is a challenging prospect for the experimentalist to identify precisely the specific site of intervention of vitamin D and/or its metabolites. It is likely that there is no single specific site of intervention of the vitamin D steroids. Historically the problem has been simplified to involve one of two questions. (a) Does vitamin D and/or its metabolites affect bone matrix formation and mineral deposition; or (b) Does vitamin D and/or its metabolites effect bone mineral mobilization and matrix degradation? In view of the complex interrelationships between vitamin D and its metabolites and parathyroid hormone and calcitonin, an additional challenge is to assess whether any putative vitamin D "effect" is permissive in that it allows other essential regulators to act, or whether it is direct, i.e., is mediated solely by the steroid molecule itself.

The two chief changes in bone tissue that occur concomitantly with a severe vitamin D deficiency are (a) a failure of normal mineralization of bone matrix, ultimately leading to an increased accumulation of unmineralized osteoid, and (b) a decrease in bone resorption activity and the number of osteoclast cells present.

In rickets the primary deficiency is caused by a defective calcification process. Since calcification along the column of hypertrophied cartilage cells in the bone does not occur, there is a disorderly invasion by blood vessels and the usual zone of provisional calcification is not resorbed. With time, the cartilage cells continue to proliferate into the zone of provisional calcification; therefore, the cartilage plate becomes wider than normal (an example of this is seen in Fig. 4-1, which illustrates the classic rat line test bioassay for vitamin D). Elsewhere in the skeleton, new osteoid or collagen tissue is laid down on bone surfaces, but it too fails to calcify. For the adult with osteomalacia, endochondrial growth has been completed and the epiphyseal abnormalities characteristic of rickets discussed above are not apparent. In adult osteomalacia, however, there is an excess of osteoid seams, and bone surfaces along the osteoid are not resorbed. Also, the remodeling of the bone that normally occurs is greatly diminished.

When either vitamin D_3 or its metabolite $25(OH)D_3$ is administered to a vitamin D-deficient animal, one of the earliest changes seen at the morphological level in the bone is the reestablishment of a normal calcification front in the osteoid surfaces (see Fig. 4-1). The fact that vitamin D treatment may lead to a reestablishment in the osteoid surface of a normal calcification front before there is any detectable change in the circulating concentration of calcium and phosphorus has been taken by some investigators as unequivocal evidence that vitamin D and/or its metabolites act directly on bone. Preliminary evidence supports the existence of a specific high-affinity binding protein for $1,25(OH)_2D_3$

in the cytosol of fetal rat bone (Kream *et al.,* 1977). The assumption is that vitamin D, or more likely one of its metabolites, is acting in bone tissue as a steroid hormone in a manner analogous to that which has been documented to occur in the intestinal mucosa cells.

The following sections review the various aspects of bone morphology and metabolism in which vitamin D or its metabolites are reported to have effects.

II. EFFECTS ON BONE COLLAGEN

The primary connection between vitamin D and collagen is the disease state rickets. The rachitic state is characterized in growing animals by an accumulation of cartilage matrix, which not only fails to mineralize but also is resorbed only with difficulty (Park, 1939). As reported by Canas *et al.* (1969), a vitamin D deficiency results in less organic matrix, which is less heavily mineralized than normal bone; associated with this in the rachitic tissue is a modest accumulation of water. As a result, vitamin D-deficient bone appears to be more porous than that obtained from normal animals.

However the primary question is whether vitamin D has any effect on the many steps associated with collagen biosynthesis. There is as yet no definitive answer to this question; undoubtedly this is due to the many separate steps associated with collagen biosynthesis, secretion, and maturation (see Table 12-1). Canas *et al.* (1969) were the first to report concrete biochemical data suggesting an effect of vitamin D in increasing the incorporation of tritiated proline into bone collagen measured *in vivo* in rats. This increased rate of proline incorporation mediated by vitamin D was not found to occur in the skin obtained from the same animals. These results suggested that one of the early consequences of vitamin D administration to rachitic chicks might be a stimulation of synthesis of bone collagen, which would serve as a new matrix for the deposition of mineral made available by increased intestinal absorption of calcium. Patterson and Fourman (1968), Baylink *et al.* (1970), Kivirriko (1970), and Oliver *et al.* (1972) all presented evidence of an effect of vitamin D on the metabolism of bone collagen present in osteoid. Morava *et al.* (1970) also reported evidence that vitamin D administered to rats *in vivo* stimulated the production of hydroxyproline under *in vitro* conditions by the proximal metaphysis of the tibia.

In later studies, Barnes *et al.* (1973) found, on the basis of radioisotope studies, that collagen synthesized in the shaft of bones from rachitic rats was similar in chain composition to that normally synthesized by bone samples obtained from vitamin D-replete, normal rats. A more interesting aspect of the report of Barnes *et al.* (1973) was that the extent of lysine hydroxylation in the α-$_1$ and α-$_2$ chains of collagen isolated from bone shafts of vitamin D-deficient rats had increased by 15–30%, whereas that of vitamin D-deficient chick bones had increased by 50%. It was felt that this reflected an altered metabolic activity in the tissue which arose as a consequence of the vitamin D deficiency and might have been in some way related to the balance that must occur between the rate of collagen protein synthesis and the subsequent associated activity of lysine hydroxylation. A major problem of interpretation in studies of this type is whether the observed change is due simply to the immediate consequences of a vitamin D or metabolite deficiency at the molecular level or whether the effect is produced by a change in calcium metabolism. That is, perturbations of calcium metabolism at the osteoclast level might also produce the reported changes.

Mechanic *et al.* (1972, 1975) studied the relation of vitamin D status to the "cross-link pattern" in the various chains of mature bone collagen. They found changes in the proportions of the major reducible cross-links, dihydroxylysinonorleucine, and hydroxylysinonorleucine; this could affect the rate of maturation of bone collagen. Again, it was not possible to determine unequivocally whether the observation was attributable to the hypocalcemia associated with vitamin D deficiency or to an absence of vitamin D or its metabolites per se. However, these workers proposed that, in the absence of vitamin D or its metabolites, more immature collagen is synthesized and the organization, packing, and structure of the resulting matrix is insufficient to support normal bone mineralization and related turnover activities. They further proposed that the structure of the collagen matrix must mature by a series of metabolic turnover steps, which are essential to ensure normal mineralization, and that vitamin D is essential for this process.

More recently, Gonnerman *et al.* (1976) from the same research group measured directly the activity of lysyl oxidase, an enzyme responsible for the production of aldehydic precursors for lysine-derived collagen cross-links in tibial metaphyses from either vitamin D-replete or vitamin D-deficient chicks. These workers reported that lysyl oxidase activity was increased twofold in the vitamin D-deficient chicks as compared to activities measured in birds receiving physiological doses of vitamin D. They further noted that an increased dietary level of calcium in the vitamin D-deficient state had no effect on the measured lysyl oxidase activity.

It is possible to envison a steroid hormonelike action of $1,25(OH)_2D_3$ or another vitamin D metabolite, possibly $24,25(OH)_2D_3$, acting directly in the bone osteoid stimulating the production of key enzymes related to the production of procollagen. Observations consistent with this suggestion are the reports of Russell *et al.* (1975) and Hahn and Avioli (1970) that the experimental generation of uremia and consequent renal osteodystrophy produces a pattern of bone collagen reminiscent of a vitamin D deficiency without any changes being manifest in the collagen present in the skin of the same animals. Their data (particularly those of Russell *et al.*, 1975) indicate that the osteodystrophy associated with chronic renal insufficiency is characterized by alteration of the quantitative relations between cross-links and aldehydic precursors of bone collagen.

III. EFFECTS ON BONE MINERAL METABOLISM

A. Bone Accretion

An early review of the possible role of vitamin D in bone formation was given by Nicolaysen and Jansen (1939). By that time it was well appreciated that vitamin D played a prominent role in stimulating intestinal absorption of calcium from the intestine. However, no definitive data had been put forth concerning possible effects of vitamin D on bone formation. An important point is that most workers in the field at this time were impressed by the potent effects of vitamin D in preventing the characteristic lesions of rickets. In fact, Robinson and Rosenheim (1934) had already reported that vitamin D added to an *in vitro* suspension of hypertrophic cartilage cells had no effect on calcification. Another interesting experiment was carried out by Fischmann (1937), who cultivated osteogenic tissue *in vitro* and observed that, in a medium containing plasma from a normal chick, calcified bone was formed but that a similar tissue grown in a medium containing plasma from a vitamin D-deficient chick formed only abnormal osteoid tissue and additional cartilage. Furthermore, the addition to the growth medium of both calcium and phosphorus salts, either separately or together, did not fully compensate for the vitamin D deficiency. Thus, one is faced with the important question of whether the effects of vitamin D on bone accretion are the result of direct intervention of the steroid or its metabolites or whether they are due to a secondary effect produced indirectly by changes in peripheral calcium and/or phosphorus metabolism. Accordingly, investigators carried out a series of experiments in which efforts were made to elevate the serum calcium and phosphorus levels of vitamin D-deficient animals so that measurements could be made on bone accretion; these results were then compared to bone accretion resulting from the dietary administration of vitamin D.

In a notable series of papers, Nicolaysen and co-workers (Nicolaysen and Jansen, 1939; Malm *et al.*, 1955; Haavaldsen and Nicolaysen, 1955; Haavaldsen *et al.*, 1955) compared the effects of dietary vitamin D versus manipulations of both dietary and blood calcium and phosphorus levels. The primary conclusion was that vitamin D was required for normal calcium metabolism at all ages, not only in the rat but also in man. Furthermore, it was clearly established that the intestinal absorption of calcium throughout life is subject to regulation and adaptation and is a process in which vitamin D was postulated to be integrally involved. They also concluded that there is a continuing requirement for vitamin D to effect normal bone accretion and remodeling throughout life. Thus, they implied that vitamin D has a direct effect on bone mineral formation. Two excellent reviews of this era are given by Nicolaysen and Eeg-Larsen (1953) and Nicolaysen *et al.* (1953).

One important consequence of the work of Nicolaysen was the postulation of the existence of an "endogenous factor," which in some way transmitted from the bone to the intestine a signal that indicated a need for increased intestinal absorption of calcium (Nicolaysen, 1943; Haavaldsen and Nicolaysen, 1955). It has been claimed by some (DeLuca, 1974; Norman and Henry, 1974) that the isolation and chemical characterization of $1,25(OH)_2D_3$ represented the identification of the "endogenous factor" of Nicolaysen. Clearly, the steroid $1,25(OH)_2D_3$ has many of the properties of the "endogenous factor" that pertain to adaptation of intestinal calcium absorption; what remains to be elucidated are possible direct effects of the steroid on bone mineral accretion.

Migicovsky (1957; Migicovsky and Emslie, 1950) was one of the first to apply the use of radioactive calcium to the study of vitamin D effects on calcium metabolism. After administering either oral or intramuscular doses of $^{45}Ca^{2+}$ (to obviate effects of vitamin D on intestinal calcium absorption), Migicovsky concluded that vitamin D increases the rate of calcium accretion into bone. However, he was not able to determine whether this increased movement of calcium into bone was a primary and direct effect of the vitamin or its metabolites or was due to an increased flow of calcium to the bone.

A further evaluation of the putative actions of vitamin D on bone accretion was reported by Dikshit and Patwardhan (1952). These workers carried out *in vivo* incubations with rat tibia obtained from either normal or rachitic animals in a "calcifying medium" that either was devoid of or contained supplemental vitamin D. They could show no *in vitro* effect of vitamin D in promoting calcification of the rat tibia obtained from either rachitic or normal animals. However, rachitic bones from animals previously administered vitamin D *in vivo* but not exhibiting any calcification *in vivo* did show a much greater calcification *in vitro*. The calcifying capacity of the rachitic bones appeared to increase with the increase in time after vitamin D administration. In fact, these investigators reported that the maximal effect *in vitro* coincided with the first evidence of calcification having commenced *in vivo*.

A similar approach was taken by Lamm and Neuman (1958) and Crenshaw *et al.* (1974), who studied the effects of dietary vitamin D levels on the *in vitro* mineralization of chick and rat metaphysis. The experiments were based on the premise that formation of bone calcium hydroxyapatite can be determined by the solubility product (K_{sp} for Ca and P; when this constant is exceeded, crystallization may occur. The primary purpose of both studies was to determine whether vitamin D and/or normal serum calcium levels are necessary for the formation of bone matrix that is competent for mineral deposition. Undermineralized metaphyseal slices from rachitic chicks that were incubated for 5 days *in vitro* in media with four different $Ca^{2+} \times HPO_4^{2-}$ ion products had significantly less mineral deposited than slices from vitamin D-replete chicks or, importantly, from chicks that had a rachitogenic diet supplemented with high levels of dietary calcium. These data support the concept that hypomineralization of rachitic bone *in vivo* is due mainly to a reduced serum calcium level and thus suggest that vitamin D does not have a direct effect on bone mineral accretion. A similar conclusion was reached by Yoshiki *et al.* (1974), who studied the role of vitamin D in the mineralization of dentin in rats made rachitic. Their results supported the view that recovery of mineralization of the rachitic dentin depended primarily on the elevation of the serum calcium level and that vitamin D played only an indirect role in the dentin mineralization process.

Table 12-2 summarizes the relative potencies of vitamin D metabolites and analogues in supporting bone ash development *in vivo* in the chick. Although it cannot be concluded from these data that vitamin D or the relevant analog participated directly in bone accretion events, it is apparent that some analogs are strikingly more effective than others in providing "the optimal environment" for mineralization.

It would be expected that, if vitamin D or its metabolites have direct effects on bone, the relevant cells would have stereospecific receptors for binding of the steroids. Kream *et al.* (1977) reported the presence of a $1,25(OH)_2D_3$-binding protein in fetal rat bone. Thus, it ultimately should be possible to define the architecture of bone cell receptors for vitamin D metabolites and to compare their

TABLE 12-2
Relative Effects *in Vivo* of Vitamin D Metabolites and Analogs on Chick Tibia Ash Weight[a]

Metabolite	Dose for 50% increase[b] (ng/chick/day)	Relative potency
$1,25(OH)_2D_3$	8	7.5
$1\alpha(OH)D_3$	11	5.5
$25(OH)D_3$	30	2.0
D_3	60	1.0
$1,24(R),25(OH)_3D_3$	70	0.8
$24(R),25(OH)_2D_3$	120	0.5
$25(OH)$-5,6-*trans*-D_3	160	0.4
$1,24(S),25(OH)_3D_3$	440	0.1
5,6-*trans*-D_3	720	0.08
$24(S),25(OH)_2D_3$	1300	0.05

[a] Abstracted from Boris *et al.* (1977). See also Larsson *et al.* (1977) for an evaluation of the effects of $25(OH)D_3$ and $1,25(OH)_2D_3$ on bone mass in the adult rat.

[b] Oral dose in nanograms per chick per day required to produce over a 21-day test period 50% of the maximum attainable tibia ash content. Ash content of vitamin D-deficient control tibia was 85 mg, and this was increased maximally to 211 mg by vitamin D_3 or $1,25(OH)_2D_3$ treatment.

specificities with the intestinal receptor for $1,25(OH)_2D_3$ (see Chapter 7). There is no *a priori* reason why they should have identical functional group requirements. Hibberd and Norman (1969) proposed that vitamin D steroids with the side chain of D_3 as compared to the side chain of D_2 act preferentially in "bone events" over "intestinal events." A similar conclusion was reached by Reeve *et al.* (1978), who evaluated the activity of $1\alpha(OH)D_2$ on bone in comparison with vitamin D_3-related analogs and metabolites. Also, Okamura *et al.* (1975) in studies evaluating the biological activity of 3-deoxy-$1,25(OH)_2D_3$ reported that the presence of the 3β-hydroxyl was more essential for bone responses than for intestinal responses. This suggests that in principle it should be possible to chemically synthesize analogs with preferential activity in either the intestine or the bone.

B. Bone Resorption

Certainly the most clearly demonstrable effect of vitamin D on bone is its ability to carry out calcium mobilization. This effect can be documented *in vivo* where it is usually assessed by elevation of serum calcium, and *in vitro* via release of $^{45}Ca^{2+}$ from bone that has been prelabeled with the isotope *in vivo*. Table 12-3 summarizes many of the reported effects of vitamin D and its metabolites on bone calcium mobilization.

The first clear evidence of an action of vitamin D in the mobilization of bone calcium was obtained by Carttar *et al.* (1950). They noted that administration of toxic doses of vitamin D resulted in bone calcium mobilization as measured by elevation of serum calcium levels. Their results are subject to the criticism that perhaps the effect they were observing is attributable to the pharmacological doses of the vitamin they administered. Carlsson and co-workers (Carlsson, 1952, 1954; Carlsson and Lindquist, 1955) were the first to demonstrate clearly that physiological doses of vitamin D could result in bone calcium mobilization, even under experimental circumstances in which no intestinal absorption of calcium could occur. The presumption was that serum calcium elevation then could occur only via bone calcium mobilization. This observation has since been confirmed by virtually all laboratories concerned with the actions of vitamin D.

From Table 12-3 it is apparent that not only the parent vitamin but also the metabolites $25(OH)D_3$, $1,25(OH)_2D_3$, and $24,25(OH)_2D_3$ have a capability of mobilizing bone calcium that can be measured *in vivo*. In this regard, $25(OH)D_3$ and the parent vitamin D are approximately equally potent, and $24,25(OH)_2D_3$ has one-half the activity of the parent vitamin; $1,25(OH)_2D_3$, however, is the most active of all compounds that have been studied to date.

The most quantitative method for evaluating bone calcium mobilization is through the use of an *in vitro* system. Pregnant mice or rats or newborn mice are injected with a massive dose of $^{45}Ca^{2+}$, and several days later paired half-calvaria

TABLE 12-3
Effects of Vitamin D and Its Metabolites on Bone Calcium Mobilization

Steroid studied	Comment	Reference
A. *In vivo* system		
Vitamin D	Bone mobilization after toxic doses of D	Carttar *et al.* (1950)
	Serum Ca^{2+} elevation in rats	Carlsson (1952), Carlsson and Lindquist (1955)
	^{45}Ca kinetics in chick	Migicovsky (1957)
	Calcium release from calvaria, measured *in vivo*	Au and Bartter (1966)
	Serum Ca elevation in chicks	Hibberd and Norman (1969)
	Enhanced osteoclastic bone resorption at vascular canals	Baylink *et al.* (1974), Liu *et al.* (1974)
$25(OH)D_3$	Serum Ca^{2+} elevation in anephric rats	Pavlovitch *et al.* (1973)
$1,25(OH)_2D_3$	Serum Ca^{2+} elevation in rats	Tanaka and DeLuca (1971)
	Serum Ca^{2+} elevation in chicks	Wong *et al.* (1972)
	Serum Ca^{2+} elevation in anephric rats	Holick *et al.* (1972)
	Serum Ca^{2+} elevation in TPTX rats	Garabedian *et al.* (1974)
	Serum Ca^{2+} elevation in hypophosphatemic rats	Castillo *et al.* (1975)
$24,25(OH)_2D_3$	Serum Ca^{2+} elevation in chicks and rats	Henry *et al.* (1976)
$1\alpha(OH)D_3$	Serum Ca^{2+} elevation	Pechet and Hesse (1974), Peacock *et al.* (1974)
$25(OH)DHT_3$	Serum Ca^{2+} elevation in TPTX rats	Seymour and DeLuca (1974)
B. *In vitro* system		
Vitamin D_3		Davidson (1975)
$25(OH)D_3$	Fetal rat bones	Trummel *et al.* (1969), Raisz *et al.* (1972)
$1,25(OH)_2D_3$	Fetal rat bones	Raisz *et al.* (1972)
	Mice bone explants	Reynolds *et al.* (1973, 1974), Reynolds (1974)
$24,25(OH)_2D_3$	Fetal rat long bones	Stern *et al.* (1975)

are explanted and placed in organ culture medium (Reynolds and Dingle, 1970). These half-calvaria are then either treated with the test steroid at the required dose level for 48 hr or not treated, and the release of $^{45}Ca^{2+}$ into the medium is measured and compared with its control (Fig. 12-3). In a variation of the assay protocol, the test substance is injected *in vivo* into the animal prior to explanting the calvaria to the organ culture medium. One interesting observation is that the parent steroid, vitamin D, is inert in these *in vitro* systems; it has no capability of mobilizing bone calcium. This is the most direct evidence that a metabolite of vitamin D, rather than the parent vitamin, is active in bone events. When vitamin D is administered *in vivo,* however, and the bone calvaria are evaluated under *in*

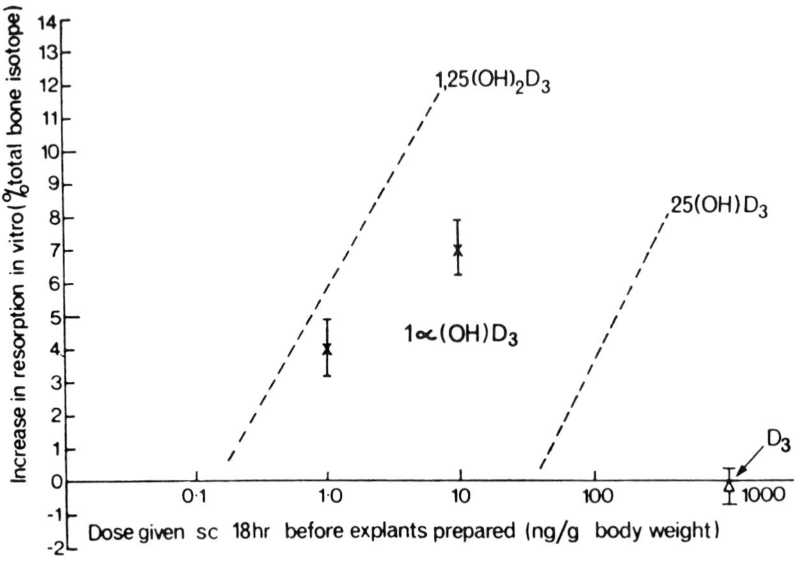

Figure 12-3. Comparison of bone mobilizing actions of 25(OH)D_3 and 1,25$(OH)_2D_3$ added *in vitro* to bone explants. Paired half-calvaria from 6-day-old mice prelabeled with $^{45}Ca^{2+}$ were either treated with the indicated steroid at the indicated doses for 48 hr or not treated. The response is plotted as the increase in resorption expressed as the difference (treated half − control half) in percent release of bone isotope into the medium. The points are mean ± S.E.M. From Reynolds (1974); reproduced with permission of the author.

vitro conditions for bone calcium mobilization, there is definitive evidence for mobilization activities, and this is assumed to be due to metabolism of the parent vitamin to the appropriate metabolites. Figure 8-4 presents a comparison the relative biological potencies of 1,25$(OH)_2D_3$, 25(OH)D_3, and 1α(OH)D_3 as determined by Reynolds *et al.* (1974). These data are discussed in Chapter 8 in the context of the use of this bone calcium mobilization assay as a biological activity measurement. The most striking observation is that the structural feature that enhances the activity of vitamin D_3 with regard to bone calcium mobilization is the simultaneous presence of both a 1α-hydroxyl and a 25-hydroxyl group. Reynolds (1974) commented that "the most potent bone mobilizer known to man is 1,25$(OH)_2D_3$."

C. Morphological and Histological Alterations

There are definitive morphological changes in bone tissue in a vitamin D deficiency as compared with a normal vitamin D-replete state. However, it is difficult to gain specific insight into the molecular mechanism of action of vitamin D and/or its metabolites in bone tissue from an evaluation of these morphological changes. Nonetheless, such observations may provide information as to the appropriate areas of focus for biochemical studies.

Certainly the most characteristic lesion of vitamin D deficiency is the wide epiphyseal growth plates that are associated with increased numbers of hypertrophic cartilage cells (Kember and Walker, 1971; Simmons and Kunin, 1970) (also see Fig. 4-1). It should be noted that in the rat these lesions occur only if the vitamin-D deficient animal has been raised on a low-phosphate diet; the morphological changes can be largely ameliorated by administration of dietary phosphate alone. Accordingly, this morphological defect may be related to perturbations in mineralization and subsequent failure of bone resorption or of the growth plate rather than to the specific presence or absence of vitamin D and/or its metabolites.

Bélanger and Migicovsky (1958) reported the early morphological changes occurring at the epiphysis of rachitic chicks following vitamin D administration *in vivo*. They followed the presence and changes in content of neutral polysaccharides and sulfated mucopolysaccharides. Their work suggests that alterations in the metabolism of carbohydrates, specifically bone mucopolysaccharides, are under the influence, either directly or indirectly, of vitamin D. Perhaps related to the foregoing observation is the report of Lindquist (1952), who found that vitamin D stimulated the uptake of radioactive inorganic sulfate into bone matrix material. Along similar lines, Cruess and Clark (1965) reported that toxic doses of vitamin D altered the total lipid, phospholipid, total and free fatty acid, and free and esterified cholesterol contents of the long bones of rats. If vitamin D has the capability of altering sulfate as well as phospholipid metabolism, it is possible to envision how histological and morphological changes may accordingly ensue. Garabedian (1977) in a preliminary study found that both $1,25(OH)_2D_3$ and $24,25(OH)_2D_3$ were effective *in vitro* in stimulating the incorporation of $^{35}SO_4$ into chondrocyte proteoglycans.

Ramalingaswami *et al.* (1954) reported results of an extensive histochemical study of rachitic epiphyseal cartilage during healing in the rat. Their study included the evaluation of changes in glycogen, lipid, nucleoproteins, alkaline phosphatase, and the glycoproteins of the matrix. Their principal observation was that the administration of vitamin D brought about a marked increase in the glycogen content of the proliferative zone of the cartilage plate immediately prior to the onset of calcification. They suggested that the failure of rachitic cartilage to calcify was due to a disturbance in glycogen metabolism. This work provided the foundation for their further explorations of glycogenolysis and organic acid metabolism in bone tissue (see following section).

Until 1960 only decalcified bone specimens were used for routine histological studies. Since that time it has been possible to evaluate sections of undecalcified bone and to quantitate several additional parameters including the resorptive surface, amount of osteoid, decalcification front, and osteocytic osteolysis. Bordier and colleagues have made pioneering contributions to the understanding of the quantitative histology of bone (Bordier and Tun Chot, 1972; Rasmussen and Bordier, 1974). It is from such studies that the current understanding of bone dynamics and its associated morphological changes have resulted (for a detailed discussion, see Rasmussen and Bordier, 1974). Bordier and Tun Chot (1972) reported that in osteomalacia related to vitamin D deficiency there are certain quantitative changes in several histological parameters; these are summarized in Table 12-4. It is clear that a vitamin D deficiency causes major morphological changes in bone tissue.

An additional development in technique is that of microradiography (Jowsey, 1966). Bone sections are prepared and, from the microradiographic appearance, bone resorption surface and new bone formation can be quantitated. The technique is somewhat difficult to apply because unusually thin sections (5–10 μm) are necessary.

Capen and colleagues (Weisbrode *et al.*, 1973, 1974; Weisbrode and Capen, 1974) carried out an ultrastructural evaluation of the effects of vitamin D, vitamin D deficiency, and calcitonin treatment on bone from normal, uremic, and thyroparathyroidectomized rats. Their primary observation was that pharmacological doses of vitamin D given to uremic rats were capable of producing ultrastructural changes in osteoblasts and osteocytes compared to placebo-treated uremic rats (Weisbrode *et al.*, 1974). Osteocytes in vitamin D-treated animals

TABLE 12-4
Quantitative Histological Changes Occurring in Vitamin D Deficiency Osteomalacia[a]

Parameter measured	Normal controls (28 cases)	Severe osteomalacia (28 cases)
Osteocytic osteolysis (% of total osteocytic lacunae)	3.9±0.6	9.3±0.6
Bone resorption surface (% of calcified bone surface)	12.2±4	33.8±5.6
Calcification front (% of osteoid surface)	83±10	19.2±8.3
Osteoid surface extent (% of total bone surface)	14.6±6	67.6±13.7
Amount of osteoid (% of cancellous bone tissue)	5.7±2	20.9±7.7
Amount of cancellous bone tissue (% of total bone volume)	19.3±4	27.8±3.8

[a] Abstracted by permision of the authors from Table 3 of Bordier and Tun Chot (1972). Values are the mean ± S.D.

were stated to have increased amounts of rough endoplasmic reticulum, whereas osteoblasts appeared to have reduced amounts of rough endoplasmic reticulum but increased levels of ribosomes and amorphous mineral deposits along plasma membranes. Weisbrode *et al.* (1978) recently completed an ultrastructural evaluation of the effects of chronic $1,25(OH)_2D_3$ administration on bone of thyroparathyroidectomized rats.

Preparations of growth plate cartilage from normal and rachitic animals have been widely employed over the years to study factors related to the process of mineralization (Robinson and Rosenheim, 1934; Sevastikoglou and Ray, 1970). From these studies it was learned that the matrix of rachitic cartilage maintained *in vitro* retained its ability to calcify and could be induced to do so by administration of phosphate *in vivo* (Howell *et al.*, 1968) or by exposure *in vitro* to metastable calcium phosphate solutions (Robinson and Rosenheim, 1934; Hirschman and Shapiro, 1960) or to normal rat serum (Yendt *et al.*, 1955). Calcification of the rachitic cartilage *in vitro* was inhibited by the presence of fluoride, cyanide, and iodoacetate; thus, Robinson and Rosenheim (1934) proposed that mineralization of cartilage is associated with or dependent on energy metabolism.

Anderson (1969), Anderson *et al.* (1970), and Bonucci (1970) identified via microscopic techniques the presence of extracellular membrane vesicles in the matrices of cartilage, bones, and teeth. Particularly in cartilage the vesicles occurred in a distribution pattern closely paralleling matrix calcification (Anderson, 1969). An exciting observation was the deposition of crystals of hydroxyapatite inside the matrix vesicles followed sequentially by the appearance of apatite spherules on the outer surface of the vesicles (Anderson, 1969; Anderson *et al.*, 1970). These matrix vesicles were found to contain alkaline phosphatase, ATPase, and inorganic pyrophosphatase (Matuzawa and Anderson, 1971; Ali *et al.*, 1970); each of these enzymes has been implicated in the general calcification process.

Thus, the prospect exists that these matrix vesicles possess enzymes that play a role in initiating calcification, perhaps by inducing local accumulation of calcium and phosphate. Anderson and colleagues (Anderson *et al.*, 1975; Anderson and Sajdera, 1976) compared histologically, histochemically, and electron microscopically the appearance of cartilage matrix vesicles obtained from rachitic and normal rats. The concentration of matrix vesicles and their distribution was found to be normal in rachitic growth plate, but rachitic cartilage matrix vesicles did not contain circumvesicular clusters of apatite as did the vesicles from normal cartilage. These investigators also developed a technique of collagenase digestion and differential centrifugation to isolate the vesicles (Anderson and Sajdeva, 1976). These vesicles were capable of accumulating $^{45}Ca^{2+}$ *in vitro* by a process that could be disrupted by heating or freezing and thawing. The results suggest that vesicle calcification is dependent on the structural and enzymatic integrity of the vesicle membrane. It will be important to learn what role, if any, vitamin D metabolites have in this system.

IV. EFFECTS ON BONE ORGANIC ACID METABOLISM

The relationship between vitamin D and citrate metabolism in bone was first observed by Dickens (1941), who fou¬d that the citrate content of bones from vitamin D-deficient animals was approximately 50% of that of normal animals. It should be recalled that 90% or more of the body citrate is found in the skeleton, where it is associated with the mineral fraction. This relationship between vitamin D and citric acid metabolism was subsequently confirmed by Nicolaysen and Nordbo (1943), Wassjo and Eeg-Larsen (1951a,b), Steenbock and Bellin (1953), and Carlsson and Hollunger (1954). Table 12-5 summarizes

TABLE 12-5
Summary of Vitamin D Effects on Citrate Metabolism

System studied	Comment	Reference
Bone citrate levels	First observation that vitamin D treatment increased bone citrate levels	Dickens (1941)
	Vitamin D treatment increased citrate level in many tissues	Steenbock and Bellin (1953)
	A comprehensive paper; vitamin D treatment elevates citrate in many tissues	Carlsson and Hollunger (1954)
	Measured many bone organic acids	Lees and Kuyper (1957)
	Through use of cortisol treatment could dissociate antirachitic action of vitamin D and its effect on citrate	Harrison *et al.* (1957)
	Measured effect of PTH and cortisol	Harrison *et al.* (1958)
Percent bone ash	Dietary citrate is not an antirachitic factor	Nicolaysen and Nordbo (1943)
Citrate as an antirachitic factor		Pileggi *et al.* (1956)
Urinary citrate excretion	Vitamin D treatment increased citraturia	Bellin and Steenbock (1952)
Bone citrogenase activity	Vitamin D treatment increased activity	Dikshit *et al.* (1956), Joshi *et al.* (1957)
Bone isocitrate dehydrogenase	No effect of vitamin D noted	Van Reen (1959)
Bone synthesis of citric acid	Vitamin D treatment decreases breakdown of citrate rather than stimulates biosynthesis	Meyer *et al.* (1959) Norman and DeLuca (1964)

TABLE 12-6
Effects of Vitamin D Status on Rat Tissue Citrate Levels[a]

Tissue examined	Vitamin D status[b] −D	+D	Increase (%)
Blood (μg/ml)	13	21	61
Heart (μg/g)	43	53	23
Kidney (μg/g)	18	38	111
Small intestine (μg/g)	61	76	25
Liver (μg/g)	13	12	—
Bone (mg/g)	3.59	5.23	54

[a] Data taken from Steenbock and Bellin (1953).

[b] Both groups of rats were fed nonrachitogenic diet 11 (see Appendix B); +D rats received 6.5 nmoles (100 IU) three times weekly.

various aspects of the relationship between vitamin D and citrate metabolism. A historical note concerns the contribution by Nicolaysen and Nordbo (1943), who demonstrated unequivocally that citric acid was not capable of curing rickets. Thus, in their view citrate did not qualify as the ''endogenous factor'' of bone.

There had been some previous nutritional data which suggested that citrate might be capable of functioning as an antirachitic agent. The antirachitic effect of citrate on rats fed cereal diets high in calcium was first reported by Shohl (1937) and also by Hamilton and Dewar (1937), but this view was put to rest by the report of Pileggi *et al.* (1956), who also found no antirachitic actions of citrate. Dietary citrate, however, was capable of mediating an increased hydrolysis of phytic acid in a noncereal, high-calcium diet so that more inorganic phosphate was available to the animals.

In other work it was shown that dietary vitamin D increases the citric acid content of many body tissues (Freeman and Chang, 1950; Steenbock and Bellin, 1953) (see Table 12-6) as well as induces citraturia, (Harrison and Harrison, 1951; Harrison *et al.*, 1957, 1958; Bellin and Steenbock, 1952).

Two hypotheses were put forward to explain possible actions of vitamin D on citric acid metabolism. On the one hand, it was felt that, since rachitic tissue had reduced levels of citrate, vitamin D enhanced the biosynthesis of citric acid. On the other hand, DeLuca and co-workers (1957a,b) proposed that in the presence of vitamin D there was a diminished rate of further metabolism or oxidation of citric acid with a concomitant increase in steady-state levels. Ramalingaswami *et al.* (1954), Dikshit *et al.* (1956), and Meyer *et al.* (1959) all obtained data which they interpreted as being consistent with the view that vitamin D increased the synthesis of citrate from acetate in bone. Particularly Joshi *et al.* (1957) claimed that vitamin D treatment resulted in an elevation in the activity of the cartilage enzyme citrogenase. However, their results were based on conclusions obtained from indirect experiments that did not directly measure metabolic activity of the organic acids of the tricarboxylic acid cycle in bone tissues.

In studies carried out with rat kidney tissue homogenates or mitochondrial preparations DeLuca and co-workers clearly showed that administration of vitamin D *in vivo* lowered the oxidation rate of citrate and isocitrate but not that of any other tricarboxylic acid cycle intermediates. Surprisingly, this observation could be repeated by the addition *in vitro* of vitamin D to kidney mitochondria preparations (DeLuca and Steenbock, 1957). Further electron microscopic evaluation of isolated rat kidney mitochondria revealed that dietary vitamin D had a marked protective effect on the structural integrity of these organelles (DeLuca *et al.,* 1960) (see Fig. 11-3). It was then felt that the diminished oxidation of citrate observed previously could be explained in terms of a physical inhibition of citrate penetration into the mitochondria. In confirmation of this Norman and DeLuca (1964) found that the *in vivo* administration of vitamin D to rachitic animals resulted in an increase in the amount of [^{14}C]acetate converted to citrate by isolated bone segments *in vitro*. Also there was a corresponding decrease in the amount of radioactivity in the other organic acids of bone. Most importantly, in bone fragments obtained from vitamin D-treated animals, there was a decrease in the amount of $^{14}CO_2$ produced. Similar results were mentioned briefly by Meyer *et al.* (1959). Collectively, these results demonstrate that vitamin D does not increase the synthesis of citrate from acetate in bone and are consistent with the view that the vitamin decreases the rate of conversion of citrate to subsequent intermediates in the tricarboxylic acid cycle in bone tissue as well as in kidney.

The observation of a relationship between vitamin D and bone citric acid levels suggested to some investigators that increased bone citrate levels might facilitate bone calcium mobilization, probably via the chelation of the calcium ion by citrate. Thus, there was a possibility that citric acid was the mediator of vitamin D action on bone. However, the results of Harrison *et al.* (1957) clearly rule out this possibility. These workers were able to dissociate the effects of vitamin D on citric acid metabolism from those on bone in rats by feeding cortisol. Although the tibias of vitamin D-deficient cortisol-fed rats gave evidence of an increased calcification in response to administration of the vitamin, there was no corresponding elevation in either serum citrate levels or bone citrate levels. Clearly, in the presence of cortisol there was a dissociation of these two separate actions of vitamin D.

In view of the prominent role of energy metabolism in the growth and development of cartilage (Section III,C), Kunin and co-workers (Balogh and Kunin, 1968; Meyer and Kunin, 1969a,b) initiated a study of the effects of vitamin D and dietary phosphorus on oxidative enzymes in the ephiphyseal cartilage of rachitic rats. Kunin and Krane (1965) demonstrated that the development of rickets in rats resulted in an increased rate of lactate production by cartilage slices and that there was an increased level of the enzyme lactate dehydrogenase in rachitic cartilage extracts. The prominent role of glycolysis in the metabolism of growth cartilage was emphasized by the reports of Kunin and Meyer (1969) and Meyer and Kunin (1969a,b). They demonstrated that cortisone administration to rats substantially lowered the rate of lactate production by isolated epiphyseal cartilage slices and also produced a depression of glycolytic enzyme activity.

Thus, there are biochemical data that support the previously discussed evidence for histological changes in cartilage tissue. However, at present there is no clear understanding of the molecular basis of the actions of vitamin D or its metabolites in mediating these changes. These effects, however, are reminiscent of those of some steroid hormones in terms of differentiation and proliferation of the tissues.

Certainly one of the major problems in evaluating the biochemical actions of any hormones, including vitamin D metabolites, is the multiplicity of cell types present in this tissue. From animal experiments *in vivo* or bone organ culture experiments *in vitro* it is not always possible to discern which bone cell type is producing the response under study. Clearly, what is required is the development of appropriate tissue cell culture techniques that will make it possible to study selected bone cell populations. The biochemical characterization by Luben *et al.* (1976) of bone cells grown in tissue culture that are differentially responsive to parathyroid and calcitonin hormones may represent an important methodological breakthrough.

V. DIFFERENTIAL ACTIONS OF VITAMIN D METABOLITES

As emphasized earlier, the multiplicity of steps associated with bone accretion and resorption suggest many sites for the intervention of vitamin D and its metabolites. Although $1,25(OH)_2D_3$ has been advanced as "the hormonally active form of vitamin D" (Norman and Henry, 1974; DeLuca, 1974), there are very few data to support the validity of this statement with regard to the actions of vitamin D on bone. The issue relevant to bone is whether vitamin D and its metabolites improve bone mineralization simply by raising the level of ion product of $P_i \times Ca$ in the extracellular fluids, and if so whether this change is mediated by a single metabolite, e.g., $1,25(OH)_2D_3$, upon intestinal phosphate and calcium absorption and upon the resorption of these ions from bone, or whether other vitamin D metabolites play a role. Indeed, there are some preliminary data suggesting that $25(OH)D_3$, $24,25(OH)_2D_3$, $25,26(OH)_2D_3$, and $1,25(OH)_2D_3$ all have unique actions on bone.

If $1,25(OH)_2D_3$ is the only hormonally active form of vitamin D, it should be capable of supporting all the actions of vitamin D both in bone and in other target tissues to permit the normal development of the animal from birth to sexual maturity. Yet Henry and Norman (1978) reported that in the chick *both* 24,25$(OH)_2D_3$ and 1,25$(OH)_2D_3$ were required for the growth and development (over a period of 9 months from the day of hatching) as well as the production of fertile eggs capable of hatching normally. When 1,25$(OH)_2D_3$ alone was administered, the fertile eggs were virtually incapable of hatching. Clearly, in this experimental system two vitamin D metabolites were required. Similarly, Bordier *et al.* (1977) reported clinical evidence that 1,25$(OH)_2D_3$ alone was incapable of stimulating a normal rate of bone mineralization in vitamin D-deficient adult males, whereas in combination with 25$(OH)D_3$ it elicited this response. They concluded (Bordier *et al.*, 1977) that "25$(OH)D_3$ or a further metabolite of this compound, other than 1,25$(OH)_2D_3$, plays a role in the mineralization of bone in man."

In separate studies Miravet *et al.* (1978) evaluated the actions of various vitamin D metabolites on the bone of vitamin D-deficient rats. They reported that the bone phosphorus content was increased only by 25,26$(OH)_2D_3$ administration and not by 1,25$(OH)_2D_3$ or 24,25$(OH)_2D_3$ treatment.

Lieberherr *et al.* (1977, 1978) found different responses for rat bone acid and alkaline phosphatase activities after the separate administration of either acute or chronic small doses of 25$(OH)D_3$, 1,25$(OH)_2D_3$, or 24,25$(OH)_2D_3$. They further noted that 25$(OH)D_3$ treatment elevated these enzymatic activities, whereas 24,25$(OH)_2D_3$ decreased the activity.

It is to be anticipated that much greater insight into the actions of vitamin D and its metabolites on bone will be obtained in coming years. An intriguing possibility is that specific biochemical roles for other vitamin D metabolites, such as 24,25$(OH)_2D_3$, 25,26$(OH)_2D_3$, or 25$(OH)D_3$, may be formulated.

REFERENCES

Ali, S. Y., Sajdera, S. W., and Anderson, H. C. (1970). *Proc. Natl. Acad. Sci. U.S.A.* **67,** 1513.

Anderson, H. C. (1969). *J. Cell Biol.* **41,** 59.

Anderson, H. C., and Sajdera, S. W. (1976). *Fed. Proc., Fed. Am. Ser. Exp. Biol.* **35,** 148.

Anderson, H. C., Matuzawa, T., Sajdera, S. W., and Ali, S. Y. (1970). *Trans. N.Y. Acad. Sci.* [2] **32,** 619.

Anderson, H. C., Cecil, R., and Sajdera, S. W. (1975). *Am. J. Pathol.* **79,** 237.

Au, W. Y. W., and Bartter, F. C. (1966). *Endocrinology* **78,** 1100.

Avioli, L. V., and Krane, S. M., eds. (1977). "Metabolic Bone Disease," Vol. 1. Academic Press, New York.

Balogh, K., and Kunin, A. S. (1968). *Lab. Invest.* **18,** 782.

Barnes, M. J., Constable, B. J., Morton, L. F., and Kodicek, E. (1973). *Biochem. J.* **132,** 113.

Baylink, D., Stauffer, M., Wergedal, J., and Rich, D. (1970). *J. Clin. Invest.* **49,** 1122.

Baylink, D., Sipe, J., Wergedal, J., and Whittemore, O. J. (1974). *Am. J. Physiol.* **224,** 1345.

Bélanger, L. F., and Migicovsky, B. B. (1958). *J. Exp. Med.* **107,** 821.

Bellin, S. A., and Steenbock, H. (1952). *J. Biol. Chem.* **194,** 311.

Bonucci, E. (1970). *Z. Zellforsch. Mikrosk. Anat.* **103,** 192.
Bordier, P. J., and Tun Chot, S. (1972). *Clin. Endocrinol. Metab.* **1,** 197.
Bordier, P. J., Ryckwaert, A., Marie, P., Miravet, L., Norman, A. W., and Rasmussen, H. (1977). *In* "Proceedings of The Third Workshop on Vitamin D: Biochemical, Chemical and Clinical Aspects Related to Calcium Metabolism" (A. W. Norman *et al.*, eds.), p. 897. de Gruyter, Berlin.
Boris, A., Hurley, J. F., and Traml, T. (1977). *J. Nutr.* **107,** 194.
Bourne, G. H., ed. (1957). "The Biochemistry and Physiology of Bone," Vol. 1. Academic Press, New York.
Bourne, G. H., ed. (1971). "The Biochemistry and Physiology of Bone," Vol. 2. Academic Press, New York.
Bourne, G. H., ed. (1977). "The Biochemistry and Physiology of Bone," Vol. 3. Academic Press, New York.
Canas, F., Brand, J. S., Neuman, W. F., and Terepka, A. R. (1969). *Am. J. Physiol.* **216,** 1092.
Carlsson, A. (1952). *Acta Physiol. Scand.* **26,** 212.
Carlsson, A. (1954). *Acta Physiol. Scand.* **31,** 121.
Carlsson, A., and Hollunger, G. (1954). *Acta Physiol. Scand.* **31,** 317.
Carlsson, A., and Lindquist, B. (1955). *Acta Physiol. Scand.* **35,** 53.
Carttar, M. S., McLean, F. C., and Urist, M. R. (1950). *Am. J. Pathol.* **26,** 307.
Castillo, L., Tanaka, Y., and DeLuca, H. F. (1975). *Endocrinology* **97,** 995.
Crenshaw, M. A., Ramp, W. K., Gonnerman, W. A., and Toverud, S. U. (1974). *Proc. Soc. Exp. Biol. Med.* **146,** 488.
Cruess, R. L., and Clark, I. (1965). *Biochem. J.* **96,** 262.
Davidson, W. (1975). *Pharmacol. & Ther., Part C* **2,** 223.
DeLuca, H. F. (1974). *Fed. Proc., Fed. Am. Soc. Exp. Biol.* **33,** 2211.
DeLuca, H. F., and Steenbock, H. (1975). *Science* **126,** 258.
DeLuca, H. F., Gran, F. C., and Steenbock, H. (1957a). *J. Biol. Chem.* **224,** 201.
DeLuca, H. F., Gran, F. C., Steenbock, H., and Reiser, S. (1957b). *J. Biol. Chem.* **228,** 469.
DeLuca, H. F., Reiser, S., Steenbock, H., and Kaesberg, P. (1960). *Biochim. Biophys. Acta* **40,** 526.
Dickens, F. (1941). *Biochem. J.* **35,** 1011.
Dikshit, P. K., and Patwardhan, V. N. (1952). *Indian J. Med. Sci.* **6,** 107.
Dikshit, P. K., Joshi, J. G., and Patwardhan, V. N. (1956). *Indian J. Med. Res.* **44,** 719.
Dixon, T. F., and Perkins, H. R. (1952). *Biochem. J.* **52,** 260.
Fischmann, P. (1937). *Arch. Exp. Zellforsch. Besonders Gewebezuecht.* **19,** 211.
Freeman, S., and Chang, T. S. (1950). *Am. J. Physiol.* **160,** 341.
Frost, H. M. (1964). "Bone Biodynamics." Little, Brown, Boston, Massachusetts.
Garabedian, M. (1977). *Abstr., Parathyroid Conf., 6th, 1977* Int. Congr. Ser. No. 421.
Garabedian, M., Tanaka, Y., Holick, M. F., and DeLuca, H. F. (1974). *Endocrinology* **94,** 1022.
Glisson, F. (1650). "De Rachitide Sive Morbo Puerili Qui Valgo." The Rickets Diciteur, London.
Gonnerman, W. A., Toverud, S. U., Ramp, W. K., and Mechanic, G. L. (1976). *Proc. Soc. Exp. Biol. Med.* **151,** 453.
Grant, M. E., and Prokop, D. J. (1972a). *N. Engl. J. Med.* **286,** 194.
Grant, M. E., and Prokop, D. J. (1972b). *N. Engl. J. Med.* **286,** 242.
Grant, M. E., and Prokop, D. J. (1972c). *N. Engl. J. Med.* **286,** 291.
Haavaldsen, R., and Nicolaysen, R. (1955). *Acta Physiol. Scand.* **36,** 103.
Haavaldsen, R., Egnund, K. M., and Nicolaysen, R. (1955). *Acta Physiol. Scand.* **36,** 109.
Hahn, T. J., and Avioli, L. V. (1970). *Arch. Intern. Med.* **126,** 882.
Hamilton, B., and Dewar, M. M. (1937). *Am. J. Dis. Child.* **54,** 548.
Harrison, H. C., and Harrison, H. E. (1951). *Yale J. Biol. Med.* **24,** 273.

Harrison, H. C., Harrison, H. E., and Park, E. A. (1957). *Proc. Soc. Exp. Biol. Med.* **96,** 768.
Harrison, H. C., Harrison, H. E., and Park, E. A. (1958). *Am. J. Physiol.* **192,** 432.
Henry, H. L., and Norman, A. W. (1978). *Science* **201,** 835.
Henry, H. L., Norman, A. W., Taylor, A. N., Hartenbower, D. L., and Coburn, J. W. (1976). *J. Nutr.* **106,** 724.
Hess, A. (1929). "Rickets, Osteomalacia, and Tetany." Lea & Febiger, Philadelphia, Pennsylvania.
Hibberd, K. A., and Norman, A. W. (1969). *Biochem. Pharmacol.* **18,** 2347.
Hirschman, A., and Shapiro, S. H. (1960). *Proc. Soc. Exp. Biol. Med.* **104,** 659.
Holick, M. F., Garabedian, M., and DeLuca, H. F. (1972). *Science* **176,** 1146.
Howell, D. S., Peta, J. C., Marquez, J. F., and Madruga, J. E. (1968). *J. Clin. Invest.* **47,** 1121.
Hunter, R. (1972). *Lancet* **1,** 1972.
Joshi, J. G., Dikshit, P. K., and Patwardhan, V. N. (1957). *Indian J. Med. Res.* **45,** 439.
Jowsey, J. (1966). *Am. J. Med.* **40,** 485.
Kember, N. F., and Walker, K. V. R. (1971). *Nature (London)* **229,** 428.
Kivirikko, K. E. (1970). *Int. Rev. Connect. Tissue Res.* **5,** 93.
Kream, B. E., Jose, M., Yamada, S., and DeLuca, H. F. (1977). *Science* **197,** 1086.
Kunin, A. S., and Krane, S. M. (1965). *Biochim. Biophys. Acta* **107,** 203.
Kunin, A. S., and Meyer, W. L. (1969). *Arch. Biochem. Biophys.* **129,** 421.
Lamm, M., and Neuman, W. F. (1958). *AMA Arch. Pathol.* **66,** 204.
Larsson, S., Lorentzon, R., and Boquist, L. (1977). *Clin. Orthop. Relat. Res.* **127,** 228.
Lees, H., and Kuyper, A. C. (1957). *J. Biol. Chem.* **225,** 641.
Lieberherr, M., Pezant, E., Garabedian, M., and Balsan, S. (1977). *Calcif. Tissue Res.* **23,** 235.
Lieberherr, M., Garabedian, M., Guillozo, H., and Balsan, S. (1978). *Ann. Biol. Anim., Biochim., Biophys.* **18,** 181.
Lindquist, B. (1952). *Acta Paediatr. (Stockholm)* **41,** Suppl. 86.
Liu, C.-C., Baylink, D. J., and Wergedal, J. (1974). *Endocrinology* **95,** 1011.
Luben, R. A., Wong, G. L., and Cohn, D. V. (1976). *Endocrinology* **99,** 526.
MacLean, M., and Urist, M. R. (1961). "Bone, an Introduction to the Physiology of Skeletal Tissue." Univ. of Chicago Press, Chicago, Illinois.
Malm, O. J., Nicolaysen, R., and Skjelkvale, L. (1955). *Ciba Found. Colloq. Ageing* **1,** 109.
Matuzawa, T., and Anderson, H. C. (1971). *J. Histochem. Cytochem.* **19,** 801.
Mechanic, G. L., Toverud, S. U., and Ramp, W. K. (1972). *Biochem. Biophys. Res. Commun.* **47,** 760.
Mechanic, G. L., Toverud, S. U., Ramp, W. K., and Gonnerman, W. A. (197[illegible]). *Biochim. Biophys. Acta* **393,** 419.
Mellanby, E. (1921). *Med. Res. Counc. (G.B.), Spec. Rep. Ser.* **SRS-61.**
Mellanby, E. (1923). "Experimental Rickets." HM Stationery Office, London.
Meyer, J., Bolen, R. J., and Antin, J. (1959). *Arch. Biochem. Biophys.* **81,** 340.
Meyer, W. L., and Kunin, A. S. (1969a). *Arch. Biochem. Biophys.* **129,** 431.
Meyer, W. L., and Kunin, A. S. (1969b). *Arch. Biochem. Biophys.* **129,** 438.
Migicovsky, B. B. (1957). *Can. J. Biochem. Physiol.* **35,** 1267.
Migicovsky, B. B., and Emslie, A. R. G. (1950). *Arch. Biochem. Biophys.* **28,** 324.
Miravet, L., Queille, M. L., Carré, M., Bordier, P., and Redel, J. (1978). *Ann. Biol. Anim., Biochim. Biophys.* **18,** 187.
Morava, E., Hegyi, Z., Winter, M., and Tarjan, R. (1970). *Acta Physiol. Acad. Sci. Hung.* **39,** 279.
Neuman, W. F., and Neuman, M. W. (1958). "The Chemical Dynamics of Bone Mineral." Univ. of Chicago Press, Chicago, Illinois.
Nicolaysen, R. (1943). *Acta Physiol. Scand.* **5,** 200.
Nicolaysen, R., and Eeg-Larsen, N. (1953). *Vitam. Horm. (N.Y.)* **11,** 29.
Nicolaysen, R., and Jansen, J. (1939). *Acta Paediatr. (Stockholm)* **23,** 405.

Nicolaysen, R., and Nordbo, R. (1943). *Acta Physiol. Scand.* **5,** 212.
Nicolaysen, R., Eeg-Larsen, N., and Malm, O. J. (1953). *Physiol. Rev.* **33,** 424.
Norman, A. W., and DeLuca, H. F. (1964). *Biochem. J.* **91,** 124.
Norman, A. W., and Henry, H. L. (1974). *Recent Prog. Horm. Res.* **30,** 431.
Okamura, W. H., Mitra, M. N., Procsal, D. A., and Norman, A. W. (1975). *Biochem. Biophys. Res. Commun.* **65,** 24.
Oliver, W. M., Leaver, A. G., and Scott, P. G. (1972). *J. Periodontal Res.* **7,** 29.
Park, E. A. (1939). *Bull. N.Y. Acad. Med.*[2] **15,** 495.
Patterson, C. R., and Fourman, P. (1968). *Biochem. J.* **109,** 101.
Pavlovitch, H., Garabedian, M., and Balsan, S. (1973). *J. Clin. Invest.* **52,** 2656.
Peacock, M., Gallagher, J. C., and Nordin, B. E. C. (1974). *Lancet* **1,** 385.
Pechet, M. M., and Hesse, R. H. (1974). *Mol. Cell. Endocrinol.* **1,** 305.
Pileggi, V. J., DeLuca, H. F., Cramer, J. W., and Steenbock, H. (1956). *Arch. Biochem. Biophys.* **60,** 52.
Raisz, L. G., Trummel, C. L., Holick, M. F., and DeLuca, H. F. (1972). *Science* **175,** 768.
Ramalingaswami, V., Sriramachari, S., Dikshit, P. K., Tulpule, P. G., and Patwardhan, V. N. (1954). *Indian J. Med. Sci.* **8,** 509.
Rasmussen, H., and Bordier, P. (1974). "The Physiological and Cellular Basis of Metabolic Bone Disease." Williams & Wilkins, Baltimore, Maryland.
Reeve, L. E., Schnoes, H. K., and DeLuca, H. F. (1978). *Arch. Biochem. Biophys.* **186,** 164.
Reynolds, J. J. (1974). *Biochem. Soc. Spec. Publ.* **3,** 91.
Reynolds, J. J., and Dingle, T. J. (1970). *Calcif. Tissue Res.* **4,** 339.
Reynolds, J. J., Holick, M. F., and DeLuca, H. F. (1973). *Calcif. Tissue Res.* **12,** 295.
Reynolds, J. J., Holick, M. F., and DeLuca, H. F. (1974). *Calcif. Tissue Res.* **15,** 333.
Robinson, R., and Rosenheim, A. H. (1934). *Biochem. J.* **28,** 684.
Russell, J. E., Avioli, L. V., and Mechanic, G. (1975). *Biochem. J.* **145,** 119.
Sevastikoglou, J. A., and Ray, R. D. (1970). *Acta Orthop. Scand , Suppl.* **136,** 43.
Seymour, J. L., and DeLuca, H. F. (1974). *Endocrinology* **94,** 1009.
Shohl, A. (1937). *J. Nutr.* **14,** 69.
Simmons, D. J., and Kunin, A. S. (1970). *Clin. Orthop. Relat. Res.* **68,** 251.
Steenbock, H., and Bellin, S. A. (1953). *J. Biol. Chem.* **205,** 985.
Stern, P. H., DeLuca, H. F., and Ikekawa, N. (1975). *Biochem. Biophys. Res. Commun.* **67,** 965.
Tanaka, Y., and DeLuca, H. F. (1971). *Arch. Biochem. Biophys.* **146,** 574.
Tanaka, Y., Frank, H., and DeLuca, H. F. (1972). *J. Nutr.* **102,** 1569.
Toole, B. P., Kang, A. H., Trelstad, R. L., and Gross, J. (1972). *Biochem. J.* **127,** 715.
Trummel, C. L., Raisz, L. G., Blunt, J. W., and DeLuca, H. F. (1969). *Science* **163,** 1450.
Van Reen, R. (1959). *J. Biol. Chem.* **234,** 1951.
Vaughan, J. M. (1970). "The Physiology of Bone." Oxford Univ. Press (Clarendon), London and New York.
Wassjo, E., and Eeg-Larsen, N. (1951a). *Acta Physiol. Scand.* **25,** Suppl. 84, 1.
Wassjo, E., and Eeg-Larsen, N. (1951b). *Acta Physiol. Scand.* **25,** Suppl. 89, 1.
Weisbrode, S. E., and Capen, C. C. (1974). *Am. J. Pathol.* **77,** 455.
Weisbrode, S. E., Capen, C. C., and Nagode, L. A. (1973). *Int. Acad. Pathol.* **28,** 29.
Weisbrode, S. E., Capen, C. C., and Nagode, L. A. (1974). *Am. J. Pathol.* **76,** 359.
Weisbrode, S. E., Capen, C. C., and Norman, A. W. (1978). *Am. J. Pathol.* **93,** 459.
Whistler, D. (1645). "Morbo Puerli Anglorum, Quem Patrio Idiomate Indigenae Vocant. The Rickets, Lugduni Batavosum.
Wong, R. G., Myrtle, J. F., Tsai, H. C., and Norman, A. W. (1972). *J. Biol. Chem.* **247,** 5728.
Yendt, E. R., Conner, T. B., and Howard, J. E. (1955). *Bull. Johns Hopkins Hosp.* **96,** 1.
Yoshiki, S., Yanagisawa, T., and Suda, T. (1974). *Calcif. Tissue Res.* **15,** 295.

CHAPTER

13

Vitamin D and Its Clinical Relationships

I. INTRODUCTION

A. Background

Preceding chapters in this book have documented in detail the elaborate metabolic pathway required for the conversion of vitamin D_3 to its metabolites $25(OH)D_3$, $24,25(OH)_2D_3$, and $1,25(OH)_2D_3$. The sophisticated endocrine mechanisms involving parathyroid hormone as well as serum calcium and vitamin D status that affect and regulate the conversion of $25(OH)D_3$ to its biologically active forms $1,25(OH)_2D_3$ and $24,25(OH)_2D_3$ as well as our current understanding of the steroid hormonelike mode of action of $1,25(OH)_2D_3$ in the intestinal mucosa are now firmly established. The reader is referred to Fig. 5-1 for a review of the metabolic pathway of vitamin D, to Figs. 9-3 and 9-8 for a summary of the regulatory processes affecting the production of $1,25(OH)_2D_3$, and to Fig. 1-5 for a review of the action of $1,25(OH)_2D_3$ at the molecular level in the intestinal mucosa. In view of the complex metabolic scheme for vitamin D and its interactions with multiple endocrine systems, it is apparent that there are many potential vitamin D-related perturbances or disease states that may arise.

B. Serum Levels of Vitamin D and Its Metabolites and Their Rates of Production and Turnover

Before considering the relation of various disease states to vitamin D action one should recall the discussion in Chapter 6 concerning vitamin D metabolism in man. It is also essential to have a working knowledge of the circulating concentrations of vitamin D metabolites in normal man, their rates of turnover, and the requirements of the target tissues for these various metabolites. It will then be possible to consider in greater detail how various disease states may arise and affect the action of vitamin D and its metabolites. Table 13-1 lists the circulating levels of vitamin D metabolites and their respective turnover times.[1] It is apparent that reasonably high concentrations of vitamin D, 25(OH)D, and

[1]In this chapter the subscript 2 or 3 will be omitted from vitamin D and its metabolites whenever reference is being made to the plasma concentrations of these steroids. As discussed in Chapter 8, the steroid competition assays employed for these determinations cannot distinguish between vitamins D_2 and D_3 or $1,25(OH)_2D_2$ and $1,25(OH)_2D_3$ or $25(OH)D_2$ and $25(OH)D_3$, etc.

TABLE 13-1
Plasma Concentrations and Turnover Times of Vitamin D and its Principal Metabolites in Man

	Approximate metabolite concentration (pg/ml)	Molarity (M)	Turnover time ($t_{\frac{1}{2}}$)
D	35,000[a]	9.1×10^{-8}	4.5 days[e]
25(OH)D	35,000[b]	8.7×10^{-8}	31 days[e]
24,25$(OH)_2$D	3,000[c]	7.2×10^{-9}	$1/n$
1,25$(OH)_2$D	30–50[d]	1.0×10^{-10}	1-5 hr[e,f]

[a]Belsey *et al.* (1971).
[b]Haddad and Chyu (1971); see Table 8-5, this volume.
[c]Taylor *et al.* (1976) and Haddad *et al.* (1976).
[d]Haussler *et al.* (1976) and Eisman *et al.* (1976); see Table 8-7, this volume.
[e]See Table 5A and 5B in Norman and Henry (1974).
[f]See Gray *et al.* (1977) and Mawer *et al.* (1976).

24,25$(OH)_2$D are normally present, e.g., 10–30, 10–30, and 1–5 ng/ml serum, respectively. In contrast, the circulating level of 1,25$(OH)_2$D is remarkably low, i.e., 30–50 pg/ml. The circulating level of 1,25$(OH)_2$D is one of the lowest for all known steroid hormones. Only estradiol and aldosterone have circulating levels that are normally as low as that of 1,25$(OH)_2$D.

From the data presented in Table 13-1 it is possible to calculate the estimated daily production of 25$(OH)D_3$ and 1,25$(OH)_2D_3$ in man (Norman and Henry, 1974). It is likely that some 4900 pmoles (equivalent to 1.7 μg) of 25$(OH)D_3$ are produced each day, whereas 300–1500 pmoles (0.14–0.68 μg) of 1,25$(OH)_2D_3$ must be produced daily by the kidney to maintain a steady state in normal man. Mawer *et al.* (1976) and Gray *et al.* (1977), who studied directly the plasma kinetics of [tritiated] 1,25$(OH)_2D_3$ in man came to virtually identical conclusions.

An interesting comparison can be made between the need for 1,25$(OH)_2D_3$ as estimated from plasma turnover times and circulating concentrations and the calculated capacity of the renal enzyme to produce 1,25$(OH)_2D_3$ based on *in vitro* measurements (Norman and Henry, 1974). The circulating concentration of 25$(OH)D_3$ of 10 to 20 ng/ml will support a rate of 1-hydroxylation that is about 5% of the maximal velocity of the 25$(OH)D_3$ 1-hydroxylase. Thus, it can be extrapolated that a 70-kg man might produce approximately 2000 pmoles of 1,25$(OH)_2D_3$ per day. As stated above, however, as little as 250 pmoles of 1,25$(OH)_2D_3$ per day may be normally produced by the human kidneys. From such calculations and the results of measurements in other species, Henry and Norman (1975) suggested that the relative concentration of 25$(OH)D_3$ 1-hydroxylase activity in the human kidney is considerably below that present in other species. This has the possible implication that man may be unusually susceptible to environmental or disease-related factors that can damage the kidney or alter its enzymatic machinery. There may be little margin for error in the capacity to produce this important steroid hormone. Indeed there may be a delicate balance between the demand for the steroid by the target tissues and the output by the kidney. This appears to be the case in the chick (Friedlander *et al.*, 1977).

Alternatively, $1,25(OH)_2D_3$ may be subject to an unusually rapid catabolism or turnover. Thus, the 2000 pmoles estimated to be produced per day might be turned over three or four times ($t_{\frac{1}{2}}$ 6–8 hr) per day, which would be consistent with a serum pool of 500 to 600 pmoles. With these considerations in mind various disease states related to vitamin D can be fruitfully reviewed.

C. Normal Man and Vitamin D

1. Adaptation of Intestinal Calcium and Phosphorus Absorption

A partial discussion of studies concerned with the intestinal absorption of calcium and phosphorus in man is presented in Chapter 10. In addition, Fig. 9-1 is a schematic diagram illustrating calcium and phosphorus dynamics and turnover in man. It should be recalled that the daily calcium intake varies from 500 to 1000 mg and is derived principally from milk products, flour with added calcium, and some vegetables. The average daily intake of phosphate expressed as milligrams of phosphorus is of the order of 800 to 1500 mg. Both calcium and phosphate ions are absorbed by specific mechanisms under the influence of vitamin D in the intestinal mucosa (see Chapter 10).

One of the important physiological aspects of intestinal absorption of both calcium and phosphorus is that the process is adaptive. As the dietary content of calcium and phosphorus decreases there is an increased efficiency of absorption of both calcium and phosphorus. These relationships for man are documented in Fig. 13-1 (calcium absorption) and Fig. 13-2 (phosphorus absorption). It is apparent that the extent or efficiency of absorption of both calcium and phosphorus by the intestine in normal man is closely regulated by the dietary level of these substances. These considerations are extensively reviewed by Coburn *et al.* (1973b) and Stanbury and Lumb (1962).

2. Photochemical Production of Vitamin D and Its Intestinal Absorption

Vitamin D from two prime sources is available to man: vitamin D produced photochemically and that in the diet. Vitamin D is normally produced in the epidermal layer of the skin, where ultraviolet radiation is absorbed by the precur-

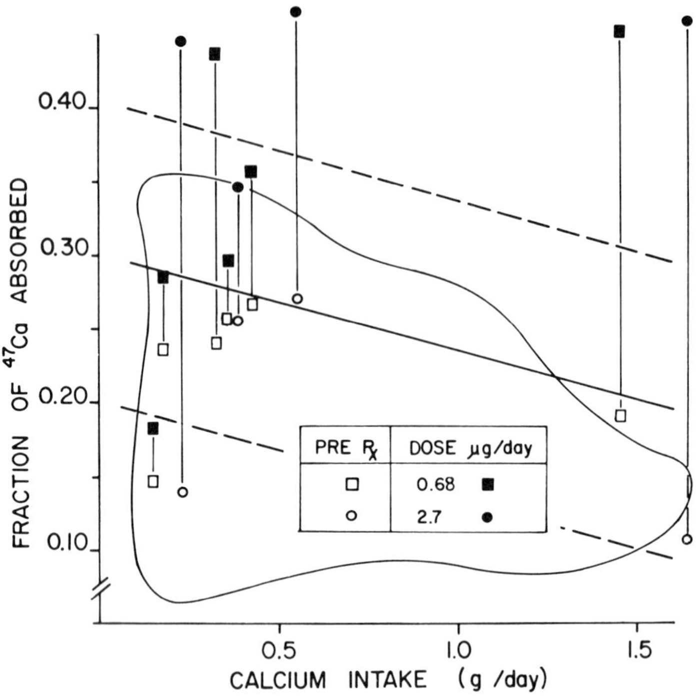

Figure 13-1. Adaptive response of the intestinal absorption of ^{47}Ca in man. Results are shown in relation to each individual's habitual dietary intake of calcium. The dashed lines outside the solid line (mean) indicate the 95% confidence limits of variation of absorption in normal man. The curved line encompasses all observations carried out in 96 patients with advanced renal failure. The vertical lines represent studies before and after treatment of uremic patients with $1,25(OH)_2D_3$. Taken from Coburn *et al.* (1973a) with permission of the author and publisher.

sor 7-dehydrocholesterol. Wheatley and Reinertson (1958) as well as Rauschkolb *et al.* (1969) documented the abundance of 7-dehydrocholesterol in the epidermis of man. Very little information, however, is available concerning the actual pathways of transmittance of light to the site of the photochemical conversion in the epidermis. It is presumed that the overall process follows that which can be carried out chemically as described in Chapter 3 (see Fig. 3-9). The vitamin D_3 content of nonirradiated human skin has been determined to be approximately 3.2 ng per gram of skin or approximately 17 IU/cm^2 by Rauschkolb *et al.* (1969) using gas–liquid chromatography techniques. No precise quantitation of the maximal endogenous rate of production of vitamin D in man is available. However, it must be of the order of the minimal daily requirement (i.e., 200–400 IU daily) since Bunker and Harris (1937) determined that ultraviolet irradiation of the skin was capable of completely curing rickets.

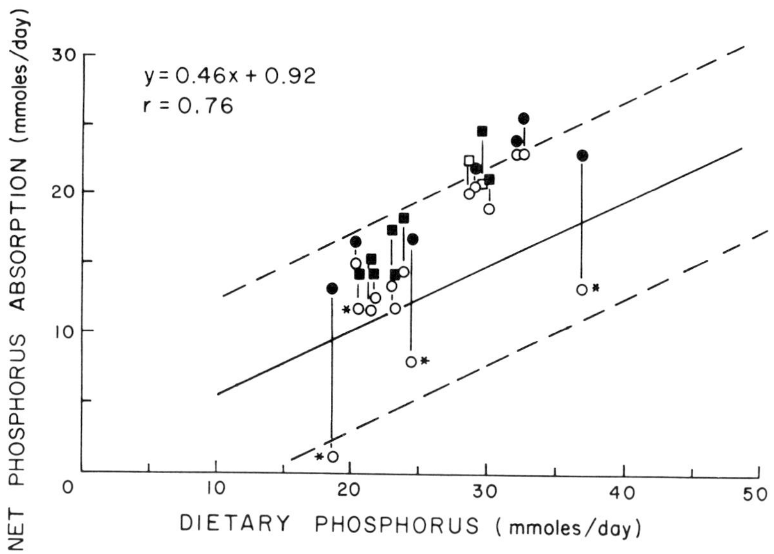

Figure 13-2. Relationship between net phosphorus absorption and dietary phosphorus intake in patients with advanced renal failure receiving either $1,25(OH)_2D_3$ or $1\alpha(OH)D_3$. Open symbols represent control measurements; closed symbols indicate measurements during treatment with either $1,25(OH)_2D_3$ (circles) or $1\alpha(OH)D_3$ (squares). The asterisk indicates those patients receiving constant daily amounts of aluminum hydroxide. The regression line for uremic patients is adapted from personal cases and studies taken from the literature. Reproduced from Coburn *et al.* (1977) with permission of the authors and publishers.

Minimal data are available on the penetration of uv light through the stratum cornea to the epidermis. Everett *et al.* (1966) estimated that approximately 30% of light of wavelength 290–300 nm was capable of penetrating the stratum corneum, and as much as 8% of the incident uv light of this wavelength was capable of penetrating the epidermis to the dermis. Doboszynska and Datsenko (1966) failed in their efforts to isolate vitamin D directly from skin. More recently, Holick *et al.* (1977) isolated and chemically characterized previtamin D from uv-irradiated rat skin.

Following the photochemical conversion of 7-dehydrocholesterol to vitamin D, the preformed vitamin D is assumed to be absorbed into the subepidermal microcirculation and transported in plasma to the liver, where it undergoes the first step of metabolism.

It is not clear whether vitamin D becomes bound to its circulating carrier protein at the site of the epidermis or whether this is a process that can take place only in the liver. In view of the limited solubility of vitamin D it would seem logical that it certainly does not diffuse in a "free" form through the circulatory system. It is known from the work of Peterson (1971) and Smith and Goodman

(1971) that vitamin D is bound to a specific globulin of molecular weight 50,000–60,000 (see Table 8-2).

Dietary forms of vitamin D, i.e., cholecalciferol and ergocalciferol, are known to be absorbed primarily from the duodenum and jejunum of the small intestine into lymphatic channels by a process that is also employed for bile salts and intraluminal lipids (Thompson *et al.*, 1969). The specific mode of absorption is via the lymphatic system and its associated chylomicrons; this has been shown to be the case in the rat (Schachter *et al.*, 1964) and in man (Avioli and Haddad, 1973). The site of transfer of vitamin D from the chylomicrons to specific globular proteins has not yet been determined. The absorbed vitamin D_2 or vitamin D_3 mixes with the endogenously synthesized vitamin D_3 in the plasma to form one common pool of provitamin D activity, which is available for further processing by the endocrine system. As discussed in Chapter 7, adipose tissue and muscle have been identified as major storage sites for vitamin D (Mawer and Schaefer, 1969; Rosenstreich *et al.*, 1971a,b). The muscle and adipose tissue presumably serve as a reservoir of prohormone activity, which can buffer the organism during periods of lack of sunlight exposure or dietary deprivation of vitamin D.

3. *Nutritional Requirement for Vitamin D*

The vitamin D requirement of healthy adults has never been clearly defined but according to Dent and Smith (1969) probably does not exceed 100 IU/day. The current allowance of vitamin D_3 recommended by the National Research Council (NRC) is 400 IU/day. It should be emphasized that in ordinary circumstances this amount of vitamin D can be readily obtained largely through casual exposure to sunshine plus consumption of normal dietary constituents. It should also be appreciated that the requirement for vitamin D and sensitivity to potential toxic effects may vary considerably from one individual to another. It is felt that the NRC recommendations incorporate a safety factor beyond the absolute minimal daily requirement (National Academy of Sciences, 1964). This is undoubtedly true, if an individual receives some exposure to sunlight.

The major food sources of vitamin D are given in Table 13-2. A complete listing of the vitamin D values of food is given by Booher *et al.* (1942). The prime sources of vitamin D are animal-derived foods. As discussed in Chapter 3, little or no vitamin D is present in the plant world. Yendt (1970) discusses in some detail vitamin D nutrition, food supplementation, and pharmacology.

D. Etiology of Clinical Disorders That May Be Related to Vitamin D

Conceptually, human clinical disorders related to vitamin D can be considered as those arising because of (a) altered availability of vitamin D, (b) altered

TABLE 13-2
Vitamin D Content of Unfortified Foods[a]

Food source	Vitamin D content (IU/100 g)
Butter	35
Cheese	12
Cod	85
Cream	50
Egg yolk (per yolk)	25
Halibut	44
Herring (canned)	330
Liver	
Beef (raw)	9–40
Calf (raw)	0–15
Pork (raw)	40
Chicken (raw)	50–65
Lamb (raw)	20
Mackerel	120
Milk	
Cow (100 ml)	0.3–4
Human (100 ml)	0–10
Salmon (canned)	220–440
Sardines	1500
Shrimp	150

[a]Abstracted from Booher *et al.* (1942).

conversion of vitamin D to $25(OH)D_3$; (c) altered conversion of $25(OH)D_3$ to $1,25(OH)_2D_3$ or $24,25(OH)_2D_3$, (d) conditions that may be due to variations in end organ responsiveness to $1,25(OH)_2D_3$ or possibly $24,25(OH)_2D_3$, and (e) other conditions of uncertain relation to vitamin D. Thus, the clinician-biochemist is faced with a problem, in a diagnostic sense, of identifying parameters of hypersensitivity, antagonism, or resistance (including genetic aberrations) to vitamin D or one of the other of its metabolites as well as identifying perturbations of metabolism that result in problems in production and/or delivery of the hormonally active form $1,25(OH)_2D_3$.

Table 13-3 lists human disease states that are believed to be related to altered metabolism or action of vitamin D. This can be considered to be a systems analysis of disorders of calcium metabolism related to vitamin D.

An alternative method of analysis is given in Fig. 13-3, which presents a schematic diagram of the metabolic processing of vitamin D via its endocrine systems. Listed under each of the substeps of the various metabolic or regulatory steps are disease states that are clinically focused at that particular locus. Thus, it is possible to identify diseases that are focused in the intestine, e.g., sarcoidosis

TABLE 13-3
Disorders of Calcium Metabolism in Man That May Involve Altered Metabolism or Action of Vitamin D

I. Availability of D_3	IV. Altered end organ response
Malabsorption syndromes	Cortisone treatment
Dietary deficiency	Sarcoidosis (?)
Absence of exposure to uv light	Uremia (?)
II. Availability of $25(OH)D_3$	V. Other disorders of uncertain relation to vitamin D
Anticonvulsant therapy	Idiopathic hypercalciuria
Hepatic disease	Sex-linked hypophosphatemic rickets
Biliary cirrhosis	Fibrogenesis imperfecta ossium
Pesticide exposure (?)	Idiopathic hypercalcemia of infancy
III. Availability of $1,25(OH)_2D_3$	VI. Hypersensitivity
Definite	Sarcoidosis
Chronic renal failure	Idiopathic hypercalciuria
Vitamin D-dependent rickets	Idiopathic hypercalcemia of infancy
Possible	VII. Antagonism
Hypoparathyroidism	Glucocorticoid therapy
Pseudohypoparathyroidism	Anticonvulsant therapy
Hyperparathyroidism	VIII. Resistance
Phosphate depletion	Vitamin D-resistant rickets (VDRR)
Diphosphonate therapy	Familial hypophosphatemia
Acute renal failure	Hypoparathyroidism
Cadmium toxicity	Adult coeliac disease
Strontium toxicity	Biliary cirrhosis
	Chronic renal disease
	Fibrogenesis imperfecta ossium

and tropical sprue, or diseases of the parathyroid gland, e.g., hyper- and hypoparathyroidism, diseases of the bone, e.g., osteomalacia, osteoporosis and rickets, or diseases of the kidney, such as chronic renal failure. All of these in their own way reflect a disturbance in or a malfunctioning of the body's normal endocrine processing of vitamin D. Inasmuch as $1,25(OH)_2D_3$ and $24,25(OH)_2D_3$ are the biologically active forms of vitamin D, it is possible that virtually all of these disease states represent in essence either an inhibition of the production of $24,25(OH)_2D_3$ or $1,25(OH)_2D_3$ or modification of their transport to target tissues and subsequent interaction to produce biological responses. Thus, any disease state that directly impairs the production of $1,25(OH)_2D_3$ by the kidney interferes with any of the steps involved in calcium and phosphorus homeostasis, leading to an abnormal feedback signal to the kidney, will result in an altered production of this hormone. The kidney plays an unusually critical role in vitamin D endocrine actions, and, accordingly, the kidney can be implicated directly or indirectly in a wide variety of metabolic diseases. In either case if a deficiency in the biologically active forms of vitamin D ensues, ultimately a large

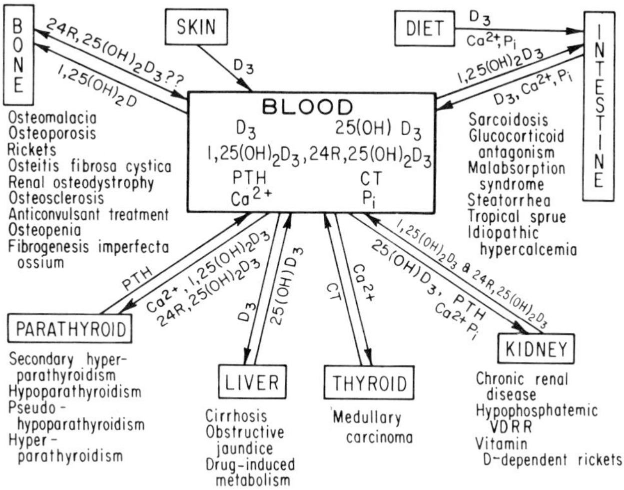

Figure 13-3. Human disease states related to vitamin D.

spectrum of bone diseases may develop; however, these conditions may occur for any of a wide variety of reasons. From the viewpoint of a clinician it is often a difficult and challenging task to analyze and predict the nature of the primary disorder. In the following sections, a detailed status report of each of the disease states shown in Fig. 13-3 or Table 13-3 is discussed in relation to its interaction with vitamin D. Table 13-4 lists recently published reports related to studies on vitamin D metabolism and action in man. It is apparent from the vast scope of subjects listed—from the vitamin D content of human milk to vitamin D and ischemic heart disease—that the endocrine system for vitamin D is a topic of concern for many clinicians.

E. Clinical Applications of Vitamin D Metabolites

With the isolation and chemical characterization of the vitamin D metabolites, followed by their chemical synthesis, a whole new era of vitamin D-related clinical study was initiated. In view of the numerous vitamin D-related human disease states, clinicians were eager to test the therapeutic efficacy of the new vitamin D metabolites. Since the causes of many of these diseases are not clearly defined, it has been difficult to precisely determine in advance which metabolite or analog would be most effective in which abnormality. Thus, the data currently available must be considered only provisional.

Table 13-5 summarizes many of the clinical trials employing $25(OH)D_3$. Since $25(OH)D_3$ was the first metabolite discovered (1968) it is surprising that it has not been more widely evaluated. However, this may be due to the fact that there

TABLE 13-4
Studies on Vitamin D Metabolism and Action in Man

Subject of paper	Reference
Absorption of vitamin D in normal individuals and patients with intestinal malabsorption	Thompson *et al.* (1966)
Skin pigment regulation of vitamin D biosynthesis in man	Loomis (1967)
Vitamin D and cardiovascular, renal, and brain damage in infancy	Seelig (1969)
Pharmacological activities of vitamin D	Yendt (1970)
Calcium-binding proteins in the duodenum of chick, rat, pig, and man	Hitchman and Harrison (1972)
Metabolism of [^{3}H]vitamin D_3 in normal, uremic, and anephric subjects	Schaefer *et al.* (1972)
Effect of combined therapy with sodium fluoride, vitamin D, and Ca in osteoporosis	Jowsey *et al.* (1972)
Treatment of osteoporosis with vitamin D_3	Buring *et al.* (1974)
Vitamin D—current clinical concepts	Avioli and Haddad (1973)
Role of kidney in metabolism of vitamin D	Coburn and Norman (1973)
Vitamin D deficiency among Asian immigrants to Britain	Preece *et al.* (1973)
Metabolism of vitamin D in relation to diseases of calcium homeostasis	Coburn *et al.* (1974)
Hazards of overuse of vitamin D	Food and Nutrition Board (1974)
Multiple sclerosis—vitamin D and Ca as environmental determinants of prevalence	Goldberg (1974a,b)
Metabolism of vitamin D and 25(OH)D in normal and anephric human beings	Gray *et al.* (1974)
Vitamin D—mode of action and biomedical applications	Haussler (1974)
Vitamin D and myocardial infarction	Linden (1974)
Plasma 25(OH)D levels in geriatric patients	Corless *et al.* (1975)
Fatal vitamin D intoxication	Laubenthal *et al.* (1975)
Vitamin D status after resection of the ileum in childhood	Preece and Valman (1975)
Ischemic heart disease and vitamin D	Seelig (1975)
Protracted vitamin D intoxication	Shetty *et al.* (1975)
Vitamin D and 25(OH)D requirements of the newborn	Wolf *et al.* (1975)
Dietary phosphate deprivation in women and men; effects of mineral, acid balances, PTH, and the metabolism of 25(OH)D	Dominguez *et al.* (1976)
Radioligand receptor assay for 25(OH)D and $1,25(OH)_2D$ and its application to hypervitaminosis D	Hughes *et al.* (1976)
Vitamin D and $25(OH)D_3$ inhibition of cholesterol biosynthesis	Philippot *et al.* (1976)
Familial hypophosphatemic rickets	Walton (1976)
Lack of effect of chronic metabolic acidosis on 25(OH)D metabolism and serum iPTH in human beings	Weber *et al.* (1976)
Effects of oral Ca and vitamin D in osteoporosis	Riggs *et al.* (1976)
Metabolic fate of $1,25(OH)_2[^3H]D_3$ in normal and hypoparathyroid patients	Mawer *et al.* (1976)

(*continued*)

TABLE 13-4 (*Continued*)

Subject of paper	Reference
Vitamin D in human milk	Lakdawala and Widdowson (1977)
$25(OH)D_3$ to $1,25(OH)_2D_3$—conversion impaired by systemic metabolic acidosis	Lee *et al.* (1977)
Altered vitamin D metabolism in pregnancy	Turton *et al.* (1977)
Absorption, hydroxylation, and excretion of vitamin D in biliary cirrhosis	Krawitt *et al.* (1977)
Anticonvulsant drugs and rickets	Stiles and Odland (1977)
Comparison of plasma 25(OH)D in hospitalized and normal adults	Fridez *et al.* (1977)
Correlation between vitamin D intake, sunlight exposure, and plasma levels of $25(OH)D_3$	Nayal *et al.* (1978)
Significance of plasma $25(OH)D_3$ levels in gastrointestinal disease	Schoen *et al.* (1978)
Hypophosphatemic nonrachitic bone disease	Scriver *et al.* (1977)
Lack of response to vitamin D therapy in a hypoparathyroid patient receiving anticonvulsants	Asherov *et al.* (1977)
Association of osteopetrosis and vitamin D-resistant rickets	Zamboni *et al.* (1977)
Oncogenic osteomalacia due to a $1,25(OH)_2D$ deficiency	Drezner and Feinglos (1977)
Calciopenic rickets in South Africa	Pettifor *et al.* (1978)
Vitamin D status of Asian infants	Singleton and Tucker (1978)
Sunlight, ozone, and vitamin D	Beadle (1977)
Evaluation of vitamin D metabolism in osteoporosis	Davies *et al.* (1977b)
Vitamin D status in different subgroups of British Asians	Neat *et al.* (1978)
Eczema, rickets, and food allergy	Bierman *et al.* (1978)
Clinical significance of disordered vitamin D metabolism (in German)	Flury (1978)

is no disease state in which it has been clearly established that $25(OH)D_3$ administration is more effective than vitamin D_3 administration. Since vitamin D is rapidly metabolized to $25(OH)D_3$ (see Chapter 6), any deficiency of $25(OH)D_3$ can probably be remedied by administration of vitamin D. It should be noted that clinically effective doses of $25(OH)D_3$ are large, of the order of 100 to 200 μg/day. It is not clear whether its effectiveness is due to increased substrate "pressure" on the renal $25(OH)D_3$ 1-hydroxylase and 24-hydroxylase or to the ability of elevated concentrations of $25(OH)D_3$ to serve as an analog of $1,25(OH)_2D_3$ by binding to its receptors. $25(OH)D_3$ is being developed by the Upjohn Company for commercial distribution in chronic renal failure.

With the discoveries of $1,25(OH)_2D_3$ and the fact that it is produced by the kidney, clinicians immediately were attracted to the concept that the absence of this steroid was the causative factor in calcium problems associated with chronic renal failure. Accordingly, many trials were initiated employing biologically synthesized $1,25(OH)_2D_3$ (Norman and Wong, 1972) and chemically synthesized $1\alpha(OH)D_3$ (Barton *et al.*, 1973). Initially it was felt that $1,25(OH)_2D_3$ would be

TABLE 13-5
Clinical Studies with $25(OH)D_3$

Disease state	Dosage (μg/day)	Duration	*n*	Comment	Reference
Chronic renal failure	250	2 weeks	1	Improved intestinal Ca absorption	DeLuca and Avioli (1970)
VDRR			5		Earp *et al.* (1970)
Hypoparathyroidism	15–125		6		Pak *et al.* (1970)
VDRR			—		Seely *et al.* (1970)
VDRR	50–150				Pak *et al.* (1972)
Vitamin D-dependent rickets					Rosen and Finberg (1972)
VDRR			3		Balsan and Garabedian (1972)
Chronic renal failure			8	Evaluated by quantitative histology	Bordier *et al.* (1975)
Chronic renal failure	100	1–12 weeks	10	Compared with $1\alpha(OH)D_3$	Fournier *et al.* (1975a,b)
Chronic renal failure			10		Slatopolsky *et al.* (1975)
Vitamin D deficiency			2	Compared with $1,25(OH)_2D_3$	Koch *et al.* (1975)
Cushing's syndrome	50–100	15–30 days	4	$25(OH)D_3$ treatment improved intestinal Ca absorption	Caniggia and Gennari (1974)
Osteoporosis, steroid induced				Reduction of osteopenia	B. Hahn and Hahn (1976), T. Hahn and Hahn (1976)
Normal subjects	100–1000	1 day	27	Measured plasma kinetics of 25(OH)D	Haddad and Rojanasathit (1976)
Chronic renal failure	40–100	3–9 months	5	Extensive quantitative histology	Teitelbaum *et al.* (1976)
Chronic renal failure	25–200	6–24 months	5	Compared D_2 and $25(OH)D_3$; carried out quantitative histology	Witmer *et al.* (1976)
Chronic renal failure	86	29 weeks	63	Evaluated by quantitive histology	Frost *et al.* (1977), Recker *et al.* (1977)
Hypoparathyroidism	100–200	3–28 months	2		Parfitt (1977)
Chronic renal failure and normal subjects	20–1000	7–10 days	34	Carried out a dose–response study	Colodro *et al.* (1978)

TABLE 13-6
Clinical Studies with $1\alpha(OH)D_3$

Disease state	Dosage (μg/day)	Duration	*n*	Comment	Reference
Chronic renal failure	2.0	7 days	12	Evaluated jejunal and ileal Ca absorption	Marini *et al.* (1976)
Chronic renal failure	2.5–30	3–10 days	3	Elevated serum Ca	Chalmers *et al.* (1973)
Chronic renal failure	1.0–4.0	6–260 days	8	Roentgenographic improvement noted	Chan *et al.* (1975)
Chronic renal failure	4.0	1–12 weeks	10	Compared with $25(OH)D_3$	Fournier *et al.* (1975a,b)
Chronic renal failure	2.5–10.0	1–3 weeks	3	Improved intestinal Ca absorption	Hirooka *et al.* (1975)
Vitamin D deficiency	0.5		2	Compared with $25(OH)D_3$	Kooh *et al.* (1975)
Chronic renal failure	1.5	1 year	4	Decrease in serum iPTH, positive Ca and P balance	Davies *et al.* (1976)
Chronic renal failure	0.25–10.0	7 months	3	Bone mineral content rose	Nielsen *et al.* (1976)
Chronic renal failure + anticonvulsant treatment	2–3	8 months	2	Anticonvulsant drugs may antagonize action of $1\alpha(OH)D_3$	Pierides *et al.* (1976)
Pseudohypoparathyroidism	0.5–1.0	10 months	1	Compared with $1,25(OH)_2D_3$	Werder *et al.* (1976)
Uremic and normal man		2–5 months	41	Compared with $1,25(OH)_2D_3$	Brickman *et al.* (1976)
Osteoporosis, senile	0.5–1.0	3 months	72		Lund *et al.* (1975)
Uremic and normal man	0.14–2.7	6–25 days	20	Measured effects on intestinal phosphorus absorption and compared with $1,25(OH)_2D_3$	Brickman *et al.* (1977)
Hypoparathyroidism	2–5	7 months	2	Restored serum Ca to normal	Jorgensen and Vogt (1977)
Chronic renal failure and magnesium metabolism	2.0	8–548 days	2	$1\alpha(OH)D_3$ has little effect on effect on intestinal Mg absorption	Kanis and Russell (1977)
Diseases resistant to vitamin D	1.0–2.0	6 months	14	Compared with $1,25(OH)_2D_3$	Kanis and Russell (1977)

TABLE 13-7
Clinical Studies with $1,25(OH)_2D_3$

Disease state	Dosage (μg/day)	Duration	*n*	Comment	Reference
Chronic renal failure	2.7	6–10 days	3	Intestinal Ca absorption increased	Brickman *et al.* (1972)
Chronic renal failure	2.5	25 days	5	Intestinal Ca absorption and Ca balance increased	Brickman *et al.* (1973a)
Hypophosphatemic VDRR	1.3–2.7	5–15 days	4	Did not correct renal tubular resorption of phosphate	Brickman *et al.* (1973b), Glorieux *et al.* (1973)
Chronic renal failure	0.027–2.7	7–16 days	12	Compared dose response in CRF and normal man	Coburn *et al.* (1973a)
Vitamin D-dependent rickets	0.5–1.0				Fraser *et al.* (1973)
Vitamin D-dependent rickets					Balsan and Garabedian (1974)
Chronic renal failure	0.027–2.7	7–16 days	12	Compared dose response in normal and CRF patient	Brickman *et al.* (1974a)
Chronic renal failure	0.14–0.68	8–17 weeks	8	Fall in plasma iPTH, bone biopsy analysis	Brickman *et al.* (1974a)
Chronic renal failure	0.37–2.7	4–150 days	11	Improvement of muscle myopathy	Henderson *et al.* (1974)

Chronic renal failure	0.7–2.7	4–8 days	11	Increased serum Ca	Russell *et al.* (1974a)
Hypoparathyroidism	0.67–2.7	25–50 days	2	Compared to $1\alpha(OH)D_3$	Russell *et al.* (1974b)
Chronic renal failure	0.54–1.35	28	2	Evaluation of effects on osteomalacia (dose given iv)	Eastwood *et al.* (1975)
Chronic renal failure	1.0–2.0	5 months	1	Patient with medullary cystic disease	Silverberg *et al.* (1975)
Pseudohypoparathyroidism	0.5–1.0	10 months	1	Compared with $1\alpha(OH)D_3$	Werder *et al.* (1976)
Normal adults	0.14–5.4	7–12 days	41	Comprehensive study, compared with $1\alpha(OH)D_3$	Brickman *et al.* (1974c, 1976)
Chronic renal failure	0.14–5.4	2–5 months	72	Comprehensive study, compared with $1\alpha(OH)D_3$	Brickman *et al.* (1974c, 1976)
Uremic and normal man	0.14–2.7	6–25 days	20	Measured effects on intestinal phosphate absorption and compared with $1\alpha(OH)D_3$	Brickman *et al.* (1977)
Hypoparathyroidism	0.25–1.0	4–24 months	8	Restoration of normal serum Ca	Davies *et al.* (1977a)
Diseases resistant to vitamin D	1.0–2.0	6 months	14	Compared with $1\alpha(OH)D_3$	Kanis and Russell (1977)
Idiopathic hypoparathyroidism in children	0.5–0.8	6–14 months	3	Achieved normocalcemia	Rosen *et al.* (1977)
Childhood renal osteodystrophy	0.25–0.6	7–26 months	6	Remineralization of bone; increase in growth velocity	Chesney *et al.* (1978)

TABLE 13-8
Clinical Trials with 25(OH)-5,6-*trans*-D_3

Disease state	Dosage[a] (μg/day)	Duration	*n*	Comment	Reference
Chronic renal failure	2.5 iv	6 days	5	Increased intestinal Ca absorption and elevated serum Ca	von Herrath *et al*. (1973a)
Chronic renal failure	5–12	13 days	8	Increased intestinal Ca absorption and elevated serum Ca	von Herrath *et al*. (1973b)
Chronic renal failure	50	9–11 months	10	Elevated serum Ca	Schulz *et al*. (1975)
Prednisolone-treated patients	100	4 weeks	7	Increased intestinal Ca absorption	Miravet *et al*. (1977)
Chronic renal failure	450	14 days	7	Increased serum Ca	Kraft and Offermann (1977)
Hypoparathyroidism	450	14 days	9	Increased intestinal Ca absorption	Kraft and Offermann (1977)
Chronic renal failure	500	14 months	58	Bone mineral content increased	Samizadeh *et al*. (1977)
Hypoparathyroidism	250–500	2–3 weeks	3	Normalized serum Ca	Kruse and Offermann (1977)
Chronic renal failure	12–200	31 weeks	73	Bone histology remained static or improved in 79% of subjects	Grigoleit *et al*. (1977)

[a] Doses unless indicated were administered orally.

"too expensive" to synthesize on a scale required to support widespread clinical usage. However, Uskokovic and co-workers at Hoffmann-La Roche (Nutley, New Jersey) (Partridge *et al.*, 1974; Narwid *et al.*, 1974) made a major breakthrough with their route of chemical synthesis of 1,25$(OH)_2D_3$ (see Chapter 5). Their method is capable of supplying 1,25$(OH)_2D_3$ on the kilogram scale required to support worldwide clinical and veterinarian usage of this steroid. 1,25$(OH)_2D_3$ preparations produced by Hoffmann-La Roche have been approved by the U.S. Food and Drug Administration for use in chronic renal failure.

Table 13-6 summarizes the clinical trials with 1α(OH)D_3; this vitamin D analog is commercially available in Europe from Leo Laboratories and in Japan from Teijin Pharmaceuticals, Ltd. Table 13-7 summarizes the clinical trials with 1,25$(OH)_2D_3$. Both 1α(OH)D_3 and 1,25$(OH)_2D_3$ are biologically active in doses of 0.25 to 1.0 μg/day. As discussed in Chapter 6 it has been established that the analog 1α(OH)D_3 is metabolized to the natural steroid hormone 1,25$(OH)_2D_3$. To date the principal clinical application of both of these steroids has been in chronic renal failure and hypoparathyroidism. It is to be anticipated, however, that their use in the treatment of many other vitamin D-related diseases will be evaluated in the near future.

The pseudo 1α analog 25(OH)-5,6-*trans*-D_3 (structure **43** in Fig. 5-9) has also been clinically evaluated, particularly with respect to chronic renal failure. The chemical synthesis of 25(OH)-5,6-*trans*-D_3 is relatively simple and inexpensive since it can be produced by isomerizing 25(OH)D_3. Doses of 50 to 600 μg/day were required to obtain biological responses in man. Schaefer *et al.* (1974) studied the tissue distribution of 25(OH)-5,6-*trans*-[26,27-^{3}H]D_3 in the rat whereas Offermann *et al.* (1975) studied the pharmacokinetics of the pseudo 1α-OH analog in man. In comparison to 25(OH)D_3, the half-life was shorter and serum levels were lower after oral or intravenous doses of tritiated 25(OH)-5,6-*trans*-D_3. This vitamin D analog is now available commercially in Europe from the Albert–Roussel Pharma GMBH. Table 13-8 summarizes the clinical trials conducted with 25(OH)-5,6-*trans*-D_3.

II. HUMAN DISEASE STATES RELATED TO VITAMIN D

The remainder of this chapter is devoted to a topic-by-topic evaluation of the human disease states known, presumed, or postulated to be related to vitamin D (see Fig. 13-3).

A. Liver

1. Cirrhosis and Obstructive Jaundice

The liver is involved in several important aspects of vitamin D function in man. Principally, the liver is the site of 25-hydroxylation of vitamin D. However, the liver also is the source of bile salts, which may be important in the intestinal absorption of dietary sources of vitamin D. It is also believed to be the site of binding or association of both vitamin D_3 and $25(OH)D_3$ to their specific plasma carrier proteins, and it is possible that these binding proteins are actually synthesized in the liver. Thus, any kind of hepatic malfunction may potentially interfere not only with the metabolism of vitamin D but also with its absorption and subsequent plasma transport. Atkinson *et al.* (1956) reported on the malabsorption of calcium and the associated bone disease that are present in prolonged obstructive jaundice. Similar reports of bone disease and calcium absorption in primary biliary cirrhosis were described by Kehayoglou *et al.* (1968). The latter investigators noted a poor response to vitamin D in subjects with primary biliary cirrhosis. Thompson *et al.* (1966) found that bile salts were essential for the normal absorption of both the vitamin and calcium in clinical studies of patients with cirrhosis in which radioactive vitamin D was employed. Avioli *et al.* (1967a) studied the metabolism of radioactive vitamin D both in normal man and in cirrhosis and found that there was a delayed disappearance in the plasma of radioactive vitamin D in patients with a hepatocellular dysfunction. In contrast, Krawitt *et al.* (1977) found that patients with primary biliary cirrhosis had no impairment of their 25-hydroxylation process but had an increased urinary excretion of vitamin D-related breakdown products in comparison to control normal subjects. Also, Haddad and Chyu (1971) reported reduced plasma levels of 25(OH)D in patients with biliary cirrhosis. Thus, it would appear that cirrhosis is capable of interfering both with the intestinal absorption of vitamin D and its subsequent metabolism to 25(OH)D. This hypothesis is consistent with the observation of Avioli and Haddad (1973), who found an immediate improvement in subjects treated with $25(OH)D_3$.

2. *Metabolism Induced by Drugs (Particularly Anticonvulsants)*

Recently, evidence has accumulated that prolonged use of anticonvulsant drugs such as diphenylhydantoin or phenobarbital may lead to an impaired response to vitamin D as determined by the appearance of rickets and osteomalacia. Significant hypocalcemia and hyperphosphatasia have been reported in 20–30% of the epileptic population (Hahn *et al.*, 1972a,b; Dent *et al.*, 1970; Richens and Rowe, 1970; Hunter *et al.*, 1971; Borgstedt *et al.*, 1972; Stamp *et al.*, 1972). The studies of Dent *et al.* (1970), who obtained bone biopsies, clearly demonstrated the existence of rampant osteomalacia; these workers further noted that the osteomalacia responded to simple dietary vitamin D supplementation.

From studies with experimental animals it has been inferred that chronic administration of phenobarbital or diphenylhydantoin may stimulate the levels of hepatic microsomal cytochrome *P*-450 enzymes; this then could lead to an erroneous catabolism of $25(OH)D_3$ and induction of a vitamin D deficiency with resulting osteomalacia (Hahn *et al.*, 1972b; Norman *et al.*, 1976). However, the situation is possibly more complicated than was first proposed. In more recent studies Norman *et al.* (1976) administered to rachitic chicks a chronic dose of phenobarbital for 2 weeks and then evaluated the biological response as well as the metabolism of vitamin D to $25(OH)D_3$ and $1,25(OH)_2D_3$. We noted that prior chronic administration of phenobarbital impaired or greatly blunted the biological response (intestinal calcium transport and bone calcium mobilization) to small physiological doses of both vitamin D and $25(OH)D_3$. Furthermore, this inhibition could be overcome by the administration of small quantities of $1,25(OH)_2D_3$. These results suggest that the metabolism and/or action not only of vitamin D but also of $25(OH)D_3$ might be impaired in situations of chronic anticonvulsant treatment. These results, however, are not in agreement with the report of Jubiz *et al.* (1977), who evaluated circulating levels of $1,25(OH)_2D_3$ in normal individuals as well as those receiving chronic anticonvulsants. They noted no differences in the circulating level of the hormonally active form of vitamin D. It is apparent that further work is needed in order to resolve at the biochemical and molecular levels the specific effects of chronic anticonvulsant treatment on the vitamin D endocrine system. However, in view of the widespread use of anticonvulsants, various sedatives, tranquilizers, and oral antidiabetic compounds, all of which are capable of inducing increased microsomal cytochrome *P*-450 hydroxylase activity (Conney, 1967), it is apparent that there is a large potential for the development of a number of drug-induced vitamin D-deficient states.

B. Kidney

1. Chronic Renal Disease

a. Etiology. Chronic renal failure (CRF) characteristically involves severe derangements in skeletal metabolism and in the homeostatic control of calcium, inorganic phosphate, and magnesium. Chronic renal insufficiency also is an important pathophysiological state believed to adversely affect the metabolism of vitamin D (Avioli *et al.*, 1968, 1970; Kimberg *et al.*, 1970; Kleeman *et al.*, 1967; Liu and Chu, 1943; Lumb *et al.*, 1971). Although an association between renal disease, skeletal abnormalities, and hyperplasia of the parathyroid glands has been known for several decades, the incidence and clinical significance of abnormalities of divalent ion metabolism, soft-tissue calcification, and osseous pathology has become even more clearly recognized with the advent of renal transplantation, hemodialysis, and improved therapy of individuals with renal failure (Rubini *et al.*, 1969). The term "renal osteodystrophy" has been used to denote the skeletal abnormalities occurring in patients with chronic renal failure. These include growth retardation, osteitis fibrosa, osteomalacia, osteoporosis, and osteosclerosis. Hyperphosphatemia, hypocalcemia, and secondary hyperparathyroidism have been considered by some to play a major role in the pathogenesis of the deranged divalent ion metabolism characteristic of uremia. Many of the clinically identifiable symptoms of chronic renal insufficiency are similar to those present in vitamin D deficiency and include an impaired gastrointestinal absorption of calcium, parathyroid overactivity, e.g., hyperparathyroidism, and an acquired resistance to the biological actions of physiological levels of vitamin D as well as a steadily progressive form of bone disease (Stanbury and Lumb, 1962; Dent *et al.*, 1961; Follis, 1950). The bone disease is also characterized by maturational defects in both collagen and mineral metabolism (Russell and Avioli, 1972). A list of pertinent papers relating calcium, vitamin D, and chronic renal failure is given in Table 13-9.

As shown in Fig. 13-4 one of the hallmarks of patients with chronic renal failure is marked malabsorption of intestinal calcium. The first example of this malabsorption was found by Liu and Chu (1943), who reported a negative calcium balance in patients suffering from renal insufficiency. In patients with renal failure, diminished intestinal absorption of calcium has been suggested by results of metabolic balance studies which indicated that fecal calcium levels were equal to or exceeded the levels of calcium ingested in the diet (Stanbury and Lumb, 1962; Liu and Chu, 1943; Dent *et al.*, 1961). With the use of radioisotopic methods, the intestinal absorption of calcium was found by numerous investigators to be reduced in uremic patients (Kaye and Silverman, 1965; Ogg, 1968; Coburn *et al.*, 1973a,b,c). De Wardener and colleagues (McDonald *et al.*, 1964; Clarkson *et al.*, 1973) found that such an impaired intestinal absorption can to some degree to minimized or overcome by a very large dietary intake of calcium. Despite this apparent inconsistency, however, most studies carried out to date show an impaired absorption of calcium in uremic patients, particularly when they are evaluated while receiving their usual calcium intake (Coburn *et al.*, 1973a,b,c). Thus, as shown in Fig. 13-1, it is quite apparent that, despite the level of habitual dietary intake of calcium, patients with chronic renal failure have a highly significant malabsorption of this cation.

Figure 13-2 (Stanbury and Lumb, 1962) illustrates that patients with chronic renal failure also have an inhibition of intestinal phosphate absorption. Since it is not known at present whether the molecular pathway for phosphate absorption is completely independent of that of calcium, it is not clear whether the malabsorption of this anion in chronic renal failure is a direct indication of malfunctioning of vitamin D or is related in some complex fashion to the mishandling of calcium. cium.

The concept that uremia may impair the response to vitamin D was pioneered by Liu and Chu (1943), who found no improvement of osteomalacia or calcium absorption in uremic patients treated with the usual oral doses of vitamin D.

TABLE 13-9
Papers Relating Calcium, Vitamin D, and Chronic Renal Failure

Subject of paper	Reference
Studies of Ca and P metabolism with special reference to pathogenesis and effect of DHT and iron	Liu and Chu (1943)
Divalent ion metabolism and osteodystrophy in CRF	Kleeman *et al.* (1967)
Metabolic fate of vitamin D in CRF	Avioli *et al.* (1968)
Osteodystrophy developing spontaneously in the course of CRF	Stanbury *et al.* (1969)
Nature of vitamin D resistance of patients with CRF	Avioli *et al.* (1970)
Effect of renal insufficiency on the active transport of calcium by the small intestine	Baerg *et al.* (1970)
Plasma PTH, Ca, and P in patients with CRF	Genuth *et al.* (1970)
Nature of vitamin D resistance in experimental uremia	Kimberg *et al.* (1970)
Causes of hypocalcemia in CRF	Cochran and Nordin (1971)
Skeletal complications of kidney disease	Crutchlow and David (1971)
Etiology of hyperparathyroidism and bone disease during chronic hemodialysis	Fournier *et al.* (1971); Goldsmith *et al.* (1973)
Metabolic fate of tritiated 25(OH)D in normal, uremic, and rachitic rats	Schaefer *et al.* (1971)
Effects of DHT on calcium absorption in uremia	Kaye and Sagar (1972)
Renal osteodystrophy; pathogenesis, clinical features, and treatment	Massry and Coburn (1972)
Serum PTH levels and renal handling of phosphorus in patients with CRF	Popovitzer *et al.* (1972)
Dihydrotachysterol and vitamin D resistance in renal failure	Sagar *et al.* (1972)
Hypocalcemia and bone disease in renal failure	Cochran *et al.* (1973)
Contrasting effects on bone histology of vitamin D and calcium carbonate in osteomalacia of CRF	Eastwood *et al.* (1973)
Calcium metabolism of brain in acute renal failure	Arieff and Massry (1974)
Role of the kidney and vitamin D metabolism in health and disease	Norman and Henry (1974)
Influence of dialysate calcium concentration and vitamin D on iPTH during repetitive dialysis	Bouillon *et al.* (1974)
Vitamin D intoxication in an anephric child	Counts *et al.* (1975)
Disappearance of vascular calcifications during treatment of CRF	Verberckmoes *et al.* (1975)
Vitamin D metabolism in CRF	Wake and Maddock (1975)
Evaluation of 25(OH)D, PTH, and digitoxin levels in patients with chronic hemofiltration	Schaefer *et al.* (1977)
	Schaefer *et al.* (1977)
Vitamin D metabolism in the nephrotic syndrome	Barragry *et al.* (1977)
A diuretic effect of $1,25(OH)_2D_3$	Andrea *et al.* (1977)
Vitamin D resistance in osteomalacia after uretosigmoidostomy	Perry *et al.* (1977)

However, the intestinal malabsorption of calcium could be overcome to some degree by the administration of enormous levels of vitamin D, e.g., 100,000–300,000 IU (2.5–7.5 mg) per day (Stanbury and Lumb, 1962; Dent *et al.*, 1961). With this increased absorption of calcium, the rickets or osteomalacia of chronic renal failure is generally overcome. Such observations led to the speculation that the intestinal absorptive mechanism for calcium was unresponsive unless the

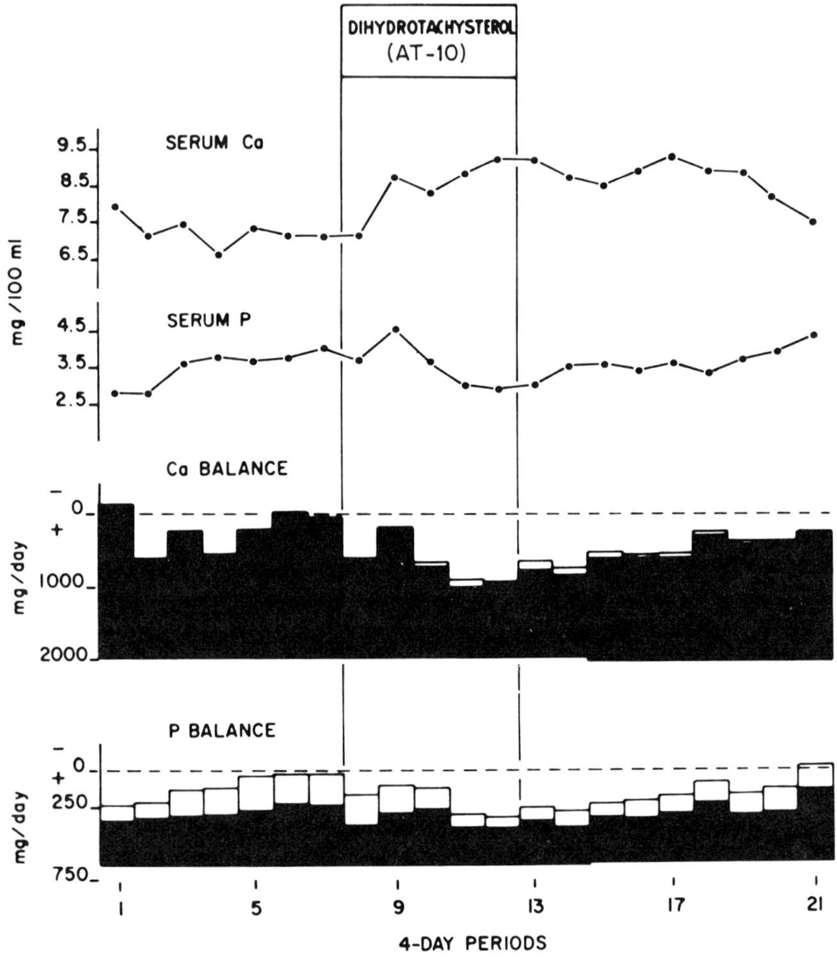

Figure 13-4. Metabolic balance changes and serum changes of calcium and phosphorus in a patient with advanced renal failure who was treated with dihydrotachysterol. Fecal losses are designated by solid columns, and urinary excretion is represented by open columns. Data adapted from Liu and Chu (1943).

total vitamin D "activity" in the plasma was increased to very high levels (Stanbury *et al.*, (1969).

Studies have been carried out to explore experimentally the cause or pathogenesis of abnormal vitamin D action in uremia with the resulting intestinal malabsorption of calcium. Avioli and co-workers (1967a,b) originally suggested that the turnover of vitamin D itself proceeds unusually rapidly in uremic subjects. Plasma levels of $25(OH)D_3$ were claimed to be lower in uremic rats than in pair-fed sham-operated controls (Russell and Avioli, 1972). In contrast, Lumb *et al.* (1971) and Mawer and co-workers (1971) compared the metabolism of [^{3}H]- or [^{14}C]vitamin D_3 in normal subjects and in uremic patients; they concluded that the production and turnover of $25(OH)D_3$ were normal in both groups.

In further support of this view are the observations by Avioli and Haddad (1973), Shen *et al.*, (1973), and Bec *et al.* (1972) that there is no difference in the circulating plasma level of 25(OH)D in the serum of uremic patients as compared with normal individuals. The weight of available evidence favors the view that defective production of 25(OH)D is not primarily responsible for impaired calcium absorption in osteomalacia and in uremia.

A major breakthrough was accomplished not only in the understanding of the mode of action of vitamin D but also in the understanding of the pathogenesis of many of the abnormalities of chronic renal failure with the discovery that the kidney was the site of conversion of $25(OH)D_3$ to $1,25(OH)_2D_3$. It then became highly plausible that the abnormal calcium metabolism of patients with renal failure might be due to an impaired renal production of this steroid hormone. Considerable data are consistent with this postulation. Investigators in several laboratories showed that nephrectomized rats failed to produce $1,25(OH)_2D_3$ (Gray *et al.*, 1971; Wong *et al.*, 1972). Also consistent with this were the metabolic studies of Mawer *et al.* (1973) and Schaefer *et al.* (1972), who administered mixed doses of [1,2-^{3}H,4-^{14}C]vitamin D to patients with either normal renal function or chronic renal failure; they noted no "tritium loss" in anephric or uremic individuals.[2]

Also, Piel *et al.* (1973) found a metabolite of vitamin D_3 that they claimed to be identical to $1,25(OH)_2D_3$ in the plasma of uremic children who had undergone successful renal transplantation, whereas this metabolite was absent prior to the surgical procedure.

The steroid radiocompetition assay of Haussler and associates (see Table 8-7) has clearly documented the reduction of plasma levels of $1,25(OH)_2D_3$ that occur in chronic renal failure. In normal man the circulating level of $1,25(OH)_2D$ is of the order of 30 to 35 pg/ml, whereas in chronic renal failure the levels fall significantly to 3–6 pg/ml.

b. Vitamin D Metabolite Treatment (Short and Long Term). One of the most dramatic and satisfying aspects of the elucidation of the metabolism of vitamin D and its endocrine system has been the application of this new knowledge to treatment of the calcium disorders associated with renal osteodystrophy.

[2]When hydroxylation occurs in the metabolism of $25(OH)D_3$ to $1,25(OH)_2D_3$, displacement of the hydrogen from the specific carbon position in the α-orientation occurs; hence, the radioactive hydrogen at the 1α position is "lost" during the hydroxylation process and when compared to a reference level of ^{14}C can be quantitated as "tritium loss."

Over 30 years ago Liu and Chu (1943) demonstrated that dihydrotachysterol (DHT) was effective in patients with renal disease, whereas vitamin D_3 was not. Some of their original data are reproduced in Fig. 13-4. These early observations were confirmed and extended by Kaye *et al.* (1970). Not only has DHT been used since the 1940's for treatment of certain patients with renal failure, it was earlier marketed under the name of Hytakerol or AT-10 (antitetany compound 10) and was noted for its hypercalcemic actions. With the chemical characterization of $1,25(OH)_2D_3$ and specific insight into the location of the hydroxyl group introduced by the kidney as being in the 1α configuration, it became clear why DHT was capable of ameliorating some of the problems of calcium metabolism associated with chronic renal failure. It is now apparent that DHT satisfies certain structural requirements provided by $1,25(OH)_2D_3$. Thus, when the "A" ring of DHT (see Fig. 5-8) is rotated, the 3β-hydroxyl group of DHT is in a position equivalent to the 1α-hydroxyl group of $1,25(OH)_2D_3$. The hydroxyl at C-3 of DHT has a stereochemical orientation similar to that of the 1-hydroxyl of $1,25(OH)_2D_3$ and is commonly referred to as a "pseudo 1α-hydroxyl." It was not long before other "pseudo 1 analogs" were produced, e.g., 5,6-*trans*-vitamin D_3 and 25(OH)-5,6-*trans*-D_3, which also functioned in a manner similar to that proposed for DHT. Another analog of $1,25(OH)_2D_3$, which was synthesized relatively early in comparison with the steroid hormone, is $1\alpha(OH)D_3$. The chemical synthesis of $1\alpha(OH)D_3$ is much more difficult than the isomerization reactions used to rotate the A ring of vitamin D (as in 5,6-*trans*-D_3).

It was quickly shown by a number of researchers that those analogs containing either a 1α-hydroxyl group or a "pseudo 1α-hydroxyl group" were capable of producing biological actions characteristic of vitamin D in the absence of the kidney; (Holick *et al.*, 1972a,b, 1973). Thus, $1\alpha(OH)D_3$, and 25(OH)-5,6-*trans*-D_3 were both shown to stimulate intestinal calcium transport and bone calcium mobilization in anephric rats. Results of such studies suggested that a number of natural and synthetic analogs might eventually be useful in rectifying some of the calcium disorders of chronic renal failure.

Coburn and co-workers pioneered experiments evaluating the clinical efficacy of $1,25(OH)_2D_3$, $1\alpha(OH)D_3$, and $25(OH)D_3$ in chronic renal failure (Brickman *et al.*, 1972, 1973a, 1974a,b,c, 1975; Coburn *et al.*, 1972; Brickman and Norman, 1973). Initially their efforts focused on evaluation of short-term effects, i.e., under circumstances in which physiological levels (0.25–1.0 μg/day) were given for approximately 1 week. Because results of these studies were so encouraging it was possible to extend the periods of treatment to 6–12 months.

Figure 13-5 compares the stimulatory effects of $1,25(OH)_2D_3$ on intestinal calcium absorption in normal individuals and in patients with chronic renal failure, and Fig. 13-6 presents similar data for serum calcium elevation. It is quite apparent that $1,25(OH)_2D_3$ is remarkably effective in stimulating intestinal absorption of calcium both in normal man and the patients with uremia. The

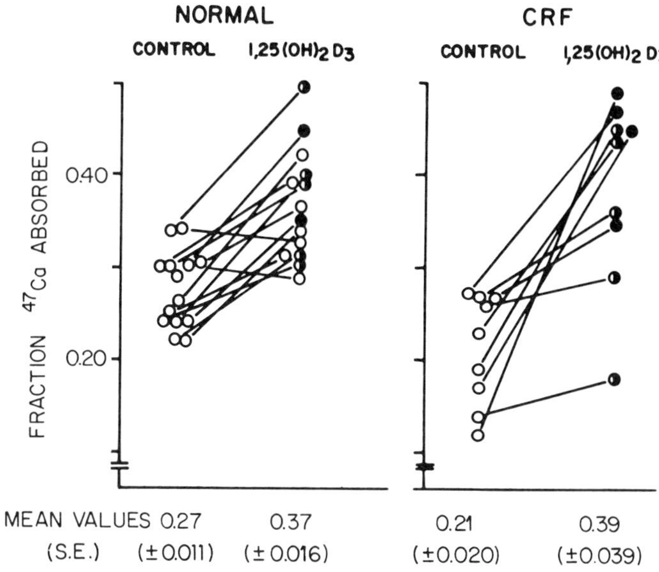

Figure 13-5. Stimulation of intestinal calcium absorption by $1,25(OH)_2D_3$ in normal and uremic man. (From Coburn *et al.*, 1974, with permission).

fractional stimulation of intestinal calcium absorption in uremic patients is usually significantly greater than that in normal control subjects ingesting an equivalent amount of dietary calcium. Before treatment, intestinal absorption of ^{47}Ca was significantly lower in the uremic patients; however, after treatment with 0.14, 0.68, and 2.7 μg/day $1,25(OH)_2D_3$ in normal subjects and 0.68 and 2.7 μg/day of $1,25(OH)_2D_3$ in patients with chronic renal failure, the mean values for the two groups were the same (Fig. 13-5). These results are compared to increases (not shown) in the mean absorption from 0.17 ± 0.015 to 0.19 ± 0.19 and from 0.25 ± 0.012 to 0.28 ± 0.16 in uremic patients and in normal patients, respectively, after 7 days of treatment with 40,000 IU (1 mg/day) of vitamin D_3.

The results of a metabolic balance study in a typical patient with chronic renal failure are shown in Fig. 13-7. During treatment with $1,25(OH)_2D_3$ there was an increased ^{47}Ca absorption with a concomitant fall in fecal calcium and phosphorus levels and a tendency toward positive balances for both calcium and phosphorus.

Comparative evaluations of the clinical efficacy of $1\alpha(OH)D_3$ and $1,25(OH)_2D_3$ were carried out by Coburn and co-workers (Brickman *et al.*, 1976) as well as by Kanis and Russell (1977). Figure 13-8 presents a dose–response study for intestinal calcium absorption in normal and uremic individuals given increasing daily doses of $1,25(OH)_2D_3$, $1\alpha(OH)D_3$, or $25(OH)D_3$. The

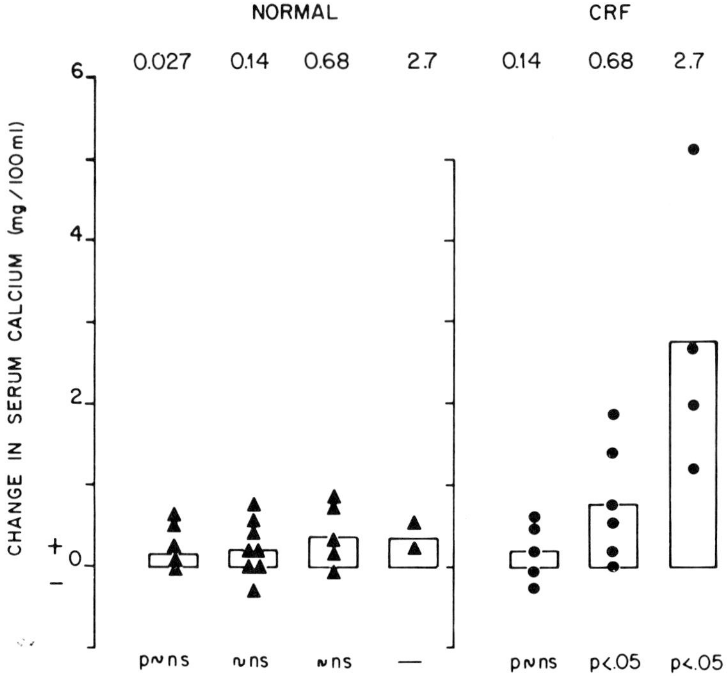

Figure 13-6. Changes in serum calcium levels in normal and uremic man in a dose-response study with $1,25(OH)_2D_3$. (Abstracted from work of Coburn *et al.*).

relative ratio of concentrations required for half-maximal stimulation are 1 : 5 : 700 in normal man and 1 : 3 : 500 in uremic man. When these values are compared with the relative biological activities derived from animal experiments reported by Boris *et al.* (1977), it is apparent that the biological activity of these three steroids in man is essentially identical to that established previously in animal studies. Clearly, $1,25(OH)_2D_3$ is the most biologically active steroid in uremic man.

There are several preliminary reports concerning the biological activity of both $24(R),25(OH)_2D_3$ and $1,24(R),25(OH)_3D_3$ in man. Kanis *et al.* (1977; 1978), Cundy *et al.* (1978), and Coburn and co-workers (Brickman *et al.*, 1978; Llach *et al.*, 1978) found, surprisingly, that doses of only 2 to 10 μg/day of $24(R),25(OH)_2D_3$ increased significantly intestinal calcium absorption in both normal and anephric subjects. Also, Cundy *et al.* (1978) found that $1,24(R),25(OH)_3D_3$ (up to 10 μg/day) given to normal subjects and patients with chronic renal failure had no consistent effect on intestinal calcium absorption. These studies suggest that $24,25(OH)_2D_3$ may have the capability of increasing intestinal calcium absorption and that in man, unlike animals, this effect is not

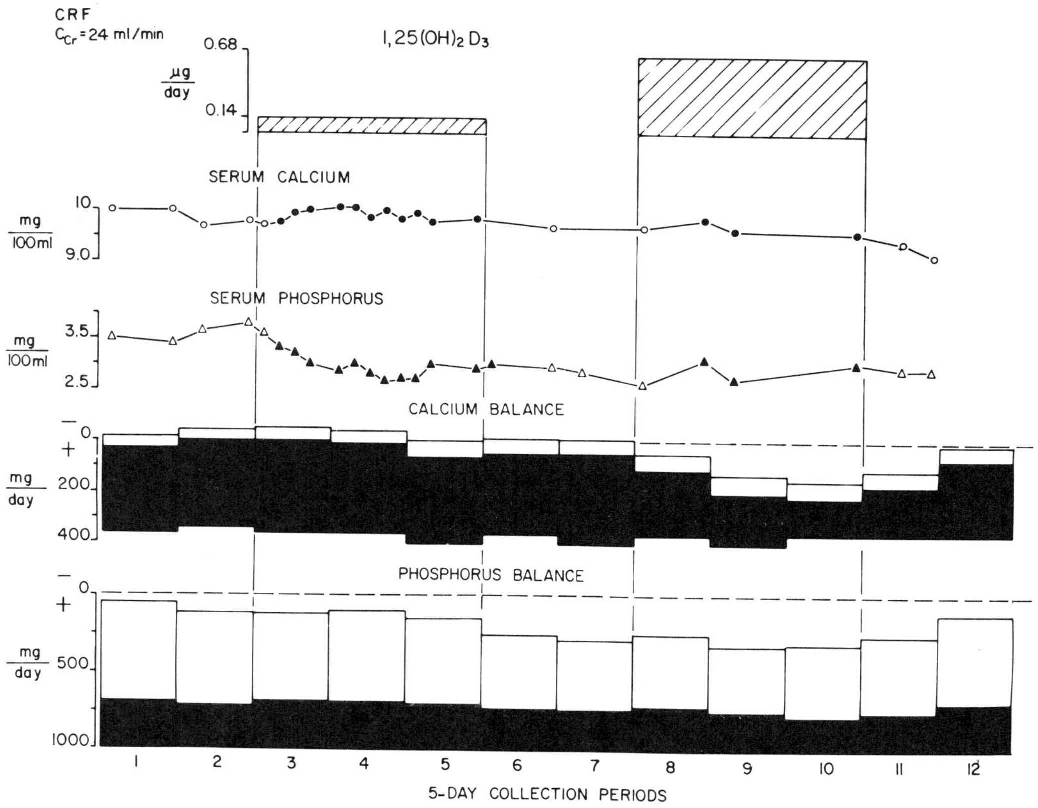

Figure 13-7. Metabolic balance study in a patient with advanced renal failure who received 0.14 and 0.68 μg $1,25(OH)_2D_3$, per day. Fecal mineral losses are designated by solid columns and urinary excretion by open columns. Reproduced by permission from Brickman *et al.* (1974b,c). C_{cr} = creatinine clearance.

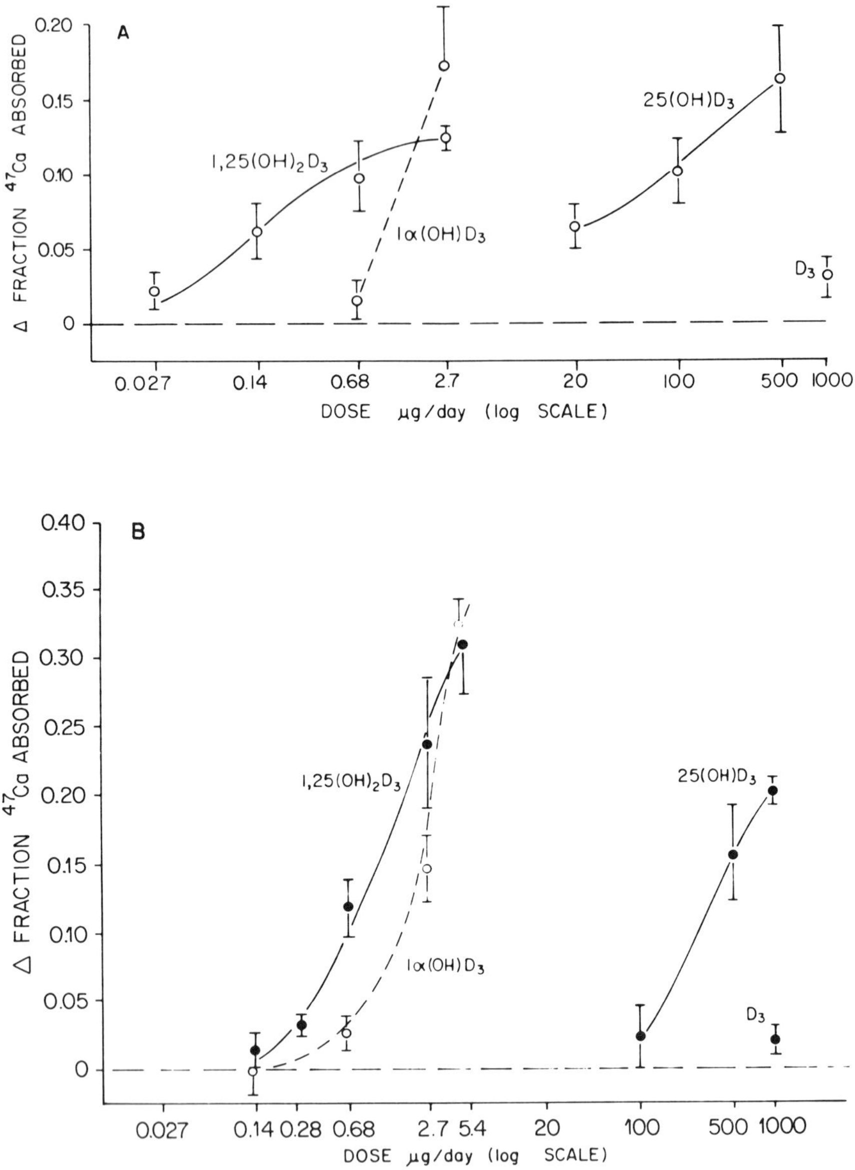

Figure 13-8. Comparative dose–response study of intestinal calcium absorption in (A) normal and (B) uremic individuals who were given 1,25(OH)$_2$D$_3$, 1α(OH)D$_3$, or 25(OH)D$_3$. (Summarized from studies of Coburn, Brickman, and Norman).

dependent on further 1α-hydroxylation or renal metabolism. However, much more work must be done to assess the clinical potential of $24(R),25(OH)_2D_3$ and $1,24,25(OH)_3D_3$. This is particularly so in light of the observations of Henry and Norman (1978) (discussed in section III,A) that demonstrate a biological role for $24,25(OH)_2D_3$.

There appear to be several instances in which $1\alpha(OH)D_3$ administration has resulted in hypercalcemia (Chalmers *et al.*, 1973; Brickman *et al.*, 1977). This may be due to the rather nonregulated metabolism of $1\alpha(OH)D_3$ to $1,25(OH)_2D_3$ (see Chapter 6). As one gives increasing doses of $1\alpha(OH)D_3$ there is, over a period of time, a slow buildup of tissue levels of this steroid. Then it is slowly and inexorably metabolized on a continuing basis to $1,25(OH)_2D_3$. In contrast, when $1,25(OH)_2D_3$ is administered alone it is cleared via normal endogenous metabolic mechanisms. It is now believed (Brickman *et al.*, 1977) that the most effective drug for management of the calcium disorders of renal osteodystrophy is $1,25(OH)_2D_3$.

Effects of $1,25(OH)_2D_3$ in patients with advanced renal failure include (a) a marked improvement in calcium and phosphorus balance, (b) enhancement of intestinal absorption of calcium, and (c) correction or improvement of hypocalcemia. In addition, Coburn *et al.* (1973a) indicated that such short-term treatment led to suppression of the levels of immunoreactive parathyroid hormone (iPTH) in uremic patients. However, these studies left unanswered the question of whether long-term treatment with $1,25(OH)_2D_3$ might cause a permanent reversal of the above parameters as well as effect remission of the skeletal lesions of renal osteodystrophy. To date there is only one published paper that addresses this important question. Skeletal abnormalities and plasma iPTH were evaluated by Brickman *et al.* (1974b) in eight patients with uremic osteodystrophy treated with 0.14–0.68 μg $1,25(OH)_2D_3$ per day for 8–17 weeks. Serum calcium levels increased in all patients but exceeded 10 mg/ml in only three; serum phosphorus changes were small and variable. Plasma iPTH levels decreased noticeably in six patients, reaching normal values in two. Bone biopsy showed a reduction in the resorptive surface for patients with skeletal lesions characteristic of secondary hyperparathyroidism. In one subject, marrow fibrosis decreased from 11.5 to 0.3%. In four persons with osteomalacic lesions predominating, osteoid width was reduced slightly in three and the calcification front improved in two. It was concluded on the basis of these observations that administration of small quantities of $1,25(OH)_2D_3$ to uremic patients can markedly reverse the hyperparathyroid manifestations of renal osteodystrophy and improve dramatically the lesions of osteomalacia.

Figure 13-9 emphasizes the dramatic ability of long-term (10–31 months) treatment with low levels of $1,25(OH)_2D_3$ to improve the extent of bone mineralization. Results such as these strikingly indicate the need for continuous availability of $1,25(OH)_2D_3$ to mediate and maintain normal skeletal metabolism.

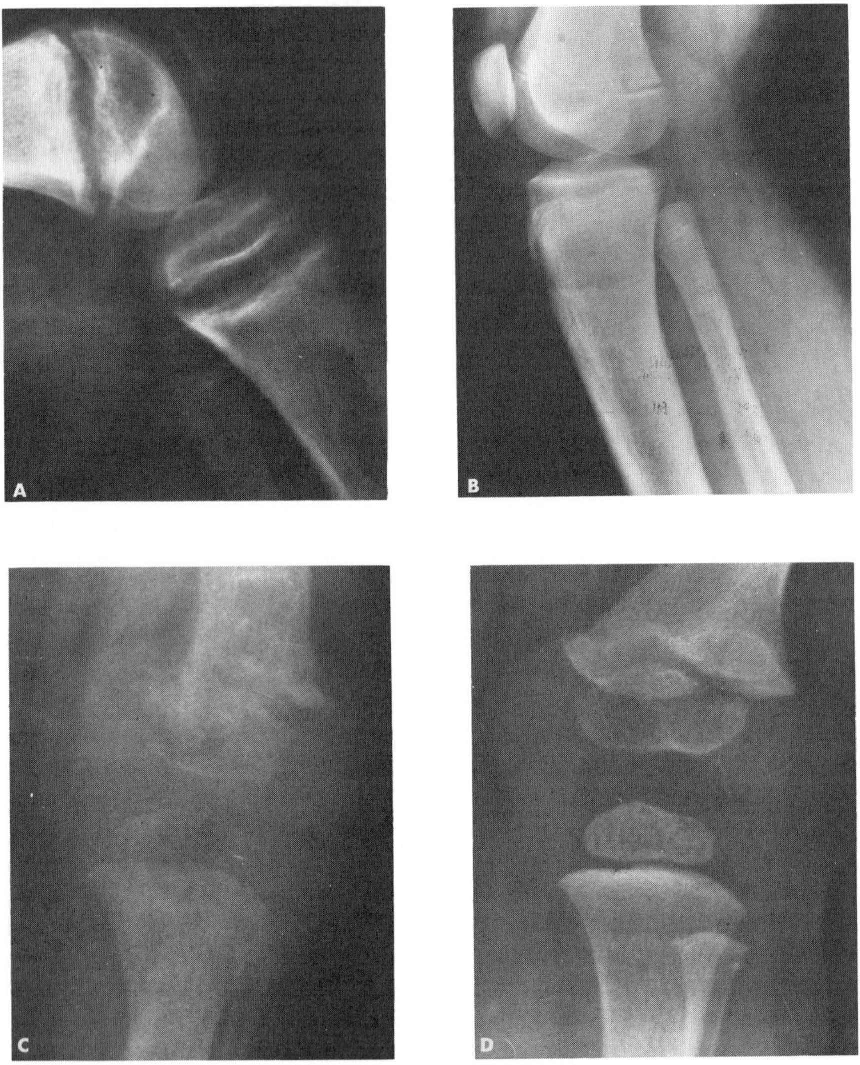

Figure 13-9. Effects of prolonged $1,25(OH)_2D_3$ therapy on X-ray appearance of long bones. A 14-year-old patient with autosomal dominant Fanconi syndrome before (A) and after (B) 31 months of therapy with 14–19 ng $1,25(OH)_2D_3$ per kilogram body weight per day. (See Chesney *et al.*, 1978, for a discussion.) A 3½-year-old boy with uremia secondary to posterior urethral valves before (C) and after (D) treatment for 10 months with $1,25(OH)_2D_3$. All figures were kindly provided by Dr. R. Chesney and are reproduced with his permission.

2. *Vitamin D-Resistant Rickets or Hypophosphatemic Rickets*

The second disease state that was originally thought to be directly related to an abnormality in the metabolism of vitamin D is the condition known as "vitamin D-resistant rickets" (VDRR). This term has been applied to a variety of clinical conditions detected during childhood because of the obvious growth retardation and skeletal deformities that are analogous to those present in rickets. These bony defects are unresponsive to normal or even massive quantities of vitamin D.

The primary clinically observable characteristic, aside from the skeletal abnormalities, is a diminished renal tubular reabsorption of phosphate (Winters *et al.*, 1958; Wilson *et al.*, 1965; Condon *et al.*, 1970; Barbour *et al.*, 1966; Burnett *et al.*, 1964). Those individuals who have VDRR are usually of short stature. Depending on the age of the individual, the bone disease is either rickets or osteomalacia. In a subject with rickets the disease usually appears between 6 months and 2 years of age. In other instances, it may defer its appearance until early adult life.

On the basis of analysis of the hypophosphatemia alone, all available genetic data, including sex ratio and segregation analysis, suggest that the disease is an X-linked dominant inheritance with complete penetrance. Males have usually been observed to have a more severe version of the skeletal disease than females, as would be predicted from the X-inactivation hypothesis of Winters. Winters *et al.* (1958) reviewed 65 documented cases of vitamin D-resistant rickets and presented evidence that the disease is almost always inherited and is usually congenital. In one instance only, the abnormality was found to follow a female sex-linked pattern wherein the females tended to have either mild deformities or no deformities whereas the males usually had moderate to severe deformities. More recently, Burnett *et al.* (1964) found that of 24 index cases eight individuals (five females and three males) were the only affected members of their respective kindreds. Such sporadic cases could conceivably be due to phenocopy, a phenomenon of an autosomal recessive trait, or to a new mutation. The same researchers felt that there were two instances in which they could identify new mutations. It was shown conclusively by Engfeldt *et al.* (1956), Villaneuva *et al.* (1966), Williams *et al.* (1960), Albright *et al.* (1937), and Harrison (1957, 1958) that individuals who have VDRR do not respond to treatment with physiological doses of vitamin D.

The hypophosphatemia of VDRR is believed to be due principally to a reduced renal tubular reabsorption of phosphate. There is disagreement as to whether decreased renal tubular reabsorption of phosphate is due to secondary overactivity of the parathyroid gland as a result of hypocalcemia or arises directly from an impairment in phosphate transport by the renal tubule. Some insight into these possibilities was obtained from measurements of the circulating levels of iPTH; however, there is no unanimity of agreement. Reitz and Weinstein (1973) as well as Lewy *et al.* (1972) reported elevated levels of iPTH in VDRR, whereas Arnaud *et al.* (1971) reported normal levels and Roof *et al.* (1973) reported reduced levels of iPTH in patients with VDRR.

Studies carried out in children with VDRR by Avioli *et al.* (1967a) employing preparations of tritiated vitamin D suggested some abnormalities in the metabolic patterns of vitamin D in these children in comparison to normal controls. However, with the knowledge that circulating levels of $25(OH)D_3$ were the same in untreated patients as in those with VDRR (Haddad *et al.*, 1973), it was suggested that the putative defect in vitamin D metabolism might occur at the metabolic sequence beyond the hepatic 25-hydroxylation.

There have been a number of reports describing attempts to clinically manage VDRR with the administration of $25(OH)D_3$. It was noted by Pak *et al.* (1972) that the impairment of intestinal calcium absorption in children with VDRR could be reversed by the administration of $25(OH)D_3$ (doses of 50 to 150 μg/day, but only limited success was achieved in terms of correction of the renal phosphate leak even with doses of $25(OH)D_3$ as high as 100–250 μg/day. Other clinical trials of $25(OH)D_3$ in VDRR have been carried out by Earp *et al.* (1970), Balsan and Garabedian (1972), and Seeley *et al.* (1970).

With the availability of $1,25(OH)_2D_3$ it was appropriate to evaluate the possibility that there is a defect in the production of $1,25(OH)_2D_3$ in VDRR. Brickman *et al.* (1973b) treated groups of patients with VDRR with doses of up to 2.7 μg/day of $1,25(OH)_2D_3$ and failed to correct the renal phosphate wasting, although there was a significant enhancement of intestinal calcium absorption.

Thus, current evidence suggests that VDRR is not due to an altered metabolism of vitamin D_3 to either $25(OH)D_3$ or $1,25(OH)_2D_3$ or to an impaired response of the intestine to the latter steroid. It is more likely that VDRR represents a specific defect in the tubular transport of phosphate.

3. Vitamin D-Dependent Rickets

The disease state known as vitamin D-dependent rickets, which was first recognized in 1961 by Prader *et al.*, is much less common than VDRR. This disorder differs from primary hypophosphatemic rickets (VDRR) in that hypocalcemia is regularly present and from nutritional rickets (a simple vitamin D deficiency) in that pharmacological doses of vitamin D are necessary to correct the osseous disease. Indeed, when afflicted children are treated with vitamin D_2 (10,000–50,000 IU/day), there is a correction of biochemical abnormalities, and even "catch-up" growth may occur. This disease state appears to have an autosomal recessive pattern of inheritance, as shown by the work of Prader *et al.* (1961) and Arnaud *et al.* (1970).

Current data suggest that this disease may arise from an altered metabolism of vitamin D at the renal level. Fraser *et al.* (1973) reported that a single patient with vitamin D-dependent rickets was highly responsive to physiological doses

(0.5–1.0 μg/day) of 1,25$(OH)_2D_3$. Similar results were obtained by Balsan and Garabedian (1974). This may be the first identified instance of a genetic mutation for a single metabolic step in the series of transformations required to convert vitamin D to its biologically active form. Consistent with these observations are the results of Rosen and Finberg (1972), who noted that a response could be obtained in patients with pseudo vitamin D deficiency rickets to much larger quantities of 25(OH)D_3. Thus, the 25(OH)D_3 was presumably acting as an analog of 1,25$(OH)_2D_3$ at appropriate receptors necessary for the biological response, or alternatively there was an increased substrate pressure on 25(OH)D_3 1-hydroxylase.

C. Parathyroid

1. *Primary Hyperparathyroidism*

The association between hyperactivity of parathyroid glands and the appearance of bone disease was first established nearly half a century ago. Interesting early descriptions of this disease state have been described by Fourman and Royer (1968) and by Albright (1970). Paterson (1974) has provided an exhaustive description of the clinical aspects of hyperparathyroidism.

Clinical evidence for the abnormal action of vitamin D in primary hyperparathyroidism was described by Woodhouse *et al.* (1971); they noted radiological improvement in the lesions of osteitis fibrosa in patients with hyperparathyroidism following treatment with vitamin D_2 (1.25 mg/day). Associated with this response was the fact that there was no related hypercalcemia, and alkaline phosphatase values fell to normal during the treatment.

Jowsey (1968) studied the histological features of bone specimens obtained via biopsy from patients with primary hyperparathyroidism and noted a frequent incidence of histological features of osteomalacia. Also, it was found by Brickman *et al.* (1975) and Birge *et al.* (1969) that the intestinal absorption of calcium is often markedly increased in patients with hyperparathyroidism. The simplest explanation for this observation is that, as discussed in Chapter 6, parathyroid hormone is a trophic factor which stimulates the production of 1,25$(OH)_2D_3$ and that the increased circulating levels of this steroid which occur in hyperparathyroidism (see Table 8-7) simply mediate an increased or hyperabsorption of intestinal calcium.

2. *Secondary Hyperparathyroidism*

There are a number of disorders of mineral and bone metabolism in which secondary hyperparathyroidism is thought to exist. By definition, secondary hyperparathyroidism is an endocrinological state of the parathyroid gland in which, due to an incoming signal, a hypersecretion of parathyroid hormone results. This stimulatory signal is usually thought to be hypocalcemia. The most important group of patients with secondary hyperparathyroidism are those suffering from either simple vitamin D deficiency or from vitamin D deficiency secondary to chronic renal failure to malabsorption of vitamin D or calcium. Thus, virtually all patients with chronic renal failure have marked secondary hyperparathyroidism; the chief clinical manifestation of this is the induction of overt "bone disease."

3. *Hypoparathyroidism*

Hypoparathyroidism is an uncommon disorder that has several possible distinct causes, which may include the following: (a) surgical damage to the parathyroid glands or their blood supply during surgery, (b) parathyroid damage by ^{131}I in the treatment of hyperthyroidism, (c) a metastatic neoplasm in the parathyroid glands, (d) hemochromatosis with iron deposits in the parathyroid glands. The main clinical features of hypoparathyroidism are hypocalcemia and a variety of neurological disorders (including anxiety and depression). There appear to be no bone symptoms overtly associated with hypoparathyroidism. Patients with hypoparathyroidism are usually well managed with massive doses of vitamin D of the order of 80,000 to 100,000 IU/day (Ireland *et al.*, 1968). Also, Pak *et al.* (1970) and Konopka *et al.* (1971) published reports describing the management of hypoparathyroidism with doses of 25(OH)D_3 (15–125 μg/day).

Since parathyroid hormone is postulated to be a trophic factor that stimulates the production of 1,25$(OH)_2D_3$ from its precursor 25(OH)D_3 and since therapy with pharmacological quantities of vitamin D or 25(OH)D_3 represents an effective form of management of hypoparathyroidism, it seems clear that the simplest explanation of most of the clinical symptoms of hypoparathyroidism is a paucity of the biologically active form of vitamin D, 1,25$(OH)_2D_3$. Haussler and colleagues and Rosen *et al.* (1977) reported (see Table 8-7) that the circulating level of 1,25$(OH)_2$D in hypoparathyroid subjects is reduced from a normal value of 33 to 28 pg/ml. One would have anticipated a marked reduction in 1,25$(OH)_2D_3$ if its absence were truly the causative factor of the hypocalcemic symptoms of hypoparathyroidism.

Russell *et al.* (1974b) treated a number of hypoparathyroid patients with 2.7 μg/day of 1,25$(OH)_2D_3$ or 1α(OH)D_3 and noted a pronounced rise in serum calcium level and an increase in urinary calcium level. These results suggest that 1,25$(OH)_2D_3$ or one of its potent analogs may eventually be a valuable therapeutic agent with which to manage this disease state.

4. *Pseudohypoparathyroidism*

The inherited disorder of pseudohypoparathyroidism was first described in 1942 by Albright and his colleagues, who identified three patients with the chemical changes consistent with hypoparathyroidism but who showed no response to the administration of parathyroid extract. Albright originally suggested that the disorder was caused by failure of the renal tubules to respond characteristically to parathyroid hormone, i.e., an induction of phosphaturia (Albright *et al.*, 1942).

The principal clinical features of pseudohypoparathyroidism are hypocalcemia and certain remarkable skeletal abnormalities (which are not present at birth); these include a shortness of stature and a reduction particularly in the lower segment of the trunk, a rounding of the face, and, most characteristically, a shortened metacarpal or metatarsal bone. The last-named abnormalities specifically afflict the fourth and fifth metacarpals without marked changes in the phalanges. Pseudohypoparathyroidism is a genetic disorder that is consistent with an autosomal dominant pattern (Weinburg and Stone, 1971). Some families include patients with the same physical signs without the characteristic hypocalcemia. Also, the circulating level of plasma iPTH is normally high in untreated patients with pseudohypoparathyroidism, and it can be suppressed by calcium infusion. It is now apparent that the basal excretion of cAMP is low in the disease state of pseudohypoparathyroidism and that there is no increase in urinary excretion of cAMP after administration of parathyroid extract (Greenberg *et al.*, 1972). The exact nature of the defect in the response to parathyroid hormone has not yet been elucidated; however, there is no deficiency of adenyl cyclase in the kidney (Marcus *et al.*, 1971) and the response to cAMP is also intact since subjects with pseudohypoparathyroidism are capable of responding to administration of dibutyryl-cAMP (Bell *et al.*, 1972).

Some intriguing recent observations linking pseudohypoparathyroidism and $1,25(OH)_2D_3$ were reported by Brickman and co-workers (1976). In these studies patients with pseudohypoparathyroidism were given moderate doses of $1,25(OH)_2D_3$ (0.5–1.0 μg/day for 5 days), and then their responsivity to PTH was assessed in terms of measurements of the urinary excretion of cAMP. Surprisingly, the prior administration of $1,25(OH)_2D_3$ markedly increased the responsivity to PTH, suggesting that in the disease state of pseudohypoparathyroidism there is a paucity of the biological form of vitamin D, $1,25(OH)_2D_3$.

D. Thyroid

Medullary Carcinoma

The disease state medullary carcinoma represents a primary disorder of thyroid C-cell function, which results in primary hypercalcitoninemia, i.e., hypersecretion of the peptide hormone calcitonin. The principal effect of long-standing hypersecretion of calcitonin is on skeletal remodeling. Quantitative histological examination of the bones of patients with medullary carcinoma indicates a very marked reduction in the rate of bone formation as well as in bone resorption.

Under most circumstances, patients have a serum calcium concentration in the normal range. The circulating plasma levels of calcitonin are quite high but are still responsive to both the infusion of EDTA, which mediates a fall, and the infusion of calcium, which mediates an increase (Deftos *et al.*, 1971).

At present there is little direct evidence suggesting a relationship between medullary carcinoma and vitamin D action.

E. Intestinal Relationships

1. Idiopathic Hypercalciuria

The major clinical significance of hypercalciuria is its relation to the genesis of urolithiasis, or renal stones; it has been reported that 20–33% of patients with renal stones may have hypercalciuria (Melick and Henneman, 1958; Albuquerque *et al.*, 1962). A large number of these patients have been characterized as having "idiopathic hypercalciuria," i.e., hypercalciuria without any known cause (Edwards and Hodgkinson, 1965; Parfitt *et al.*, 1964; Albright *et al.*, 1953; Henneman *et al.*, 1960). This would then exclude as possible explanations of idiopathic hypercalciuria the disease states relating to hyperparathyroidism, diseases causing bone resorption, excessive dietary intake of calcium or vitamin D, and various renal tubular defects. Most often these patients are males with normal levels of serum calcium, normal or slightly reduced serum phosphorus concentrations, and renal stones that usually consist of calcium oxalate. The most informative clinical symptom is an increased intestinal absorption of calcium, as was reported by Liberman *et al.* (1968) and Wills *et al.* (1970). It has been proposed that the increased intestinal absorption of calcium may be the pathogenetic mechanism underlying the consequent hypercalciuria. It was shown by Nordin *et al.* (1967) as well as Dent and Watson (1965) that, when dietary calcium intake is restricted, its renal excretion also falls; also, Peacock *et al.* (1967) found that urinary calcium increased when dietary calcium intake was augmented. These observations suggest that in idiopathic hypercalciuria there may be made available to the intestine increased levels of $1,25(OH)_2D_3$. Consistent with this are the observations of Kaplan *et al.* (1977) (see Table 8-7), who found elevated circulating levels of $1,25(OH)_2D_3$ in idiopathic hypercalciuria.

Another possible explanation for the hypercalciuria is a defective renal tubular reabsorption of calcium. In support of this, Edwards and Hodgkinson (1965) found an increased renal clearance of calcium while its filtered load was below normal. Also consistent was the observation of Coe *et al.* (1971), who reported increased plasma levels of PTH in patients with this disorder. They proposed that primary losses of urinary calcium led to small decrements in plasma calcium, which in turn stimulated the release of PTH, with a concomitant increase in calcium absorption produced by increased production of $1,25(OH)_2D_3$; also, low levels of serum phosphorus occurred secondary to the action of PTH.

The observations by Nordin *et al.* (1967) and Dent and Watson (1965) that urinary calcium returns to normal following dietary restriction of calcium intake and the finding by Finn *et al.* (1970) of a normal urinary excretion of calcium in a transplant recipient who had received a kidney from a donor with idiopathic hypercalciuria are inconsistent with the proposal that a renal tubular defect of calcium reabsorption is the primary factor in the genesis of hypercalciuria. From calcium balance and kinetic studies with radioactive calcium, Liberman *et al.* (1968) reported an increased rate of calcium turnover in bone and suggested that a fundamental disturbance of calcium metabolism was occurring, which led to the markedly high rate of calcium turnover.

It is likely that idiopathic hypercalciuria may represent more than one disorder. It is possible that certain patients with this disorder could have either an increased renal production of $1,25(OH)_2D_3$ or, alternatively, an enhanced intestinal sensitivity to this steroid.

2. *Sarcoidosis*

Sarcoidosis is a disease characterized by hypercalcemia and hypercalciuria in patients receiving normal quantities of vitamin D. Hypercalcemia was first noted in patients with sarcoidosis by Harrell and Fisher (1939). It has been posposed that sarcoidosis results because of an unusual sensitivity to vitamin D. The reported frequency of hypercalcemia in sarcoidosis varies widely, with the reported incidence ranging from 2 to 60% (Goldstein *et al.*, 1971; Jasper and Denny, 1968). Although most individuals have minimal elevations of serum calcium levels, which are responsive to therapy, occasionally the hypercalcemia is life-threatening or is capable of inducing progressive metastatic calcification with eventual death due to uremia. In some instances serum calcium levels may be as high as 20 mg per 100 ml. As shown by Bell *et al.* (1964) and Bell and Bartter (1967) the hypercalcemia may appear in patients with sarcoidosis who have received only relatively modest doses of vitamin D. It is also possible that the hypercalcemia may be exacerbated following greater seasonal exposure to sunlight in the summer, as was documented by Taylor *et al.* (1963). Furthermore, it has been possible to induce remission of hypercalcemia by eliminating exposure to ultraviolet light (Hendrix, 1967).

Observations of this kind provide evidence for the theory that there is an "increased sensitivity" to vitamin D in the disorder of sarcoidosis. The cause(s) of such an increased sensitivity remains obscure; plasma levels of total vitamin D as determined via measurement of antirachitic activity (the rat line test; see Chapter 4) were found by Bell *et al.* (1964) to be normal. Similarly, Avioli and Haddad (1973) reported normal plasma levels of 25(OH)D in sarcoidosis. Also,

Avioli *et al.* (1965) studied the fate of intraveneously administered tritiated vitamin D in normal subjects and in patients with sarcoidosis and noted no differences in the metabolic turnover in these two states.

It is well known that the hypercalcemia of sarcoidosis responds readily to treatment with cortisone or other glucocorticoids (Anderson *et al.*, 1954; Bell *et al.*, 1964). Glucocorticoids inhibit the action of vitamin D steroids both in enhancing the intestinal transport of calcium (Harrison and Harrison, 1960; Kimberg, 1969; Kimberg *et al.*, 1971) and in stimulating bone resorption (Raisz *et al.*, 1972). Therefore, it is attractive to propose that steroids such as hydrocortisone ameliorate the hypercalcemia of sarcoidosis by inhibiting the action of vitamin D. Unfortunately, however, the mechanism whereby glucocorticoids inhibit vitamin D-stimulated intestinal transport of calcium remains unknown (see Chapter 9).

3. Glucocorticoid Antagonism

The inhibitory action of glucocorticoids on the functioning of vitamin D in the intestine has been well documented. A detailed discussion of this subject appears in Chapter 9, where reference is also made to the glucocorticoid antagonism of calcium absorption as an effective means of managing the hypercalcemia and increased intestinal absorption of calcium associated with the disease state sarcoidosis.

4. Sprue (Coeliac Disease)

Sprue or coeliac disease is a gluten-sensitive enteropathy. Because of the associated malabsorption of vitamin D, individuals with sprue or coeliac disease often develop osteomalacia. Nassim *et al.* (1959) carried out balance studies on patients with gluten-sensitive enteropathy and found that vitamin D given either orally or parenterally was without effect on calcium absorption until gluten was totally excluded from the diet. In the absence of gluten there was a marked improvement in calcium intestinal absorption, but it was not clearly determined whether there was an increased absorption of vitamin D or loss of an inhibitor of the absorption of vitamin D related to the absence of gluten. Rose (1967) demonstrated that ultraviolet light was capable of causing a marked increase in phosphorus absorption in patients with coeliac disease and osteomalacia. These results are consistent with the view that there is a true vitamin D deficiency associated with coeliac disease and that patients with this disorder may be resistant to oral vitamin D, whereas when vitamin D is given parenterally it is normally metabolized.

As yet no clinical trials have been carried out with vitamin D metabolites in this disease state.

F. Bone

1. *Rickets/Osteomalacia*

Rickets in children and osteomalacia in adults are the characteristic bone disorders induced by a vitamin D deficiency. As discussed in other chapters of this book the identification of rickets as a disease state and the ability of Mellanby (1919, 1921, 1923) to experimentally induce rickets in puppies via nutritional withholding of vitamin D provided key information in efforts to elucidate the actions of vitamin D. As can be noted in Fig. 13-3, there are a number of obvious causes of osteomalacia and rickets. These include (a) any nutritional vitamin D deficiency, whether in the infant, the adolescent, or the adult, (b) any disorders of the intestinal absorption of vitamin D, which may occur in coeliac disease and biliary obstruction under circumstances of partial gastrectomy, and (c) any defects in vitamin D metabolism such as those that occur in chronic renal failure, liver disease, and vitamin D-dependent rickets.

The clinical features of rickets and osteomalacia depend on the age of onset, and therefore it is appropriate to consider these two similar diseases separately. The classic skeletal disorders of rickets include enlargement of the bone, especially in the knees, wrists, and ankles as well as associated changes in the costochondrial junctions, which have been termed by some the "rachitic rosary." If rickets develop in the first 6 months of life, infants may suffer from convulsions or develop tetany, but have only minor skeletal changes; however, after 6 months, bone abnormalities, pain, as well as tetany, are likely to be present. Figure 13-10 shows a classic example of rickets in the child.

The main symptoms of osteomalacia are muscular weakness and bone pain. Osteomalacia is usually present only after growth development of the skeleton is complete, i.e., in the adult stage of life. Only a few adults with osteomalacia ever develop tetany.

A characteristic feature of both osteomalacia and rickets is the failure of new bone to calcify. This leads to the appearance of excessive quantities of uncalcified bone matrix, termed osteoid. An example of osteoid is presented in Fig. 4-1, where the width of the osteoid, which is reflective of the severity of the vitamin D deficiency, is quantitatively determined in the offical "rat line test." A more detailed discussion of the bone abnormalities associated with osteomalacia and rickets is given in Chapter 12.

Almost all subjects with osteomalacia or rickets have a characteristic low serum calcium level, usually of the order of 5 to 7 mg per 100 ml. In addition there is often a high serum level of alkaline phosphatase enzyme activity. In fact, the elevation of this enzyme activity is often used clinically to diagnose the presence of osteomalacia. Also as shown by Bayard *et al.* (1972) and others

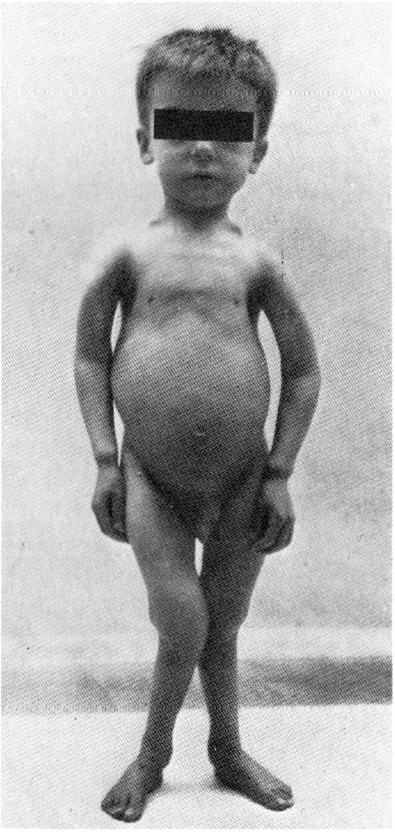

Figure 13-10. Classic appearance of rickets in a child.

there is a marked reduction in the circulating level of 25(OH)D in individuals with osteomalacia.

Drezner and Feinglos (1977) reported the clinical details of a case of osteomalacia occurring in a patient with a giant cell tumor of bone. This subject was shown to have low circulating levels of $1,25(OH)_2D_3$ (16 pg/ml). Oral administration of $1,25(OH)_2D_3$ resulted in a healing of the osteomalacia. These intriguing results suggest that the tumor secreted a factor that inhibited the production of $1,25(OH)_2D_3$, thus leading to a vitamin D deficiency and resulting osteomalacia.

2. *Osteoporosis*

Osteoporosis is the most common generalized disorder of bone. It is most simply characterized as a state of insufficient calcified bone and is the end result of a number of disease states that affect the skeleton. Some of the causes of osteoporosis that have been recognized include (a) adrenal cortical hyperfunction, (b) acromegaly, (c) a prolonged calcium deficiency, (d) a prolonged immobilization, and (e) a reduced level of estrogen, as in postmenopausal women. The chief clinical symptom of osteoporosis is a thinning of the bones with a concomitant increase in the number of fractures. Osteoporosis is often characterized by a crushed fracture of the vertebra with associated back pain.

Two theories have been advanced to account for the development of osteoporosis. (a) There is a stimulation of bone resorption; or (b) there is a decreased rate of new bone formation. Accordingly, there may result an imbalance, on a long-term basis, of the rates of bone formation versus bone resorption, so that resorptive activity is favored. It was shown (Gallagher *et al.*, 1973; Horsman and Nordin, 1973) that from the age of 35 to 40 and above there is a progressive loss of skeletal mass. In view of this normal age-related loss of skeletal calcium, it is not clear whether senile osteoporosis represents a distinct disease entity or merely an exaggeration of the normal physiological changes. It is quite apparent, however, that the disease preferentially appears in women, particularly postmenopausal women. Of course, these individuals have a reduced circulation of estrogens, and as age increases there is also a marked reduction in physical activity. It was shown clearly by Nordin and co-workers (Horsman and Nordin, 1973; Horsman and Simpson, 1975) using photon-absorption spectrometry that there is a quantitative documentable loss in bone density in postmenopausal women as compared with age-matched male controls. It was originally proposed that the onset of osteoporosis was stimulated by an increasing reduction in the rate of bone formation. However, this view has not been entirely supported by more modern bone histological techniques.

A variety of therapeutic approaches to the management of osteoporosis that include some form of vitamin D treatment have been proposed. Buring *et al.* (1974) proposed an increased intake of vitamin D to stimulate intestinal calcium absorption. Jowsey *et al.* (1972) extensively evaluated the consequences of the combined therapy of sodium fluoride, calcium, and vitamin D_3. Riggs *et al.* (1976) summarized the biochemical theory of such combined treatment. In general, it is hoped that increased intestinal absorption of calcium, which is enhanced by a higher dietary intake of both calcium and vitamin D, will lead to an increased rate of bone formation, which is claimed to be stimulated by fluoride. However, since there is no uniform agreement that any of these therapies will always lead to a prevention or reversal of the bone lesions of osteoporosis, they will not be discussed in further detail here. The reader should consult the following for a detailed analysis: Riggs *et al.* (1967), with an excellent review of the literature, and Nordin (1971).

Davies *et al.* (1977b) measured the pharmacokinetics of administered [^{3}H]vitamin D_3 in osteoporotic woman and age-matched controls; they concluded that there was no significant difference in the rate of appearance or levels of $1,25(OH)_2D_3$ in these two groups.

One intriguing possibility in terms of the potential relation of osteoporosis to vitamin D is that with the aging process there is a mild degree of inhibition of the renal $25(OH)D_3$ 1-hydroxylase so that somewhat reduced levels of $1,25(OH)_2D_3$ are available to the physiological system. Although there are no direct data suggesting that there is malabsorption of intestinal calcium in osteoporosis, there is the report of Lund *et al.* (1975) suggesting the possible efficacy of treatment of osteoporosis with low levels of $1,25(OH)_2D_3$. Although these results are only very preliminary, they indicate a possible dramatic clinical application of $1,25(OH)_2D_3$.

3. *Osteitis Fibrosa Cystica*

Osteitis fibrosa cystica is the classic disorder of bone related to hyperparathyroidism. Osteitis fibrosa is most important in the portions of the skeleton where bone turnover is enhanced; thus, the trabeculae of the vertebra, the phalanges, the ends of the long bone, and parts of the skull exhibit the most clearly demonstrable changes. The bone shows an increased activity with a deposition of excessive fibrous tissue in the marrow and an increased number of osteoclasts lying in the lacunae of bone surfaces that are undergoing resorption.

There are four identifiable causes of osteitis fibrosa cystica: (a) primary or secondary hyperparathyroidism, (b) severe acidosis, (c) thyrotoxicosis, and (d) neoplasms, which may produce a parathyroid-like polypeptide.

Thus, the relationship between vitamin D and the bone disease osteitis fibrosa cystica may occur because of the effects of parathyroid hormone on vitamin D metabolism.

4. *Osteopenia–Osteopetrosis*

Osteopenia, or osteopetrosis, is a rare disease that appears shortly after birth in a severe form or in a milder version during adolescence. This disorder was first described in 1904 by a German radiologist, Heinrich Albers-Schonberg, and has sometimes been referred to as the Albers-Schonberg disease or marble bone disease. Characteristics of osteopetrosis include a generalized increase in bone density, often associated with multiple fractures and anemia. Johnston *et al.* (1968) evaluated some 300 cases and divided them into approximately two equal groups: those that were severe and resulted in death early in childhood and those that were more benign and permitted survival into old age.

Histological examination of osteopetrotic bone indicates that there are virtually no osteoclasts present and that the bone structure is highly "immature." Evaluation by quantitative histology suggests that although the rate of bone formation is normal there is a marked reduction in bone resorption. An interesting relationship that has possible signficance to the functioning of vitamin D is that many affected individuals characteristically absorb greater than usual levels of calcium from the diet and excrete very little calcium into the urine. However, no studies have as yet clearly outlined the aberrations in vitamin D function that may occur in this disease state; see, however, Zamboni *et al.* (1977).

5. *Fibrogenesis Imperfecta Ossium*

Fibrogenesis imperfecta ossium is a rare disorder characterized by the appearance in adults of osteomalacia with marked bone pain and tenderness, as originally described by Baker *et al.* (1966). There is a normal intestinal absorption of calcium, and serum levels of both phosphorus and calcium are also normal. Skeletal biopsy shows histological evidence of osteomalacia with an associated defective formation of collagen (Frame *et al.*, 1971). In one case the administration of vitamin D was followed by an initial response but later resistance ensued. Dihydrotachysterol was shown by Baker and Turnbull (1950) to be effective throughout the period of their study. Whether this disease is due to defective metabolism or action of vitamin D is unknown. The response to DHT may represent a pharmacological action of the steroid that does not occur with physiological quantities of vitamin D_2 or D_3 because of regulation of their metabolism. One might anticipate that $1,25(OH)_2D_3$ might also be effective but that doses larger than "physiological" may be required. Clearly, much more information is needed for clarification of the cause and proper management of this very rare disorder.

III. ANIMAL HEALTH APPLICATIONS

The purpose of this section is not to provide an in-depth review of poultry nutrition vis-à-vis egg production and hatchability or postparturient paresis. Rather, the objective is to relate the modern developments in our understanding of vitamin D to these subjects.

A. Poultry Nutrition

One of nature's natural but extreme stresses of calcium homeostasis is the effort required to generate an eggshell (Romanoff and Romanoff, 1949). The shell gland of the avian oviduct supplies vast amounts of calcium and carbonate for formation of the eggshell even though significant quantities of these minerals are not stored in the uterine mucosa. Approximately 5 g of $CaCO_3$ are secreted by the oviduct mucosa in a period of 14 to 20 hr. The principal source of this calcium is medullary bone, where it is mobilized via estrogen stimulation. During the course of eggshell formation, serum calcium levels in the hen may increase to 25–50 mg per 100 ml. There is, however, no increase in plasma ionized calcium levels, the increase occurring solely in protein-bound Ca^{2+}. After the egg has been laid, it is essential for the bird to replace its medullary bone calcium stores via an increased intestinal absorption of calcium. Thus, it is understandable that the endocrine system for vitamin D plays an integral role in achieving calcium homeostasis during eggshell formation. This may involve the actions of the dihydroxylated metabolites at the intestine, kidney, bone, and possibly the shell gland.

A number of investigators have studied the nature of the calcium transport process across the avian shell gland. This gland is exceedingly efficient at extracting calcium from the plasma. Winget *et al.* (1958) reported a 20% efficiency for removal of plasma calcium; e.g., the venous concentration is about 20% less than the arterial concentration. Ehrenspeck *et al.* (1971) reported that the major flux of Ca^{2+} across the shell gland was by an active transport process; however, the essentiality of vitamin D or its metabolites for this transport was not established. It should be recalled that Corradino *et al.* (1968), Lippello and Wasserman (1975), and Bar and Hurwitz (1975) (see Table 10-10) clearly demonstrated the presence of a vitamin D-dependent calcium-binding protein (CaBP) in the avian shell gland. Thus, it appears likely that $1,25(OH)_2D_3$ is involved in some aspect of this calcium transport system.

Hurwitz, Bar, and colleagues evaluated the changes in intestinal calcium absorption that occur during the different phases of egg production. They proposed (Hurwitz and Bar, 1965; Hurwitz *et al.*, 1973) the existence of two types of regulatory mechanisms: (a) an increase in calcium absorption associated with an increase in CaBP observable either under conditions of calcium depletion or at the onset of egg production and (b) a higher calcium absorption during eggshell calcification than during shell gland inactivity (Bar and Hurwitz, 1972). Bar *et al.* (1976) concluded on the basis of daily feeding of $1\alpha(OH)D_3$ to egg-laying birds, thus bypassing the regulated production of $1,25(OH)_2D_3$ by the kidney, that the higher calcium absorption during eggshell formation occurred independently of any changes in the specific activity of the renal $25(OH)D_3$ 1-hydroxylase.

Britton and Wyatt (1978) evaluated the effects of dietary aflatoxin[3] on vitamin D metabolism. They noted only minor alterations in the patterns of radioactive metabolites occurring in the blood 6–24 hr after administration of $[^3H]$vitamin D_3 or $25(OH)[^3H]D_3$.

Various laboratories have reported over the years the essential requirement of vitamin D for successful reproduction in both mammals, e.g., the rat (Richter and Rice, 1943a,b) and cow (Wallis, 1938), and birds, e.g., the chicken (Hart *et al.*, 1925; Carver *et al.*, 1934). There were suggestions in some of these studies

[3]Aflatoxin is an antibiotic that is often included in chicken diets at a low level to prevent mycotoxicoses.

that the action of vitamin D in the reproductive process is different from its role in preventing rickets. Turk and McGinnis (1964), particularly, found that White Leghorn pullets raised from 8 to 24 weeks on a suboptimal intake of vitamin D_3 failed to show a normal onset and increase in egg production even though they developed the secondary sexual characteristics of birds in normal egg production. Thus, vitamin D is clearly required in the adult hen for normal egg production.

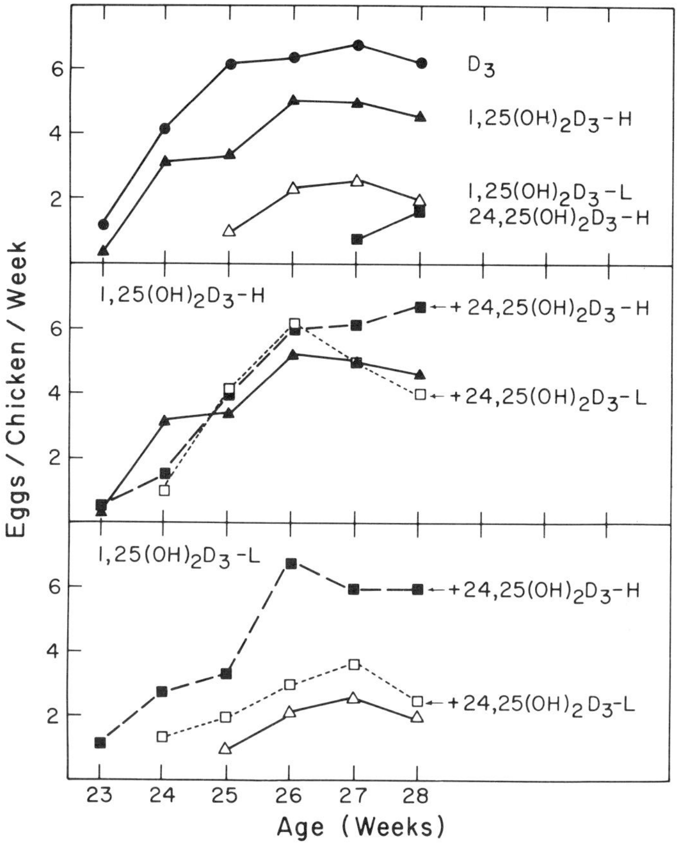

Figure 13-11. Onset of egg production in hens given dihydroxylated vitamin D metabolites. White Leghorn hens were raised from hatching to sexual maturity (23–28 weeks) on a rachitogenic diet and received as their sole source of vitamin D one of the following daily doses (in nanomoles steroid per day per kilogram body weight), which were administered orally: $1,25(OH)_2D_3$-L, 0.24; -H, 1.2; $24,25(OH)_2D_3$-L, 3.2; -H, 16.0; vitamin D_3, 10. The top panel shows the group receiving only vitamin D_3 (●—●) and the other groups receiving either $1,25(OH)_2D_3$-H and -L, or $24,25(OH)_2D_3$-H alone, not in combination. The middle panel shows the groups that received $1,25(OH)_2D_3$-H alone (▲—▲) or in combination with $24,25(OH)_2D_3$-H or -L. The bottom panel shows the groups of birds that received $1,25(OH)_2D_3$-L alone (△—△) or in combination with $24,25(OH)_2D_3$-H or -L. From the unpublished work of A. W. Norman and H. Henry, 1978.

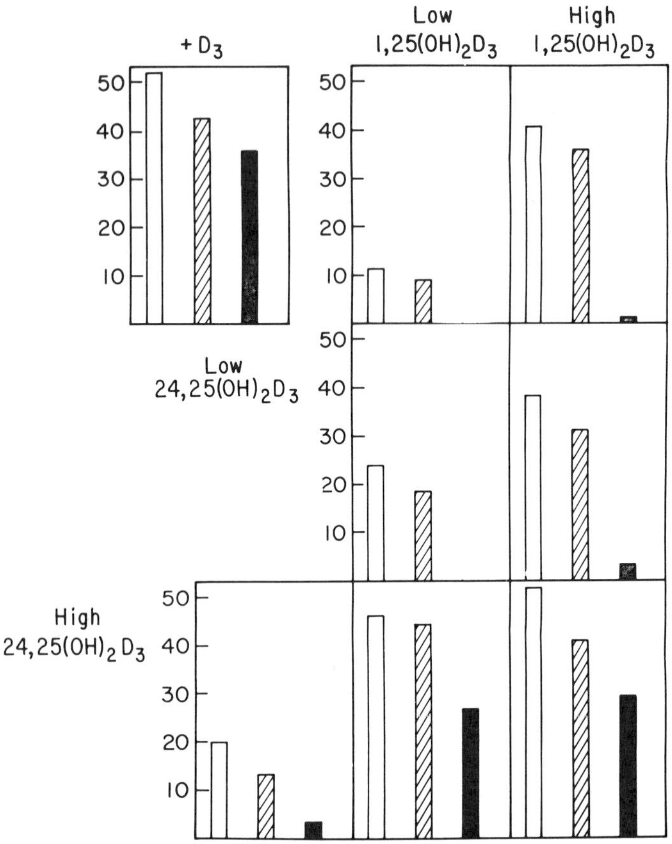

Figure 13-12. Influence of vitamin D or its dihydroxylated metabolites on egg production, fertility, and hatchability. White leghorn hens raised on doses (marked high and low on the figure) as described in the legend to Fig. 13-11 were artificially inseminated at the beginning of weeks 34 and 35. The open bars indicate the number of eggs collected per group during the 2-week period of fertility (1 week following each insemination). The striped bars indicated the number of eggs judged to be fertile 1 week after incubation. The solid bars indicate the number of chicks that hatched. Taken from Henry and Norman (1978) with permission. (Copyright by the American Association for the Advancement of Science.)

In light of our understanding of the vitamin D endocrine system and the existence of the three principal metabolites, $25(OH)D_3$, $1,25(OH)D_2D_3$, and $24,25(OH)_2D_3$, the important question is, Which of these metabolites singly or in combination can satisfy the vitamin D requirements for normal sexual maturity—onset of egg production and fertile eggs that are capable of hatching in a normal manner? Henry and Norman (1978) raised White Leghorn chicks from hatching to sexual maturity on a rachitogenic diet for a period of 9 months. Over this entire period, groups of hens received daily oral doses of either 1,25$(OH)_2D_3$ or 24,25$(OH)_2D_3$ singly or in combination as their sole source of vitamin D. Figure 13-11 shows the dramatic differences in the ability of the various vitamin D metabolites to initiate egg production. Only the combination doses of 24,25$(OH)_2D_3$ and 1,25$(OH)_2D_3$ in comparison to vitamin D_3 supported a completely normal onset of egg production.

More interesting, however, was the clear requirement of 24,25$(OH)_2D_3$ in the presence of 1,25$(OH)_2D_3$ to support normal hatchability of the fertile eggs. Figure 13-12 indicates that, although hens which received only 1,25$(OH)_2D_3$ laid approximately the same number of fertile eggs as the vitamin D_3-treated birds, these eggs were incapable of hatching. A similar observation was made by Sunde *et al.* (1978). However, as reported by Henry and Norman (1978), when both 24,25$(OH)_2D_3$ and 1,25$(OH)_2D_3$ were supplied to the hens, the fertile eggs were capable of hatching in a normal manner. This represents the first clear-cut demonstration of a biological requirement for 24,25$(OH)_2D_3$. The biochemical bases of the actions mediated by 24,25$(OH)_2D_3$ are not yet known.

Manley *et al.* (1978) found that addition of 25$(OH)D_3$ to a diet containing normal levels of vitamin D_3 did not influence the hatchability of turkey eggs. Since vitamin D_3 is normally metabolized rapidly to 25$(OH)D_3$ this is not an unexpected finding.

B. Postparturient Paresis (Milk Fever)

Postparturient paresis, or milk fever, is a metabolic disease occurring at or near parturition principally in dairy cows and sheep. In dairy animals the incidence rate of milk fever is 4.7%. As summarized in Table 5-1, there were 11.9 million dairy cows in the United States in 1976. Of these, approximately 6.7 million were bred annually; thus, 314,000 animals per year were afflicted with this disease.

Capen (1972) has reviewed the problems of endocrine control of calcium metabolism in dairy cattle. The onset of paresis is associated with the initiation of lactation and is marked by a rapid decline in the blood concentration of calcium and phosphorus. Eventually the animal develops a low-calcium tetanic state, which can be corrected by the infusion of calcium gluconate. However, if the clinical condition is not promptly treated, at least 60–70% of the animals will die (Weighton, 1958).

Because of the dramatic hypocalcemia with its expected effects in stimulating parathyroid hormone release and mobilizing bone calcium, it has been fruitful to carry out ultrastructural evaluations of the parathyroid (Black *et al.*, 1973a) and thyroid glands (Black *et al.*, 1973b) as well as bone (Yarrington *et al.*, 1976).

The feeding of massive doses of vitamin D (20–30 million IU, or 500–750 mg) shortly before parturition can prevent approximately 80% of milk fever occurrences (Hibbs and Conrad, 1960; Gurtler *et al.*, 1977; Seidel and Seidel, 1977). However, the administration of these large doses of vitamin D_3 is not uniformly effective in preventing the disease. Also, there is the inherent danger that inordinately high levels of vitamin D will be transmitted to the milk.

Thus, with the development of our current understanding of vitamin D metabolism it was appropriate to evaluate the efficacy of 25(OH)D_3 and 1,25$(OH)_2D_3$ analogs in preventing postparturient paresis. Olson *et al.* (1974) found, however, that administration of doses of 320,000 U (8 mg) of 25(OH)D_3 daily to animals shortly before parturition was not uniformly effective in preventing hypocalcemia. This is undoubtedly due to the fact that 25(OH)D_3 itself is not particularly potent with regard to mobilizing bone calcium or stimulating intestinal calcium absorption. As discussed in Chapter 6, Section III,A, the further metabolism of 25(OH)D_3 is stringently regulated. Thus, little 1,25$(OH)_2D_3$ would be produced in these animals even though large doses of 25(OH)D_3 were given.

Much more impressive effects have been obtained in preventing milk fever by administration of the potent 1,25$(OH)_2D_3$ analog 1α(OH)D_3. Gast *et al.* (1977) as well as Sansom *et al.* (1976) reported that administration of as little as 250–600 μg of 1α(OH)D_3 intramuscularly 24 hr before to 2 hr after calving dramatically reduced the incidence of milk fever. Associated with this beneficial response was a significant elevation in serum calcium levels. Capen *et al.* (1977), using 1,25$(OH)_2D_3$, also reported preliminary evidence consistent with these findings. Thus, there is now the realistic possibility that these 1α-OH-containing steroids can be used in a straightforward treatment of milk fever.

In spite of the favorable findings of Gast *et al.* (1977), the same group subsequently reported (Horst *et al.*, 1977) that the plasma concentration of 1,25$(OH)_2D_3$ as measured by steroid competition assay (see Chapter 8) was not reduced in animals with postparturient paresis. This puzzling result will require further evaluation before its significance is understood.

REFERENCES

Albright, F. (1970). *Arch. Interm. Med.* **126,** 558.
Albright, F., Butler, A. M., and Bloomberg, E. (1937). *Am. J. Dis. Child.* **54,** 529.
Albright, F., Burnett, C. H., Smith, P. H., and Parson, W. (1942). *Endocrinology* **30,** 922.
Albright, F., Henneman, P., and Benedict, P. H. (1953). *J. Clin. Endocrinol. Metab.* **13,** 860.
Albuquerque, P. F., Forster, R., and Zanandrea, B. (1962). *Trans. Am. Assoc. Genito-Urinary Surg.* **54,** 45.
Anderson, J., Dent, C. E., and Harper, C. (1954). *Lancet* **2,** 720.
Andrea, M., Holmlund, D. E. W., Larsson, S.-E., Lindqvist, B., and Lorentzon, R. (1977). *Lancet* **2,** 8047.
Arieff, A. I., and Massry, S. G. (1974). *J. Clin. Invest.* **53,** 387.
Arnaud, C. D., Maijer, R., Reade, T., Scrivner, C. R., and Whelan, D. T. (1970). *Pediatrics* **46,** 871.

Arnaud, C., Glorieux, F., and Scriver, C. (1971). *Science* **173,** 845.
Asherov, J., Weinberger, A., and Pinkhas, J. (1977). *Helv. Paediatr. Acta* **32,** 369.
Atkinson, M., Nordin, B. E. C., and Sherlock, S. (1956). *Q. J. Med.* **25,** 299.
Avioli, L. V., and Haddad, J. G. (1973). *Metab., Clin. Exp.* **22,** 507.
Avioli, L. V., McDonald, J. E., Lund, J., and DeLuca, H. F. (1965). *J. Clin. Invest.* **44,** 1026.
Avioli, L. V., Lee, S. W., McDonald, J. E., Lund, J., and DeLuca, H. F. (1967a). *J. Clin. Invest.* **46,** 983.
Avioli, L. V., Williams, T. F., Lund, J. and DeLuca, H. F. (1967b). *J. Clin. Invest.* **46,** 1907.
Avioli, L. V., Birge, S. J., Lee, S. W., and Slatopolsky, E. (1968). *J. Clin. Invest.* **47,** 2239.
Avioli, L. V., Birge, S. J., and Slatopolsky, E. (1970). *Proc. Int. Congr. Nephrol., 4th, 1969* Vol. 2, p. 175.
Backhouse, J., Lumb, G. A., and Mawer, E. B. (1971). *Nature (London), New Biol.* **232,** 188.
Baerg, R. D., Kimberg, D. V., and Gershon, E. (1970). *J. Clin. Invest.* **49,** 1288.
Baker, S. L., and Turnbull, H. M. (1950). *J. Pathol. Bacteriol.* **62,** 132.
Baker, S. L., Dent, C. E., and Friedman, M. (1966). *J. Bone Jt. Surg., Br. Vol.* **48,** 804.
Balsan, S., and Garabedian, M. (1972). *J. Clin. Invest.* **51,** 749.
Balsan, S., and Garabedian, M. (1974). *Endocrinol., Proc. Int. Symp., 4th, 1973* p. 147.
Bar, A., and Hurwitz, S. (1972). *Comp. Biochem. Physiol. B* **41,** 735.
Bar, A., and Hurwitz, S. (1975). *Poult. Sci.* **54,** 1325.
Bar, A., Eisner, U., Montecuccoli, G., and Hurwitz, S. (1976). *J. Nutr.* **106,** 1336.
Barbour, B. H., Kronfield, S. J., and Pawlicki, A. M. (1966). *Nephron* **3,** 40.
Barragry, J. M., France, M. W., Carter, N. D., Auton, J. A., Beer, M., Boucher, B. J., and Cohen, R. D. (1977). *Lancet* **1,** 629.
Barton, O. H., Hesse, R. H., Pechet, M. M., and Rizzardo, E. (1973). *J. Am. Chem. Soc.* **95,** 2748.
Bayard, F., Bec, P., and Louvet, J. P. (1972). *Eur. J. Clin. Invest.* **2,** 195.
Beadle, P. C. (1977). *Br. J. Dermatol.* **97,** 585.
Bec, P., Louvet, J., and Bayard, F. (1972). *Clin. Res.* **19,** 732.
Bell, N. H., and Bartter, F. C. (1967). *Acta Endocrinol. (Copenhagen)* **54,** 173.
Bell, N. H., Gill, J. R., and Bartter, F. C. (1964). *Am. J. Med.* **36,** 500.
Bell, N. H., Avery, S., Sinha, T., Clark, C. M., Allen, D. O., and Johnston, C. (1972). *J. Clin. Invest.* **51,** 816.
Belsey, R., DeLuca, H. F., and Potts, J. T., Jr. (1971). *J. Clin. Endocrinol. Metab.* **33,** 554.
Bierman, C. W., Shapiro, G. G., Christie, D. L., VanArsdel, P. P., Jr., Furukawa, C. T., and Ward, B. H. (1978). *J. Allergy Clin. Immunol.* **61,** 119.
Birge, S. J., Peck, W. A., Berman, M., and Whedon, G. D. (1969). *J. Clin. Invest.* **48,** 1705.
Black, H. E., Capen, C. C., and Arnaud, C. D. (1973a). *Lab. Invest.* **29,** 173.
Black, H. E., Capen, C. C., Yarrington, J. T., and Rowland, G. N. (1973b). *Lab. Invest.* **29,** 437.
Booher, L. E., Hartzler, E. R., and Hewston, E. M. (1942). *U.S., Dep. Agric., Circ.* **638.**
Bordier, P., Marie, J. P., and Arnaud, L. D. (1975). *Kidney Int., Suppl.* **2,** 510.
Borgstedt, A. D., Bryson, M. F., Young, L. W., and Forbes, G. B. (1972). *J. Pediatr.* **81,** 9.
Boris, A., Hurley, J. F., and Trmal, T. (1977). *J. Nutr.* **107,** 194.
Bouillon, R., Verberckmoes, R., and Moor, P. D. (1974). *Kidney Int.* **7,** 422.
Brickman, A. S., and Norman, A. W. (1973). *Kidney Int.* **4,** 161.
Brickman, A. S., Coburn, J. W., and Norman, A. W. (1972). *N. Engl. J. Med.* **287,** 891.
Brickman, A. S., Coburn, J. W., and Norman, A. W. (1973a). *Clin. Aspects Metab. Bone Dis., Proc. Int. Sump., 1972* Int. Congr. Ser. No. 270, p. 367.
Brickman, A. S., Coburn, J. W., Kurokawa, K., Bethune, J. E., Harrison, H. E., and Norman, A. W. (1973b). *N. Engl. J. Med.* **289,** 495.
Brickman, A. S., Coburn, J. W., Massry, S. G., and Norman, A. W. (1974a). *Ann. Intern. Med.* **80,** 161.

Brickman, A. S., Coburn, J. W., Norman, A. W., and Massry, S. G. (1974b). *Am. J. Med.* **57,** 28.
Brickman, A. S., Sherrard, D. J., Jowsey, J., Singer, F. R., Baylink, D. J., Maloney, N., Massry, S. G., Norman, A. W., and Coburn, J. W. (1974c). *Arch. Intern. Med.* **134,** 883.
Brickman, A. S., Jowsey, J., Sherrard, D. J., Friedman, G., Singer, F. R., Baylink, D. J., Maloney, N., Massry, S. G., Norman, A. W., and Coburn, J. W. (1975). *In* "Proceedings of the Second Workshop on Vitamin D and Problems Related to Uremic Bone Disease" (A. W. Norman *et al.,* eds.), p. 241. de Gruyter, Berlin.
Brickman, A. S., Coburn, J. W., Friedman, G. R., Okamura, W. H., Massry, S. G., and Norman, A. W. (1976). *J. Clin. Invest.* **57,** 1540.
Brickman, A. S., Hartenbower, D. L., Norman, A. W., and Coburn, J. W. (1977). *Am. J. Clin. Nutr.* **30,** 1064.
Brickman, A. S., Gerzi, K., Norman, A. W., and Coburn, J. W. (1978). *Clin. Res.* **26,** 411a.
Britton, W. M., and Wyatt, R. D. (1978). *Poult. Sci.* **57,** 163.
Bunker, J. W. M., and Harris, R. S. 1937). *N. Engl. J. Med.* **216,** 165.
Buring, K., Hilth, A. G., Nilsson, B. E., Westlin, N. E., and Wikland, P. E. (1974). *Acta Med. Scand.* **195,** 471.
Burnett, C. H., Dent, C. E., Harper, C., and Warland, B. J. (1964). *Am. J. Med.* **36,** 222.
Caniggia, A., and Gennari, C. (1974). *Helv. Med. Acta* **37,** 221.
Capen, C. C. (1972). *In* "The Bovine Practitioner" (E. I. Williams, ed.), p. 181. Heritage Press, Stillwater, Oklahoma.
Capen, C. C., Hoffsis, G. G., and Norman, A. W. (1977). *In* "Vitamin D: Biochemical, Chemical and Clinical Aspects Related to Calcium Metabolism" (A. W. Norman *et al.,* eds.), p. 565. de Gruyter, Berlin.
Carver, J. S., Robertson, E. I., Brazie, D., Johnson, R. H., and St. John, J. L. (1934). *Wash., Agric. Exp. Stn., Bull.* **299.**
Castells, S., Shai, F., Gauthier, B., Hashemi, S., Reddy, C. M., and DeLuca, H. F. (1976). *Curr. Ther. Res., Clin. Exp.* **19,** 410.
Chalmers, T. M., Hunter, J. O., Davie, M. W., Szaz, K. F., Pelc, B., and Kodicek, E. (1973). *Lancet* **1,** 696.
Chan, J. C. M., Oldham, S. B., Holick, M. F., and DeLuca, H. F. (1975). *J. Am. Med. Assoc.* **234,** 47.
Chesney, R. W., Moorthy, A. V., Eisman, J. A., Jax, D. K., Mazess, R. W., and DeLuca, H. F. (1978). *N. Engl. J. Med.* **298,** 238.
Clarkson, E. M., Eastwood, J. B., Koutsaimanis, K. G., and de Wardener, H. E. (1973). *Kidney Int.* **3,** 258.
Coburn, J. W., and Norman, A. W. (1973). *Clin. Nephrol.* **1,** 273.
Coburn, J. W., Brickman, A. S., Rowe, P. H., Massry, S. G., and Norman, A. W. (1972). *Proc. Dial. Transplant Forum* **2,** 112 and 118.
Coburn, J. W., Brickman, A. S., Massry, S. G., Singer, F. R., and Norman, A. W. (1973a). *Trans. Eur. Dial. Transplant Soc., 1973* p. 210.
Coburn, J. W., Hartenbower, D. L., and Massry, S. G. (1973b). *Kidney Int.* **4,** 96.
Coburn, J. W., Koppel, M. H., Brickman, A. S., and Massry, S. G. (1973c). *Kidney Int.* **3,** 264.
Coburn, J. W., Hartenbower, D. L., and Norman, A. W. (1974). *West. J. Med.* **121,** 22.
Coburn, J. W., Brickman, A. S., Hartenbower, D. L., and Norman, A. W. (1977). *In* "Phosphate Metabolism" (S. G. Massry and E. Ritz, eds.), p. 549. Plenum, New York.
Cochran, M., and Nordin, B. E. C. (1971). *Clin. Sci.* **40,** 305.
Cochran, M., Bulusu, L., Horsman, A., Stasiak, L., and Nordin, B. E. C. (1973). *Nephron* **10,** 113.
Coe, F. L., Canterbury, J., and Reiss, E. (1971). *Trans. Assoc. Am. Physicians* **84,** 152.
Colodro, I. H., Brickman, A. S., Coburn, J. W., Osborn, T. W., and Norman, A. W. (1978). *Metab., Clin. Exp.* **27,** 745.

Condon, J. R., Nassim, J. R., and Rutter, A. (1970). *Br. J. Med.* **3,** 138.
Conney, A. H. (1967). *Pharmacol. Rev.* **19,** 317.
Corless, D., Boucher, B. J., Beer, M., Gupta, S. P., and Cohen, R. D. (1975). *Lancet* **1,** 1404.
Corradino, R. A., Wasserman, R. H., Publos, M. H., and Chang, S. I. (1968). *Arch. Biochem. Biophys* **125,** 378.
Counts, S. J., Baylink, D. J., Shen, F. H., Sherrard, D. J., and Hickman, R. O. (1975). *Ann. Intern. Med.* **82,** 196.
Crutchlow, W. P., and David, D. S. (1971). *Clin. Orthop. Relat. Res.* **74,** 209.
Cundy, T., Kanis, J. A., Paton, S., Russell, R. G. G., and Warner, G. T. (1978). *Med. Res. Soc.* p. 23.
Davies, M., Taylor, C. M., Hill, L. F., and Stanbury, S. W. (1977a). *Lancet* **1,** 55.
Davies, M., Mawer, E. B., and Adams, P. H. (1977b). *J. Clin. Endocrinol. Metab.* **45,** 199.
Davies, M. W. J., Chalmers, T. M., Hunter, J. O., Pelc, B., and Kodicek, E. (1976). *Ann. Intern. Med.* **84,** 281.
Deftos, L. J., Bury, A. E., Habener, J. F., Singer, F. R., and Potts, J. T. (1971). *Metab., Clin. Exp.* **20,** 1129.
DeLuca, H. F., and Avioli, L. V. (1970). *Arch. Intern. Med.* **126,** 896.
DeLuca, H. F., Lund, J., Rosenbloom, A., and LoBeck, C. C. (1967). *J. Pediatr.* **70,** 828.
Dent, C. E., and Smith, R. (1969). *Q. J. Med.* **38,** 195.
Dent, C. E., and Watson, L. (1965). *Br. Med. J.* **2,** 449.
Dent, C. E., Harper, C. N., and Philpot, G. R. (1961). *Q. J. Med.* **30,** 1.
Dent, C. E., Richens, A., Rowe, D. J. F., and Stamp, T. C. B. (1970). *Br. Med. J.* **4,** 69.
Doboszynska, B., and Datsenko, Z. M. (1966). *Bull. Acad. Pol. Sci., Ser. Sci. Biol.* **14,** 199.
Dominguez, J. H., Gray, R. W., and Lemann, J. (1976). *J. Clin. Endocrinol. Metab.* **43,** 1056.
Drezner, M. K., and Feinglos, M. N. (1977). *J. Clin. Invest.* **60,** 1046.
Earp, H. S., Ney, R. L., Gitelman, H. J., Richman, R., and DeLuca, H. F. (1970). *N. Engl. J. Med.* **283,** 627.
Eastwood, B., Bordier, P. J., Clarkson, E. M., Tun Chot, S., and deWardener, H. E. (1973). *Clin. Sci. Mol. Med.* **47,** 23.
Eastwood, J. B., Phillips, M. E., de Wardener, H. E., Bordier, P., Arnaud, C. D., and Norman, A. W. (1975). *In* "Proceeding of The Second Workshop on Vitamin D and Problems Related to Uremic Bone Disease" (A. W. Norman *et al.*, eds.), p. 595. de Gruyter, Berlin.
Edwards, N. A., and Hodgkinson, A. (1965). *Clin. Sci.* **29,** 327.
Ehrenspeck, G., Schraer, H., and Schraer, R. (1971). *Am. J. Physiol.* **220,** 967.
Eisman, J. A., Hamstra, A. J., Kream, B. E., and DeLuca, H. F. (1976). *Science* **193,** 1021.
Engfeldt, B., Zetterström, R., and Winberg, J. (1956). *J. Bone/Jt. Surg., Am. Vol.* **38,** 1323.
Everett, M. A., Yeagers, E., Sayre, R. M., and Olson, R. L. (1966). *Photochem. Photobiol.* **5,** 533.
Favus, M. J., Kimberg, D. V., Millar, G. N., and Gershon, E. (1973). *J. Clin. Invest.* **52,** 1328.
Finn, W. F., Cerilli, G. J., and Ferris, T. F. (1970). *N. Engl. J. Med.* **283,** 1450.
Flury, W. (1978). *Schweiz. Med. Wochenschr.* **108,** 129.
Follis, R. H. (1950). *Bull. Johns Hopkins Hops.* **87,** 593.
Food and Nutrition Board (1974). *J. Am. Diet. Assoc.* **66,** 453.
Fourman, P., and Royer, P. (1968). "Calcium Metabolism and the Bone." Blackwell, Oxford.
Fournier, A. E., Johnson, W. J., Taves, D. R., Béabout, J. W., Arnaud, C. D., and Goldsmith, R. S. (1971). *J. Clin. Invest.* **50,** 592.
Fournier, A. E., Bordier, P., Guéris, J., Chanard, J., Bedrossian, J., Ossario, M., and DeLuca, H. F. (1975a). *Kidney Int.* **8,** 126.
Fournier, A. E., Bordier, P. J., Guéris, J., Chanard, J., Marie, P., Ferriere, C., Osario, M., Bedrossian, J., and DeLuca, H. F. (1975b). *Endocrinol., Proc. Int. Symp., 1975* p. 227.

Frame, B., Frost, H. M., Pak, C. Y. C., Reynolds, W., and Argen, R. J. (1971). *N. Engl. J. Med.* **285,** 769.
Fraser, D., Kooh, S. W., Kind, H. P., Holick, M. F., Tanaka, Y., and DeLuca, H. F. (1973). *N. Engl. J. Med.* **289,** 817.
Fraser, D. R., and Kodicek, E. (1970). *Nature (London)* **228,** 764.
Fridez, C., Barras, C., and Garcia, B. (1977). *Schweiz. Med. Wochenschr.* **107,** 764.
Friedlander, E. J., Henry, H. L., and Norman, A. W. (1977). *J. Biol. Chem.* **252,** 8677.
Frost, H. M., Jee, W. S. S., Kimmel, D., and Teitelbaum, S. (1977). *In* "Vitamin D: Biochemical, Chemical and Clinical Aspects Related to Calcium Metabolism" (A. W. Norman *et al.*, eds.), p. 885. de Gruyter, Berlin.
Gagnon, R., Ogden, G. W., Just, G., and Kaye, M. (1974). *Can. J. Physiol. Pharmacol.* **52,** 272.
Gallagher, J. C., Aaron, J., Horsman, A., Marshall, D. H., Wilkinson, R., and Nordin, B. E. C. (1973). *Clin. Endocrinol Metab.* **2,** 293.
Gast, D. R., Marquardt, J. P., Jorgensen, N. A., and DeLuca, H. F. (1977). *J. Dairy Sci.* **60,** 1910.
Genuth, S. M., Sherwood, L. M., and Vertes, V., and Leonards, J. R. (1970). *J. Clin. Endocrinol. Metab.* **30,** 15.
Glorieux, F. H., Scriver, C. R., Holick, M. F., and DeLuca, H. F. (1973). *Lancet* **2,** 287.
Goldberg, L. D. (1972). *Lancet* **2,** 732.
Goldberg, P. (1974a). *Int. J. Environ. Stud.* **6,** 19.
Goldberg, P. (1974b). *Int. J. Environ. Stud.* **6,** 121.
Goldsmith, R. S., Furszyfer, J., Johnson, W. J., Fournier, A. E., Sizemore, G. W., and Arnaud, C. D. (1973). *J. Clin. Invest.* **52,** 173.
Goldstein, R. A., Israel, H. L., Becker, K. L., and Moore, C. F. (1971). *Am. J. Med.* **51,** 21.
Gray, R. W., Boyle, I., and DeLuca, H. F. (1971). *Science* **172,** 1232.
Gray, R. W., Weber, H. P., Dominguez, J. E., and Lemann, J. (1974). *J. Clin. Endocrinol. Metab.* **39,** 1045.
Gray, R. W., Wilz, D. R., Caldas, A., Lemann, J., and DeLuca, H. F. (1977). *In* "Vitamin D: Biochemical, Chemical and Clinical Aspects Related to Calcium Metabolism" (A. W. Norman *et al.*, eds.), p. 123. de Gruyter, Berlin.
Greenberg, S. R., Karabell, S., and Sade, G. A. (1972). *Arch. Intern. Med.* **129,** 633.
Grigoleit, H.-G., Schaefer, K., Kraft, D., Offerman, G., von Herrath, D., and Dalling, G. (1977). *In* "Vitamin D: Biochemical, Chemical and Clinical Aspects Related to Calcium Metabolism" (A. W. Norman *et al.*, eds.), p. 701. de Gruyter, Berlin.
Gruson, P. M., and Miravet, L. (1974). *Sco. Biol.* **168,** 948.
Gurtler, H., Seidel, H., and Liebaugh, E. (1977). *Monatsh. Veterinaermed.* **32,** 664.
Haddad, J. G., and Chuy, K. Y. (1971). *J. Clin. Endocrinol. Metab.* **33,** 992.
Haddad, J. G., and Rojanasathit, S. (1976). *J. Clin. Endocrinol. Metab.* **42,** 284.
Haddad, J. G., Walgate, J., and Hahn, T. (1976). *J. Clin. Endocrinol. Metab.* **43,** 712.
Haddad, J. G., Jr., Chyu, K. J., Hahn, T. J., and Stamp, T. C. B. (1973). *J. Lab. Clin. Med.* **81,** 22.
Hahn, B., and Hahn, T. (1976). *Arthritis Rheum.* **19,** 800.
Hahn, T. J., and Hahn, B. (1976). *Semin. Arthritis* **2,** 165.
Hahn, T. J., Birge, S. J., Scharp, C. R., and Avioli, L. V. (1972a). *J. Clin. Invest.* **51,** 741.
Hahn, T. J., Hendin, B. A., Scharp, C. R., and Haddad, J. G., Jr. (1972b). *N. Engl. J. Med.* **287,** 900.
Harrell, G. T., and Fisher, S. (1939). *J. Clin. Invest.* **18,** 687.
Harrison, H. E. (1957). *Clin. Orthop.* **9,** 61.
Harrison, H. E. (1958). *J. Chronic Dis.* **7,** 346.
Harrison, H. E., and Harrison, H. C. (1960). *Am. J. Physiol.* **199,** 265.

Hart, E. B., Steenbock, H., Lepkovsky, S., Kletzeen, S. W. F., Halpen, J. G., and Johnson, O. N. (1925). *J. Biol. Chem.* **65,** 579.

Haussler, M. R. (1974). *Nutr. Rev.* **32,** 257.

Haussler, M. R., Baylink, D. J., Hughes, M. R., Brumbaugh, P. F., Wergedal, G. E., Shen, F. H., Nillsen, R. L., Counts, S. J., Bursac, K. M., and McCain, T. A. (1976). *Clin. Endocrinol. (London)* **5,** 1515.

Henderson, R. G., Russell, R. G. G., Ledingham, J. G. G., Smith, R., Oliver, D. O., Walton, R. J., Small, D. G., Preston, C., Warner, G. T., and Norman, A. W. (1974). *Lancet* **1,** 379.

Hendrix, J. Z. (1967). *Clin. Res.* **11,** 220.

Henneman, P. H., Benedict, P. H., and Forbes, A. P. (1960). *N. Engl. J. Med.* **259,** 802.

Henry, H. L., and Norman, A. W. (1975). *Comp. Biochem. Physiol.* **50,** 431.

Henry, H. L., and Norman, A. W. (1978). *Science* **201,** 835.

Hibbs, J. W., and Conrad, H. R. (1960). *J. Dairy Sci.* **43,** 1124.

Hirooka, M., Wako, H., Kaneko, C., Ishikawa, M., Sasaki, S., and Suda, T. (1975). *J. Nutr. Sci. Vitaminol.* **21,** 277.

Hitchman, A. J. W., and Harrison, J. E. (1972). *Can. J. Biochem.* **50,** 758.

Holick, M. F., Garabedian, M., and DeLuca, H. F. (1972a). *Biochemistry* **11,** 2715.

Holick, M. F., Garabedian, M., and DeLuca, H. F. (1972b). *Science* **176,** 1247.

Holick, M. F., Semmler, E. J., Schnoes, H. K., and DeLuca, H. F. (1973). *Science* **180,** 190.

Holick, M. F., Frommer, J., McNeill, S., and Potts, J. T. (1977). *In* "Vitamin D: Biochemical, Chemical and Clinical Aspects Related to Calcium Metabolism" (A. W. Norman *et al.*, eds.), p. 135. de Gruyter, Berlin.

Horsman, A., and Nordin, B. E. C. (1973). *Proc. Eur. Symp. Calcif. Tissues, 9th 1974* p. 185.

Horsman, A., and Simpson, M. (1975). *Br. J. Radiol.* **48,** 471.

Horst, R. L., Eisman, J. A., Jorgensen, N. A., and DeLuca, H. F. (1977). *Science* **196,** 662.

Hughes, M. R., Baylink, D. J., Jones, P. G., and Haussler, M. R. (1976). *J. Clin. Invest.* **58,** 61.

Hunter, J., Maxwell, M. D., Stewart, D. A., Parsons, V., and Williams, R. (1971). *Br. Med. J.* **4,** 202.

Hurwitz, S., and Bar, A. (1965). *J. Nutr.* **86,** 433.

Hurwitz, S., Bar, A., and Cohen, I. (1973). *Am. J. Physiol.* **225,** 150.

Ireland, A. W., Clubb, J. S., Neale, F. C., Posen, S., and Reeve, T. S. (1968). *Ann. Intern. Med.* **69,** 81.

Jasper, P. L., and Denny, F. W. (1968). *J. Pediatr.* **73,** 499.

Johnston, C. C., Lavy, N., Lord, T., Vellios, F., Merritt, A. D., and Deiss, W. P. (1968). *Medicine (Baltimore)* **47,** 149.

Jorgensen, H., and Vogt, J. H. (1977). *Acta Med. Scand.* **201,** 3.

Jowsey, J. (1968). *In* "Parathyroid Hormone and Thyrocalcitonin (Calcitonin)" (R. V. Talmage and L. F. Bélanger, eds.), Int. Congr. Ser. No. 159, p. 137. Exerpta Med. Found., Amsterdam.

Jowsey, J., Riggs, B. L., Kelley, P. J., and Hoffman, D. L. (1972). *Am. J. Med.* **53,** 43.

Jubiz, W., Haussler, M. R., McCain, T. A., and Tobman, G. (1977). *J. Clin. Endocrinol. Metab.* **44,** 617.

Kanis, J. A., and Russell, R. G. G. (1977). *Br. Med. J.* **1,** 78.

Kanis, J. A., Heynen, G., Russell, R. G. G., Smith, R., Walton, R. J., and Warner, G. T. (1977). *In* "Vitamin D: Biochemical, Chemical and Clinical Aspects Related to Calcium Metabolism" (A. W. Norman *et al.*, eds.), p. 793. de Gruyter, Berlin.

Kanis, J. A., Cundy, T., Bartlett, M., Smith, R., Heynen, G., Warner, G. T., and Russell, R. G. G. (1978). *Br. Med. J.* **1,** 1382.

Kaplan, R. A., Haussler, M. R., Deftos, L. J., Bone, H., and Pak, C. Y. C. (1977). *J. Clin. Invest.* **59,** 756.

Kaye, M., and Sagar, S. (1972). *Metab., Clin. Exp.* **21,** 815.
Kaye, M., and Silverman, M. (1965). *J. Lab. Clin. Med.* **66,** 535.
Kaye, M., Chatterjee, G., Cohen, G. F., and Sagar, S. (1970). *Ann. Intern. Med.* **73,** 225.
Kehayoglou, A. K., Agnew, J. E., Holdsworth, C. D., Whelton, M. J., and Sherlock, S. (1968). *Lancet* **1,** 715.
Kimberg, D. V. (1969). *N. Engl. J. Med.* **280,** 1396.
Kimberg, D. V., Baerg, R. D., and Gershon, E. (1970). *Arch. Intern. Med.* **126,** 891.
Kimberg, D. V., Baerg, R. D., Gershon, E., and Graudusius, R. T. (1971). *J. Clin. Invest.* **50,** 1309.
Kleeman, C. R., Better, O., Massry, S. G., and Maxwell, M. H. (1967). *Yale J. Biol. Med.* **40,** 1.
Konopka, P., Benhamou, T., and Klotz, H. P. (1971). *Ann. Endocrinol. (Paris)* **32,** 906.
Kooh, S. W., Fraser, D., DeLuca, H. F., Holick, M. F., Belsey, R. E., Clark, M. B., and Murray, T. M. (1975). *New Engl. J. Med.* **293,** 840.
Kraft, D., and Offermann, G. (1977). *Naunyn-Schmiedeberg's Arch. Pharmacol.* **297,** 75.
Krawitt, E. L., Grundman, M. J., and Mawer, E. B. (1977). *Lancet* **2,** 1246.
Kruse, K., and Offermann, G. (1977). *Monatsschr. Kinderheilkd.* **125,** 489.
Lakdawala, D. R., and Widdowson, E. M. (1977). *Lancet* **1,** 167.
Laubenthal, F., Reichenberger, M., and Reinwein, D. (1975). *Dtsch. Med. Wochenschr.* **100,** 412.
Lee, S. W., Russell, J., and Avioli, L. V. (1977). *Science* **195,** 994.
Lewy, J. E., Cabana, E. C., Repetto, H. A., Canterbury, M. S., and Reiss, E. (1972). *J. Pediatr.* **81,** 294.
Liberman, U. A., Sperling, O., and Atsmon, A. (1968). *J. Clin. Invest.* **47,** 2580.
Linden, V. (1974). *Br. Med. J.* **562,** 647.
Lippiello, L., and Wasserman, R. H. (1975). *J. Histochem. Cytochem.* **23,** 110.
Liu, S. H., and Chu, H. I. (1943). *Medicine (Baltimore)* **22,** 103.
Llach, F., Brickman, A. S., Gerzi, K., Norman, A. W., and Coburn, J. W. (1978). *Clin. Res.* **26,** 543a.
Loomis, W. (1967). *Science* **157,** 501.
Lumb, G. A., Mawer, E. B., and Stanbury, S. W. (1971). *Am. J. Med.* **50,** 421.
Lund, B., Hjorth, L., Kjaer, I., Reimann, I., Friis, T., Andersen, R. B., and Sorensen, O. H. (1975). *Lancet* **2,** 1168.
McDonald, S. J., Clarkson, E. M., and de Wardener, H. E. (1964). *Clin. Sci.* **26,** 27.
Madsen, S., and Olgaard, K. (1976). *Acta Med. Scand.* **200,** 1.
Manley, J. M., Voitle, R. A., and Harms, R. H. (1978). *Pout. Sci.* **57,** 290.
Marcus, R., Wilbur, J. F., and Aurbach, G. D. (1971). *J. Clin. Endocrinol. Metab.* **33,** 537.
Marini, P. V., Parker, T. F., Pak, C. Y. C., Hull, A. R., DeLuca, H. F., and Fordtran, J. S. (1976). *J. Clin. Invest.* **57,** 861.
Massry, S. G., and Coburn, J. W. (1972). *Natl. Kidney Found.* **5,** 1.
Mawer, E. B., and Schaefer, K. (1969). *Biochem. J.* **114,** 74.
Mawer, E. B., Lumb, G. A., Schaefer, K., and Stanbury, S. W. (1971). *Clin. Sci.* **40,** 39.
Mawer, E. B., Backhouse, J., and Taylor, C. M. (1973). *Lancet* **1,** 626.
Mawer, E. B., Backhouse, J., Davies, M., Hill, L. F., and Taylor, C. M. (1976). *Lancet* **1,** 1203.
Melick, R. A., and Henneman, P. H. (1958). *N. Engl. J. Med.* **259,** 307.
Mellanby, E. (1919). *Med. Res. Counc. (G. B.), Spec. Rep. Ser.* **38.**
Mellanby, E. (1921). *Med. Res. Counc. (G. B.), Spec. Rep. Ser.* **61.**
Mellanby, E. (1923). "Experimental Rickets." HM Stationery Office, London.
Miravet, L., Guéris, J., Rousselet, F., and Ryckewaert, A. (1977). *Nouv. Presse Med.* **6,** 1847.
Narwid, T. A., Blounti, J. F., Iacobelli, J. A., and Uskoković, M. R. (1974). *Helv. Chim. Acta* **57,** 781.

Nassim, J. R., Saville, P. D., Cook, P. B., and Mulligan, L. (1959). *Q. J. Med.* [n.s.] **28,** 141.

National Academy of Sciences (1964). *N.A.S.—N.R.C., Bull.*

Nayal, A. S., MacLennan, W. J., Hamilton, J. C., Rose, P., and Kong, M. (1978). *Gerontology* **24,** 117.

Neat, G. E., Nash, A. H., Hunt, S. P., and Truswell, A. S. (1978). *Br. Med. J.* **1,** 304.

Nielsen, S. P., Binderup, E., Godtfredsen, W. O., Jensen, H., and Ladefoged, J. (1976). *Nephron* **16,** 359.

Nordin, B. E. C. (1971). *Br. Med. J.* **1,** 571.

Nordin, B. E. C., Hodgkinson, A., and Peacock, M. A. (1967). *Clin. Orthop., Relat. Res.* **52,** 293.

Norman, A. W., and Henry, H. L. (1974). *Clin. Orthop. Relat. Res.* **98,** 258.

Norman, A. W., and Wong, R. G. (1972). *J. Nutr.* **102,** 1709.

Norman, A. W., Midgett, R. J., Myrtle, J. F., and Nowicki, H. G. (1971). *Biochem. Biophys. Res. Commun.* **42,** 1082.

Norman, A. W., Bayless, J. D., and Tsai, H. C. (1976). *Biochem. Pharmacol.* **25,** 163.

Offermann, G., Schaefer, K., Grigoleit, H.-G., and Dittmar, F. (1975). *Eur. J. Clin. Pharmacol.* **8,** 255.

Ogg, C. S. (1968). *Clin. Sci.* **34,** 467.

Olson, W. G., Jorgensen, N. A., Bringe, A. N., Schultz, L. H., and DeLuca, H. F. (1974). *J. Dairy Sci.* **57,** 677.

Pak, C. Y. C., DeLuca, H. F., Chavez de los Rios, J. M., Suda, T., Ruskin, B., and DeLea, C. S. (1970). *Arch. Intern. Med.* **126,** 239.

Pak, C. Y. C., DeLuca, H. F., Bartter, F. C., Henneman, D. H., Frame, B., Simopoulos, A., and DeLea, C. S. (1972). *Arch. Intern. Med.* **129,** 894.

Parfitt, A. M. (1977). *In* "Vitamin D: Biochemical, Chemical and Clinical Aspects Related to Calcium Metabolism" (A. W. Norman *et al.*, eds.), p. 809. de Gruyter, Berlin.

Parfitt, A. M., Higgins, B. A., and Nassim, J. R. (1964). *Clin. Sci.* **27,** 463.

Partridge, J. J., Faber, S., and Uskoković, M. R. (1974). *Helv. Chim. Acta* **57,** 764.

Paterson, C. R. (1974). "Metabolic Disorders of Bone," p. 79. Blackwell, Oxford.

Peacock, M. A., Hodgkinson, A., and Nordin, B. E. C. (1967). *Br. Med. J.* **3,** 469.

Perry, W., Allen, L. N., Stamp, T. C. B., and Walker, P. G. (1977). *N. Engl. J. Med.* **297,** 1110.

Peterson, P. A. (1971). *J. Biol. Chem.* **246,** 7748.

Pettifor, J., Ross, F. P., Wang, J., Moodley, G., and Couper-Smith, J. (1978). *J. Pediatr.* **92,** 320.

Philippot, J. R., Cooper, A. G., and Wallach, D. F. H. (1976). *Biochem. Biophys. Res. Commun.* **72,** 1035.

Piel, C. F., Roof, B. S., and Avioli, L. V. (1973). *J. Clin. Endocrinol. Metab.* **37,** 944.

Pierides, A. M., Simpson, W., Ward, M. K., Ellis, H. A., Deward, J. H., and Kerr, D. N. S. (1976). *Lancet* **1,** 1092.

Popovitzer, M. M., Pinggera, W. F., Hutt, M. P., Robinette, J., Halgrimson, C. G., and Starzl, T. E. (1972). *J. Clin. Endocrinol. Metab.* **35,** 213.

Prader, A., Illig, R., and Heierli, E. (1961). *Helv. Paediatr. Acta* **16,** 452.

Preece, M. A., and Valman, H. B. (1975). *Arch. Dis. Childh.* **50,** 283.

Preece, M. A., McIntosh, W. B., Tomlinson, S., Ford, J. A., Dunnigna, M. G., and O'Riordan, J. L. H. (1973). *Lancet* **2,** 907.

Raisz, L. G., Trummel, C. L., and Wener, J. A. (1972). *Endocrinology* **90,** 961.

Rauschkolb, E. W., Davis, H. W., Fenimore, D. C., Black, H. S., and Fabre, L. F. (1969). *J. Invest. Dermatol.* **53,** 289.

Recker, R. R., Schoenfeld, P., Letteri, J., Slatopolsky, E., Martin, K., Kleinman, L., Hartenbower, D., Brickman, A., Goldsmith, R., Frost, H., Jee, W., Teitebaum, S., Kimmel, D., Arnaud, C., Arnaud, S., and Heaney, R. (1977). *In* "Vitamin D: Biochemical, Chemical and Clinical

Aspects Related to Calcium Metabolism'' (A. W. Norman *et al.*, eds.), p. 649. de Gruyter, Berlin.
Reitz, R. E., and Weinstein, R. L. (1973). *Clin. Aspects Metab. Bone Dis., Proc. Int. Symp., 1972* Int. Congr. Ser. No. 270, 247.
Richens, A., and Rowe, D. J. F. (1970). *Br. Med. J.* **4,** 73.
Richter, C. P., and Rice, K. K. (1943a). *Am. J. Physiol.* **139,** 147.
Richter, C. P., and Rice, K. K. (1943b). *Am. J. Physiol.* **139,** 693.
Riggs, B. L., Kelly, P. J., Kinney, V. R., Scholz, D. A., and Bianco, A. (1967). *J. Bone Jt. Surg., Am. Vol.* **49,** 915.
Riggs, B. L., Jowsey, J., Kelly, P. J., Hoffman, D. L., and Arnaud, C. D. (1976). *J. Clin. Endocrinol. Metab.* **42,** 1139.
Romanoff, A. L., and Romanoff, A. J. (1949). ''The Avian Egg.'' Wiley, New York.
Roof, B. S., Piel, C. F., and Gordan, G. S. (1973). *Trans. Assoc. Am. Physicians* 221.
Rose, G. A. (1967). *Sci. Basis Med.* p. 252.
Rosen, J. F., and Finberg, L. (1972). *Pediatr. Res.* **6,** 552.
Rosen, J. F., Fleischman, A. R., Finberg, L., Eisman, J., and DeLuca, H. F. (1977). *J. Clin. Endocrinol. Metab.* **45,** 457.
Rosenstreich, S. J., Rich, C., and Volwiler, W. (1971a). *J. Clin. Invest.* **50,** 679.
Rosenstreich, S. J., Volwiler, W., and Rich, C. (1971b). *J. Clin. Nutr.* **24,** 897.
Rubini, M. E., Coburn, J. W., and Massry, S. G. (1969). *Arch. Intern. Med.* **124,** 663.
Russell, J. E., and Avioli, L. V. (1972). *J. Clin. Invest.* **51,** 3072.
Russell, R. G. G., Henderson, R. G., Ledingham, D. O., Oliver, D., Preston, C., Smith, R., Warner, G. T., Walten, R. J., and Norman, A. W. (1974a). *Endocrinol., Proc. Int. Symp., 1973* p. 393.
Russell, R. G. G., Walton, R. J., Smith, R., Preston, C., Basson, R., Henderson, R. G., and Norman, A. W. (1974b). *Lancet* **2,** 14.
Sagar, S., Estrada, R. L., and Kaye, M. (1972). *Arch. Intern. Med.* **130,** 768.
Samizadeh, A., Loew, H., Busch, G., Muller, H., and Losse, H. (1977). *Klin. Wochenschr.* **55,** 1005.
Sansom, B. F., Allen, W. M., Davies, D. C., Hoare, M. N., Stenton, J. R., and Vagg, M. J. (1976). *Vet. Rec.* **99,** 310.
Schachter, D., Finkelstein, J. D., and Kowarski, S. (1964). *J. Clin. Invest.* **43,** 787.
Schaefer, K., von Herrath, D., Opitz, A., Koch, H. U., and Stratz, R. (1971). *Eur. J. Clin. Invest.* **2,** 133.
Schaefer, K., von Herrath, D., and Stratz, R. (1972). *Isr. J. Med. Sci.* **8,** 80.
Schaefer, K., Kraft, D., von Herrath, D., and Grigoleit, H.-G. (1974). *IRCS, Res. Biochem. Connect. Tissue Skin Bone* **2,** 1112.
Schaefer, K., Offermann, G., von Herrath, D., Asmus, G., and Hufler, M. (1977). *J. Dial.* **1,** 619.
Schoen, M. S., Lindenbaum, J., Roginsky, M. S., and Holt, P. R. (1978). *Dig. Dis.* **23,** 137.
Schulz, W., Heidler, R., Gessler, U., Offermann, G., Schulz, A., and Delling, A. (1975). *Proc. Dtsch. Ges., Inn. Med.* **81,** 976.
Scriver, C. R., MacDonald, W., Reade, T., Glorieux, F., and Nogrady, B. (1977). *Am. J. Med. Genet.* **1,** 101.
Seelig, M. S. (1969). *Ann. N.Y. Acad. Sci.* **147,** 539.
Seelig, M. S. (1975). *Br. Med. J.* **1,** 647.
Seeley, J. R., Coussons, H., Smith, J. D., and DeLuca, H. F. (1970). *Pediatr. Res.* **4,** 451.
Seidel, H., and Seidel, R. (1977). *Monatsh. Veterinaermed.* **32,** 568.
Shen, F. H., Baylink, D. J., Sherrard, D. J., Shen, L., Maloney, N. A., and Wergedal, J. E. (1975). *J. Clin. Endocrinol. Metab.* **40,** 1009.
Shen, L., Baylink, C. D., and Sherrard, D. J. (1973). *Clin. Res.* **21,** 204.

Shetty, K. R., Ajlouni, K., Rosenfeld, P. S., and Hagen, T. C. (1975). *Arch. Intern. Med.* **135,** 986.
Silverberg, D. S., Bettcher, K. B., Dossetor, J. B., Overton, T. R., Holick, M. F., and DeLuca, H. F. (1975). *CMA Journal* **112,** 190.
Singleton, N., and Tucker, S. M. (1978). *Br. Med. J.* **1,** 607.
Slatopolsky, E., Hruska, K., and Rutherford, W. E. (1975). *Kidney Int.,* Suppl. 2, 590.
Smith, J. E., and Goodman, D. S. (1971). *J. Clin. Invest.* **50,** 2159.
Sorensen, E., Smith, R., Tougard, L., Neilsen, S. P., and Randall, R. E. (1976). *Br. Med. J.* **1,** 211.
Stamp, T. C. B., Round, J. M., Rowe, D. J. F., and Haddad, J. G. Jr. (1972). *Br. Med. J.* **4,** 9.
Stanbury, S. W., and Lumb, G. A. (1962). *Medicine (Baltimore)* **41,** 1.
Stanbury, S. W., Lumb, G. A., and Mawer, E. B. (1969). *Arch. Intern Med.* **124,** 274.
Stiles, F. C., and Odland, P. K. (1977). *Wis. Med. J.* **76,** S139.
Sunde, M. L., Turk, C. M., and DeLuca, H. F. (1978). *Science* **200,** 1067.
Taylor, C. M., Hughes, S. E., and DeSilva, P. (1976). *Biochem Biophys. Res. Commun.* **70,** 1243.
Taylor, R. L., Lynch, H. J., and Wysor, W. G. (1963). *Am. J. Med.* **34,** 221.
Teitelbaum, S. L., Bone, J. M. Stein, P. M., Gilden, J. J., Bates, M., Boisseau, V. C., and Avioli, L. V. (1976). *J. Am. Med. Assoc.* **235,** 164.
Thompson, G. R., Lewis, B., and Booth, C. C. (1966). *J. Clin. Invest.* **45,** 94.
Thompson, G. R., Ockner, R. K., and Isselbacher, K. J. (1969). *J. Clin. Invest.* **48,** 87.
Turk, J. L., and McGinnis, J. (1964). *Poult. Sci.* **43,** 539.
Turton, C. W. G., Stamp, T. C. B., Stanley, P., and Maxwell, J. D. (1977). *Lancet* **1,** 222.
Valentzas, C., Oreopoulos, D. G., Brandes, L., Wilson, D. R., and Marquez-Julio, A. (1976). *Ann. Intern. Med.* **86,** 198.
Verberckmoes, R., Bouillon, R., and Krempien, B. (1975). *Ann. Intern. Med.* **82,** 529.
Villanueva, A. R., Illnicki, L., Frost, H. M., and Arnstein, R. (1966). *J. Lab. Clin. Med.* **67,** 973.
von Herrath, D., Schaefer, K., Kraft, D., Grigoleit, H.-G., and Koeppe, P. (1973a). *Klin. Wochenschr.* **51,** 979.
von Herrath, D., Kraft, D., Grigoleit, H., and Schaefer, K. (1973b). *Ger. Med. Mon.* **3,** 93.
Wake, C. J., and Maddock, L. (1975). *Lancet* **1,** 120.
Wallis, G. C. (1938). *J. Dairy Sci.* **21,** 315.
Walton, J. (1976). *Clin. Pediatr.* **11,** 1007.
Weber, H. P., Gray, R. W., Dominquez, J. H., and Lemann, J. (1976). *J. Clin. Endocrinol. Metab.* **43,** 1047.
Weighton, C. (1958). *Vet. Rec.* **70,** 1006.
Weinburg, A. G., and Stone, R. T. (1971). *J. Pediatr.* **79,** 996.
Werder, E. A., Kind, H. P., Egert, F., Fischer, J., and Prader, A. (1976). *J. Pediatr.* **89,** 266.
Wheatley, V. R., and Reinertson, R. P. (1958). *J. Invest. Dermatol.* **31,** 51.
Williams, T. F., Winters, R. W., and Burnett, C. H. (1960). *In* "The Metabolic Basis of Inherited Disease" (J. B. Stanbury, J. B. Wyngaarden, and D. S. Frederickson, eds.), p. 1177. New York.
Wills, M. R., Zisman, E., and Wortsman, J. (1970). *Clin. Sci.* **39,** 95.
Wilson, D. R., York, S. E., Jaworski, Z. F., and Yendt, E. R. (1965). *Medicine (Baltimore)* **44,** 99.
Winget, C. M., Smith, A. M., and Hoover, G. N. (1958). *Pout. Sci.* **37,** 1325.
Winters, R. W., Graham, J. B., Williams, T. F., McFalls, V. W., and Burnett, C. H. (1958). *Medicine (Baltimore)* **37,** 97.
Witmer, G., Margolis, A., Fontaine, O., Fritsch, J., Lenoir, G., Broyer, M., and Balsan, S. (1976). *Kidney Int.* **10,** 395.
Wolf, H., Kerstan, B., and Kerstan, J. (1975). *Klin. Paediatr.* **187,** 331.
Wong, R. G., Norman, A. W., Reddy, C. R., and Coburn, J. W. (1972). *J. Clin. Invest.* **51,** 1287.

Woodhouse, N. J. Y., Doyle, F. H., and Joplin, G. F. (1971). *Lancet* **2,** 283.
Yarrington, J. T., Capen, C. C., Black, H. E., Re, R., Potts, J. T., and Geho, W. B. (1976). *Am. J. Pathol.* **83,** 559.
Yendt, E. R. (1970). *Int. Encycl. Pharmacol. Thersp.* **1,** Sect. 51, 139.
Zamboni, G., Cecchettin, M., Marradi, P., Foradori, M., and Zoppi, G. (1977). *Helv. Paediatr. Acta* **32,** 363.

Appendix

A. MOLECULAR WEIGHTS, UNITS, AND MOLE-EQUIVALENTS FOR VITAMIN D, ITS METABOLITES, AND IMPORTANT ANALOGS[a]

Substance	Molecular weight	nmoles/ 1.00 μg	units/ 1.00 μg[b]	ng/unit[b]	nmoles/unit[b]		
					10 units	50 units	100 units
Cholecalciferol series							
D	384.3	2.60	40.0	25.0			
$25(OH)D_3$	400.3	2.49	38.4	26.0			
$1,25(OH)_2D_3$	416.3	2.40	36.9	27.1	0.65	3.25	6.50
$24,25(OH)_2D_3$	416.3	2.40	36.9	27.1			
$25,26(OH)_2D_3$	416.3	2.40	36.9	27.1			
$1,24,25(OH)_3D_3$	432.3	2.31	35.5	28.1			
Ergocalciferol series							
D_2	396.3	2.52	38.8	25.8			
$25(OH)D_2$	412.3	2.42	37.3	26.8			
$1,25(OH)_2D_2$	428.3	2.33	35.8	27.8	0.65	3.25	6.50
$24,25(OH)_2D_2$	428.3	2.33	35.8	27.8			
$25,26(OH)_2D_2$	428.3	2.33	35.8	27.8			
$1,24,25(OH)_3D_2$	444.3	2.25	34.6	28.9			
Analogs							
$1\alpha(OH)D_3$	400.3	2.49	38.4	26.0			
Dihydrotachysterol$_3$	385.3	2.59	39.9	25.0	0.65	3.25	6.5
5,6-*trans*-D_3	384.3	2.60	40.0	25.0			
25(OH)-5,6-*trans*-D_3	400.3	2.49	38.4	26.0			

[a] From A. W. Norman, *J. Nutr.* **102,** 1243 (1972); League of Nations; Memorandum on the International Standard for Vitamin D and its application. *League Nations, Bull Health Organ.* **4,** No. 3, 540 (1935).

[b] 1.00 unit has been proposed by Norman (1972) to be 65.0 pmoles for all vitamin D compounds. For vitamin D_3 1.0 IU is by definition (League of Nations, 1935) 0.025 μg, which is exactly equivalent to 65.0 pmoles.

B. DIETS USED TO RAISE VITAMIN D-DEFICIENT ANIMALS

Constituents[a]	Rats[b] Nonrachitogenic (% by weight)	Rats[b] Rachitogenic (% by weight)	Chicks,[c] rachitogenic (% by weight)
Cerelose	63.8	62.8	—
Casein	18.0	18.0	8.0
Corn	—	—	35.4
Wheat middlings	—	—	30.0
Soybean meal	—	—	16.0
Cottonseed oil	10.0	10.0	1.0
L-Cysteine	0.2	0.2	—
Roughage (Alphacel)	3.0	3.0	—
Alfalfa	—	—	6.0
Calcium carbonate	1.1	3.7	—
Equimolar phosphate[d]	1.6	—	—
Choline chloride	0.2	0.2	—
Charcoal	—	—	0.46
$CaHPO_4 \cdot 2H_2O$	—	—	2.0
Water-soluble vitamins[e]	0.1	0.1	0.1
Ca- and P-free salts[f,g]	2.0[g]	2.0[g]	1.04[f]
Calcium content (%)	0.47	0.30	0.60
Phosphorus content (%)	1.20	0.10	0.40

	Rats for "line test" assay[h] (% by weight)
Yellow corn	76.0
Gluten (from wheat flour)	20.0
$CaCO_3$	3.0
NaCl	1.0

	Chicks for 21-day prophylactic test[h] (% by weight)
Yellow corn, ground	58.0
Wheat flour middlings	27.0
Casein, crude acid precipitated	12.0
Iodized NaCl	1.0
Yeast (nonirradiated; 7% minimum nitrogen content)	2.0
$MnSO_4 \cdot 4H_2O$	0.02

(*continued*)

B. (*Continued*)

[a]In addition all animals should receive weekly 100 μg of tocopherol, 125 μg of menadione, and 100 μg of β-carotene.

[b]From H. Steenbock, and D. C. Herting, *J. Nutr.* **57,** 449 (1955).

[c]From A. W. Norman and R. G. Wong, *J. Nutr.* **102,** 1243 (1972).

[d]Equimolar phosphate mix: $Na \cdot H_2PO_4 + Na_2\ HPO_3$, equimolar quantities.

[e]Water-soluble vitamin mix (percentage): cerelose, 63.7; ascorbic acid, 10.0; thiamine, 0.5; riboflavin, 0.5; pyridoxine, 0.5; nicotinamide, 2.0; cyanocobalamin, 0.002; calcium pantothenate, 2.8; myoinositol, 20.0; folic acid, 0.02; biotin, 0.01.

[f]Calcium- and phosphorus-free salts for chicks (percentage): NaCl, 35.3; KCl, 34.2; $MnSO_4 \cdot H_2O$, 1.6; KI, 0.004; $MgSO_4$, 25.6; $Fe(C_6H_5O_7) \cdot 5H_2O$, 2.4; $CuSO_4$, 0.15; $ZnCl_2$, 0.69.

[g]Calcium- and phosphorus-free salts for rats (percentage): NaCl, 20.9; KCl, 57.7; $MgSO_4$, 17.9; $FeSO_4 \cdot 7H_2O$, 3.22; $CuSO_4 \cdot 5H_2O$, 0.078; $Al(SO_4)_3K_2SO_4 \cdot 24H_2O$, 0.018; NaF, 0.113; $Na_2HAsO_4 \cdot 7H_2O$, 0.0014; $CoCl_2$, 0.004; KI, 0.01; $MnSO_4 \cdot H_2O$, 0.04.

[h]From "Official Methods of Analysis," 9th ed., p. 675. Assoc. Off. Agric. Chem., Washington, D.C., 1960; also 12th ed., p. 885 (1975).

C. IUPAC NOMENCLATURE RULES FOR VITAMIN D

1. Nomenclature Rules for Vitamin D

The following rules are abstracted from a report of the IUPAC–IUB Commission on Biochemical Nomenclature report entitled "Trivial Names for Miscellaneous Compounds of Importance in Biochemistry"[1] (only the relevant sections are reproduced).

Section M-1

2.1 Compound III (R = $-\underset{H}{\overset{Me}{C}}-C{=}C-\underset{H}{\overset{Me}{C}}-C-Me_2$)

9,10-secoergosta-5,7,10(19),22-tetraen-3β-ol, also known as vitamin D_2 or calciferol, should be designated *ergocalciferol*.

2.2 Compound III (R = $-C-CH_2-CH_2-CH_2-C-Me_2$)

9,10-secocholesta-5,7,10(19)-trien-3β-ol, also known as vitamin D_3, should be designated *cholecalciferol*.

[1]Taken from IUPAC–IUB Commission on Biochemical Nomenclature, *J. Biol. Chem.* **241,** 2987 (1966).

2. The Nomenclature of Steroids

The molecule vitamin D is derived from a steroid nucleus—either cholesterol or ergosterol. Technically vitamin D is a secosteroid. Accordingly, it is appropriate to apply the guidelines of the Revised Tentative Rules for Nomenclature of Steroids prepared by the IUPAC–IUB Commission on Biochemical Nomenclature.[2]

The rule defining the term "seco" is produced below; the rules provide the structure of vitamin D_3 as particular example.

Rule 25-8

8.1 Fission of a ring, with addition of a hydrogen atom at each terminal group thus created, is indicated by the prefix "seco-", the original steroid numbering being retained.

3. Nomenclature concerning:

A. Asymmetric centers

The configuration at the asymmetric centers in a vitamin D molecule is indicated in a fashion identical to that of any other compound. They are designated according to the R,S notation by application of the sequence-rule scheme of Cahn, *et al.*[3]

Thus, the orientation of the hydroxyl on C-24 of the naturally occurring metabolite is $24R,25(OH)_2D_3$. Similarly, the correction notation for the naturally occurring $25,26(OH)_2D_3$ metabolite is $25R,26(OH)_2D_3$.

B. Configuration about double bonds

Configurations about double bonds are now most correctly specified by the E,Z notation.[4] The Z notation is usually a *cis* configuration while the E notation is a *trans* configuration, however the official procedures should be consulted for detailed understanding. Thus, the most correct notation for vitamin D_3 is 9,10-seco(5Z,7E)-5,7,10(19)-cholestatriene-3β-ol.

D. BIBLIOGRAPHY: REVIEW ARTICLES AND BOOKS RELATED TO VITAMIN D

1. Books

Comar, C. L. and Bronner, F., eds. (1964). "Mineral Metabolism," Vol. 2, Part A. Academic Press, New York.

[2]IUPAC–IUB Commission on Biochemical Nomenclature *Biochim. Biophys. Acta* **164,** 453–486 (1968).

[3]Cahn, R. S., Ingold, C., and Prelog, V. (1966). *Angew. Chem. Internat. Ed. Engl.* **5,** 385.

[4]Blackwood, J. E., Gladys, C. L., Loening, K. L., Petarca, A. E., and Rush, J. E. (1968). *J. Am. Chem. Soc.* **90,** 509.

Comar, C. L., and Bronner, F., eds. (1969). "Mineral Metabolism," Vol. 3. Academic Press, New York.

Czitober, H., and Eschberger, J., eds. (1974). "Calcified Tissue: Proceedings of the Ninth European Symposium on Calcified Tissue." Facta Publication, Vienna.

DePalma, A. F., ed. (1960). "Clinical Orthopaedics." Lippincott, Philadelphia, Pennsylvania.

DePalma, A. F., ed. (1965). "Clinical Orthopaedics and Related Research." Lippincott, Philadelphia, Pennyslvania.

DeLuca, H. F., and Suttie, J. W. (1969). "The Fat Soluble Vitamins," Uni. of Wisconsin Press, Madison.

Deuel, H. J., Jr. (1957). "The Lipids," Vol. III. Wiley (Interscience), New York.

Dick, J. L. (1922). "Rickets." Heinemann, London.

Dyke, S. F. (1965). "The Chemistry of the Vitamins." Wiley (Interscience), New York.

Fieser, L. F., and Fieser, M. (1959). "Steroids," Chapter 3. Van Nostrand: Reinhold, Princeton, New Jersey.

Freudenthal, P. (1927). "Experimental Rickets." Munksgaard, Copenhagen.

Greep, R. O., and Talmage, R. V., eds. (1961). "The Parathyroids." Thomas, Springfield, Illinois.

Hess, A. F. (1929). "Rickets: Including Osteomalacia and Tetany." Lea & Febiger, Philadelphia, Pennsylvania.

Irving, J. T. (1957). "Calcium Metabolism." Methuen, London.

Irving, J. T. (1973). "Calcium and Phosphorus Metabolism." Academic Press, New York.

James, V. H. T., and Martini, L., eds. (1971). "Hormonal Steroids," Int. Congr. Ser. No. 219. Excerpta Med. Found., Amsterdam.

Kuhlencordt, F., and Kruse, H. P., eds. (1975). "Calcium Metabolism, Bone and Metabolic Bone Disease." Springer-Verlag, Berlin and New York.

Lawson, D. E. M., ed. (1978). "Vitamin D," Academic Press, London.

McLean, F. C., and Urist, M. R. (1961). "Bone." Univ. of Chicago Press, Chicago, Illinois.

Medical Research Council (1923). "Studies of Rickets in Vienna 1919–1922." HM Stationery Office, London.

Mellanby, E. (1923). "Experimental Rickets." HM Stationery Office, London.

Menczel, J., and Harel, A., eds. (1971). "Calcified Tissue: Structural, Functional and Metabolic Aspects." Academic Press, New York.

Moore, N. (1884). "History of the First Treatise on Rickets." St. Bartholomew's Hospital Reports.

Nielsen, S. P., and Hjorting-Hansen, E. (1975). "Calcified Tissues 1975: Proceedings of the XIth European Symposium on Calcified Tissues." FADL's Forlag, Copenhagen.

Norman, A. W. (1979). "Vitamin D: Nutritional and Clinical Aspects." Dekker, New York.

Norman, A. W., Schaefer, K., Grigoleit, H.-G., von Herrath, D., and Ritz, E., eds. (1975). "Vitamin D and Problems Related to Urenic Bone Disease." de Gruyter, Berlin.

Norman, A. W., Schaefer, K., Coburn, J. W., DeLuca, H. F., Fraser, D., Grigoleit, H. G., and von Herrath, D., eds. (1977). "Vitamin D: Biochemical, Chemical and Clinical Aspects Related to Calcium metabolism." de Gruyter, Berlin.

Norman, A. W., Schaefer, K., von Herrath, D., Grigoleit, H.-G., Mawer, E. B., Suda, T., DeLuca, H. F., and Coburn, J. W., eds. (1979). "Vitamin D: Recent Basic Advances and their Clinical Application (Proceedings of the Fourth Workshop on Vitamin D)" Walter de Gruyter Publishing Company, Elmsford, New York.

Paterson, C. R. (1974). "Metabolic Disorders of Bone." Blackwell, Oxford.

Rasmussen, H., and Bordier, P. (1974). "The Physiological and Cellular Basis of Metabolic Bone Disease." Williams & Wilkins, Baltimore, Maryland.

Reed, C. I., Struck, H. C., and Steck, I. E. (1939). "Vitamin D." Univ. of Chicago Press, Chicago, Illinois.

Schraer, H., ed. (1970). "Biological Calcification: Cellular and Molecular Aspects." Appleton, New York.

Sebrell, W. H. Jr., and Harris, R. H. (1974). "The Vitamins," Vol. 3. Academic Press, New York.

Vaughan, J. M. (1970). "The Physiology of Bone." Oxford Univ. Press (Clarendon), London and New York.

Wasserman, R. H., ed. (1963). "The Transfer of Calcium and Strontium Across Biological Membranes." Academic Press, New York.

Whistler, D. (1645). "Inaugural Medical Disputation on the Disease of English Children Which is Popularly Termed the Rickets." University of London, London.

2. Review Articles

Arnaud, S. B., and Stickler, G. B. (1974). Recent developments in vitamin-D research. *Clin. Pediatr.* **13,** 444-456.

Avioli, L. V. (1972). Vitamin D, the kidney and calcium homeostasis. *Kidney Int.* **2,** 241-246.

Avioli, L. V., and Haddad, J. G. (1973). Progress in endocrinology and metabolism—Vitamin D: Current concepts. *Metab., Clin. Exp.* **22,** No. 3, 507-531.

Bartter, F. C. (1973). Vitamin D, parathyroid hormone, and the kidney. *Kidney* **4,** 249-270.

Beale, M. G., Chan, J. C. M., Oldham, S. B., and DeLuca, H. F. (1976). Vitamin D-Discovery of its metabolites and their therapeutic applications. *Pediatrics* **57,** 729-741.

Bekemeier, H. (1969). Evolution der Hautfarbe und Kutane Vitamin-D-Photosynthese. *Dtsch. Med. Wochenschr.* **4,** 185-189.

Best, C. H., and Taylor, N. B. (1843). The physiological basis of medical practice. *Univ. Toronto Text Appl. Physiol.* pp. 1098-1106.

Bianchi, C. P. (1968). "Cell Calcium." Appleton, New York.

Bijvoet, O. L. M., and Froehling, P. G. A. N. (1973). Renal actions of parathyroid hormone and calcitonin. *In* "Endocrinology" (R. O. Scow, ed.), Int. Congr. Ser. No. 273, pp. 474-479. Excerpta Med. Found., Amsterdam.

Bills, C. E. (1954). Chemistry. *In* "The Vitamins" (W. H. Sebrell, Jr. and R. S. Harris, eds.), Vol. 2, pp. 132-209. Academic Press, New York.

Bills, C. E. (1954). Industrial preparations. *In* "The Vitamins" (W. H. Sebrell, Jr., and R. S. Harris, eds.), Vol. 2, pp. 210-215. Academic Press, New York.

Bills, C. E. (1954). Estimation. *In* "The Vitamins" (W. H. Sebrell, Jr. and R. S. Harris, eds.), Vol. 2, pp. 215-221. Academic Press, New York.

Bills, C. E. (1954). Standardization of activity. *In* "The Vitamins" (W. H. Sebrell, Jr. and R. S. Harris, eds.), Vol. 2, pp. 221-223. Academic Press, New York.

Blunt, J. W., and DeLuca, H. F. (1969). *In* "The Fat-Soluble Vitamins" (H. F. DeLuca and J. W. Suttie, eds.), pp. 67-79. Univ. of Wisconsin Press, Madison.

Boyle, I. T. (1974). Vitamin D an old hormone rediscovered. *Scott. Med. J.* **19,** 247-249.

Briggs, M. H., and Briggs, M. (1974). Vitamin D hormones. Part 1. *Med. J. Aust.* **1,** 838-896.

Briggs, M. H., and Briggs, M. (1974). Vitamin D hormones. Part 2. *Med. J. Aust.* **1,** 891-896.

Bronner, F. (1973). Calcium homeostasis. *Eng. Princ. Physiol.* **1,** 227-248.

Bronner, F. (1973). *In* "Calcium and Phosphorus Metabolism" (J. T. Irving, ed.), pp. 149-186. Academic Press, New York.

Coburn, J. W., and Norman, A. W. (1973). Role of the kidney in the metabolism of calciferol (vitamin D). *Clin. Nephrol.* **1,** 273-283.

Coburn, J. W., Hartenbower, D. L., and Massry, S. G. (1973). Intestinal absorption of calcium and the effect of renal insufficiency. *Kidney Int.* **4,** 96-104.

Cooper, C. W., McGuigan, J. E., Ontjes, P. A., Hennessy, J. F., Schwesinger, W. H., and Gray, T. K. (1973). Control of secretion of parathyroid hormone and thyrocalcitonin. *In* "Endocrinology" (R. O. Scow, ed.), Int. Congr. Ser. No. 273, pp. 494-500. Exerpta Med. Found., Amsterdam.

DeLuca, H. F. (1967). Mechanism of action and metabolic fate of vitamin D. *Vitam. Horm. (N.Y.)* **25,** 315–366.

DeLuca, H. F. (1969). Metabolism and function of vitamin D. *In* "The Fat-Soluble Vitamins" (H. F. DeLuca and J. W. Suttie, eds.), pp. 3–20. Univ. of Wisconsin Press, Madison.

DeLuca, H. F. (1969). 25-Hydroxycholecalciferol: The probable metabolically active form of vitamin D_3: Its identification and subcellular site of action. *Arch. Intern. Med.* **124,** 442–450.

DeLuca, H. F. (1969). Recent advances in the metabolism and function of Vitamin D. *Fed. Proc., Fed. Am. Soc. Exp. Biol.* **28,** 1678–1689.

DeLuca, H. F. (1969). 25-Hydroxycholecalciferol, the probable metabolically active form of vitamin D: Isolation, identification and subcellular location. *Am. J. Clin. Nutr.* **22,** 412–424.

DeLuca, H. F. (1971). Active compounds. *In* "The Vitamins" (W. H. Sebrell, Jr. and R. S. Harris, eds.), Vol. 3, pp. 230–247. Academic Press, New York.

DeLuca, H. F. (1971). Vitamin D: A new look at an old vitamin. *Nutr. Rev.* **29,** 179–181.

DeLuca, H. F. (1973). The kidney as an endocrine organ for the production of 1,25-dihydroxyvitamin D_3, a calcium-mobilizing hormone. *N. Engl. J. Med.* **289,** 359–365.

DeLuca, H. F. (1975). Calcium metabolism. *Acta Orthop. Scand.* **46,** 286–314.

DeLuca, H. F. (1975). Function of the fat-soluble vitamins. *Am. J. Clin. Nutr.* **28,** 339–345.

DeLuca, H. F. (1975). The kidney as an endocrine organ involved in the function of vitamin D. *Am. J. Med.* **58,** 39–47.

DeLuca, H. F. (1975). Recent advances in our understanding of the metabolism of vitamin D and its regulation. *Clin. Endocrinol. (Oxford)* **58,** 97s–119s.

DeLuca, H. F. (1976). Recent advances in our understanding of the vitamin D endocrine system. *J. Lab. Clin. Med.* **87,** 7–26.

DeLuca, H. F., and Kleiner-Bossaller, A. (1973). II. Hauptthema: Vitamin D-Stoffwechsel. Metaboliten von Vitamin D als Hormone in der Regulation des Calcium-und Phosphatstoffwechsels. *Monatsschr. Kinderheilkd.* **121,** 329–337.

DeLuca, H. F., and Melancon, M. J., Jr. (1972). 25-Hydroxycholecalciferol: A hormonal form of vitamin D. *In* "Biochemical Actions of Hormones" (G. Litwack, ed.), Vol. 2, pp. 338–383. Academic Press, New York.

DeLuca, H. F. and Schnoes, H. K. (1976). Metabolism and mechanism of action of vitamin D. *Annu. Rev. Biochem.* **45,** 631–642.

DeLuca, H. F., Blunt, J. W., and Rikkers, H. (1971). Biogenesis. *In* "The Vitamins" (W. H. Sebrell, Jr. and R. S. Harris, eds.), Vol. 3, pp. 213–230. Academic Press, New York.

Denayer, P. (1975). Mode of action of vitamin D—recent progress. *Louvain Med.* **94,** 449–456.

Edelstein, S. (1974). Vitamin D binding proteins. *In* "International Symposium on Fat-Soluble Vitamins" (R. S. Harris *et al.*, eds.), p. 407–428. Academic Press, New York.

Edelstein, S., Sapir, R., and Harell, A. (1975). The action of vitamin D on bone. *Clin. Endocrinol. (Oxford)* **5s,** 145s–150s.

Frederick, A. (1965). La vitamine D. Metabolisme, actions physiologiques et pharmacodynamiques. *Pathol.-Biol.* **13,** 434–457.

Harris, R. S. (1954). Nomenclature and formulas. *In* "The Vitamins" (W. H. Sebrell, Jr. and R. S. Harris, eds.), Vol. 2, p. 132. Academic Press, New York.

Harris, R. S. (1971). *In* "The Vitamins" (W. H. Sebrell, Jr. and R. S. Harris, eds.), Vol. 3, pp. 156–157. Academic Press, New York.

Harrison, H. E. (1958). The Fanconi syndrome. *J. Chronic Dis.* **7,** 346–355.

Harrison, H. E. (1961). Vitamin D and calcium and phosphate transport. *Pediatrics* **28,** 531–544.

Harrison, H. E., and Harrison, H. C. (1969). *In* "The Fat Soluble Vitamins" (H. F. DeLuca and J. W. Suttie, eds.), pp. 39–54. Univ. of Wisconsin Press, Madison.

Haussler, M. R. (1974). Vitamin D: Mode of action and biomedical applications. *Nutr. Rev.* **32**(9), 257–266.

Haussler, M. R., and McCain, T. A. (1977). *N. Engl. J. Med.* **297**, 974–983 and 1041–1050.
Haussler, M. R., Baylink, D. J., Hughes, M. R., Brumbaugh, P. F., Wergedal, J. E., Shen, F. H., Nielsen, R. L., Counts, S. J., Bursac, K. M., and McCain, T. M. (1975). The assay of 1,25-dihydroxyvitamin D_3: Physiologic and pathologic modulation of circulating hormone levels. *Clin. Endocrinol. (Oxford)* **5s**, 151s–165s.
Havinga, E. (1973). Vitamin D, example and challenge. *Sep. Exp.* **29**, 1181.
Holick, M. F., and DeLuca, H. F. (1974). Vitamin D metabolism. *Annu. Rev. Med.* **25**, 349–367.
Kodicek, E. (1956). Metabolic studies on vitamin D. *Bone Struct. Metab., Ciba Found. Symp., 1955* pp. 161–205.
Kodicek, E. (1960). The metabolism of vitamin D. *Proc. Int. Congr. Biochem., 4th, 1958* Vol. 11, pp. 198–208.
Kodicek, E. (1969). Studies on Vitamin D Metabolism. *In* "The Fat Soluble Vitamins" (H. F. DeLuca and J. W. Suttie eds.), pp. 81–91. Univ. of Wisconsin Press, Madison.
Kodicek, E. (1971). Mode of action of vitamin D. *Acta Vitaminol. Enzymol.* **25**, 153–157.
Kodicek, E. (1972). Recent advances in vitamin D metabolism: 1,25—Dihydroxycholecalciferol, a kidney hormone controlling calcium metabolism. *Clin. Endocrinol. Metab.* **1**, 305–323.
Kolata, G. B. (1975). Vitamin-D: Investigations of a new steroid-hormone. *Science* **187**, 635–636.
Lawson, D. E. M. (1969). Studies on the mode of action of vitamin D. *Nutr. Metab.* **13**, 6–16.
Lawson, D. E. M., and Emtage, J. S. (1974). *In* "International Symposium on Fat-Soluble Vitamins" (R. S. Harris *et al.*, eds.), pp. 277–298. Academic Press, New York.
Loomis, W. F. (1970). Rickets. *Sci. Am.* **223**, 77–91.
MacIntyre, I. (1973). *In* "Endocrinology" (R. O. Scow, ed.), Int. Congr. Ser. No. 273, pp. 485–588. Excerpta Med. Found., Amsterdam.
MacIntyre, I., Colston, K. W., Evans, I. M., Lopez, E., MacAuley, S. J., Piegnoux-Deville, J., Spanos, E. and Szelke, E. (1975). *Clin. Endocrinol. (Oxford)* **5s**, 85s–95s.
McLean, F. C. (1941). Glandular physiology and therapy. Activated sterols in the treatment of parathyroid insufficiency. *J. Am. Med. Assoc.* **117**, 609–619.
Melançon, M. J., Jr., Morii, H., and DeLuca, H. F. (1969). Physiologic effects of vitamin D, parathyroid hormone and calcitonin. *In* "The Fat-Soluble Vitamins" (H. F. DeLuca and J. W. Suttie, eds.), pp. 111–123. Univ. of Wisconsin Press, Madison.
Murad, F., and Weitzman, R. (1973). *In* "Endocrinology" (R. O. Scow, eds.), Int. Congr. Ser. No. 273, pp. 468–473. Excerpta Med. Found., Amsterdam.
Neer, R. M. (1974). Evolutionary significance of vitamin D skin pigment, and ultraviolet light: A review. *Am. J. Phys. Anthropol.* **41**, 496.
Nichols, G., Jr., and Wasserman, R. H., eds. (1971). "Cellular Mechanism for Calcium and Homeostasis," Academic Press, New York.
Nicolaysen, R., and Eeg-Larsen, N. (1953). Vitamin D. *Vitam. Horm. (N.Y.)* **11**, 29–60.
Nicolaysen, R., Eeg-Larsen, N., and Malm, O. J. (1953). Physiology of calcium metabolism. *Physiol. Rev.* **33**, 424–444.
Norman, A. W. (1967). Recent studies on vitamin D and parathyroid hormone regulation of calcium and phosphorus metabolism. *Clin. Orthop. Relat. Res.* **52**, 249–266.
Norman, A. W. (1968). The mode of action of vitamin D. *Biol. Rev. Cambridge Philos. Soc.* **43**, 97–137.
Norman, A. W. (1973). *In* "Endocrinology: Congress of Endocrinology" (R. O. Scow, ed.), Int. Congr. Ser. No. 273, pp. 501–506. Excerpta Med. Found., Amsterdam.
Norman, A. W. (1974). The hormone-like action of 1,25-dihydroxycholecalciferol. *In* "International Symposium on Fat-Soluble Vitamins" (R. S. Harris *et al.*, eds.), Vitamins and Hormones, *32,* pp. 325–284. Academic Press, New York.
Norman, A. W. (1974). Gegenwartige Vorstellungen zum biochemischen Wirkungsmechanismus von Vitamin D. *Muench. Med. Wochenschr.* **116**, 1585–1598.

Norman, A. W. (1974). 1,25-dihydroxyvitamin D_3: A kidney-produced steroid hormone essential to calcium homeostasis. *Am. J. Med.* **57,** 21–27.

Norman, A. W., and Henry, H. (1974). The role of the kidney and vitamin D metabolism in health and disease. *Clin. Orthop. Relat. Res.* **98,** 258–287.

Norman, A. W., and Henry, H. L. (1974). 1,25-dihydroxycholecalciferol—A hormonally active form of vitamin D_3. *Recent Prog. Horm. Res.* **30,** 431–480.

Norman, A. W., and Roberts, P. A. (1973). Vitamin D: Vitamin or hormone? *In* "Applied Nutrition in Clinical Practice" (M. Walczak, ed.), pp. 89–120. Intercontinental Med. Book Corporation, New York.

Norman, A. W., and Wecksler, W. R. (1977). Vitamin D. Receptors and biologic responses. *In* "Receptors and Hormone Action" (B. W. O'Malley and L. Birnbaumer, eds.), Vol. 2, pp. 533–571. Academic Press, New York.

Norman, A. W., Haussler, M. R., Adams, T. H., Myrtle, J. F., Roberts, P., and Hibberd, K. A. (1969). Basic studies on the mechanism of action of vitamin D. *Am. J. Clin. Nutr.* **22,** 396–411.

Norman, A. W., Coburn, J. W., and Hartenbower, D. (1974). Vitamin D and calcium homeostasis. *West. J. Med.* **121,** 508.

Norman, A. W., Johnson, R. L., Osborn, T. W., Procsal, D. A., Carey, S. C., Hammond, M. L., Mitra, M. N., Pirio, M. R., Rego, A., Wing, R. M., and Okamura, W. H. (1976). The chemistry and conformational and biological analysis of vitamin D_3, its metabolites and analogues. *Clin. Endocrinol. (Oxford)* **5s,** 121s–143s.

Oberiter, V. (1972). New discoveries about the vitamin D metabolism. *Lijec. Vjesn.* **94,** 468–470.

Omdahl, J. L., and DeLuca, H. F. (1973). Regulation of vitamin D metabolism and function. *Physiol. Rev.* **53,** 327–372.

Schachter, D. (1969). Calcium Transport, vitamin D and the molecular basis of active transport. *In* "The Fat-Soluble Vitamins" (H. F. DeLuca and J. W. Suttie, eds.), pp. 55–65. Univ. of Wisconsin Press, Madison.

Schnoes, H. K., and DeLuca, H. F. (1974). Vitamin D Metabolism. *In* "International Symposium on Fat-Soluble Vitamins" (R. S. Harris *et al.*, eds.), pp. 385–406. Academic Press, New York.

Shaw, J. H. (1955). Effect of nutritional factors on bones and teeth. *Ann. N.Y. Acad. Sci,* **60,** 733–762.

Stanbury, S. W., Mawer, E. B., Lumb, G. A., Hill, L. F., Holman, C. A., Jones, M., and Van Den Berg, C. J. (1972). Some aspects of vitamin D metabolism in man. *Endocrinol., Proc. Int. Symp., 3rd, 1971* pp. 487–499.

Steendijk, R. (1974). Metabolism of vitamin D: Recent developments and their clinical relevance. *Neth. J. Med.* **17,** 131–139.

Talmage, R. V., and Munson, P. L., eds. (1972). "Calcium, Parathyroid Hormone and the Calcitonins," Int. Congr. Ser. No. 243. Excerpta Med. Found., Amsterdam.

Talmage, R. V., Owen, M., and Parsons, J. A., eds. (1975). "Calcium-Regulating Hormones," Int. Congr. Ser. No. 386. Excerpta Med. Found., Amsterdam.

Wasserman, R. H. (1968). Calcium transport by the intestine: A model and comment on vitamin D action. *Calcif. Tissue Res.* **2,** 301–313.

Wasserman, R. H., Corradino, R. A., Fullmer, C. S., and Taylor, A. N. (1974). Vitamin D-dependent calcium binding protein. *In* "International Symposium on Fat-Soluble Vitamins" (R. S. Harris *et al.*, eds.), pp. 299–324. Academic Press, New York.

Winters, R. W., Graham, J. B., Williams, T. F., McFalls, V. W., and Burnett, C. H. (1958). A genetic study of familial hypophosphatemia and vitamin D resistant rickets with a review of the literature. *Medicine (Baltimore)* **37,** 97–141.

Wright, D. R. (1975). The pieces of a vitamin D puzzle fall into place - almost! *N. Engl. J. Med.* **17,** 872–873.

Index

B

N

W

X